D1315003

THE KIDNEY AND HYPERTENSION IN DIABETES MELLITUS

FIFTH EDITION

THE KIDNEY AND HYPERTENSION IN DIABETES MELLITUS

Fifth Edition
Year 2000

EDITED BY

CARL ERIK MOGENSEN
Medical Department M
(Diabetes & Endocrinology)
Aarhus Kommunehospital
Aarhus University Hospital
Aarhus C, Denmark

Editorial Secretary

Anna Honoré

KLUWER ACADEMIC PUBLISHERS
Boston/Dordrecht/London

Distributors for North, Central and South America:
Kluwer Academic Publishers
101 Philip Drive
Assinippi Park
Norwell, Massachusetts 02061 USA

Distributors for all other countries:
Kluwer Academic Publishers Group
Distribution Centre
Post Office Box 322
3300 AH Dordrecht, THE NETHERLANDS

Library of Congress Cataloging-in-Publication Data

The kidney and hypertension in diabetes mellitus / edited by Carl Erik Mogensen ;
editorial secretary, Anna Honoré.-- 5th ed.
   p. ; cm.
  Includes bibliographica references and index.
  ISBN 0-7923-7901-2
   1. Diabetic nephropathies. 2. Renal hypertension. 3. Diabetes--Complications. I.
  Mogensen, Carl Erik.
  [DNLM: 1. Diabetic Nephropathies. 2. Diabetes Mellitus--complications. 3.
  Hypertension, Renal. 4. Kidney Disease--etiology. WK 835 K458 2000]
  RC918.D53 K53 2000
  616.4'62--dc21
                                         00-040548

Printed on acid-free paper.

Printed in the United States of America

This book is dedicated to the memory of Knud Lundbæk (born 1912 - †1995), distinguished diabetologist, my friend and mentor, and a great inspiration for all of us. He also became strongly engaged in exciting and penetrating new studies in the field of sinology, his second science.

CEM

TABLE OF CONTENTS

TABLE OF CONTENTS

Chapters from the 4th edition (1998) not included in this edition:

(Readers may contact the editor regarding the chapters from the 4ᵗʰ edition)

(Readers may contact the editor regarding the chapters from the 4ᵗʰ edition)

SOME KEYS TO THE LITERATURE

S.-E. Bachman, ed. *Le Rein des Diabétiques* (Thesis). Paris: Librairie J.-B. Baillière et Fils, 1936.

H. Rifkin, L. Leiter, J. Berkman, eds. *Diabetic Glomerulosclerosis. The specific renal disease of diabetes mellitus.* Springfield, Illinois, USA: Charles C. Thomas Publisher, 1952.

L. Scapellato, ed. *La Nefropatia Diabetica.* Roma: Luigi Pozzi, 1953

K. Lundbæk, ed. Long-Term Diabetes. The clinical picture in diabetes mellitus of 15-25 years' duration with a follow-up of a regional series of cases. Copenhagen: Ejnar Munksgaard, 1953.

Å.Chr. Thomsen, ed. *The Kidney in Diabetes Mellitus. A clinical and histological investigation base on renal biopsy material* (Thesis). Copenhagen: Munksgaard, 1965.

G. Ditscherlein, ed. *Nierenveränderungen bei Diabetikern.* Jena: VEB Gustav Fischer Verlag, 1969

JS Cameron, JT Ireland and PJ Watkins. The kidney and Renal Tract in (eds.) Harry Keen and John Jarrett: Complications of Diabetes. Edward Arnold, 1975; 99-150.

D.E. McMillan, J. Ditzel, eds. Proceedings of a Conference on Diabetic Microangiopathy. April 6-10, 1976. Santa Ynez Valley, California. Diabetes 1976; 25: Suppl. 2.

C.E. Mogensen, ed. Diabetes Mellitus and the Kidney. Kidney Int 1982; 21: 673-791.

H. Keen, M. Legrain, eds. *Prevention and treatment of Diabetic Nephropathy.* Boston, The Hague, Dordrecht, Lancaster: MTP Press Limited, 1983.

D.E. McMillan, J. Ditzel, ed.. Proceedings of a Conference on Diabetic Microangiopathy. Diabetes 1983; 32: Suppl. 2: 1-104.

P. Weidmann, C.E. Mogensen, E. Ritz, eds. Diabetes and Hypertension. Proceedings of the First International Symposium on Hypertension Associated with Diabetes Mellitus. June 22-23, 1984. Hypertension 1985; 7: Part II: S1-S174.

P. Passa, C.E. Mogensen, eds. Microalbuminuria in Diabetes Mellitus. Proceedings of an international workshop. Chantilly, France, May 8-9, 1987. Diabete Metab 1988; 14: Suppl.: 175-236.

H.U. Janka, E. Standl, eds. Hypertension in Diabetes Mellitus: Pathogenesis and clinical impact. Proceedings of an International Symposium. Munich, Germany, May 3, 1989. Diabete Metab 1989; 15: Suppl.: 273-366.

R.A. DeFronzo, ed. Diabetic Nephropathy. Semin Nephrol 1990; 10: 183-304.

W.J. Howard, G.C. Viberti, eds. When to treat? A workshop to address the threshold of treatment of hypertension in diabetes. Diabetes Care 1991; 14: Suppl. 4: 1-47.

Proceedings of the International Symposium on Diabetic Nephropathy, July 24-25 1990, Otsu, Japan. J Diabetic Complications 1991; 5: 49-203.

B. Charbonnel, J.M. Mallion, A. Mimran, Ph. Passa, P.F. Plouin, G. Tchobroutsky, eds. Hypertension, diabète et systèmes rénine-angiotensine tissulaires. Aspects fondamentaux et conséquences thérapeutiques. Diabete Metab 1992; 18: 127-186.

A.S. Krolewski, ed. Third International Symposium on Hypertension Associated with Diabetes Mellitus. J Am Soc Nephrol 1992; 3: Suppl.: S1-S139.

G.C. Viberti, W.B. White, eds. What to treat? The structural basis for renal and vascular complications and hypertension, and the role of angiotensin converting enzyme inhibition. J Hypertens 1992; 10: Suppl. 1: S1-S51.

S. M. Mauer, C.E. Mogensen, G.C. Viberti, eds. Symposium on the Progress in Diabetic Nephropathy. Kidney Int 1992: 41: 717-929

G. Crepaldi, R. Nosadini, R. Mangili, eds. Proceedings of the International Meeting »State of the art and new perspective sin Diabetic Nephropathy« University of Padua, 6-7 March, 1992. Acta Diabetol 1992; 29: 115-279.

C.E. Mogensen, C. Berne, E. Ritz, G.-C. Viberti, eds. Proceedings of the Symposium Diabetic Renal Disease in Type 2 Diabetic Patients. A major worldwide health problem. Prague, 7 September, 1992. Diabetologia 1993; 36: 977-1117.

F. Belfiore, R.N. Bergman, G.M. Molinatti, eds. *Current Topics in Diabetes Research. 4th International Diabetes Conference, Florence, March 18-20, 1992. Frontiers in Diabetes, Vol. 12.* Basel, Freiburg, Paris, London, New York, New Delhi, Bangkok, Singapore, Tokyo, Sydney: Karger, 1993.

M.M. Avram, S. Klahr, eds. Proceedings from the Long Island College Hospital. Symposium on Lipids and Vasoactive Agents in Renal Disease. Am J Kidney Dis 1993; 22: 64-239.

E. Ferrannini, ed. Insulin Resistance Syndrome. Cardiovasc Risk Factors 1993; 3: 1-81.

D. Batlle, ed. The Diabetes/Hypertension Connection. Cardiovasc Risk Factors 1993; 3: 145-187.

C. Hasslacher, C.G. Brilla, eds. Renin-angiotensin-system and collagen metabolism in diabetes mellitus and arterial hypertension. Clin Investig 1993; 71: Suppl.: S1-S50.

E. Ferrannini, ed. *Insulin Resistance and Disease. Baillière's Clinical Endocrinology and Metabolism. International Practice and Research. Vol. 7.* London, Philadelphia. Sydney, Tokyo, Toronto: Baillière Tindall, 1993.

C.E. Mogensen, E. Standl, eds. *Research Methodologies in Human Diabetes. Part 1*, Berlin, New York: Walter de Gruyter, 1994.

P.T. Sawicki, ed. *Hemmung der Progression diabetischer Nephropathie.* Mainz: Verlag Kirchheim, 1994.

W.F. Keane, B.M. Brenner, H.H. Parving, eds. Progression of Renal Disease. Kidney Int 1994; Suppl. 45: S1-S180.

Journal of Diabetes and Its Complications. Special Issue: Selected presentations from Epidemiology of Microalbuminuria, Mortefontaine, France, 13 November 1993. July-September 1994; 8: No. 3.

H.J.G. Bilo, G.C. Viberti, eds. *Diabetic Nephropathy. de Weezenlanden Series, No. 2. Zwolle 1994.* Den Haag: CIP-Gegevens Koninklijke Bibliotheek, 1994.

Ch. Hasslacher, ed. *Der Hypertensive Typ-II-Diabetiker. Pathophysiologie, Diagnostik, Komplikationen und Differentialtherapie.* Berlin/New York: Walter de Gruyter, 1994.

L.M. Ruilope et al. Microalbuminuria in clinical practice. Kidney: A current survey of world literature 1995; 4: 211-216.

C.E. Mogensen, E. Standl, eds. *Research Methodologies in Human Diabetes. Part 2*, Berlin, New York: Walter de Gruyter, 1995.

Journal of Diabetes and Its Complications. Special Section: Proteinuria and Progressive Renal disease. Second International Symposium, Vienna, Austria, 2 July 1994. January-March 1995; 9: No. 1.

Journal of Diabetes and Its Complications. Special Issue: Proceedings of the Fourth International Symposium on Hypertension Associated with Diabetes Mellitus, A Satellite Symposium of the 15th International Diabetes Fedration Congress, Otsu, Japan, 4-5 November 1994. October-December 1995; 9: No. 4.

R. Nosadini, ed. Symposium on diabetic nephropathy. Diab Nutr Metab 1995; 8: 129-185.

H.B. Lee, ed. Pathogenesis of Diabetic Nephropathy: Experimental approaches. Kidney Int 1995; Suppl. 51.

E. Ritz, P.U. Weidmann, eds. Hypertension and the Kidney. 29th Deidesheimer Gespräch, April 29, 1995. Nephrol Dial Transplant 1995; 10: Suppl. 9.

H.-H. Parving, R. Østerby, P.W. Anderson, W.A. Hsueh. »Diabetic nephropathy.« In *The Kidney.* Brenner BM, Rector F, eds. W.B. Saunders Co., 1995; pp 1864-1892.

R.A. DeFronzo. Diabetic nephropathy: etiologic and therapeutic considerations. Diabetes Rev 1995; 3: 510-564.

H. Koide, I. Ichikawa, eds. *Progression of Chronic Renal Diseases. International Symposium, Shizuoka, May 20-23, 1995.* Contributions to Nephrology, vol. 118. Basel, Freiburg, Paris, London, New York, New Delhi, Bangkok, Singapore, Tokyo, Sydney: Karger, 1996.

C.E. Mogensen, R. Turner, eds. Proceedings of the Symposium: Improving Prognosis in NIDDM. Stockholm, 11-12 September, 1995. Diabetologia Diabetologia 1996; 39: 1539-1678.

Grossman E, Messerli FH. Diabetic and hypertensive heart disease. Ann Intern Med 1996; 125: 304-310.

R. Østerby. Lessons from Kidney Biopsies. Diabetes/Metabolism Reviews 1996; 12: 151-174.

Chronic Complications of Diabetes. Endocrinology and Metabolism Clinics of North America 1996; 25: 217-438.

Journal of Diabetes and Its Complications. Special Section: Diabetic Complications and Early Treatment using ACE Inhibitors. May-June 1996; 10: No. 3: 124-153

C.E. Mogensen, ed. *Microalbuminuria. A Marker for Organ Damage.* 2nd ed. London: Science Press, 1996.

A.H. Barnett, P.M. Dodson, eds. *Hypertension and Diabetes*. 2nd ed. London: Science Press, 1996.

M. Mauer, C.E. Mogensen. »Diabetic nephropathy.« In *Diseases of the Kidney*, vo. III, R.W. Schrier, C.W. Gottschalk. eds. Boston: Little, Brown and Company, 1996; Chapter 73: p. 2019-2062.

R. Pedrinelli. Microalbuminuria in hypertension (Editorial). Nephron 1996; 73: 499-505.

R. Pontremoli. Microalbuminuria in essential hypertension - its relation to cardiovascular risk factors (Editorial Comment). Nephrol Dial Transplant 1996; 11: 2113-2115.

C.E. Mogensen, ed. Over-Mortality in NIDDM. Journal of Diabetes and Its Complications 1997; 11: 59-143.

C.E. Mogensen, P. Weidmann, eds. Hypertension and Diabetes: a risky alliance. How can drug therapy improve clinical outcome? Am J Hypertens 1997; 10: no. 9, pt. 2, suppl.: 171S-217S.

P.E. de Jong, Dick de Zeeuw, C.E. Mogensen, eds. Proteinuria and Progressive Renal Disease. June 1996. Amsterdam, The Netherlands. Nephrol Dial Transplant 1997; 12: suppl. 2: 1-85.

F.A. Gries, T. Koschinsky, D. Tschöpe, D. Ziegler, eds. Current State and Perspectives of Diabetes Research: Chronic Complications. Diabetes 1997; 46: suppl. 2: S1-S134.

R.W. Bilous, P. Fioretto, P. Czernichow, K. Drummond. Growth factors and diabetic nephropathy: kidney structure and therapeutic interventions. Diabetologia 1997; 40: B68-B73.

T. Baba, S. Neugebauer, T. Watanabe. Diabetic Nephropathy. Its relationship to hypertension and means of pharmacological intervention. Durgs 1997; 54: 197-234.

E.J. Lewis, ed. Prevention of Diabetic Nephropathy. Sem Nephrol 1997; 17: 77-147.

H.B. Lee, H. Ha, eds. Experimental Approaches to Diabetic Nephropathy. The Third Hyonam Kidney Laboratory International Symposium. Seoul, South Korea, January 24-25, 1997. Kidney Int 1997; 51: suppl. 60: 1-103.

W.F. Keane, B.M. Brenner, K. Kurokawa, eds. Progression of Renal Disease: Clinical Patterns, Therapeutic Options, and Lessons from Clinical Trials, Coolum, Australia, May 31-June 3, 1997. Kidney Int 1997; 52: suppl. 63: 1-243.

D.J. Barnes, J.R. Pinto, G.-C. Viberti. The Kidney in systemic disease. The patient with diabetes mellitus. In A.M. Davision, J.S. Cameron, J.-P. Grünfeld, D.N.S. Kerr, E. Ritz, C.G. Winearls, eds. Oxford Textbook of Clinical Nephrology, 2nd ed. Oxford, New York, Tokyo; Oxford University Press 1998; 723-776.

American Diabetes Association. Diabetic Nephropathy. Diabetes Care 1999: 22: S-66-69

L.P. Aiello, T.W. Gardner, G.L. King, G. Blankenship, J.D. Cavallerano, F.L. Ferris III, R. Klein. Diabetic Retinopathy. Diabetes Care 1998; 21: 143-156.

C.E. Mogensen, ed. Proceedings from 4th Symposium on Proteinuria and Progressive Renal Disease. September 1997. Montreux, Switzerland. Nephrol Dial Transplant 1998; 13: 1056-1079.

C.E. Mogensen. Microalbuminuria and diabetic renal disease. Origin and development of ideas. Diabetologia, 1999; 42: 263-285.

G. Crepaldi, A. Tiengo, S. Del Prato, eds. Insulin resistance, metabolic diseases and diabetic complications. Proceedings of the 7th European Symposium on Metabolism, Padova, September 30-October 3, 1998. Amsterdam, Lausanne, New York, Oxford, Shannon, Singapore, Tokyo.: Elsevier, 1999.

E. Ritz. Nephropathy in type 2 diabetes. Journal of Internal Medicine, 1999; 245: 111-126.

R. Mangili. Microalbuminuria in Diabetes. Clin Chem Lab Med., 1998; 36(12):941-946.

T.C. Fagan, J. Sowers. Type 2 Diabetes Mellitus. Greater cardiovascular risks and greater benefits of therapy. Arch Intern Med, 1999; 159: 1033-134.

Guidelines Subcommittee. 1999 World Health Organization – International Society of Hypertension Guidelines for the Management of Hypertension. Journal of Hypertension, 1999; 17: 151-183.

N. Ismail, B. Becker, P. Strzelczyk, E. Ritz. Renal disease and hypertension in non-insulin-dependent diabetes mellitus. Kidney International, 1999; 55: 1-28.

L. Groop, R. DeFronzo, eds. Diabetes and research and clinical practice. vol. 39 (suppl. (1998)). Hypertension and NIDDM – Doubling the risk Elsevier, 1998.

P. Ruggenenti, G. Remuzzi. Nephropathy of Type-2 Diabetes Mellitus. J Am Soc Nephrol, 1998; 9: 2157-2169.

H.-H. Parving. Renoprotection in diabetes: Genetic and non-genetic risk factors and treatment. Review. Diabetologia, 1998; 41: 745-759.

G. Jerums. Differences in renal outcomes with ACE-inhibitors in Type 1 and Type 2 diabetic patients: Possible explanations. Miner Electrolyte Metab, 1998; 24: 423-437.

A Salevetti, P Mattei, I. Sudana. Renal Protection and antihypertensive drugs. Current status. Drugs, 1999; 57(5): 665-693.

C.E. Mogensen, G. Scherntaner (eds.) Improving Prognosis in Type 1 diabetes. Proceedings from an official Satellite Symposium of the 16th International Diabetes Federation Congress. Helsinki, Finland, 19-20 July 1997, Diabetes Care, 1999; 22(2).

S.M. Marshall and P.H. Winocour. Microalbuminuria, biochemistry, epidemiology and clinical practice. Cambridge University Press, 1998.

E. Ritz and I. Rychlík. Nephropathy in type 2 diabetes. Oxford Clinical Nephrology Series, 1999.

M.F. Lokhandwala, K. Abe, B.S. Jandhyala, J.P. Chalmers and M. Paul. Proceedings of the WHO/ISH International expert meeting on hypertension. Clinical and Experimental Hypertension, 1999; vol. 21 nos. 5&6.

G. A. Fleming, S.S. Jhee, R.F. Coniff, H.J. Riordan, M.F. Murphy, N.M. Kurtz, N.R. Cutler. Optimizing therapeutic developments in diabetes. Greenwich Medical Media Ltd., 1999.

E. Ritz, S. R. Orth. Nephropathy in patients with type 2 diabetes mellitus. New Engl J Med, 1999; 341: 1127-1133.

S. M. Marshall. Blood pressure control, microalbuminuria and cardiovascular risk in type 2 diabetes mellitus. Diabetic Medicine, 1999; 16: 358-372.

M. Marre. Genetics and the prediction of complications in type 1 diabetes. Diabetes Care, 1999; 22(2): B53-B58

A.S. Krolewski. Genetics of diabetic nephropathy: Evidence for major and minor gene effects. Kidney International, 1999; 55: 1582-1596.

Gerald M. Reaven, Ami Laws (eds.). Insulin resistance, The metabolic syndrome. Humana Press, Totowa, New Jersey, 1999

Groffen AJA, Veerkamp JH, Monnens LAH, LPWJ van den Heuvel. Recent insights into the structure and functions of heparan sulfate proteoglycans in the human glomerular basement membrane. Nephrol Dial Transplant, 1999; 14: 2119-2129.

Nyengaard JR. Stereological methods and their application in kidney research. J Am Soc Neprhol, 1999; 10: 1100-1123.

Yvo M. Smulders. Microalbuminuria and cardiovascular risk factors in type 2 diabetes mellitus. Thesis, University of Amsterdam, 1999.

Ramsey LE, Williams B, Johnston CD, Macgregor GA, Poston L, Potter JF, Poulter NR, Russell G. Guidelines for management of hypertension – report of the 3rd working party of the British Hypertension Society (Review). Journ. Hum Hypertension, 1999; 13: 569-592.

Chiarell F, Casani A, Tumini S, Kordonou O, Danne T. Diabetic nephropathy in childhood and adolescents (review). Diabetic nutr, 1999; 12: 144-153.

Patterson JE, Andriole V. Bacterial urinary tract infections in diabetes. Infectious Disease Clinics of North America, 1997; 11: 735-750.

Diabetes and metabolism. La prise en charge des diabétiques urémiques. Règles de bonnes pratiques cliniques. Rapport des experts de l'ALFEDIAM et de la Société de Néphrologie, 25(s.5), 1999

Keller C, Ritz E, Pommer W, Stein G, Frank J, Schwarzbeck A. Behandlungsqualität Niereninsuffizienter Diabetiker in Deutschland. Deutsche Medizinische Wochenschrift, 2000. In press.

Psaty BM, Furberg CD (1999). British guidelines on managing hypertension. Provide evidence, progress, and an occasional missed opportunity. BMJ, 1999; 319: 589-90.

Ramsay LE, Williams B, Johnston GD, MacGregor GA, Poston L, Potter JF, Poulter NR, Russell G. British Hypertension Society Guidelines for hypertension management 1999: Summary. BMJ, 1999; 319: 630-635.

Marshall SM. Blood pressure control in diabetes. Diabetic Medicine, 1999; 16:358-372.

Hartland A, Gosling P. Microalbuminuria – yet another cardiovascular risk factor (editorial). Ann Clin Bi, 1999; 36: 700-703.

Schafers RF, Lutkes P, Ritz E, Philipp T. Guidelines for the treatment of arterial hypertension in diabetics – consensus recommendations of the German league for the fight against high blood pressure, the German diabetes society and the nehprological society (Review). Deut Med Woche, 1999; 124: 1356-1372.

Nosidini R, Fioretto P. Renal involvement in type 2 diabetes mellitus: prognostic role of proteinuria and morphological lesions. J Nephrol, 1999; 12:329-46.

An Ace in the hole? (editorial) Diabetic Med, 1999; 16: 887-888.

Belfiore F, Mogensen CE (eds). New Concepts in Diabetes and its Treatment, Karger, Basel, 2000

Passa Ph, Mogensen CE (eds.) Supplementum on Data, Results and Consequences of Major Trials with Focus on Type 2 Diabetes. Diabetes Care, april 2000.

Vanderwoude FJ. Heparins in diabetic microangiopathy –rationale and preliminary clinical results. Haemostatis 29 (S1): 61-67, 1999

Bianchi S, Bigazzi R, Campese VM. Microalbuminuria in essential hypertension: Significance, pathophysiology, and therapeutic implications. Am J Kidney Dis, 1999; 34: 973-95.

Opie LH. Angiotensin-converting enzyme inhibitors: The advance continues, 3rd ed. University of Cape Town Press, 1999.

Fokko J van der Woude. Heparins in diabetic microangiopathy: rationale and preliminary clinical results. Haemostatis, 1999; 29(s1):61-67.

J. S. Cameron. Villain and victim: the kidney and high blood pressure in the nineteenth century. J R Coll Physicians Lond, 1999; 33-382-394

O. Gambaro, FJ Vanderwo. Glycosaminoglycans – use in treatment of diabetic nephropathy (Review), JASN, 2000; 11: 359-368.

SM Thomas, GC Viberti. Is it possible to predict diabetic kidney disease (review). J Endoc Inv. 2000; 23: 44-53.

R.B Goldberg. Cardiovascular disease in diabetic patients. Medical clinics of North America, 2000; 84: 81-93

CJ Raats, J Vandenbo, Berden JHM. Glomerular heparan-sulfate alterations – mechanisms and relevance for proteinuria (review). Kidney Int, 2000; 57: 385-400.

SC Bain, TA Chowdhur. Genetics sf diabetic nehropathy and microalbuminuria (review). J Roy S Med, 2000; 93: 62-66.

GC Viberti, S Thomas. Should we screen for microalbuminuria in essential hypertension (editorial). Am J Kidn. Dis., 1999; 34: 1139-41.

Report of a WHO Consultation. Definition, diagnosis and classification of diabetes mellitus and its complications. World Health Organization. Department of noncumminicable disease surveillance, Geneva, 1999.

E Faloia, G Giacchetti, F Mantero. Obesity and hypertension. J Endocrinol. Invest, 2000; 23: 54-62.

E.A. Friedman, F.A. L'Esperance Jr. (eds). Diabetic renal-retinal syndrome. 21st Century Management Now, Kluwer Academic Publ., 1998

E. Ritz, I Rychlik (eds). Nephropathy in type 2 diabetes. Oxford Clinical Nephrology Series. Oxford University Press Inc., New York 1999

Relevant review articles in DIABETES ANNUAL

E.N. Ellis, S.M. Mauer. »Diabetic nephropathy.« In *The Diabetes Annual/1*. Alberti KGMM, Krall LP, eds. Amsterdam, New York, Oxford: Elsevier Science Publishers B.V., 1985; pp 309-322.

C.E. Mogensen. »Early diabetic renal involvement and nephropathy. Can treatment modalities be predicted from identification of risk factors?« In *The Diabetes Annual/3*. Alberti KGMM, Krall LP, eds. Amsterdam, New York, Oxford: Elsevier Science Publishers B.V., 1987; pp 306-324.

A.R. Christlieb, A.S. Krolewski, J.H. Warram. »An update on hypertension in patients with diabetes mellitus.« In *The Diabetes Annual/4*. Alberti KGMM, Krall LP, eds. Amsterdam, New York, Oxford: Elsevier Science Publishers B.V., 1988; pp 384-393.

C.E. Mogensen. »Diabetic renal involvement and disease in patients with insulin-dependent diabetes.« In *The Diabetes Annual/4*. Alberti KGMM, Krall LP, eds. Amsterdam, New York, Oxford: Elsevier Science Publishers B.V., 1988; pp 411-448.

G.C. Viberti. »New insights into the genesis of diabetic kidney disease in insulin-dependent diabetic patients.« In *The Diabetes Annual/5*. Alberti KGMM, Krall LP, eds. Amsterdam, New York, Oxford: Elsevier Science Publishers B.V., 1990; pp 301-311.

P.L. Drury. »Hypertension in diabetes.« In *The Diabetes Annual/5*. Alberti KGMM, Krall LP, eds. Amsterdam, New York, Oxford: Elsevier Science Publishers B.V., 1990; pp 362-372.

S.M. Marshall. »Diabetic nephropathy.« In *The Diabetes Annual/6*. Alberti KGMM, Krall LP, eds. Amsterdam, London, New York, Tokyo: Elsevier Science Publishers B.V., 1991; pp 302-325.

H.-H. Parving. »Hypertension and diabetes.« In *The Diabetes Annual/7*. Marshall SM, Home PD, Alberti KGMM, Krall LP, eds. Amsterdam, New York, Oxford: Elsevier Science Publishers B.V., 1993; pp 301-311.

G. Jerums, R. Gilbert. »Renal tubular dysfunction in diabetes mellitus.« In *The Diabetes Annual/7*. Marshall SM, Home PD, Alberti KGMM, Krall LP, eds. Amsterdam, New York, Oxford: Elsevier Science Publishers B.V., 1993; pp 146-165.

H. Vlassara, R. Bucala. »Advanced glycation and diabetes complications: an update.« In *The Diabetes Annual/9*. Marshall SM, Home PD, Rizza RA, eds. Amsterdam, Lausanne, New York, Oxford, Shannon, Tokyo: Elsevier Science B.V., 1995; pp 227-244.

A.S. Reddi. »The basement membrane in diabetes.« In *The Diabetes Annual/9*. Marshall SM, Home PD, Rizza RA, eds. Amsterdam, Lausanne, New York, Oxford, Shannon, Tokyo: Elsevier Science B.V., 1995; pp 245-263.

P. Ruggenenti, G. Remuzzi. »Anti-hypertensive agents and incipient diabetic nephropathy.« In *The Diabetes Annual/9*. Marshall SM, Home PD, Rizza RA, eds. Amsterdam, Lausanne New York, Oxford, Shannon, Tokyo: Elsevier Sci ence Publishers B.V., 1995; pp 295-317.

G. Jerums and R.E. Gilbert. »Microalbuminuria in non-insulin-dependent diabetes: significance and management. » In *The Diabetes Annual/11*. Marshall SM, Home PD, Rizza RA, eds., Amsterdam, Lausanne, New York, Oxford, Shannon, Tokyo: Elsevier Science Publishers B.V., 1998, pp. 141-168.

S.M. Marshall. »Diabetic nephropathy and insulin-dependent diabetes mellitus« In » In *The Diabetes Annual/11*. Marshall SM, Home PD, Rizza RA, eds., Amsterdam, Lausanne, New York, Oxford, Shannon, Tokyo: Elsevier Science Publishers B.V., 1998, pp. 169-194.

Kohner E.M. Prevention of visual loss in diabetic retinopathy. In the *Diabetes Annual/12.* Marshall SM, Home PD, Rizza RA, eds. Elsevier Science Publishers B.V., 1999 pp 329-339.

AUTHORS

Sharon Anderson, M.D.
Division of Nephrology and Hypertension
PP262
Oregon Health Sciences University
3314 SW US Veterans Hospital
Portland, OR 97201
USA
Tel: +1-503-494-8490
Fax: +1-503-721-7810
e-mail: anderssh@ohsu.edu

George L. Bakris, MD, F.A.C.P
Rush University Hypertension Center
Rush-Presbyterian-St. Luke's Medical Center
1700 W. Van Buren
Suite #470
Chicago, IL 60612-3833
USA
Tel: +1 312 563 2195
Fax: +1 312 942 4464
gbakris@rush.edu

Hans-Jacob Bangstad, M.D.
Unit of Nephrology
Pediatric Department
Aker Diabetes Research Center
Ullevål University Hospital
0407 Oslo
Norge
Tel: +47 2211 7954
Fax: +47 2211 8663
e-mail: h.j. bangstad@ioks.uio.no

Rudy W. Bilous, MD, FRCP
Consultant Physician
South Tees Undergraduate
Medical centre
Marton Road, Middlesbrough
Cleveland TS4 3BW
United Kingdom
Tel: +44 1 642 854 145
Fax: +44 1 642 854 148
e-mail: r.w.bilous@ncl.ac.uk

Geoffrey Boner, M.B.B.Ch.
Department of Medicine,
Sackler Faculty of Medicine
Tel Aviv University, Tel Aviv
Institute of Hypertension and Kidney Diseases
Rabin Medical Center – Beilinson Campus
Petah Tikva 49100
Tel: +972 3 93 77414
Fax: +972 3 9223212
e-mail: gboner@post.tau.ac.il

Knut Borch-Johnsen, M.D.
Steno Diabetes Center
Niels Steensens Vej 2
2820 Gentofte
Tel: +45 4443 9415
Fax: +45 4443 8233
e-mail: kbjo@novo.dk

Vito M. Campese, M.D.
LAC/USC Medical Center
1200 North State St.
Los Angeles, CA 90033
USA
Tel: +1 213 226 7307
Fax: +1 213 226 5390
e-mail: campese@hsc.usc.edu

Nishi Chaturvedi, M.D.
Department of Primary Care and General
Practice
Imperial College of Medicine at St Mary's
Norfolk Place
London W2 1PG, UK
Tel: +44 20 7594 3381
Eurodiab fax: +44 20 7706 8426
e-mail: n.chaturvedi@ic.ac.uk

Sheldon Chen, MD.
Nephrology Fellow
700 Clinical Research Building
Renal-Electrolyte & Hypertension Div.
University of Pennsylvania
415 Curie Blvd.
Philadelphia, PA 19104-6144
Tel: (215) 898-0192
Fax: (215) 898-0189
e-mail:chens@mail.med.upenn.edu

Per K. Christensen
Steno Diabetes Center
Niels Steensens Vej 2
2820 Gentofte
tel: +45 3968 0800
fax: +45 3968 1048
e-mail:pkc@novo.dk

Mark Cooper, M.D.
The University of Melbourne
Department of Medicine
Austin and Repatriation Medical Centre -
Repatriation Campus
West Heidelberg 3081
Australia
Tel: +61 3 9496 2347
Fax: +61 3 9497 4554
e-mail cooper@austin.unimelb.edu.au

Bo Feldt-Rasmussen, M.D.
Medical Department P 2132
Rigshospitalet
DK-2100 København Ø
Denmark
Tel: +45 3545 2135
Fax: +45 3545 2240
e-mail: bfr@rh.dk

Ele Ferrannini, M.D.
Istituto di Fisiologia Clinica del CNR
CNR Institute of Clinical Physiology
Consiglio Nazionale delle Ricerche - C.N.R.
c/o Università di Pisa
Via Savi, 8
I-56100 Pisa
Italy
Tel: +39 50 500087
Fax: +39 50 553235
e-mail: ferranni@ifc.pi.cnr.it

Paola Fioretto, M.D.
Istituto di Medicina Interna
Università di Padova
Via Giustiniani, 2
I-35128 Padova
Italy
Tel: +39 49 821 2150
Fax: +39 49 821 2151
e-mail: fiorep@uxl.unipd.it

G. Alexander Fleming, MD
Vice President, Regulatory Affairs
Worldwide Clinical Trials
5454 Wisconsin Avenue, Suite 810
Chevy Chase, MD 20815
Washington D.C
Tel: +1 301 986 0553
Fax: +1 301 986 5788
e-mail: afleming@usa.wctrials.com

Allan Flyvbjerg, MD. D.Sc.
Ass. Professor
Medical Department M
Diabetes & Endocrinology
Aarhus Kommunehospital
Aarhus University Hospital
DK-8000 Aarhus C
Denmark
Tel: +45 8949 2161
Fax: +458949 2010/86 56 00 87
e-mail: allan.flyvbjerg@dadlnet.dk

Amy L. Friedman
Department of Surgery, Yale University
College of Medicine,
New Haven, Connecticut
USA

Eli A. Friedman, M.D.
Division of Renal Disease
Department of Medicine
State University of New York Health Science
Center at Brooklyn
450 Clarkson Avenue, Box 52
Brooklyn, NY 11203
USA
Tel: +1 718 270 1584
Fax: +1 718 270 3327
e-mail: elifriedmn@aol.com

Annarita Gabriele
Endocrinology Division
Department of Clinical Science
La Sapienza University
Rome 00161
Italy

Lennart Hansson, MD.
Clinical Hypertension Research
Dept. Of Public Health and Social Sciences
University of Uppsala
Box 609
S-75 125 Uppsala
Tel: +46 18-101384
Fax: +46 18-177973

Andy I.M. Hoepelman
Department of Internal Medicine
Division Infectious Diseases & Aids
Utrecht
Tel: +31 30 2506288
Fax: +31 302523741
e-mail: i.m.hoepelman@digd.azu.nl

Norman K. Hollenberg, M.D., Ph.D.
Brigham and Women's Hospital
75 Francis Street
Boston, MA 02115
USA
Tel: +1 617 732 6682
Fax: +1 617 232 2869
e-mail: daprice@bics.bwh.harvard.ed'

Klavs Würgler Hansen, M.D.
Medical Department M
Aarhus Kommunehospital
Aarhus University Hospital
DK-8000 Aarhus C
Denmark
Tel: +45 8949 2023
Fax: +45 8949 2010
e-mail: kwh@dadlnet.dk

Guiseppina Imperatore, MD, PhD
Diabetes and Arthritis Epidemiology Section
National Institute of Diabetes
and Digestive Kidney Diseases
1550 East Indian School Road
Phoenix, Arizona, 85014, USA

Susan E. Jones
Department of medicine
The Medical school
Framlington Place
Newcastle Upon Tyne NE2 4HH, UK
Tel: +44 (0) 191 2227 019
Fax: +44 (0) 191 2220 723
e-mail: susan.jones@ncl.ac.uk

John L. Kitzmiller, M.D.
Chief, Maternal Fetal Medicine
Good Samaritan Health System
Perinatal Associates of Santa Clara Valley
2425 Samaritan Drive
San Jose, California 95124
USA
Tel: +1 408 559 2258
Fax: +1 408 559 2658
e-mail: kitz@batnet.com

William C. Knowler, M.D., Dr.P.H.
Diabetes and Arthritis Epidemiology Section
Department of Healthy & Human Services
National Institutes of Health
National Institute of Diabetes and Digestive
and Kidney Diseases
1550 East Indian School Road
Phoenix, Arizona 85014
USA
Tel: +1 602 263-1610
Fax: +1 602 263-1577
e-mail: kcw@cu.nih.gov

Michel Marre, M.D.
Service de Diabétogie – Endocrinologie-
Metabolisme
Hôpital Bichat
46, rue Henri Huchard
F-75877 Paris Cedex 18
Tel: +33 140 2573 01
Fax: +33 140 2588 43
e-mail: michel.marre@bch.ap-hop-paris.fr

Carl Erik Mogensen, M.D.
Medical Department M
Diabetes & Endocrinology
Aarhus Kommunehospital
Aarhus University Hospital
DK-8000 Aarhus C
Denmark
Tel: +45 8949 2011
Fax: +45 8613 7825/8949 2010
e-mail: cem@afdm.au.dk

Henrik Bindesbøl Mortensen, M.D.
Pediatric Department L
Amtssygehuset i Glostrup
Ndr. Ringvej
DK-2600 Glostrup
Denmark
Tel: +45 4323 2967
Fax: +45 43233964
e-mail: hbm@dadlnet.dk

Gerjan J. Navis, M.D.
Department of Medicine
Division of Nephrology
University Hospital
Hanzeplein 1
9700 RB Groningen
The Netherlands
Fax: +31 50 3169310
e-mail: g.j.navis@int.azg.nl

Søren Nielsen, M.D.
Medical Department M
Diabetes & Endocrinology
Aarhus Kommunehospital
Aarhus University Hospital
DK-8000 Aarhus C
Denmark
Tel: +45 8949 2019
Fax: +45 8949 2010
e-mail: Nielsen.Soren@dadlnet.dk

Jens Randel Nyengaard, M.D.
Stereological Res. Lab.
Ole Worms Allé
Building 182
University of Aarhus
DK-8000 Aarhus C
Denmark
Tel: +45 8942 2955
Fax: +45 8942 2952
e-mail: lfjrn@svfcd.au.dk

Unini Odama, MD
Fellow in Hypertension
Rush University Hypertension Center
1700 W. Van Buren St, Suite 470
Chicago, IL 60612

Steen Olsen, M.D.
Professor Emeritus
Department of Pathology
Herlev Hospital
DK-2730 Herlev, Denmark
Tel: (home: 45 3976 2520)
e-mail: steeno@dadlnet.dk

Margrethe Mau Pedersen, M.D.
Randers Centralsygehus
Medical Dept.
DK-8900 Randers
Denmark
e-mail: JD@hi.au.dk

David J. Pettitt, M.D.
Sansum Medical Research Foundation
2219 Bath Street
Santa Barbara, CA 93105
USA
Tel: +1 805 682 7640
Fax: +1 805 682 3332
e-mail: dpettitt@sansum.org

Per Løgstrup Poulsen, M.D.
Medical Department M
Diabetes & Endocrinology
Aarhus Kommunehospital
Aarhus University Hospital
DK-8000 Aarhus C
Denmark
Tel: +45 8949 2019
Fax: +45 8949 2010
e-mail: logstrup@dadlnet.dk

Bruce L Riser, AB, MS, PhD
Senior staff Investigator
Henry Ford Hospital
Division of Nephrology and Hypertension
2799 West Grand Boulevard
Detroit, Michigan 48202-2689
USA
e-mail: riserb@usa.net

Eberhard Ritz, M.D.
Sektion Nephrologie
Klinikum der Universität Heidelberg
Medizinische Klinik
Bergheimer Strasse 56a
D-69115 Heidelberg
Germany
Tel: +49 6221 91120
Fax: +49 6221 162476
e-mail: Prof.E.Ritz@T-online.de

Peter Rossing, M.D.
Steno Diabetes Center
Niels Steensensvej 2
DK-2820 Gentofte
Denmark
Tel: +45 3968 0800
Fax: +45 4443 8232
e-mail: prossing@dadlnet.dk

Dr. Piero Ruggenenti
Mario Negri Institute for Pharmacological
Research
Via Gavazzeni 11
24125 Bergamo, Italy
Tel: +39 035 319 888
Fax: +39 035 319 331
e-mail: ruggenenti@irfmn.mnegri.it

Erwin Schleicher, M.D.
Institute of Internal Medicine
Dep. Of Endocrinology, Metabolism and
Pathobiochemistry
University of Tübingen
Otfried-Müller-Str. 10
D-72076 Tübingen
Germany
Tel: +49 7071 29 87599
Fax: +49 7071 29 5974
e-mail: enschlei@med.uni-tuebingen.de

Anita Schmitz, M.D.
Medical dept.
Horsens Sygehus
DK-8700 Horsens
Denmark
Tel: +45 7927 4444
Fax: +45 7927 4484
e-mail: Schmitz@mail1.stofanet.dk

Coen D.A. Stehouwer, M.D.
Department of Internal Medicine
Free University Hospital
De Boelelaan 1117
1081 HV Amsterdam
The Netherlands
Tel: +31 20 444 0531
Fax: +31 20 444 0502
e-mail: cda.stehouwer@azvu.nl

GianCarlo Viberti, M.D.
Division of Medicine
Guy's and St Thomas's Medical and Dental
School
Unit for Metabolic Medicine
Diabetes, Endocrinology, Metabolism
Floor 5 Hunt's House, Guy's Hospital
London Bridge, London SE1 9RT
United Kingdom
Tel: +44 1 71 955 4826
Fax: +44 1 71 955 2985
e-mail: giancarlo.viberti@kcl.ac.uk

James Walker, M.D.
Department of Diabetes
The Royal Infirmary of Edinburgh
Lauriston Place
Edinburgh EH3 9YW
Scotland
Tel: +44 1 31 536 1000
Fax: +44 1 31 536 1001
e-mail: jdwalker@mcmail.com

Bryan Williams. M.D.
Cardiovascular Research Institute
University of Leicester
Faculty of Medicine and Biological Sciences
PO Box 65
Leicester Royal Infirmary
Leicester LE2 7LX, UK
Tel: +44 116 252 3182
Fax: +44 116 252 5847
e-mail: bw17@le.ac.uk

Fuad N. Ziyadeh, M.D.
Renal-Electrolyte and Hypertension Division
700 Clinical Research Building
University of Pennsylvania Medical Center
415 Curie Boulevard
Philadelphia, PA 19104-6144
USA
Tel: +1 215 573 1837
Fax: +1 215 898 0189
e-mail: ziyadeh@mail.med.upenn.edu

Giulio Zuanetti, M.D.
Department of Cardiovascular Research
Istituto Mario Negri
via Eritrea 62
I-20157 Milan
Italy
Tel: +39 2 3901 4454
Fax: +39 2 3320 004
e-mail: zuanetti@irfmn.mnegri.it

Ruth Østerby
Electron Microscopy Laboratory
Building 3
Aarhus Kommunehospital
Aarhus University Hospital
DK-8000 Aarhus C
Tel: +45 8949 2141
Fax: +45 8949 2150
e-mail: ro@em.au.dk

The first sporadic observations describing renal abnormalities in diabetes were published late in the 19th century, but systematic studies of the kidney in diabetes started only half a century ago after the paper by Cambier in 1934 and the much more famous study by Kimmelstiel and Wilson in 1936. These authors described two distinct features of renal involvement in diabetes: early hyperfiltration and late nephropathy. Diabetic nephropathy is, despite half a century of studies, still a very pertinent problem, renal disease in diabetes now being a very common cause of end-stage renal failure in Europe and North America and probably throughout the world. It is a very important part of the generalized vascular disease found in long-term diabetes as described by Knud Lundbæk in his monograph *Long-term Diabetes* in 1953, published by Munksgaard, Copenhagen.

Surprisingly, there has not been a comprehensive volume describing all aspects of renal involvement in diabetes, and the time is now ripe for such a volume summarizing the very considerable research activity within this field during the last decade and especially during the last few years.

This book attempts to cover practically all aspects of renal involvement in diabetes. It is written by colleagues who are themselves active in the many fields of medical research covered in this volume: epidemiology, physiology and pathophysiology, laboratory methodology, and renal pathology. New studies deal with the diagnosis and treatment of both incipient and overt nephropathy by metabolic, antihypertensive, and dietary invention. Considerable progress has been made in the management of end-stage renal failure and also in the management and treatment of nephropathy in the pregnant diabetic woman. Diabetic nephropathy is a world-wide problem, but it is more clearly defined in Europe and North America where facilities for the diagnosis and treatment of diabetes and its complications are readily available. Much more work needs to be done in other parts of the world, as it appears from this book.

It is hoped that we now have a handbook for the kidney and hypertension in diabetes and that further progress can be made in clinical work in diagnosing and treating diabetic patients. Much more work still needs to be done regarding patient education with respect to complications. Many diabetics have now been trained to take part in the management of their metabolic control; they should also be trained to take part in the follow-up and treatment of complications.

This volume also underlines the considerable need for future research. So far, research in this field has been carried out in relatively few countries and centres in the world. The editor is sure that this volume will also stimulate further advancement in clinical science within the field of diabetic renal disease.

In 1952, the book *Diabetic Glomerulosclerosis, The Specific Renal Disease in Diabetes Mellitus*, by Harold Rifkin and co-workers, published by Charles C. Thomas, Springfield, Illinois, USA, summarized all current knowledge on the diabetic kidney in about 100 short pages, including many case histories. Much more space is needed now and the many disciplines involved will undoubtedly attract many readers.

Carl Erik Mogensen

The sum of clinical problems caused by diabetic renal disease has been steadily increasing since the first edition of this book was published in 1988. Indeed, it is now estimated that throughout the world about 100,000 diabetic individuals are receiving treatment for end-stage renal failure. Obviously, this means a burden with respect to human suffering, disease and premature mortality, but additionally these treatment programmes are extremely costly, so costly that in many areas resources are not available for this kind of care. It is therefore clear, that every efforts should be made to prevent or postpone the development of end-stage disease.

The years since the first edition appeared we have seen a tremendous progress in research activities. Importantly, this also includes improvement in the treatment programmes to prevent end-stage renal failure. Thus it has become clear that the diabetic kidney is extremely pressure-sensitive, responding to effective antihypertensive treatment by retarded progression of disease. Some agents may be more beneficial in this respect than other, although the effective blood pressure reduction per se is crucial throughout the stages of diabetic renal disease. However, the prime cause of diabetic renal disease is related to poor metabolic control and it is now documented beyond doubt that good metabolic control is able to postpone or perhaps even prevent the development of renal disease. However, in many individuals we are not able to provide such a quality of control that will prevent complications, and therefore non-glycaemic intervention remains important. Maybe in the future non-glycaemic intervention will become the most important research area in diabetic nephropathy.

With respect to the exact mechanisms behind poor metabolic control and development of renal disease, much information is now being gained. It is likely that a combination of genetic predisposition and metabolic and haemodynamic abnormalities explain the progression to renal disease, seen in about 30% of the diabetic individuals. Much of this development probably relates to modifiable genetic factors, such as blood pressure elevation or haemodynamic aberrations. However, mechanisms related to the response to hyperglycaemia are also of clear importance as is the possibility that these metabolic or haemodynamic pathway may be inhibited.

This volume review older data as well as the progress seen within the research of diabetic nephropathy over the last five years and provides a state of the art of the development. However, we are still far from the main goal, which is the abolition of end-stage renal disease in diabetic individuals. Obviously, much work still needs to be done and one of the intentions of this book is to stimulate further research in this area where so many sub-disciplines of medical science are involved from the extremes of genetic and molecular biology to clinical and pharmacological research trials.

Carl Erik Mogensen
January 1994

PREFACE, third edition

Many new dimensions have been added to the concepts regarding diabetic renal disease in the past few years. In addition some considerably amounts of new studies have been published since the second edition of this book. Therefore, there is a clear need to update the issue on diabetic renal disease. Ever more focus is placed on pressure-induced and metabolic related aberration, in relation to genetic abnormalities and also changes developing in foetal life. New chapters also include exercise, lipidemia and retinopathy in diabetic renal disease. New data are also included regarding structural changes in NIDDM-patients. Much of the development in diabetic renal disease is also relevant to non-diabetic renal disease, and therefore chapters comparing diabetic and non-diabetic renal disease have been included.

As a result of the studies on pathogenesis of treatment of diabetic renal disease, new guidelines have been published as recently reviewed in the Lancet 1995. These guidelines are also included in this new edition, where the editor has tried to focus on all major issues relevant to diabetic renal disease.

Many groups are working within this field, but the most cited authors are the following as recently reviewed by JDF (for the years 1981-95).

Measure Diabetes Research 1981-95 - Hypertension, Nephropathy (T-10)

		Cites	Papers	C/P
USA	Brenner B	2499	33	76
DK	*Christiansen JS*	2659	115	23
DK	*Deckert T*	4229	157	27
USA	Knowler WC	2975	127	23
USA	Krolewski AS	2220	74	30
USA	Mauer SM	2307	101	23
DK	*Mogensen CE*	3456	146	24
DK	*Parving HH*	4702	216	22
F	*Passa P*	1570	196	8
UK	*Viberti GC*	2820	119	24

Carl Erik Mogensen
August 1996

PREFACE, fourth edition

We have witnessed a rapid development within the field of the kidney and hypertension in diabetes mellitus. A lot of work within the traditional areas has been published, and several new dimensions are now being developed, mostly in the experimental setting as discussed in several chapters. Therefore, there is now a need for an updated edition of this volume. A clear policy has been to have completely updated versions of the book, at disposal for the clinicians and the scientists in the area.

New guidelines are being developed within the field of hypertension and also in the field of diabetes mellitus, where new definitions are being introduced, mainly relevant for type 2 diabetes. The number of patients entering end-stage renal failure programmes are still increasing, underscoring the need for better management of these patients. The number of patients with diabetes is predicted to increased over the next decade, mainly due to changing patterns of life-style and an older population. Therefore, we need to be even more prepared to look after these patients, also with respect to renal, hypertensive and cardiovascular complications.

Since diabetic nephropathy is in most cases associated with heart disease and with retinopathy, new chapters on this aspects have been added. Very importantly, there is now more and more scientific support for early treatment in normotensive patients with microalbuminuria with ACE-inhibitors. This treatment seems beneficial also for diabetic heart disease and diabetic retinopathy according to new studies, also discussed in the book. The maxim is that diabetic nephropathy, retinopathy and heart disease often go together. The same seems to be the case regarding treatment and prevention.

Carl Erik Mogensen
January 1998

PREFACE, Fifth Edition

Over the years this volume may have developed as the OPUS MAGNUM within in diabetic renal disease and hypertension. This is a rapidly expanding area as will be seen from all the new references which have been included since the fourth edition.

Also knowledge within the field of hypertension in type 2 diabetes has developed very rapidly with the publication of many new trials, including the UKPDS. This study and other studies really emphasise the importance of good glycemic control and especially control of hypertension in these patients. Effective treatment would greatly minimise all vascular complications.

It is likely that the number of patients entering renal end-stage programs is still increasing but we can expect that this is due to better survival and postponement of the disease and also to better acceptance of patients that were earlier not allowed into this treatment programme.

The number of publications regarding microalbuminuria is continuously increasing, not only regarding diabetic nephropathy in its early phase, but also as a marker for cardiovascular disease, both in hypertension and in the general background population.

The maxim is still true that diabetic nephropathy, retinopathy, heart disease and vascular disease all go together often with neuropathy. This is also apparent in this volume, with focus on good glycemic control and the best possible antihypertensive treatment program to be implemented early.

Carl Erik Mogensen
March 2000

Few complications of systemic diseases are better understood than diabetic nephropathy. In large part, progress in this area is due to Carl Erik Mogensen's steadfast preoccupation over more than three decades with the disorder's epidemiology, pathogenesis, pathophysiology, clinical diagnosis and evolving strategies of management. Though he sparked progress in each of these areas, he generously opens the forum of discussion to many expert contributors to this latest and most comprehensive edition of his exemplary textbook. In eliciting all relevant and up-to-date views the reader, whether internist, pediatrician, or specialist in endocrinology or nephrology, is assured a thorough review of the entire subject and in a format which is exceptionally well-written, well-illustrated and easy to read.

Each of the prior editions has been an essential resource for my own work in this field and the 5th edition will no doubt continue to provide the information I and others will require to move forward in the years ahead. If only the other renal diseases were as masterfully synthesized, how much easier our task would be of achieving a comprehensive vision of all else in clinical nephrology.

Barry M. Brenner, M.D.

Samuel A. Levine Professor of Medicine
Harvard Medical School

1. PRESSURE INDUCED AND METABOLIC ALTERATIONS IN THE GLOMERULUS: ROLE IN CYTOKINE ACTIVITY AND PROGRESSIVE SCLEROSIS

Bruce L. Riser and Pedro Cortes
Henry Ford Hospital, Detroit, Michigan USA

The experimental search for mechanisms responsible for the development and progression of glomerulosclerosis has resulted in the identification of factors, broadly classified as hemodynamic and metabolic, which may be involved in both the glomerular injury of diabetes and in that occurring in the kidney remnant following subtotal nephrectomy. The hemodynamic factors include systemic arterial hypertension [1–3], glomerular hyperfunction and increased glomerular capillary hydrostatic pressure [4–6]. The metabolic factors relate to changes associated with glomerular hypertrophy [7–9], hyperlipidemia [10, 11] and, in the case of diabetes, the effects of hyperglycemia exerted either directly [12–14] or through the formation of advanced glycosylation end products and increased oxidative stress [15–19] or the increased activity of the polyol pathway [20].

Early studies on the pathogenesis of glomerulosclerosis were aimed at the identification of unique crucial alterations which could be responsible for the onset and progression of the sclerotic process. Now however, it has become apparent that hemodynamic and metabolic factors are intimately intertwined. For example, increased plasma glucose concentration directly stimulates extracellular matrix synthesis, but may also contribute to the development of glomerular hypertension and hyperfunction. The latter, in turn, is aggravated by the presence of early glycosylation products and closely associated with glomerular hypertrophy and the overexpression of cytokine [21, 22]. Not surprisingly, it is the concerted effect of multiple alterations that leads to extracellular matrix accumulation, although the relative importance of separate pathogenetic mechanisms may vary depending on the conditions of the experimental model studied or the type of human diabetes.

HYPERFUNCTION INTRAGLOMERULAR PRESSURE, AND THE ELASTIC PROPERTIES OF THE GLOMERULUS

Although increased glomerular capillary pressure is a long recognized alteration closely associated with the local deposition of extracellular matrix material, it has been only recently that information is emerging regarding the mechanisms by which the mechanical stimulus of altered hemodynamics is translated into metabolic events. Evidence has been obtained suggesting that activation or injury of the endothelium lining dilated capillaries near the glomerular vascular pole may be the initial triggering event [23]. In this case, the hemodynamic force initiating the process is likely to be shear stress induced by increased flow rates. Studies in endothelial cells in culture have shown that laminar shear stress results in generation of active pro-sclerotic growth factors and altered extracellular matrix deposition [24–26].

Additional mechanisms for the coupling of hemodynamic strain and metabolic events have emerged following the demonstration of the unique elastic properties of the glomerular structure and the response of mesangial cells when subjected to mechanical stretch in tissue culture. The elasticity of glomeruli was implied, although not so recognized, from the early observations by Bernik of spontaneous contractility/relaxation of isolated glomeruli [27] and from those by others in later studies on the angiotensin II-induced contractile response of glomeruli in suspension [28, 29]. Conclusive evidence of glomerular elasticity has been provided by studies in isolated microperfused glomeruli *ex vivo* [30]. As the intraglomerular pressure is increased from zero to levels approximating those observed in the diabetic and in the remnant kidney, glomerular volume increases by about 30% [31]. In addition, due to the high elasticity of the glomerular structure, volume changes reach their maximum within 3-4 seconds following alteration in intraglomerular pressure [32]. This elasticity, therefore, allows the occurrence of significant volume changes even with the most transient variations in intraglomerular pressure.

Glomerular expansion is, obviously, associated with the stretching of its structural components, including the extracellular matrix and the cellular constituents. Because both capillary lumina and mesangial regions equally participate in the overall increase in glomerular volume [32], endothelial, mesangial and epithelial cells will all be subjected to stretch as intraglomerular pressure increases. Due to the central location of the mesangial regions within the glomerular lobule, mesangial cells, in particular, experience substantial mechanical strain. Detailed morphological studies have demonstrated how numerous cytoplasmic projections emerging from the mesangial cell body extend between adjacent capillaries and firmly attach to the perimesangeal regions of the glomerular basement membrane [33]. Therefore, the centrifugal displacement of these regions during glomerular expansion is expected to result in marked tridimensional mesangial cell stretch.

MESANGIAL CELL MECHANICAL STRECTH AND METABOLIC RESPONSE

A vast body of information has been accumulated in recent years demonstrating remarkable morphologic and metabolic alterations resulting from the application of mechanical stimuli in various cell types. Because of the recognition of glomerular distensibility, now mesangial cells can be included among those cells which may alter their metabolism when subjected to mechanical stretch. In fact, many of the stretch-induced metabolic changes described in other cells have been also demonstrated in mesangial cells. Cyclic stretch of mesangial cells in culture stimulates the synthesis and deposition of collagen and other extracellular matrix constituents [30, 34]. This stimulation is proportional to the intensity of cellular stretch [30] and its deposition is strongly influenced by the extracellular glucose concentration. Although cyclic stretch of mesangial cells in culture stimulates collagen synthesis at all glucose concentrations, it is only at high levels of the sugar that net collagen accumulation in the medium can be demonstrated. This is the result of catabolic rates insufficient to match the increased synthesis occurring in an environment of high glucose concentration [35].

CYTOKINES, GROWTH FACTORS AND THE RESPONSE TO MECHANICAL STRAIN

A number of studies have now shown that stimulated cytokine expression is an important pathogenetic component in the excessive matrix deposition [36–38]. These cytokines, specially transforming growth factor-β (TGF-β) and platelet-derived growth factor (PDGF) are known to induce extracellular matrix deposition in glomeruli and to stimulate the mesangial cell synthesis of extracellular matrix components [39–42]. TGF-β - a growth-regulating, prosclerotic cytokine is a causal factor in various forms of glomerulosclerosis [43, 44]. New evidence indicates that the autocrine activation of specific isoforms of TGF-β may be part of the mechanism translating the stimulus of cellular stretch into alterations in extracellular matrix synthesis in mesangial cells in tissue culture. It has been shown that cyclic stretch of mesangial cells upregulates the expression, secretion and activation of TGF-β1 [45]. This response is specific since, under the same conditions, the activities of interleukin-1 (IL-1), tumor necrosis factor-β (TNF-β) and even the TGF-β isoform TGF-β2, remain unchanged [45]. Exposure of mesangial cells to high levels of glucose also increases the secretion of TGF-β1 and there is a further elevation when these two stimuli are combined [45, 46]. Thus, the potentiating effect of high glucose concentration on the stretch-induced enhancement of collagen formation may be mediated via this enhanced cytokine action. TGF-β neutralization significantly reduces baseline collagen synthesis, breakdown, and accumulation in low glucose, but has no significant effect on the metabolic changes induced by stretch. In contrast, a similar TGF-β inactivation under high glucose conditions greatly reduces the stretch-induced increase in synthesis and breakdown of collagen and totally abolishes the augmentation in collagen accumulation [46].

In cultures of mesangial cells exposed to a gradient of stretching amplitude, only those cells subjected to significant mechanical strain demonstrate intense immunostaining for the active form of TGF-β, as opposed to those in the same culture experiencing little or no strain [45]. This occurs even though all cells in the culture are exposed to a medium containing greatly increased amounts of this cytokine, as compared with unstretched control cultures. Thus, it is likely that TGF-β binding is increased in response to cyclic strain. In recent studies, it has been found that exposure to cyclic stretch significantly increases the overall number of TGF-β receptors as well as the ligand associated with TGF-β receptors (βR) I, II and III [47]. βRI and βRII are the signaling receptors, whereas, βRIII, or betaglycan increases the binding of TGFβ1 and β3 to the signaling receptors and may be necessary for an equivalent TGF-β2 binding [48]. Further studies have also shown that the stretch-induced enhancement of TGF-β binding is the result of increased receptor synthesis and expression, and is not due to a change in its binding affinity [47]. Therefore, the modulation of TGF-β receptors may be an additional control point in the mechanism of mechanical force-induced increase in ECM deposition by mesangial cells.

Another molecule that may play a role in the response of mesangial cells to mechanical strain is vascular endothelial growth factor (VEGF). A promoter of vascular permeability, VEGF is induced in mesangial cells by both TGF-β and stretching [49]. However, stretch-induced VEGF production is unaffected by the addition of TGF-β neutralizing antibody. Finally, there is a significant additive effect on VEGF production when mesangial cells are pre-exposed to stretch and then treated with angiotensin II (AII) [50].

A recently characterized cytokine, connective tissue growth factor (CTGF) has been investigated as a possible component in the response of mesangial cells to mechanical stretch and in the progression of diabetic glomerulosclerosis. The potential importance of this cytokine was originally suggested by studies demonstrating, in other cell types, its induction by TGF-β and the ability to stimulate fibrosis in the skin [51]. Cyclic stretching of cultured mesangial cells upregulates CTGF expression in a rapid (2 hours) and sustained manner [52]. This induction precedes that of TGF-β, suggesting that the stretch-induced CTGF expression may occur independently of TGF-β action. Exposure of mesangial cells in static cultures to recombinant CTGF markedly increases the production of the extracellular matrix components fibronectin and collagen I. Further, although mesangial cells express CTGF mRNA and secrete the protein in relatively low levels, these are markedly stimulated by both TGF-β and high glucose concentrations. Results of experiments with neutralizing antibodies have shown that the induction of CTGF by a high glucose concentration is mediated by TGF-β. Finally, the *in vivo* relevance of a stretch- and glucose-stimulated CTGF in the pathogenesis of diabetic glomerulosclerosis has been shown in the diabetic db/db mouse. After 3.5 months of diabetes, when mesangial expansion is mild and interstitial disease absent CTGF mRNA levels in whole kidney and microdissected glomeruli are markedly increased [52]. This overexpression of CTGF closely correlated with increased levels of fibronectin mRNA expression (Fig. 1.1). These results suggest the CTGF upregulation may be an important factor in the pathogenesis of diabetic glomerulosclerosis, acting both downstream of TGF-β stimulated by high glucose levels and stretch, but also independently of TGF-β early during cyclic strain.

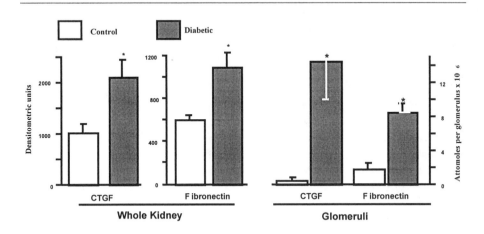

Figure 1-1. Effects of diabetes on the whole kidney and glomerular expression of CTGF and fibronectin. Studies were carried out in 5-month old diabetic *db/db* mice and results compared to nondiabetic, age-matched lean controls. RNA was extracted from whole kidneys and probed by Northern analysis. Results were quantified by densitometric analysis. Glomerular analyses were performed in samples of 50 microdissected glomeruli. After competitive reverse transcription-PCR, the amount of CTGF or fibronectin mRNA was determined and expressed per glomerulus. * P<0.01 *versus* control, n=5 in all groups.

MECHANICAL STRAIN CELL SIGNALING
In mesangial cells subjected to cyclic stretch in tissue culture, recent evidence points to the early and transient activation of specific pathways that may act as triggering mechanisms for later events. Stretch-induced activation of extracellular signal-regulated kinase (ERK) and stress-activated protein kinase/Jun terminal kinase (SAPK/JNK) has been observed between 5-10 min and 5-30 min, respectively, and DNA-binding activity of AP-1 is transiently enhanced at 60 min [53]. These early changes are apparently independent of PKC activation. However, the induction of c-*fos* and the increase in cytosolic S6 kinase, described by others between 15 and 30 min after initiating stretch, is dependent on PKC activity [54, 55]. Further, although activation of ERK after 60 min of stretch has been confirmed by a different group of investigators, they did not observe

changes in SAPK/JNK activity [56]. In summary, even though the data is fragmentary and somewhat inconsistent, the overall evidence is that transient activation of MAPKs is an early event in the response to stretch by mesangial cells.

DETERMINANTS OF GLOMERULAR EXPANSION

Because cellular mechanical strain is the consequence of cyclic variations in glomerular volume, it is important to understand which factors control glomerular expansion. These factors have been recently outlined, and their relative importance assessed [32]. As depicted in Table 1.1, the magnitude of glomerular distention will depend on the balance between elements opposing (overall stiffness) and the forces promoting (capillary wall tension) deformation. The degree of glomerular stiffness is primarily determined by the rigidity of the glomerular scaffold, i. e., peripheral basement membrane and mesangial matrix [32, 57]. The composition and distribution of the extracellular matrix is probably an important determinant of the glomerular mechanical properties because, contrary to what might have been predicted, the rigidity of the passive component of glomerular stiffness is diminished in conditions of incipient glomerulosclerosis [32]. Mesangial cells are known to maintain cell tone in tissue culture and to be responsible for the contractile activity of isolated, suspended (non perfused) glomeruli [58]. However, under conditions of physiological intraglomerular pressure levels, their maximal contraction only reduces glomerular volume by 3.8%. This, therefore, suggests that mesangial cell tone is only a small contributor to overall glomerular rigidity and volume control.

Table 1-1 Factors determining glomerular expansion

Limiting Glomerular Distention	Favoring Glomerular Distension
Glomerular Stiffness	Capillary Wall Tension

a) Passive component:
     Intrinsic elasticity of the capillary wall and mesangial matrix
	a) Glomular size:
	     Capillary diameter

b) Active component mesangial cell tone	b) Increased intraglomerular hydrostatic pressure

Increased capillary wall tension is, obviously, the force causing distention of the elastic glomerulus. This wall tension depends on the level of intraluminal hydrostatic pressure and the diameter of the vessel, as defined by the LaPlace's principle [59]. Thus, for any given pressure, glomerular expansion will be greater in large glomeruli containing capillaries with increased vessel radius than in smaller glomeruli formed by capillaries of smaller radius. However, independently of the prevalent stiffness and capillary diameter, it is the wide oscillation in intraglomerular pressure the force which ultimately may cause the repeating glomerular expansion/contraction that causes mesangial mechanical stretch. Under normal conditions these oscillations are not expected to occur. Due to the precise adjustment of afferent arteriole contractility, intraglomerular pressure is finely regulated, varying little with alterations in renal perfusion pressure [60]. It is only after this autoregulation is compromised when systemic perfusion pressure may be freely transmitted into the glomerular capillary network.

Glomerular autoregulation of pressure is impaired early in disease processes that eventually lead to glomerulosclerosis, such as in the kidney remnant [60] and in experimental insulin-deficient diabetes [61]. If systemic hypertension is present, this deficient autoregulation will permit the transmission into the glomerulus of, not only a higher mean pressure, but also the wide moment-to-moment variations in arterial pressure which are commonly observed in conditions with hypertension [1, 2, 62]. The large oscillations in intraglomerular pressure are anticipated to cause periods of glomerular distention/contraction with levels of expansion 18-fold greater than that in normal conditions (7.3% vs 0.4% distention) [32]. This large difference is likely to be of biological significance, imposing an vastly exaggerated mechanical strain on glomerular cells and thus, triggering cytokine activation and metabolic alterations.

CONCLUSION
The hemodynamic glomerular injury of diabetes is closely related to the loss of afferent arteriole autoregulation of pressure, the presence of increased mean arterial pressure and the occurrence of large moment-to-moment oscillations in systemic arterial pressure. This mechanical injury is possible due to the elasticity of the glomerular structure permitting the repeated stretch/relaxation of the cellular component. The cellular response to this mechanical stimulus is one leading to the enhanced action of growth factors and the accumulation of extracellular matrix. These processes are further aggravated by an environment of high glucose concentration. The glucose- and stretch-induced overexpression of the growth factors VEGF, TGF-β and CTGF are likely to be determinants in the stimulation of mesangial matrix formation.

REFERENCES
1. Bidani AK, Mitchel KD, Schwatz MM, Navar LG, Lewis EJ. Absence of glomerular injury or nephron loss in a normotensive rat remnant kidney model. Kidney Int 1990; 38: 28-38.
2. Bidani AK, Griffin KA, Picken M, Lansky DM. Continuous telemetric blood pressure monitoring and glomerular injury in the rat remnant kidney model. Am. J Physiol 1993; 265 (Renal Fluid Electrolyte Physiol 34): F391-F398.
3. Gaber L, Walton C, Brown S, Bakris G. Effects of different antihypertensive treatments on morphologic progression of diabetic nephropathy in uninephrectomized dogs. Kidney Int 1994; 46: 161-169.

4.   Hostetter TH, Olson JL, Rennke HG, Venkatachalam MA, Brenner BM. Hyperfiltration of remnant nephrons: a potentially adverse response to renal ablation. Am J Physiol 1981; 241(Renal Fluid Electrolyte Physiol 10): F85-F93.

5.   Miller PL, Rennke HG, Meyer TW. Hypertension and glomerular injury caused by focal glomerular ischemia. Am J Physiol 1990; 259 (Renal Fluid Electrolyte Physiol 28): F239-F245.

6.   Zatz R, Dunn BR, Meyer TW, Anderson S, Rennke HG, Brenner BM. Prevention of diabetic glomerulopathy by pharmacological amelioration of glomerular capillary hypertension. J Clin Invest 1986; 77: 1925-1930.

7.   Miller PL, Rennke HG, Meyer TW. Glomerular hypertrophy accelerates hypertensive glomerular injury in rats. Am J Physiol 1991; 262 (Renal Fluid Electrolyte Physiol 30): F459-F465.

8.   Yoshida H, Mitarai T, Kitamura M, Suzuki T, Ishikawa H, Fogo A, Sakai O. The effect of selective growth hormone defect in the progression of glomerulosclerosis. Am J Kidney Dis 1994; 23: 302-312.

9.   Østerby R, Gundersen HJG. Fast accumulation of basement membrane material and the rate of morphological changes in acute experimental diabetic glomerular hypertrophy. Diabetologia 1980; 18: 493-500.

10.   Joles JA, van Goor H, Braam B, Willekes-Koolschijn N, Jansen EHJM, van Tol A, Koomas HA. Proteinuria, lipoproteins and renal apolipoprotein deposits in uninephrectomized female analbuminemic rats. Kidney Int 1995; 47: 442-453.

11.   Kasiske BL, O'Donnell MP, Cleary MP, Keane WF. Effects of reduced renal mass on tissue lipids and renal injury in hyperlipidemic rats. Kidney Int 1989; 35: 40-47.

12.   Fumo P, Kuncio GS, Ziyadeh FN. PKC and high glucose stimulate collagen β1(IV) transcriptional activity in a reporter mesangial cell line. Am J Physiol 1994; 267 (Renal Fluid Electrolyte Physiol 36): F632-F638.

13.   Danne T, Spiro MJ, Spiro RG. Effect of high glucose on type IV collagen production by cultured glomerular epithelial, endothelial and mesangial cells. Diabetes 1993; 42: 170-177.

14.   Kreisberg JI, Garoni JA, Radnik R, Ayo SH. High glucose and TGFβ1 stimulate fibronectin gene expression through a cAMP response element. Kidney Int 1994; 46: 1019-1020.

15.   Nakamura S, Makita Z, Ishikawa S, Yasumura K, Fujii W, Yanagisawa K, Kawata T, Koide T. Progression of nephropathy in spontaneous diabetic rats is prevented by OPB-9195 a novel inhibitor of advanced glycation. Diabetes 1997; 46 :895–899.

16.   Yang C-W, Vlassara H, Striker GE, Striker LJ. Administration of AGEs in vivo induces genes implicated in diabetic glomerulosclerosis. Kidney Int 1995; 47 (Suppl 49): S55-S58.

17.   Weiss MF, Rodby RA, Justice AC, Hricik DE. Free pentosidine and neopterin as markers of progression rate in diabetic nephropathy. Kidney Int 1998; 54: 193–202.

18.   Schleicher ED, Wagner E, Nerlich AG. Increased accumulation of the glycooxidation product N□-(carboxymethyl)lysinein human tissues in diabetes and aging. J Clin Invest 1997; 99: 457–468.

19.   Suzuki D, Miyata T, Saotome N, Horie K, Inagi R, Yasuda Y, Uchida K, Izuhara Y, Yagame M, Sakai H, Kurokawa K. Immunohistochemical evidence for an increased oxidative stress and carbonyl modification of proteins in diabetic glomerular lesions. J Am Soc Nephrol 1999; 10: 822–832.

20. Goldfarb S, Ziyadeh FN, Kern EFO, Simmons DA. Effects of polyol pathway inhibition and dietary *myo*-inositol on glomerular hemodynamic function in experimental diabetes mellitus in rats. Diabetes 1991; 40: 465-471.

21. Sabbatini M, Sansone G, Uccello F, Giliberti F, Conte G, Andreucci VE. Early glycosylation products induce glomerular hyperfiltration in normal rats. Kidney Int 1992; 42: 875-881.

22. Shankland SJ, Ly H, Thai K, Scholey JW. Increased glomerular capillary pressure alters glomerular cytokine expression. Circ Res 1994; 75: 844-853.

23. Lee LK, Meyer TW, Pollock AS, Lovett DH. Endothelial cell injury initiates glomerular sclerosis in the rat remnant kidney. J Clin Invest 1995; 96: 953-964.

24. Ohno M, Cooke JP, Dzau VJ, Gibbons GH. Fluid shear stress induces endothelial transforming growth factor beta-1 transcription and production. J Clin Invest 1995; 95: 1363-1369.

25. Mitsumata M, Fishel RS, Nerem RM, Alexander RW, Berk BC. Fluid shear stress stimulates platelet-derived growth factor expression in endothelial cells. Am J Physiol 1993; 265 (Heart Circ Physiol 34): H3-H8.

26. Thoumine O, Nerem RM, Girard PR. Changes in organization and composition of the extracellular matrix underlying cultured endothelial cells exposed to laminar steady shear stress. Lab Invest 1995; 73: 565-576.

27. Bernik MB. Contractile activity of human glomeruli in culture. Nephron 1969; 6: 1-10.

28. Barnett R, Scharschmidt L, Ko Y-H, Schlondorff D. Comparison of glomerular and mesangial prostaglandin synthesis and glomerular contraction in two rat models of diabetes mellitus. Diabetes 1987; 36: 1468-1475.

29. Fujiwara Y, Kitamura E, Ueda N, Fukunaga M, Orita Y, Kamada T. Mechanism of action of angiotensin II on isolated rat glomeruli. Kidney Int 1989; 36: 985-991.

30. Riser BL, Cortes P, Zhao X, Bernstein J, Dumler F, Narins RG. Intraglomerular pressure and mesangial stretching stimulate extracellular matrix formation in the rat. J Clin Invest 1992; 90: 1932-1943.

31. Cortes P, Riser BL, Zhao X, Narins RG. Glomerular volume expansion and mesangial cell mechanical strain: mediators of glomerular pressure injury. Kidney Int 1994; 45 (Suppl 45): S11-S16.

32. Cortes P, Zhao X, Riser BR, Narins RG. Regulation of glomerular volume in normal and partially nephrectomized rats. Am J Physiol 1996; 270 (Renal Fluid Electrolyte Physiol 39): F356-F370.

33. Kriz W, Elger M, Lemley K, Sakai T. Structure of the glomerular mesangium: A biomechanical interpretation. Kidney Int 1990; 38 (Suppl 30): S2-S9.

34. Harris RC, Haralson MA, Badr KF. Continuous stretch-relaxation in culture alters rat mesangial cell morphology, growth characteristics, and metabolic activity. Lab Invest 1992; 66: 548-554.

35. Cortes P, Zhao X, Riser BL, Narins RG. Role of glomerular mechanical strain in the pathogenesis of diabetic nephropathy. Kidney Int 1997; 51: 57–68.

36. Nakamura T, Fukui M, Ebihara I, Osada S. Nagakoa I, Tomino Y, Koide H. mRNA expression of growth factors in glomeruli from diabetic rats. Diabetes 1993; 42: 450-456.

37. Sharma K, Ziyadeh FN. Hyperglycemia and diabetic kidney disease. The case for transforming growth factor-ß as a key mediator. Diabetes 1995; 44: 1139-1146.

38. Young BA, Johnson RJ, Alpers CE, Eng E, Gordon C, Floege J, Couser WG. Cellular events in the evolution of experimental diabetic nephropathy. Kidney Int 1995; 47: 935-944.

39. Isaka Y, Fujiwara Y, Ueda N, Kaneda Y, Kamada T, Imai E. Glomerulosclerosis induced by in vivo transfection of transforming growth factor-ß or platelet-derived growth factor gene into the rat kidney. J Clin Invest 1993; 92: 2597-2601.

40. Floege J, Eng E, Young BA, Alpers CE, Barret TB, Bowen-Pope DF, Johnson RJ. Infusion of platelet-derived growth factor or basic fibroblast growth factor induces selective glomerular mesangial cell proliferation and matrix accumulation in rats. J Clin Invest 1993; 92: 2952-2962.

41. Ziyadeh FN, Sharma K, Ericksen M, Wolf G. Stimulation of collagen gene expression and protein synthesis in murine mesangial cells by high glucose is mediated by autocrine activation of transforming growth factor-ß. J Clin Invest 1994; 93: 536-542.

42. Douthwaite JA, Johnson TS, Haylor JL, Watson P, El Nahas AM. Effects of transforming growth factor-β1 on renal extracellular matrix components and their regulating proteins. J Am Soc Nephrol 1999; 10: 2109–2119.

43. Yamamoto T, Noble NA, Miller DE, Border WA. Sustained expression of TGF-β1 underlies development of progressive kidney fibrosis. Kidney Int 1994, 45: 916–927.

44. Yamamoto T, Nakamura T, Noble NA, Ruoslahti E, Border WA. Expression of transforming growth factor ß is elevated in human and experimental diabetic nephropathy. Proc Natl Acad Sci USA 1993; 90: 1814-1818.

45. Riser BL, Cortes P, Heilig C, Grondin J, Ladson-Wofford S, Patterson D, Narins RG. Cyclic stretching force selectively up-regulates transforming growth factor-beta isoforms in cultured rat mesangial cells. American Journal of Pathology 1996; 148: 1915-23.

46. Riser BL, Cortes P, Yee J, Sharba AK, Asano K, Rodriguez-Barbero A, Narins RG. Mechanical strain- and high glucose-induced alterations in mesangial cell collagen metabolism: Role of TGF-β. J Am Soc Nephrol 1998; 9: 827-36.

47. Riser BL, Ladson-Wofford S, Sharba A, Cortes P, Drake K, Guerin C, Yee J, Choi ME, Segarini PR, Narins RG. TGF-β receptor expression and binding in rat mesangial cells: Modulation by glucose and cyclic mechanical strain. Kidney Int 1999; 56: 428–39.

48. Lopez-Casillas F, Wrana JL, Massague J. Betaglycan presents ligand to the TGF beta signaling receptor. Cell 1993; 73: 1435–44.

49. Gruden G, Thomas S, Burt D, Lane S, Chusney G, Sacks S, Viberti GC. Mechanical stretch induces vascular permeability factor in human mesangial cells: mechanisms of signal transduction. Proc. Natl. Acad. Sci. USA 1997; 94: 12112-1216.

50. Gruden G, Thomas S, Burt D, Zhou W, Chusney G, Gnudi L, Viberti GC. Interaction of angiotensin II and mechanical stretch on vascular endothelial growth factor production by human mesangial cells. J Am Soc Nephrol 1999; 10: 730–7.

51. Grotendorst GR, Okochi H, Hayashi N. A novel transforming growth factor beta response element controls the expression of the connective tissue growth factor gene. Cell Growth Diff 1996; 7: 469–80.

52. Riser BL, DeNichilo M, Cortes P, Baker C, Grondin J, Yee J, Narins RG. Regulation of connective tissue growth factor activity in cultured rat mesangial cells and its expression in experimental diabetic glomerulosclerosis. J Am Soc Nephrol 2000: 11:25-38.

53. Ishida T, Haneda M, Maeda S, Koya D, Kikkawa R. Stretch-induced overproduction of fibronectin in mesangial cells is mediated by the activation of mitogen-activated protein kinase. Diabetes 1999; 48: 595–602.

54. Akai Y, Homma T, Burns KD, Yasuda T, Badr KF, Harris RC. Mechanical stretch/relaxation of cultured rat mesangial cells induces protooncogenes and cyclooxygenase. Am J Physiol 1994; 267 (Cell Physiol. 36): C482–C490.

55. Homma T, Akai Y, Burns D, Harris RC. Activation of S6 kinase by repeated cycles of stretching and relaxation in rat glomerular mesangial cells. J Biol Chem 1992; 267: 23129–23135.

56. Ingram AJ, Ly H, Thai K, Kang M, Scholey JW. Activation of mesangial cell signaling cascades in response to mechanical strain. Kidney Int 1999; 55: 476–485.

57. Welling LW, Grantham JJ. Physical properties of isolated perfused renal tubules and tubular basement membranes. J Clin Invest 1972; 51: 1063-1075.

58. Iversen BM., Kvam FI, Matre K, Mørkrid L, Horvei G, Bagchus W, Grond J, Ofstad J. Effect of mesangiolysis on autoregulation of renal blood flow and glomerular filtration rate in rats. Am J Physiol 1992; 262 (Renal Fluid Electrolyte Physiol 31): F361-F366.

59. Nave CR, Nave BC. Physics for the Health Sciences. Philadelphia, London and Toronto, WB Saunders Company; 1980, p. 111.

60. Pelayo JC, Westcott JY. Impaired autoregulation of glomerular capillary hydrostatic pressure in the rat remnant nephron. J Clin Invest 1991; 88: 101-105.

61. Ohishi K, Okwueze MI, Vari RC, Carmines PK. Juxtamedullary microvascular dysfunction during the hyperfiltration stage of diabetes mellitus. Am J Physiol 1994; 267 (Renal Fluid Electrolyte Physiol 36): F99-F105.

62. Parati, G, Omboni S, Di Rienzo M, Frattola A, Albini F, Mancia G. twenty-four hour blood pressure variability: Clinical implications. Kidney Int 1992; 41 (Suppl 37): S24-S28.

2. DEFINITION OF DIABETIC RENAL DISEASE IN INSULIN DEPENDENT DIABETES MELLITUS BASED ON RENAL FUNCTION TESTS

Carl Erik Mogensen
Medical Department M, Aarhus Kommunehospital, Aarhus, Denmark

Defining renal disease and renal involvement in diabetes appeared not to be an easy task, mainly because of the wide range of changes seen. The different degree of abnormalities, often with the same duration of disease, seemingly same quality of long-term metabolic control, and the same type of diabetes, may according to older literature indeed be striking [1-2]. However, with better techniques and more well-defined patients [3] much more consistency is found, and even in the situation with very long-term diabetes and normoalbuminuria a normal GFR is usually found [4]. There can, however, be little doubt that progression in normo- and microalbuminuria is associated to level of albuminuria, including "high-normo", HbA_{1C} and BP.

The main criteria for a suitable system of definition are outlined in table 2-1: (a) the parameters should have strong prognostic or predictive power with respect to progression of disease, (b) clear pathophysiologic relevance, (c) relation to structural or ultrastructural abnormalities, and (d), because of the generalized disease process of complications, the system should be related to other microvascular and also macrovascular lesions of diabetes. (e) It should also be clinically relevant and treatment-orientated.

During the last fifteen years, a diagnostic system has been elaborated [5] that seems to fulfil the criteria indicated above. This system was mainly worked out on the basis of the predictive power of urinary albumin excretion (UAE) as well as knowledge of the pathophysiology of renal changes in diabetes. Structural changes appear still to be secondary elements in the system, but importantly microalbuminuria clearly correlate to structural lesions [6,7], and they may be stopped by antiglycemic and antihypertensive treatment [7]. The »subclinical« level of increased albumin excretion is termed microalbuminuria [8]. So far this system is mainly relevant to insulin-dependent patients, but can also be used in non-insulin-dependent diabetes.

Table 2-1. Definition of diabetic renal disease

	Hyperfiltration	Micro-albuminuria	Clinical Proteinuria	Structural lesions
Predictive power	Yes/(No)	Strong	Strong	Yes
Relationship to patho-physiology	Likely	Yes	Yes	Not yet defined
Relationship to structural damage	Not clearly	Yes	Yes	Interrelationship
Associated with other vascular lesions	?	Yes	Yes	Likely
To be controlled	HbA_{1C} [49]	HbA_{1C}/BP [51,82,84]	HbA_{1C}/BP [84]	HbA_{1C}/BP [85,86]

LONGITUDINAL AND FOLLOW-UP STUDIES IN INSULIN-DEPENDENT DIABETICS

Three centres documented the predictive power of raised UAE [8-11]. If UAE is above a certain limit, excretion rate tends to increase with time and spontaneous reversal occurs only in relatively few patients. The exact level above which albumin excretion rate tends to rise with time is not clearly defined [5], but even patients with upper-normal level tends to progress [12]. The level is likely to vary with methods of urine collection, e.g. the critical level of albumin excretion rate was 30 µg/min in a study using overnight urine collection procedure, 70 µg/min in a study using 24-h urine collection, and as low as 15 µg/min in another study using short-term collection during the daytime in hospital. Usually albuminuria is lower during night (lower BP, lower GFR and recumbency), than during the day. The procedure of urine collection seems to be more important than the method used for measuring albumin, but duration of follow-up is also likely to be of significance in these studies. Continuous follow-ups are now routine in most diabetes centres.

The risk for future clinical nephropathy over the next decade is markedly higher (≈80%) in the presence of microalbuminuria, compared with patients with a completely normal excretion rate (≈5%). Thus it is now possible to identify, early in the course of diabetes, patients prone to the development of overt renal disease. Longitudinal studies in patients with microalbuminuria have revealed a rather slow rate of progression, as measured by yearly increase in UAE. In recent longitudinal studies, the yearly percentage increase in albumin excretion on conventional insulin treatment was around 15%-20% [13,14]. The yearly increase rate in albumin excretion rate was related to BP elevation [13,14] as well as metabolic control during the observation period [14,15]. Long-term diabetic patients may have a slower course.

The recognition of the ability of microalbuminuria to predict future diabetic nephropathy (DN) leads to the definition of a new stage in the development of renal disease in diabetics, namely, incipient DN [5]. Obvious, effective antihypertensive treatment as well as intensified diabetes treatment reduces microalbuminuria or risk of development of microalbuminuria [6,14,15]. This is likely to change also long-term prognosis.

URINARY ALBUMIN EXCRETION IN YOUNG NORMAL SUBJECTS AND PROCEDURE OF URINE COLLECTION

In one study, the UAE measured in 24-h samples in 23 normal men and 20 normal women (aged 22-40 years) averaged 4.7±4.7 µg/min (SD) (range, 2.6-12.6) and 4.3±4.8 (range, 1.1-21.9), respectively [16]. The day-to-day variation in UAE of 24 normal subjects, estimated as the coefficient of variance of 24-h samples, was 31.3%. The mean UAE at rest (short-term collections over several hours, or overnight n=180) was similar (5.8±1.4 µg/min). Similar values have been obtained by other authors, but usually overnight excretion rates are somewhat lower than day-time values, even at complete rest: median daytime UAE: 6.2 µg/min; overnight 3.7 µg/min for men, and similar values for women. There is not very precise correlation between UAE and urinary albumin creatinine ratio or albumin concentration as seen in figure 2-1 [E. Vestbo et al., personal communication].

Higher values for UAE are recorded in some elderly non-diabetic individuals in population studies, as related to BP and other risk factors [17]. Because the UAE varies with posture [18] and with exercise [19] and after heavy water drinking [20], evaluation should be carried out only on urine collected under very standardized conditions.

Each of the following procedures is considered acceptable: (a) overnight (approximately 8-h) urine collection, (b) short-term collections over one or several hours in the laboratory or clinic, (c) a 24-h collection, and (d) an early morning urine sample using albumin concentration or possibly corrected for urine flow by creatinine measurements, using albumin creatinine ratio. The latter procedure is gaining more and more acceptance.Because the coefficient of variance in UAE is between 30%-45%, at least three urine collections are recommended [21]. Studies among diabetics should always include measurements in comparable healthy controls, with exactly the same procedures.

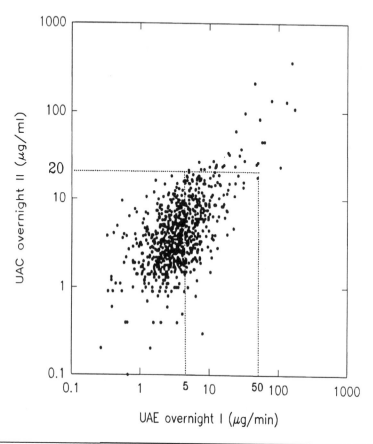

Fig. 2-1. Relationship between UAE overnight 1 and UAC overnight II. Spearmans R = 0.53. [Else Vestbo, with permission].

CRITERIA FOR DIAGNOSING MICROALBUMINURIA AND INCIPIENT DIABETIC NEPHROPATHY IN INSULIN-DEPENDENT PATIENTS

It has recently been proposed that more firm criteria should be applied, both in research projects and in the clinical setting. The following criteria have been proposed for insulin-dependent patients [21], and subsequently used in many studies.

Microalbuminuria
is present when UAE is greater than 20 µg/min and less than or equal to 200 µg/min. BP should always be carefully recorded by several measurements. Patients should be peaceful conditions while collecting urine.

Incipient diabetic nephropathy
is suspected when microalbuminuria is found in two out of three urine samples, preferably collected over a period of 6 months. Urine should be sterile in non-ketotic patients and other causes of increased excretion rate should be excluded. If duration of diabetes is less than 6 years, other causes should especially be considered. Urine collection during the typical diabetes control of the individual patient is recommended. Long-term prognosis without intensified treatment may be poor as recently confirmed in the post DCCT-study [22, 82, 84].

Overt diabetic nephropathy
is suspected when UAE rate is greater than 200 µg/min (macroalbuminuria) in at least two out of three urine samples collected within 6 months. Urine samples should be sterile in non-ketotic patients and other causes of increased UAE rate should again be excluded.

Dipsticks for urinary protein
should not be applied in the classification of renal disease in diabetes according to this proposal. The dipstick procedure is useful, however, in clinical laboratories, and new screening tests, e.g. the Micral-test® are very useful in screening for microalbuminuria.

A NEW CLASSIFICATION SYSTEM
Knowledge of the predictive power of microalbuminuria for renal disease in diabetes, and the description of glomerular hyperfiltration and hypertrophy in diabetes present already at diagnosis, have underlined the need for redefinition of renal involvement in diabetes and DN. A redefinition is most easily achieved by defining new stages in the development of renal changes. These stages, as well as their main characteristics, and outlined in table 2-2. The following stages can be defined:

1. *Glomerular hyperfunction and hypertrophy stage* present at diagnosis. It should be mentioned that certain features in this stage will also accompany diabetes of longer duration when metabolic control is not completely perfect.
2. *The silent stage with normal albumin excretion*, but with structural lesions being present. This stage may last many years; in fact, most patients will continue in this stage throughout their lifetime. Occasionally, in stress situations, e.g. during episodes of very poor metabolic control or during moderate exercise, albumin

excretion rate may increase, but this is a readily reversible phenomenon. Transition to stage 3 is seen in 2-4% of cases per year, associated with poor metabolic control, and high level of normoalbuminuria [12,23].

3. *Incipient diabetic nephropathy* is characterized by persistent and, with long observation period, usually increasing microalbuminuria, Patients with microalbuminuria have a very high risk of subsequent development of overt DN.

    However, intervention (e.g. optimized metabolic control [24, 82] as well as antihypertensive treatment [7]) may certainly change the so-called natural history, reversing functional and maybe even stabilizing structural changes [6,7]. In patients with long-standing diabetes progression may be slower [81,83].

4. *Overt diabetic nephropathy* is characterized by proteinuria, hypertension and subsequent fall in glomerular filtration rate (GFR) [25-27]. A decrease in incidence has been reported [28].

    Beta-2-microglobulin excretion starts to increase in the stage of overt DN, at UAE of around 1000 µg/min [13]. Dextran clearance is according to older as well as most recent study only abnormal with advanced proteinuria [5,29].

5. *End-stage-renal-failure* (ESRF). This entity is now the most common cause of uraemia in the US, and very common also elsewhere. Treatment options are also discussed in the final chapters of the book. Recently scepticism has been expressed about combined pancreas-kidney transplantation, which with the exception of selected patients, may be regarded as experimental medicine [30].

    Systematic screening for early renal involvement is clearly advisable in the diabetes clinic, e.g. by annual measurement of albuminuria in all ranges, or possibly at each visit; more frequent monitoring should be done if UAE is elevated.

THE TRADITIONAL CLINICAL DEFINITION OF DIABETIC NEPHROPATHY

The clinical definition can also, as by tradition, be based on measurement of total protein excretion over three 24-h periods. If mean excretion rate is more than 0.5 g over 24 h, DN is likely in a patient with more than 8-10 years' of diabetes, especially with the presence of retinopathy. This level corresponds approximately to >200 µg/min in UAE or 300 mg/24h.

With a non-typical course, e.g. short duration of diabetes in patients without retinopathy or rapid progression of disease (e.g. great fall in GFR, very rapid increase in proteinuria, or sudden onset of proteinuria) - renal biopsy would be appropriate in order to diagnose non-diabetic renal disorders. Measurement of total proteinuria is now usually being replaced by measurement specific for albuminuria. However, in my experience, biopsy readings practically never change clinical management.

Table 2.2 Microalbuminuria and diabetic nephropathy stages in diabetic renal involvement and nephropathy (DN) (**continue below**)

Stage	Designation	Main characteristics	Main structural changes	GFR (ml/min)
Stage I	Hyperfunc-tion/hypertrophy[a]	Glomerular hyperfiltration	Glomerular Hypertrophy	≈150
Stage II	Normoalbuminuria	Normal UAE	Increasing basal membrane (bm) thickness	Hyperfiltration[a]
Transition from I→ II	Transition phase	High normal UAE	Not known	Hyperfiltration
Stage III	Incipient DN, microalbuminuria	Elevated UAE	UAE correlated to structural damage	Still high GFR
Stage IV	Overt DN	Clinical proteinuria or UAE >200 g/min	Advanced structural damage	"Normal" to advanced reduction

Table 2.2 (continued from above)

Stage	UAE	Blood pressure	Suggested main pathophyiologic change
Stage I	May be increased	N	Glomerular volume and pressure increase
Stage II	N (high in stress situations)	N	Changes as indicated above but quite variable
Transition from I→II	Increasing	Increasing	Somewhat poor metabolic control
Stage III	20→200 g/min	Elevated compared to stage II	Advancing glomerular lesions. Permeability defect not located
Stage IV	>200 μg/min	Often frank hypertension increase by ≈ 5% yearly	High rate of glomerular closure advancing and severe mesangial expansion.

[a]Changes present probably in all states when control is imperfect and in stage II marker of future nephropathy (if GFR >250 ml/min.). The scheme is valid in the "untreated situation" without antihypertensive treatment. BP reduction often reduces albuminuria (Proteinuria→Microalbuminuria→Normoalbuminuria). Stage V is ESRD. Progression associated to HbA1C in all stages (incl. IV)

ABNORMALITIES ASSOCIATED WITH MICROALBUMINURIA
Several abnormalities have been documented in patients with incipient DN.

1. During the stages of incipient DN, the GFR is most often elevated above normal [4]. As microalbuminuria progresses to proteinuria, GFR returns to the »normal« range, which is in fact usually abnormally low IDDM-patients. Patients who enter the stage of clinical proteinuria exhibit gradual decreases in both GFR and renal plasma flow (RPF).
2. Several groups have recognized that elevated BP is an early accompaniment of incipient DN; the magnitude of the elevation is in the range of 10%-15% above

values in control subjects and normoalbuminuric diabetics [12,31-33]. Disturbed salt sensitivity may exist [34,35].

3.   Diabetic retinopathy is more advanced in patients with microalbuminuria than in patients with silent stage II disease. Importantly, patients at risk for proliferative diabetic retinopathy can be identified on the basis of microalbuminuria [36].

4.   Transcapillary escape rate of albumin is increased in incipient DN [37], and plasma lipid abnormalities may be found. Atherosclerotic vascular disease may be predicted [38].

5.   A multitude of other features of vascular, cardiac and neurological damage is seen in these patients [39]. Plasma prorenin may also be associated to microalbuminuria [40] but its significance is still not clearly defined [41].

At the time of diagnosis of microalbuminuria or incipient DN, HbA_{1c} is often elevated by in mean by 10%-20% compared to normoalbuminuric diabetics [4]. Patients with microalbuminuria are obviously likely to have been in poorer control, also during many years earlier in the course of diabetes [12,23,33,42,43]. A decreasing incidence has been suggested [28] but recently disputed [44].

PROBLEMS RELATED TO DIAGNOSING DIABETIC NEPHROPATHY ON THE BASIS OF URINARY ALBUMIN EXCRETION

There are a number of other causes of raised UAE rate in diabetic patients [23]. UAE may increase during very poor metabolic control [21], and it may also be slightly increased at the time of clinical diagnosis [18]. Such elevations are usually readily reversible. Urinary tract infection may also be present and may cause some elevation of UAE. Other vascular diseases such as essential hypertension and cardiac failure should also be considered [45]. Moderate exercise causes increases in UAE more readily in diabetics than in non-diabetics and is thus a confounding factor [19]. It has also been shown that UAE increases temporarily (less than one hour) after drinking large amounts of water, e.g. 1 litre [20]. Therefore, urine flow and UAE should be stable sometime after the start of water drinking (2 h are advisable) when evaluating patients during, e.g. renal clearance procedures [4].

A special problem regarding interpretation of data is borderline increase of UAE. Some patients do show an excretion rate of around 15-30 µg/min and classification may be difficult during a short observation period. The risk of progression is, however, high [12,46], but there may be regression, e.g. by better metabolic control.

PROGRESSION OF CHANGES

It is important to note that progression of nephropathy in the incipient phase is rather slow: yearly mean increase rate in UAE is around 15%-20%. GFR probably starts to decline late in this stage. Progression is more rapid in overt nephropathy without treatment and GFR declines at a mean value of 12 ml/min/year [47,48]. To have clinical relevance, studies of the spontaneous course as well as studies on the effect of intervention should be sufficiently long, e.g. at least 2-3 years or even longer. A given treatment modality may also be difficult to sustain for a prolonged period without any other intervention: e.g. can optimized insulin treatment be given without considering BP elevation? Of course the final end point would be prevention of development of ESRF. In any microalbuminuric patients under study, however, development of renal failure would last one or more decades. Therefore ESRF is not really a feasible test parameter. Increasing albuminuria and especially fall in GFR are satisfactory intermediate endpoints, but arrest of structural lesions would be convincing and has been documented, also for antihypertensive treatment.

GLOMERULAR FILTRATION RATE IN THE DEFINITION OF DIABETIC NEPHROPATHY

An isolated GFR is not a very appropriate parameter to use in the definition of DN. Both metabolic control and structural lesions have a profound effect on GFR. A low GFR (e.g. 110 ml/min), accompanied by totally normal UAE (≈ 4 µg/min), usually indicates an excellent prognosis. A similar low GFR may be found in patients with even marked proteinuria. Such a patient is likely to have experienced a decline in GFR, e.g. from 170 to 110 ml/min. However, normo- and microalbuminuria usually ensures no reduction in GFR [3,39, 81] as also observed in the post-DCCT study [82].

When optimizing metabolic control, GFR usually falls, as does an even borderline elevated UAE, whereas a completely normal UAE may not change. Progression of structural lesions also results in reduction of GFR, but in this case UAE increases considerably. Antihypertensive treatment reduces GFR acutely by 10-20 per cent and GFR may rise after stopping treatment as does microalbuminuria.

Importantly, hyperfiltration in well-defined patients with and without microalbuminuria usually carries poorer prognosis [10,49]. In the follow-up of patients, it is extremely important to *monitor* GFR along with UAE, but the definition of DN should be based upon UAE (in patients without antihypertensive treatment and in their usual glycaemic control).

The coefficient of variance in GFR measurements using a constant infusion technique with 3-6 periods may vary according to the degree of renal involvement or vascular and neuropathic damage in general. In normoalbuminuric and microalbuminuric patients, the coefficient is low, on the order of 5%-8% [4]. In some situations it is not possible to use a constant infusion technique in patients with advanced nephropathy because of voiding problems. Six or more collection periods are usually advisable in such patients and, if the coefficient of variance is high (>15%), this procedure for measuring GFR simply cannot be used. Single-shot measurement of GFR, e.g. using

[Cr]EDTA clearance, is then clearly advisable [50,51]. Importantly, Mathiesen et al recently showed that GFR and the preservation by early AHT [51]

Several more detailed reviews on different aspects of microalbuminuria and diabetic renal disease is available elsewhere [5,23,52-71]. and discussed extensively in many chapters in this book.

NEW PROPOSALS

New avenues of prevention and treatment of diabetic renal disease (and other vascular complication) are now in the horizon. Protein kinase C may be involved in genesis of renal complication and inhibitors are now developed [72]. Interestingly agents that cleave glucose-derived protein crosslinks in vitro and in vivo may offer a new potential therapeutic approach [73,74]. This is a somewhat different principle than the inhibitor aminoguanidine, earlier used in experimental diabetes, but recently explored in non-diabetic rats, preventing cardiovascular and renal pathology of ageing [75]. It is also being examined in patients on dialysis [76]. But generally results are disappointing according to a recent conference. Much enthusiasm regarding aldose reduction inhibition in diabetes, as a non-glycemic measure has now disappeared.

NEW DEFINITIONS

New definitions of diabetes has recently been developed [77], as outlined in Fig 2-2. Fasting plasma glucose is now a key parameter. Individuals with repeated values over 7.0 are now by definition diabetes and values between 6.1 and 6.9 are designated impaired fasting plasma glucose [77]. Obviously fasting plasma glucose, not related to age - unlike values during glucose tolerance tests - often is a continuum. Borderline-values and especially values higher than 6.1 are often related to syndrome X or the metabolic syndrome. The new definitions have been challenged [80], since cardiovascular disease may relate more to abnormalities in glucose tolerance tests [80]. Blood pressure abnormalities are being redefined, also for diabetics, according to the new Joint National Committee [78-79], with the sixth report. Regarding treatment the following is stated: Antihypertensive drug therapy should be initiated along with life-style modifications, especially weight loss, to reduce arterial blood pressure to below 130/85 mmHg. This is further discussed in the final chapters of this volume Angiotensin-converting enzyme inhibitors, α-blockers, calcium antagonists, and diuretics (in low doses) are preferred because of fewer adverse effects on glucose homeostasis, lipid profiles, and renal function. Although β-blockers may have adverse effects on peripheral blood flow, prolong hypoglycemia, and mask hypoglycemic symptoms, patients with diabetes who are treated with diuretics and β-blockers experience a similar or greater reduction of CHD and total cardiovascular events compared with persons without diabetes. In patients with diabetic nephropathy, ACE inhibitors are preferred. If ACE inhibitors are contraindicated or are not well tolerated, angiotensin II receptor blockers may be considered.

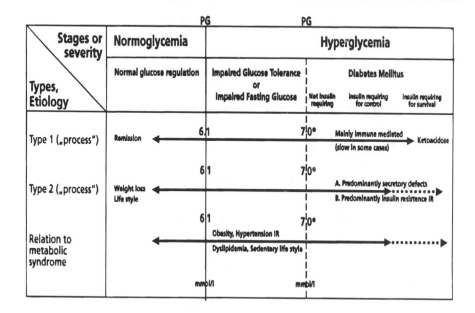

* or casual plasma glucose (PG) ≥11.1 (+symptoms) or 2h PG≥11.1 mmol/l (varies with age).
Blood glucose show lower values.

Fig. 2-2. New criteria for diagnosis according to fasting plasma glucose types, definitions and specifications in diabetes.

REFERENCES

1. Thomsen OF, Andersen AR, Christiansen JS, Deckert T. Renal changes in long-term type 1 (insulin-dependent) diabetic patients with and without clinical nephropathy: a light microscopic, morphometric study of autopsy material. Diabetologia 1984; 26: 361-365.
2. Mauer SM, Steffes MW, Ellis EN, Sutherland DER, Brown DM, Goetz FC. Structural-functional relationships in diabetic nephropathy. J Clin Invest 1984; 74: 1143-1155.
3. Hansen KW, Mau Pedersen M, Christensen CK, Schmitz A, Christiansen JS, Mogensen CE. Normoalbuminuria ensures no reduction of renal function in type 1 (insulin-dependent) diabetic patients. J Intern Med 1992; 232: 161-167.
4. Mogensen CE. Glomerular filtration rate and renal plasma flow in long-term juvenile diabetics without proteinuria. BMJ, 1974; 4: 257-59.

5.   Mogensen CE, Christensen CK, Vittinghus E. The stages in diabetic renal disease. With emphasis on the stage of incipient diabetic nephropathy. Diabetes 1983; 32: Suppl. 2: 64-78.
6.   Bangstad H-J, Østerby R, Dahl-Jørgensen K, Berg KJ, Hartmann A, Hanssen KF. Improvement of blood glucose control retards the progression of morphological changes in early diabetic nephropathy. Diabetologia 1994; 37: 483-490.
7.   Rudberg S, Østerby R, Bangstad H-J, Dahlquist G, Persson B. Effect of angiotensin converting enzyme inhibitor or beta blocker on glomerular structural changes in young microalbuminuric patients with type 1 (insulin-dependent) diabetes mellitus. Diabetologia, 1999: 42: 589-95
8.   Viberti GC, Jarrett RJ, Mahmud U, Hill RD, Argyropoulos A, Keen H. Microalbuminuria as a predictor of clinical nephropathy in insulin-dependent diabetes mellitus. Lancet 1982; i: 1430-1432.
9.   Parving H-H, Oxenbøll B, Svendsen PAA, Christiansen JS, Andersen AR. Early detection of patients at risk of developing diabetic nephropathy: a longitudinal study of urinary albumin excretion. Acta Endocrinol (Copenh) 1982; 100: 550-555.
10.   Mogensen CE, Christensen CK. Predicting diabetic nephropathy in insulin-dependent patients. N Engl J Med 1984; 311: 89-93.
11.   The Microalbuminuria Collaborative Study Group. Predictors of the development of microalbuminuria in patients with type 1 diabetes mellitus: a seven year prospective study. Diabet Med, 1999; 16: 918-925.
12.   Poulsen PL, Hansen KW, Mogensen CE. Ambulatory blood pressure in the transition from normo- to microalbuminuria. A longitudinal study in IDDM patients. Diabetes 1994; 43: 1248-1253.
13.   Christensen CK, Mogensen CE. The course of incipient diabetic nephropathy: Studies of albumin excretion and blood pressure. Diabetic Med 1985; 2: 97-102.
14.   Feldt-Rasmussen B, Mathiesen E, Deckert T. Effect of two years of strict metabolic control on the progression of incipient nephropathy in insulin-dependent diabetes. Lancet 1986; ii: 1300-1304.
15.   The Diabetes Control and Complications Trial Research Group. The effect of intensive treatment of diabetes on the development and progression of long-term complications in insulin-dependent diabetes mellitus. New Engl J Med 1993; 329: 977-986.
16.   Mogensen CE. »Microalbuminuria and kidney function in diabetes: Notes on methods, interpretation and classification.« In *Methods in Diabetes Research, volume II: Clinical Methods*, W.L. Clarke, J. Larner, S.L. Pohl, eds. New York, Chichester, Brisbane, Toronto, Singapore: John Wiley & Sons, 1986; pp 611-631.
17.   Vestbo E, Damsgaard EM, Frøland A, Mogensen CE. Urinary albumin excretion in a population based cohort. Diabetic Med 1995; 12: 488-493.
18.   Mogensen CE. Urinary albumin excretion in early and long-term juvenile diabetes. Scand J Clin Lab Invest 1971; 28: 183-193.
19.   Christensen CK, Mogensen CE. Acute and long-term effect of antihypertensive treatment on exercise-induced albuminuria in incipient diabetic nephropathy. Scand J Clin Lab Invest 1986; 46: 553-559.
20.   Viberti GC, Mogensen CE, Keen H, Jacobsen FK, Jarrett RJ, Christensen CK. Urinary excretion of albumin in normal man. The effect of water loading. Scand J Clin Lab Invest 1982; 42: 147-152.

21. Mogensen CE, Chachati A, Christensen CK, Close CF, Deckert T, Hommel E, Kastrup J, Lefebvre P, Mathiesen ER, Feldt-Rasmussen B, Schmitz A, Viberti GC. Microalbuminuria: an early marker of renal involvement in diabetes. Uremia Invest 1985-86; 9: 85-95.

22. Messent JWC, Elliott TG, Hill RD, Jarrett RJ, Keen H, Viberti GC. Prognostic significance of microalbuminuria in insulin-dependent diabetes mellitus: A twenty-three year follow-up study. Kidney Int 1992; 41: 836-839.

23. Mogensen CE, Vestbo E, Poulsen PL, Christiansen C, Damsgaard EM, Eiskjær H, Frøland A, Hansen KW, Nielsen S, Mau Pedersen M. Microalbuminuria and potential confounders. A review and some observations on variability of urinary albumin excretion. Diabetes Care 1995; 18: 572-581.

24. The Diabetes Control and Complications Trial (DCCT)/Epidemiology of Diabetes Interventions and Complications Research Group. Retinopathy and nephropathy in patients with typ 1 diabetes four years after a trial of intensive therapy, New Engl J Med, 2000; 342: 381-9.

25. Rossing P, Hommel E, Smidt UM, Parving H-H. Reduction in albuminuria predicts a beneficial effect on diminishing the progression of human diabetic nephropathy during antihypertensive treatment. Diabetologia 1994; 37: 511-516.

26. Rossing P, Hommel E, Smidt UM, Parving H-H. Reduction in albuminuria predicts diminished progression in diabetic nephropathy. Kidney Int 1994; Suppl. 45: S145-149.

27. Parving H-H, Rossing P, Hommel E, Smidt UM. Angiotensin-converting enzyme-inhibition in diabetic nephropathy - 10 years experience. Am J Kidney Dis 1995; 26: 99-107.

28. Bojestig M, Arnqvist HJ, Hermansson G, Karlberg BE, Ludvigsson J. Declining incidence of nephropathy in insulin-dependent diabetes mellitus. N Engl J Med 1994; 330: 15-18.

29. Deckert T, Kofoed-Enevoldsen A, Vidal P, Nørgaard K, Andreasen HB, Feldt-Rasmussen B. Size- and charge selectivity of glomerular filtration in IDDM patients with and without albuminuria. Diabetologia 1993; 36: 244-251.

30. Remuzzi G, Ruggenenti P, Mauer SM. Pancreas and kidney/pancreas transplants: experimental medicine or real improvement? Lancet 1994; 343: 27-31.

31. Mogensen CE, Christensen CK. Blood pressure changes and renal function changes in incipient and overt diabetic nephropathy. Hypertension 1985; 7: II-64-II-73.

32. Mogensen CE. Diabetic Renal Disease: The quest for normotension - and beyond. Diabetic Med 1995; 12: 756-769.

33. Molitch ME, Steffes MW, Cleary PA, Nathan DM. Baseline analysis of renal function in the diabetes control and complications trial. Kidney Int 1993; 43: 668-674.

34. Strojek K, Grzeszczak W, Lacka B, Gorska J, Keller CK, Ritz E. Increased prevalence of salt sensitivity of blood pressure in IDDM with and without microalbuminuria. Diabetologia 1995; 38: 1443-1448.

35. Gerdts E, Svarstad E, Myking OL. Lund-Johansen P, Omvik P. Salt sensitivity in hypertensive type-1 diabetes mellitus. Blood Pressure 1996; 5: 78-85.

36. Vigstrup J, Mogensen CE. Proliferative diabetic retinopathy: at risk patients identified by early detection of microalbuminuria. Acta Ophthalmol 1985; 63: 530-534.

37. Feldt-Rasmussen B. Increased transcapillary escape rate of albumin in type 1 (insulin-dependent) diabetic patients with microalbuminuria. Diabetologia 1986; 29: 282-286.

38.   Deckert T, Yokoyama H, Mathiesen E, Rønn B, Jensen T, Feldt-Rasmussen B, Borch-Johnsen K, Jensen JS. Cohort study of predictive value of urinary albumin excretion for atherosclerotic vascular disease in patients with insulin dependent diabetes. BMJ 1996; 312: 871-874.

39.   Mogensen CE, Christensen CK, Christensen PD, Hansen KW, Mølgaard H, Mau Pedersen M, Poulsen PL, Schmitz A, Thuesen L, Østerby R. »The abnormal albuminuria syndrome in diabetes.« In *Current Topics in Diabetes Research. Front Diabetes*, F. Belfiore, R.N. Bergman, G.M. Molinatti, eds. Basel: Karger, 1993; pp 86-121.

40.   Deinum J, Rønn B, Mathiesen E, Derkx FHM, Hop WCJ, Schalekamp MADH. Increase in serum prorenin precedes onset of microalbuminuria in patients with insulin-dependent diabetes mellitus. Diabetologia, 1999; 42: 1006-1010.

41.   Matinlauri IH, Rönnemaa T, Koskinen PJ, Aalto MA, Viikari JSA, Irjala KMA. Elevated serum total renin is insensitive in detecting incipient diabetic nephropathy. Diabetes Care 1995; 18: 1357-1361.

42.   Mathiesen ER, Rønn B, Storm B, Foght H, Deckert T. The natural course of microalbuminuria in insulin-dependent diabetes: a 10-year prospective study. Diabetic Med 1995; 12: 482-487.

43.   Krolewski AS, Laffel LMB, Krolewski M, Quinn M, Warram JH. Glycosylated hemoglobin and the risk of microalbuminuria in patients with insulin-dependent diabetes mellitus. N Engl J Med 1995; 332: 1251-1255.

44.   Rossing P, Rossing K, Jacobsen P, Parving H-H. Unchanged incidence of diabetic nephropathy in IDDM patients. Diabetes 1995; 44: 739-743.

45.   Christensen CK, Krusell LR, Mogensen CE. Increased blood pressure in diabetes: essential hypertension or diabetic nephropathy? Scand J Clin Lab Invest 1987; 47: 363-370.

46.   Microalbuminuria Collaborative Study Group UK. Risk factors for development of microalbuminuria in insulin dependent diabetic patients: a cohort study. BMJ 1993; 306: 1235-1239.

47.   Mogensen CE. Angiotensin converting enzyme inhibitors and diabetic nephropathy (editorial). BMJ 1992; 304: 227-228.

48.   Mogensen CE. Long-term antihypertensive treatment inhibiting progression of diabetic nephropathy. BMJ 1982; 285: 685-688.

49.   Rudberg S, Persson B, Dahlquist G. Increased glomerular filtration rate as a predictor of diabetic nephropathy - An 8-year prospective study. Kidney Int 1992; 41: 822-828.

50.   Brøchner-Mortensen J. Current status on assessment and measurement of glomerular filtration rate. Clin Physiol 1985; 5: 1-17.

51.   Mathisen ER, Hommel E, Hansen HP, Smidt UM, Parving H-H. Randomised controlled trial of long term efficacy of captopril on preservation of kidney function in normotensive patients with insulin dependent diabetes and microalbuminuria. BMJ, 1999; 302:210-16

52.   Mogensen CE, Hansen KW, Sommer, S, Klebe J, Christensen CK, Marshall S, Schmitz A, Mau Pedersen M, Christiansen JS, Pedersen EB. »Microalbuminuria: Studies in diabetes, essential hypertension, and renal diseases as compared with the background population.« In *Advances in Nephrology, Vol. 20*, J.P. Grünfeld, J.F. Bach, J.-L. Funck-Brentano, M.H. Maxwell, eds. St. Louis, Baltimore, Boston, Chicago, London, Philadelphia, Sydney, Toronto: Mosby Year Book, 1991; pp 191-228.

53.   Mogensen CE. Management of renal disease and hypertension in insulin-dependent diabetes, with an emphasis on early nephropathy. Curr Opin Nephrol Hypertens 1992; 1: 106-115.

54.   Mauer SM, Mogensen CE, Viberti GC. Introduction. Symposium on the Progression Diabetic Nephropathy. Kidney Int 1992; 41: 717-718.

55.   Mogensen CE, Hansen KW, Østerby R, Damsgaard EM. Blood pressure elevation versus abnormal albuminuria in the genesis and prediction of renal disease in diabetes. Diabetes Care 1992; 15: 1192-1204

56.   Mogensen CE, Damsgaard EM, Frøland A, Hansen KW, Nielsen S, Mau Pedersen M, Schmitz A, Thuesen L, Østerby R. Reduced glomerular filtration rate and cardiovascular damage in diabetes: a key role for abnormal albuminuria. Acta Diabetol 1992; 29: 201-213.

57.   Mogensen CE, Poulsen PL, Heinsvig EM. «Abnormal albuminuria in the monitoring of early renal changes in diabetes.» In *Concepts for the Ideal Diabetes Clinic. Diabetes Forum Series, Volume 4*, C.E. Mogensen, E. Standl, eds. Berlin, New York: Walter de Gruyter, 1993; pp 289-313.

58.   Mogensen CE, Hansen KW, Nielsen S, Mau Pedersen M, Rehling M, Schmitz A. Monitoring diabetic nephropathy: Glomerular filtration rate and abnormal albuminuria in diabetic renal disease - reproducibility, progression, and efficacy of antihypertensive intervention. Am J Kidney Dis 1993; 22: 174-187.

59.   Mogensen CE, Berne C, Ritz E, Viberti G-C. Preface. The kidney in Type 2 (non-insulin-dependent) diabetes mellitus. Diabetologia 1993; 36: 977.

60.   Mogensen CE. Microalbuminuria, early blood pressure elevation and diabetic renal disease. Curr Opin Endocrinol 1994; 4: 239-247.

61.   Mogensen CE. Systemic blood pressure and glomerular leakage with particular reference to diabetes and hypertension. J Intern Med 1994; 235: 297-316.

62.   Mogensen CE. Microalbuminuria in prediction and prevention of diabetic nephropathy in insulin-dependent diabetes mellitus patiens. J Diabetes and Its Complications 1995; 9: 337-349.

63.   Alzaid AA. Microalbuminuria in patients with NIDDM: An overview. Diabetes Care 1996; 19: 79-89.

64.   Gilbert RE, Cooper ME, McNally PG, O'Brien RC, Taft J, Jerums G. Microalbuminuria: Prognostic and therapeutic implications in diabetes mellitus. Diabetic Med 1994; 11: 636-645.

65.   DeFronzo RA. Diabetic nephropathy: etiologic and therapeutic considerations. Diabetes Rev 1995; 3: 510-564.

66.   Breyer JA. Medical management of nephropathy in type I diabetes mellitus: Current recommendations. J Am Soc Nephrol 1995; 6: 1523-1529.

67.   Gosling P. Microalbuminuria: a marker of systemic disease. Br J Hosp Med 1995; 54: 285-290.

68.   Raskin GS, Tamborlane WV. Molecular and physiological aspects of nephropathy in type I (insulin-dependent) diabetes mellitus. J Diabetes and Its Complications 1996; 10: 31-37.

69.   Clark CM, Lee DA. Prevention and treatment of the complications of diabetes mellitus. N Engl J Med 1995; 332: 1210-1217.

70. Mogensen CE. »Management of the diabetic patient with elevated blood pressure or renal disease. Early screening and treatment programs: albuminuria and blood pressure.« In *Hypertension: Pathology, Diagnosis & Management. 2nd ed*, J.H. Laragh, B.M. Brenner, eds. New York: Raven Press Ltd., 1995; pp 2335-2365.

71. Leese GP, Vora JP. The management of hypertension in diabetes: with special reference to diabetic kidney disease. Diabetic Med 1996; 13: 401-410.

72. Ishii H, Jirousek MR, Koya D, Takagi C, Xia P, Clermont A, Bursell S-E, Kern TS, Ballas LM, Heath WF, Stramm LE, Feener EP, King GL. Amelioration of vascular dysfunctions in diabetic rats by an oral PKC β inhibitor. Science 1996; 272: 728-731.

73. Drickamer K. Breaking the course of the AGEs. Nature 1996; 382: 211-212.

74. Vasan S, Zhang X, Zhang X, Kapurniotu A, Bernhagen J, Teichberg S, Basgen J, Wagle D, Shih D, Terlecky I, Bucala R, Cerami A, Egan J, Ulrich P. An agent cleaving glucose-derived protein crosslinks in vitro and in vivo. Nature 1996; 382: 275-278.

75. Li YM, Steffes M, Donnelly T, Liu C, Fuh H, Basgen J, Bucala R, Vlassara H. Prevention of cardiovascular and renal pathology of aging by the advanced glycation inhibitor aminoguanidine. Proc Natl Acad Sci USA 1996; 93: 3902-3907.

76. Friedman EA. Will pimagidine improve survival of diabetics on dialysis? Nephrol Dial Transplant 1996; 11: 1524-1527.

77. The Expert Committee on the Diagnosis and Classification of Diabetes Mellitus. Report of the Expert Committee on the Diagnosis and Classification of Diabetes Mellitus. Diabetes Care 1997; 20: 1183-1197.

78. The sixth report of the Joint National Committee on Prevention, Detection, Evaluation and Treatment of High Blood Pressure. Arch Intern Med 1997; 157: 2413-2446.

79. Fagan TC. Evolution of the Joint National Committee Reports, 1988-1997. Evolution of the Science of Treating Hypertension. Arch Intern Med 1997; 157: 2401-2402

80. The Decode Study group on behalf of the European Epidemiology Group.
Glucose tolerance and mortality: comparison of WHO and American Diabetes Association diagnostic criteria. Lancet, 1999; 354:617-21

81. Sackmann H, Tran-Van T, Tack I, Hanaire-Broutin H, Tauber JP, Ader JL (2000). Contrasting renal functional reserve in very long-term type I diabetic patients with and without nephropathy. Diabetologia, 43: 227-30.

82. The Diabetes Control and Complications Trial/Epidemiology of Diabetes Interventions and Complications Research Group. (2000). Retinopathy and nephropathy in patients with type 1 diabetes four years after a trial of intensive therapy. N Engl J Med, 342: 381-9.

83. Karamanos B, Porta M, Songini M, Metelko Z, Kerenyi Z, Tamas G, Rottiers R, Stevens LK, Fuller JH and the EURODIAB IDDM Complications Study Group. (2000). Different risk factors of microangiopathy in patients with type 1 diabetes mellitus of short versus long duration. The EURODIAB IDDM Complications Study. Diabetologia, 43: 348-355.

84. Sawicki PT, Bender R, Berger M, Mülhauser I (2000). Non-linear effects of blood pressure and glycosylated haemoglobin on progression of diabetic nephropathy. J Intern Med, 247: 131-38.

85. Rudberg S, Østerby R, Bangstad H-J, Dahlquist G, Persson B (1999). Effect of angiotensin converting enzyme inhibitor or beta blocker on glomerular structural changes in young microalbuminuric patients with type 1 diabetes mellitus. Diabetologia, 42: 589-95.

86. Weir MR (1999). Diabetes and Hypertension: Blood pressure control and consequences. Am J Hypertens, 12: 170S-178S.

3.   RETINOPATHY IN RELATION TO ALBUMINURIA AND BLOOD PRESSURE IN IDDM

Nish Chaturvedi[1], John H Fuller[2]

[1]Department of Primary Care and General Practice, Imperial College of Medicine at St. Mary's, Norfolk Place, London, UK And [2]EURODIAB, Department of Epidemiology and Public Health, University College London, UK

The microvascular complications of diabetes, retinopathy and nephropathy, are often considered as a single entity, with the implicit assumption of a close correlation between these complications, both in terms of occurrence, and in terms of putative risk factors 1-3. It is certainly true that patients with one complication will generally demonstrate signs of the other, and that glycaemic control and duration of diabetes are clear risk factors for each of these complications 4-10. But in contrast, current evidence indicates that while the majority of patients with IDDM will develop retinopathy (estimates vary from 70% to 100%) [11-13], only about a third of patients will develop detectable nephropathy [2,14], even when glycaemic control is poor, and the duration of diabetes is long [2,15].

Raised blood pressure is an important associated factor with even relatively early stages of diabetic renal disease [16,17]. But while blood pressure and albuminuria are unquestionably closely related [18], there is still controversy about whether increases in blood pressure result in renal damage, or whether albuminuria precedes the rise in blood pressure, or whether in fact each of these variables could be risk factors for the other [19]. Several studies have demonstrated a relationship between retinopathy and blood pressure [6,9,20-23], but whether this relationship is confounded by renal disease or is truly independent remains unclear [23-25]

This chapter will describe the relationship between retinopathy and nephropathy, and examine the role of blood pressure in this association, both in terms of aetiology and intervention. One major difficulty in assessing these relationships is the near ubiquity of retinopathy in people with diabetes. However, the EURODIAB and Diabetes Control and Complications Trial studies have shown that this need not necessarily be so [26,27]. The EURODIAB study, a cross-sectional survey of 3250 people with IDDM, drawn from 31 centres across Europe, had substantial numbers of people without retinopathy. This is probably due to several design features of that study. The first is that the

Mogensen C.E. (ed.), THE KIDNEY AND HYPERTENSION IN DIABETES MELLITUS
Copyright© 2000 by Kluwer Academic Publishers, Boston ● Dordrecht ● London. All rights reserved.

sampling of IDDM patients in all clinics was stratified by age, sex, and most importantly duration of diabetes, thus about a third of patients had a very short duration of diabetes (less than 8 years). This is in contrast with other study populations, which are generally biased towards those with a relatively long duration of diabetes. Secondly, glycaemic control in this study was relatively good. This is probably a reflection of the current clinical acceptance of the importance of tight glycaemic control in the avoidance of diabetes related complications.

Thus in the EURODIAB study, the prevalence of any retinopathy was 82%, even after 20 years duration of diabetes [26]. In contrast, only 30% of these participants had either micro- or macroalbuminuria. In those with macroalbuminuria, 89% had some degree of retinopathy, compared with 30% in the normoalbuminuric group. However, in those with proliferative retinopathy, only 63% had albuminuria, compared to 20% in those without retinopathy. This confirms that albuminuria without retinopathy is rare, while retinopathy without albuminuria is common [2].

There is now evidence that the key to understanding the association between retinopathy and nephropathy is blood pressure [2,9,15,18,23]. The EURODIAB study showed that the prevalence of retinopathy was positively correlated with blood pressure, in those with and without nephropathy, but the increase in prevalence of retinopathy with blood pressure was more marked in those with nephropathy than those without[15]. Others have claimed that this relationship is confined to those with nephropathy [23,24], but on closer inspection, this may not necessarily be true. In the study by Norgaard et al [23], in those without nephropathy, the prevalence of advanced retinopathy was 17% in the hypertensive group, and 9% in the normotensive group; a clinically important effect even if not statistically significant. Similarly, Krolewski et al claimed that there was no relationship between isolated retinopathy and blood pressure [24], but blood pressure on average was 6mmHg higher than those without complications.

More strikingly, Stephenson et al, demonstrated an important new feature in the relationship between blood pressure and albumin excretion rate (AER). In people with retinopathy, AER increased exponentially with increasing blood pressure, and the curve describing this relationship is very similar to that describing the relationship for the whole EURODIAB population (figure 3-1) [15]. However, in those without retinopathy, there was no rise in AER with increasing blood pressure. From these data, it would appear that the relationship between blood pressure and nephropathy is dependent upon retinopathy. Differences in diabetes duration or glycaemic control could not account for this observation, as these were adjusted for in the analysis. Furthermore, when retinopathy status was stratified by good or poor glycaemic control, any effect of glycaemic control was confined to those with retinopathy. The effect of blood pressure on nephropathy was most marked in those with poor glycaemic control, and attenuated (although still present) in those with good control. In people without retinopathy, the relationship between blood pressure and AER was identical in those with good and poor glycaemic control.

How can we account for this difference in relationship between blood pressure and AER by retinopathy status? and what does it mean for further research and clinical practice?

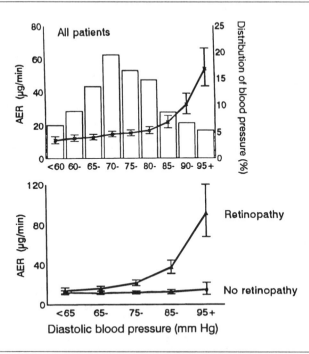

Fig. 3-1. Geometric mean AER by diastolic blood pressure in all patients (top, n=3046) and in those with (n=1098) and without (n=1280) retinopathy (bottom). Geometric means with 95% confidence intervals are adjusted for duration of diabetes and HbA_{1C}. With permission from Diabetologia.

This relationship has not been demonstrated in other studies for two reasons, firstly, others have not stratified by retinopathy status when examining the blood pressure/AER relationship, and secondly, there have not been sufficient numbers of people without retinopathy to examine the relationship in this subgroup separately. But it is unlikely that this is a chance finding, due to the large numbers of patients both with and without retinopathy in the EURODIAB study, and the clear clinical and statistical significance of these findings.

Studies of clinic based populations are often criticised because they are often prone to bias. This is an unlikely explanation for the observed findings in this case however, as one would have to postulate a rather complicated patient selection bias, i.e. patients with retinopathy were somehow selected for their propensity to show a relationship between blood pressure and nephropathy, whilst those without retinopathy were selected on the basis that they had no relationship between blood pressure and nephropathy. This seems highly unlikely, particularly as this relationship was observed in all centres which took part in the EURODIAB study, indicating that such a selection bias would have had to have taken place in each centre.

A further explanation is that this relationship could be due to confounding. People with retinopathy tend to have poorer glycaemic control, and have had diabetes for longer. Thus the relationship of blood pressure and AER could simply be a reflection of the poor control and long duration of diabetes in people with diabetes. Whilst these factors were adjusted for in the above analysis, there remains the possibility of residual confounding. It is well known that duration of diabetes is poorly estimated in studies of people with diabetes, and there is no easy way of assessing the duration of the pre-diagnostic phase. Glycaemic control was measured by a central assessment of glycated haemoglobin, which is a good measure of glycaemic control in the previous three months, and is likely to be correlated with previous glycaemic control, but is obviously not as good as repeated measures of glycaemic control throughout the history of disease. Thus adjustment for these measured variables does not fully adjust for duration and glycaemic control, and a degree of confounding remains. An indication of the likely effect of residual confounding can be obtained from comparing the unadjusted and adjusted effects. In this case, the unadjusted levels of AER by blood pressure and retinopathy status were similar to those of the adjusted effects, and residual confounding is an unlikely explanation for this observation. There may however be other confounders, such as smoking, which were not controlled for in this analysis. Again, it is unlikely that these factors can account for this relationship, as they are less strongly related to complications than duration of diabetes and glycaemic control, and would therefore have a minimal effect in any adjustment.

It is therefore possible that this may be a true and independent association. There is clear evidence that hyperglycaemia is associated with an unfavourable lipid profile and increased blood pressure, as part of a syndrome of insulin resistance[28]. Even in people with diabetes, those with glucose levels at the higher end of the spectrum were more likely to have an unfavourable lipoprotein pattern than those with relatively good control [29,30] These disturbances contribute to vascular damage, as evidenced by raised von Willebrand factor and other indicators of endothelial damage[30,32]. This vascular damage is reflected in the kidney, with resulting protein excretion in the urine [10,31,33,34]. But we hypothesise that this relationship is stronger in people with retinopathy, in other words people with retinopathy are at higher risk of renal damage, as a result of disturbances in vascular risk factors due to hyperglycaemia, than people without retinopathy. The presence of retinopathy merely acts as a marker of this increased susceptibility. When we plot the association between lipids, von Willebrand factor or glycated haemoglobin and albumin excretion rate stratified by retinopathy, we show a very similar picture to that observed for blood pressure. This supports our hypothesis that the effect of these risk factors on renal disease depends upon retinopathy status, and that changes in these risk factors occur before the onset of albuminuria. What exactly retinopathy is a marker for is unclear. A genetic predisposition to retinopathy cannot be ruled out. Those who have this predisposition will have some degree of retinopathy, even if duration of diabetes is short and glycaemic control good. Others will only develop retinopathy if glycaemic control is poor, or the duration of diabetes is long. This observation might explain why the risk of retinopathy cannot fully be accounted for by glycaemic control and duration of diabetes, and indicates that no matter how well blood glucose is controlled, retinopathy will always be found in a subgroup of people with diabetes. A candidate for this gene is not yet available, and studies of ACE gene polymorphism, the most likely candidate so far, have produced disappointing results [35].

The final, most important caveat of these findings is that they were demonstrated in a cross-sectional study, where cause and effect cannot be concluded. Further longitudinal studies are required to test these findings on different populations, with better measures of confounders. If these findings are replicated in other studies, we need to search for the pathogenetic mechanism, and consider what this means for clinical practice. With increasing recognition of the importance of tight glycaemic control in reducing the risk of retinopathy, it is likely that the proportion of people without retinopathy will increase [27]. The identification of those who develop or who are at risk of developing retinopathy, despite good control, would be of importance in ensuring that interventions are instituted early, at relatively low levels of blood pressure, and which would reduce the progression of renal disease, and thus the risk of nephropathy and perhaps even macrovascular disease.

One such important intervention which currently has clear evidence of benefit for at least nephropathy is the use of ACE inhibitors[36]. Given the relationships between blood pressure, nephropathy and retinopathy, it is reasonable to suggest that this class of agent may be of value in retinopathy as well. Trials in IDDM [37,39] as well as NIDDM patients [40] all demonstrate a clinically important effect in terms of progression of retinopathy. A combined analysis of these trials suggests that a halving in the risk of progression of retinopathy can be observed over a period as short as two years (figure 3-2). The largest trial by far in this group of studies is the EUCLID study, which together with a halving in progression of retinopathy associated with ACE inhibitor treatment also demonstrated a reduction in the incidence of retinopathy by 30% [39].

These are extremely important findings, both in terms of understanding the pathogenesis of microvascular complications, and in terms of clinical practice. It is clear that for nephropathy in IDDM, ACE inhibitors are superior to other classes of antihypertensive agent, despite similar achieved reductions in systemic blood pressure. This would indicate that other mechanisms are involved. No direct comparisons between ACE inhibitors and other classes of agent have been made in terms of retinopathy, but in the EUCLID study, adjustment for changes in systemic blood pressure had little impact on the observed beneficial treatment effect. This should not be the case if the reduction in risk of retinopathy progression in the treatment arm is solely due to changes in systemic blood pressure. A likely explanation for these findings is the existence of local renin-angiotensin systems in the eye and the kidney[41].

Thus it is hypothesised that the usually efficient blood-retina barrier is breached in the presence of diabetes[42], and that the leakage of angiotensin II has a direct effect on the genesis of diabetic retinopathy. Direct administration of ACE inhibitors reduce this leakage[42].

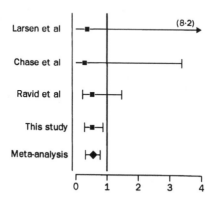

Fig. 3.2 Odds ratio (95%CI) for progression of retinopathy for both groups in EUCLID and previous studies (With permission, the Lancet).

Both EUCLID and earlier studies on retinopathy have limitations which would not support immediate changes in current prescribing. However, the implications of these findings for clinical practice are enormous. If the EUCLID findings were to be replicated in further, adequately powered clinical trials, it would not be unreasonable to suggest that all IDDM patients should receive ACE inhibitors, regardless of their complication status. The beneficial effects of ACE inhibitors on retinopathy were not restricted to patients with microalbuminuria at baseline; equivalent beneficial effects were observed in both normoalbuminuric and microalbuminuric patients. So to restrict ACE inhibitors to those patients at risk of nephropathy would exclude many patients who may stand to benefit in terms of retinopathy. The outcome of such trials is keenly awaited.

There is now accumulating evidence that ACE inhibitors may be beneficial in slowing the progression of retinopathy in type 2 diabetes. The earliest study, by Ravid and colleagues [43], indicated an approximate halving in risk of retinopathy progression due to ACE inhibition, similar to that found in the EUCLID study of type 1 diabetes [44]. But patient numbers in the Ravid study were small. More recently, two much larger studies have provided additional evidence of a beneficial effect. The UK

Prospective Diabetes Study (UKPDS), demonstrated in about 1000 newly diagnosed type 2 patients who were also hypertensive, that tight control (<150/85) with anti-hypertensive therapy over a median 7.5 year follow-up reduced progression of retinopathy by around 40%, compared with those patients on less tight control (<180/105) [45]. Similarly, the HOPE study demonstrated a reduction in need for laser therapy by 22% in 3577 high risk patients with diabetes on ramipril compared to placebo over a 5 year period, a clinically meaningful difference although not statistically significant due to the relatively small numbers affected [46]. Interestingly though, there appeared to be no difference in the treatment effect in the UKPDS in those randomised to the ACE inhibitor, captopril, compared to those randomised to the beta blocker, atenolol [47]. The dosing schedule for captopril has been criticised as being too infrequent, and therefore not providing full 24 hour coverage, and this may account for its disappointing performance compared to atenolol. But the main disadvantage of these previous studies is that none has been designed to explore the impact of anti-hypertensive therapy on retinopathy as a primary end-point. Furthermore, these previous studies have been performed in relatively high risk patients, ie those who are already hypertensive. What is now required is a properly designed study of anti-hypertensive therapy in both types of diabetes with retinopathy as a primary end point.

REFERENCES

1.   Root HF, Pote WH, Frehner H. Triopathy of diabetes: a sequence of neuropathy, retinopathy and nephropathy. Arch Intern Med 1954; 94: 931-941.

2.   Chavers BM, Mauer SM, Ramsay RC, Steffes MW. Relationship between retinal and glomerular lesions in IDDM patients. Diabetes 1994; 43: 441-446.

3.   Johansen J, Sjolie AK, Elbol P, Eshoj O. The relation between retinopathy and albumin excretion rate in insulin-dependent diabetes mellitus. From the Funen County Epidemiology of Type 1 Diabetes Complications Survey. Acta Ophthalmol Copenh 1994; 72: 347-351.

4.   Watts GF, Harris R, Shaw KM. The determinants of early nephropathy in insulin-dependent diabetes mellitus: a prospective study based on the urinary excretion of albumin. Quarterly J Med 1991; 79: 365-378.

5.   Klein R, Klein BE, Moss SE, Cruickshanks KJ. Relationship of hyperglycaemia to the long-term incidence and progression of diabetic retinopathy. Arch Intern Med 1994; 154: 2169-2178.

6.   Teuscher A, Scnhell H, Wilson PW. Incidence of diabetic retinopathy and relationship to baseline plasma glucose and blood pressure. Diabetes Care 1988; 11: 246-251.

7.   Knuiman MW, Welborn TA, McCann VJ, Stanton KG, Constable IJ. Prevalence of diabetic complications in relation to risk factors. Diabetes 1986; 35: 1332-1339.

8.   Nielsen NV. Diabetic retinopathy I. The course of retinopathy in insulin-treated diabetics. A one year epidemiological cohort study of diabetes mellitus. The Island of Falster, Denmark. Acta Ophthalmol Copenh 1984; 62: 256-265.

9.   Chase HP, Garg SK, Jackson WE. Blood pressure and retinopathy in type 1 diabetes. Ophthalmology 1990; 97: 155-159. P8`4

10.   Coonrod BA, Ellis D, Becker DJ, et al. Predictors of microalbuminuria in individuals with IDDM. P ittsburgh Epidemiology of Diabetes Complications Study. Diabetes Care 1993; 16: 1376-1383.

11.   Danielsen R, Jonasson F, Helgason T. Prevalence of retinopathy and proteinuria in type 1 diabetics in Iceland. Acta Med Scand 1982; 212: 277-280.

12.   Dwyer MS, Melton LJ3d, Ballard DJ, Palumbo PJ, Trautmann JC, Chu CP. Incidence of diabetic retinopathy and blindness: a population-based study in Rochester, Minnesota. Diabetes Care 1985; 8: 316-322.

13.   Klein R, Klein BE, Moss SE, Davis MD, DeMets DL. The Wisconsin epidemiologic study of diabetic retinopathy. II. Prevalence and risk of diabetic retinopathy when age at diagnosis is less than 30 years. Arch Ophthalmol 1984; 102: 520-526.

14.   Andersen AR, Christiansen JS, Andersen JK, Kreiner S, Deckert T. Diabetic nephropathy in type I (insulin-dependent) diabetes: an epidemiologic study. Diabetologia 1983; 25: 496-501.

15.   Stephenson JM, Fuller JH, Viberti GC, Sjolie AK, Navalesi R, EURODIAB IDDM Complications Study Group . Blood pressure, retinopathy and urinary albumin excretion in IDDM: the EURODIAB IDDM Complications Study. Diabetologia 1995; 38: 599-603.

16.   Parving HH, Smidt UM, Frisberg B, Bonnevie-Nielsen V, Andersen AR. A prospective study of glomerular filtration rate and arterial blood pressure in insulin- dependent diabetes with diabetic nephropathy. Diabetologia 1981; 20: 457-461.

17.   Mogensen CE, Christensen CK. Predicting diabetic nephropathy in insulin-dependent patients. N Engl J Med 1984; 311: 89-93.

18.   Krolewski AS, Canessa M, Warram JH. Predisposition to hypertension and susceptibility to renal disease in insulin-dependent diabetes mellitus. N Engl J Med 1988; 318: 140-145.

19.   Mogensen CE, Osterby R, Hansen KW, Damsgaard EM. Blood pressure elevation versus abnormal albuminuria in the genesis and prediction of renal disease in diabetes. Diabetes Care 1992; 15: 1181-1204.

20.   West KM, Erdreich LJ, Stober A. A detailed study of risk factors for retinopathy and nephropathy in diabetes. Diabetes 1980; 29: 501-508.

21.   Janka HU, Warram JH, Rand LI, Krolewski AS. Risk factors for progression of background retinopathy in long-standing IDDM. Diabetes 1989; 38: 460-464.

22.   Klein BE, Klein R, Moss SE, Palta M. A cohort study of the relationship of diabetic retinopathy to blood pressure. Arch Ophthalmol 1995; 113: 601-606.

23.   Norgaard K, Feldt-Rasmussen B, Deckert T. Is hypertension a major risk factor for retinopathy in type 1 diabetes? Diabetic Med 1991; 8: 334-337.

24.   Krolewski AS, Warram JH, Cupples A, Gorman CK, Szabo AJ, Christlieb AR. Hypertension, orthostatic hypotension and the microvascular complications of diabetes. J Chronic Dis 1985; 38: 319-326.

25.   Vigstrup J, Mogensen CE. Proliferative diabetic retinopathy: at risk patients identified by early detection of microalbuminuria. Acta Opthalmol 1985; 63: 530-534. P8`4

26.   The EURODIAB IDDM Complications Study Group . Microvascular and acute complications in IDDM patients: the EURODIAB IDDM Complications Study. Diabetologia 1994; 37: 278-285.

27.   The Diabetes Control and Complications Trial Research Group . The effect of intensive treatment of diabetes on the development and progression of long-term complications in insulin-dependent diabetes mellitus. N Engl J Med 1993; 329: 977-986.

28.   Reaven GM. Role of insulin resistance in human disease. Diabetes 1988; 37: 1595- 1607.

29. Sosenko JM, Breslow JL, Miettinen OS, Gabbay KH. Hyperglycaemia and plasma lipid levels: a prospective study of young insulin-dependent diabetic patients. N Engl J Med 1980; 302: 650-654.

30. Jensen T, Stender S, Deckert T. Abnormalities in plasma concentrations of lipoproteins and fibrinogen in type 1 (insulin-dependent) diabetic patients with increased urinary albumin excretion. Diabetologia 1988; 31: 142-145.

31. Jones SL, Close CF, Mattock MB, Jarrett RJ, Keen H, Viberti GC. Plasma lipid and coagulation factor concentrations in insulin dependent diabetics with microalbuminuria. Br Med J 1989; 298: 487-490.

32. Stehouwer CD, Stroes ES, Hackeng WH, Mulder PG, Den-Ottolander GJ. von Willebrand factor and development of diabetic nephropathy in IDDM. Diabetes 1991; 40: 971-976.

33. Stehouwer CD, Fischer HR, van-Kuijk AW, Polak BC, Donker AJ. Endothelial dysfunction precedes development of microalbuminuria in IDDM. Diabetes 1995; 44: 561-564.

34. Winocour PH, Durrington PN, Ishola M, Anderson DC, Cohen H. Influence of proteinuria on vascular disease, blood pressure, and lipoproteins in insulin dependent diabetes mellitus. Br Med J 1987; 294: 1648-1651.

35. Tarnow L, Cambien F, Rossing P, et al. Lack of relationship between an insertion/deletion polymorphism in the angiotensin I-converting enzyme gene and diabetic nephropathy and proliferative retinopathy in IDDM patients. Diabetes 1995; 44: 489-393.

36. Kasiske BL, Kalil RS, Ma JZ, Liao M, Keane BF. Effect of antihypertensive therapy on the kidney in patients with diabetes: a meta-regression analysis. Ann Intern Med 1993; 118: 129-138.

37. Chase HP, Garg SK, Harris S, Hoops S, Jackson WE, Holmes DL. Angiotensin Converting Enzyme Inhibitor Treatment for Young Normotensive Diabetic Subjects: A Two-Year Trial. Ann Opthalmol 1993; 25: 284-289.

38. Larsen M, Hommel E, Parving HH, Lund-Andersen H. Protective effect of captopril on the blood-retina barrier in normotensive insulin-dependent diabetic patients with nephropathy and background retinopathy. Graefes Arch Clin Exp Ophthalmol 1990; 228: 505-509.

39. Chaturvedi N, Sjolie A-K, Stephenson JM, et al. Effect of lisinopril on progression of retinopathy in normotensive people with type 1 diabetes. Lancet 1998; 351: 28-31.

40. Ravid M, Savin H, Jutrin I, Bental T, Katz B, Lishner M. long-term stabalising effect of angiotensin-converting enzyme inhibition on plasma creatinine and on proteinuria in normotensive type II diabetic patients. Ann Intern Med 1993; 118: 577-581.41. Wagner J, Danser AHJ, Derkx FHM, et al. Demonstration of renin mRNA, angiotensin mRNA, and angiotensin converting enzyme mRNA expression in the human eye: evidence for an intraocular renin-angiotensin system. Br J Ophthalmol 1996; 80: 159-163.

42. Danser AHJ, Derkx FHM, Admiraal PJJ, Deinum J, De Jong PTVM, Schalekamp MADH. Angiotensin levels in the eye. Invest Ophthalmol Vis Sci 1994; 35: 1008-1018.

43. Ravid M, Savin H, Jutrin I, Bental T, Katz B, Lishner M. Long-term stabilizing effect of angiotensin-converting enzyme inhibition on plasma creatinine and on proteinuria in normotensive type II diabetic patients. Ann Intern Med 1993; 118: 577-581.

44. Chaturvedi N, Sjolie A, Stephenson JM, et al. Effect of lisinopril on progression of retinopathy in normotensive people with type 1 diabetes.. Lancet 1998; 351: 28-31.

45. UK Prospective Diabetes Study Group. Tight blood pressure control and risk of macrovascular and microvascular complications in type 2 diabetes: UKPDS 38. BMJ 1998; 317: 703-713.

46.   Heart Outcomes Prevention Evaluation (HOPE) Study Investigators. Effects of ramipril on cardiovascular and microvascular outcomes in people with diabetes mellitus: results of the HOPE study and MICRO-HOPE substudy. Lancet 2000; 355: 253-259.
47.   UK Prospective Diabetes Study Group. Efficacy of atenolol and captopril in reducing risk of macrovascular and microvascular complications in type 2 diabetes: UKPDS 39. BMJ 1998; 317: 713-720.

4. MICROALBUMINURIA AND CARDIOVASCULAR DISEASE

S.M. Thomas, G.C. Viberti.
Department of Endocrinology, Diabetes & Internal Medicine Division of Medicine GKT School of Medicine Guy's Hospital Campus KCL, 5th Floor Thomas Guy House Guy's Hospital, London SE1 9RT

INTRODUCTION

The term microalbuminuria was first coined in 1969 by Keen and Chlouverakis in Guy's Hospital Reports 1969 [1] when following the development of a radioimmunoassay to detect low concentrations of albumin in the urine [2], urinary albumin excretion rate (AER) was determined in a population of patients with type 2 diabetes. Parving et al in 1974 described that this phenomenon was associated with essential hypertension and in the early 1980's the predictive value of microalbuminuria for overt nephropathy and renal failure in diabetes was described. Since that time there has been an explosion of interest in microalbuminuria and it's associations. Microalbuminuria is now defined as an AER of 20-200µg/min or 30 - 300 mg/day.

Microalbuminuria is not only a marker of renal involvement but rather is indicative of a systemic alteration associated with several non–renal implications.

MICROALBUMINURIA AND CARDIOVASCULAR DISEASE IN DIABETES

Type 2 Diabetes
Classical risk factors for cardiovascular disease (CVD) mortality, such as cholesterol, blood pressure and smoking operate both in diabetic and non -diabetic subjects. However the absolute risk of cardiovascular death for people with diabetes, principally Type 2 diabetes, is two to four times higher and is progressively greater with each additional risk factor than in non-diabetics [3,4].

An analysis in 1984 showed that of a cohort of 44 patients with type 2 diabetes studied in 1966-67 15 had died of CVD by 1980 and that the mortality was related to the AER [5]. The association between microalbuminuria and CVD in type 2 diabetes has now been shown in several cross-sectional and retrospective studies (Table 4-1).

Table 4-1. Multivariate risk factors associated with the development of microalbuminuria in Caucasian patients with type 2 diabetes.

	All Subjects
n	100
Fasting plasma glucose (mmol/l)	2.27 (1.33-3.88)
Log_{10}UAER (µg/min)	1.84 (1.09-3.11)
Current smoker (yes/no)	3.72 (1.23-11.3)
Pre-existing CHD (yes/no)	3.61 (1.09-11.9)

Data are OR (95% C.I.)

Several prospective studies have shown microalbuminuria to be an independent predictor of mortality [6-11] Fig 4-1. In 1988 in a 10-year follow up study of 500 patients with type 2 diabetes, microalbuminuria was shown to be associated with CVD mortality [6]. Damsgaard found microalbuminuria to be the best predictor of long term mortality in type 2 diabetes in a 8 – 9 year follow-up of 228 patients with type 2 diabetes [7].

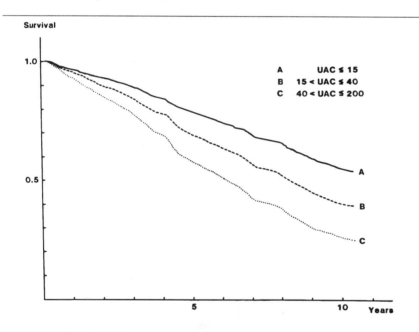

Figure 6-1. Survival curves for the three UAC groups, after correction for the other independent significant prognostic variables;age, known diabetes duration and serum creatinine. N=407,(subjects with missing value(s) excluded).

In a 8 year prospective follow up study Macleod et al compared 153 with abnormal AER and 153 UK patients with type 2 diabetes with AER in the non –diabetic range. Subjects with an abnormal AER had a higher all cause mortality (OR 1.47). The increase in risk was detectable at AER's over 10.6 µg/min. The incidence of vascular deaths was also higher at these levels of AER (OR 1.7) [8]. This has led to suggestions that in type 2 diabetes microalbuminuria should be defined as an AER > 10 µg/min. In a 9-year follow up of 134 patients with type 2 diabetes in Finland, thirty-eight patients died, 68% from CVD. The baseline predictors of death were a higher HBA1c, higher LDL-Triglycerides, lower HDL-cholesterol, higher non –esterified fatty acid concentrations and AER. 45% of the patients who died had microalbuminuria as opposed to 6% of the survivors [9].

In Europid patients with Type 2 diabetes, the presence of an elevated UAE increases the relative risk of all cause mortality to between 1.6 and 2.7-fold.

There has been recent evidence suggesting that in part the cardiovascular risk associated with microalbuminuria is related to disadvantageous alterations in conventional cardiovascular risk factors. In a recent 7 year prospective study of a hospital-based cohort, coronary heart disease (CHD) was the cause of death in 72% of patients with microalbuminuria as compared with 39% of patients with normoalbuminuria.

Microalbuminuria, in this study, was an independent predictor of early mortality if cholesterol and HBA1c were entered as categorical variables but not when these same parameters were analysed as continuous variables (Table 4-2) [12]. Whether under all circumstances microalbuminuria is an independent predictor of CHD has also been questioned by other investigators. In a ten year prospective study of patients with newly diagnosed type 2 diabetes urinary AER measured at 5 years predicted independently of serum lipid abnormalities 10 year CVD mortality but was not an independent predictor when adjusted for plasma glucose [13].

In South Asian populations microalbuminuria is more common than in Europid patients [14] and is associated with more ischaemic heart disease in these populations but maybe less retinopathy and neuropathy [15] and peripheral vascular disease [16]. In Japanese populations however the relationship between microalbuminuria and cardiovascular disease appears weaker. In a six-year follow up of 297 Japanese patients with type 2 diabetes, 96 of whom had microalbuminuria, the all cause mortality was higher in those with microalbuminuria but there was no difference in cardiovascular death [17]. Similar results were seen in a ten-year follow up study of 47 Japanese patients ~ 60% of whom had microalbuminuria at baseline [18].

A combined analysis using all available studies in 1995 yielded a pooled odds ratio of 2.5 (95% Confidence Interval 1.8 - 3.60) for total mortality [19]. In non - European Type 2 Diabetes, where the diabetes often develops at a younger age, this relationship persists although as the prevalence of large vessel disease in these studies has been lower, microalbuminuria is a predictor predominantly of renal disease (Knowler et al. 1997).

Table 4-2. Multivariate analysis of risk factors for coronary heart disease mortality in type 2 diabetes (After Mattock et al)

	CHD Mortality
Age	2.0 (0.94-4.30)
Sex	3.8 (1.16-12.6)
Pre-existing CHD	2.7 (0.93-7.94)
HbA1	1.5 (1.01-2.32)
Serum cholesterol	2.5 (1.50-4.17)
Microalbuminuria (Y/N)	1.8 (0.56-6.04)

Risk ratio (95% confidence level)

MICROALBUMINURIA AND CARDIOVASCULAR DISEASE IN TYPE 1 DIABETES

Microalbuminuria is strongly predictive of the development of overt diabetic nephropathy and its associated excess of coronary, cerebrovascular and peripheral arterial disease in type 1 diabetes [20]. In prospective studies those with microalbuminuria have a significantly higher risk of dying from a cardiovascular cause. In a twenty three year follow up study of patients with type 1 diabetes and microalbuminuria those with microalbuminuria had a significantly higher mortality from a cardiovascular cause (Relative Risk 2.94 95% Confidence Interval 1.18 - 7.34) [21]. Rossing et al confirmed this in a ten-year observational follow up of 939 patients with type 1 diabetes, 593 with normal AER, 181 with microalbuminuria and 165 with overt nephropathy [22]. Age, smoking, microalbuminuria and overt nephropathy were significant predictors of cardiovascular mortality [22]. Myocardial involvement may even be present at the stage of microalbuminuria, aerobic work capacity is reduced in patients with microalbuminuria [23] and significant coronary lesions may be present [24]. There is also evidence that in addition to microalbuminuria the presence of significant neuropathy may be an extra risk factor for CVD [24].

Microalbuminuria is associated with LVH in type 1 diabetes [25] and this effect seems independent of clinic measured blood pressure [26].

MICROALBUMINURIA IN THE NON-DIABETIC POPULATION

In Europid non - diabetic individuals the prevalence of microalbuminuria is quoted around 2 – 10% and in non –European populations may be higher.

Several population based studies have suggested a link between microalbuminuria , blood pressure and cardiovascular disease [27,28]. In the Islington heart study an elevated AER was found in 9% of non - diabetic patients over 40 years of age. Those with an elevated AER had more coronary disease (73% versus 32% odds ratio 5.7), more peripheral vascular disease (PVD) (44 versus 9% odds ratio 7.45) and an increased mortality after 3.6 years (33% versus 2% odds ratio 24.3) [29]. The relationship between microalbuminuria and cardiovascular end-points such as blood pressure and ischaemic heart disease have been confirmed in other population-based studies [30,31].

ESSENTIAL HYPERTENSION

Microalbuminuria is attracting increasing interest in essential hypertension. Several observations have been made suggesting that those with essential hypertension and microalbuminuria differ from those with normal AER.

The prevalence of microalbuminuria varies between 5 and 25% in treated hypertension and up to 40% in untreated hypertension [32-35].

Those with essential hypertension and microalbuminuria have certain distinguishing features. They have an altered blood pressure circadian rhythm with less nocturnal reduction in pressure [36]. They have salt-sensitive hypertension, a condition whereby derangements of renal haemodynamics in response to salt intake result in raised intraglomerular pressure [37], which itself may be associated with a greater prevalence of renal and cardiovascular disease [38,39].

There is some debate as to whether microalbuminuria is best associated with diastolic or systolic hypertension. In some studies non –diabetic subjects with microalbuminuria have higher DBP (Pontremoli et al. 1995)while in others both systolic blood pressure (SBP) and DBP were higher (Haffner et al. 1990). Several studies have shown the correlation to be best with 24 hour ambulatory blood pressure monitoring. Patients with microalbuminuria have higher 24 hour mean levels, lower day: night ratios and greater variability of pressure readings [40,41].

As in diabetes, microalbuminuria in essential hypertension is associated with a cluster of metabolic abnormalities, which range from impaired glucose tolerance to a disadvantageous lipid profile with uric acid disturbances and insulin resistance [42-44]. How all these different anomalies relate to each other is still unclear but the suggestion has been made that endothelial cell dysfunction may be an underlying explanation for these defects [45,46].

Possibly as a result of these characteristics hypertensive patients with microalbuminuria show more evidence of target organ damage. In a cross-sectional study of 333 treated hypertensive men aged 50 –72 years 47.6% of those with microalbuminuria had organ damage, as evidenced by a cardiovascular event or ECG changes as compared with 30.9% of those with a normal AER [47]. Patients withessential hypertension and microalbuminuria are also more prone to increased carotid artery thickness which correlates with the degree of microalbuminuria [48], retinopathy [49] and left ventricular hypertrophy [50,51].

Several cross-sectional studies have observed that the prevalence of coronary artery disease and cardiovascular disease in general is significantly higher in hypertensive patients with microalbuminuria [47,52, 27, 53] compared to hypertensive patients without microalbuminuria. Retrospective longitudinal studies and cross-sectional studies have confirmed that microalbuminuria is an independent, predictor of cardiovascular disease events [54]. In contrast, however a prospective study of median 6.3-year duration including hypertensive men with and without diabetes, found that microalbuminuria was a risk factor only in those with diabetes. In hypertensive patients without diabetes the presence of macroalbuminuria (AER > 200mg/24h) increased the risk of cardiovascular events [55].

A major potential confounder of the relationship between microalbuminuria and cardiovascular disease is the use of anti-hypertensive treatment, which by lowering AER [56], may modify the level of the risk indicator.

To address this, Calviño et al studied cross-sectionally 319 non-diabetic patients with essential hypertension but never drug treated. 40% of the patients had microalbuminuria and that subgroup had greater left ventricular mass index and more retinopathy.

The significance of the development of microalbuminuria for renal disease in essential hypertension is currnetly less clear. There have been few histological studies performed, and no specific renal lesion has been seen in patients with essential hypertension and microalbuminuria as compared with those with normoalbuminuria [57,58].

Functionally one prospective study over 5 years reported a faster rate of decline of creatinine clearance in 24 hypertensive patients with microalbuminuria when compared with 49 hypertensive patients with a normal AER [49]. In addition, a retrospective analysis of 141 individuals with essential hypertension over seven years showed that microalbuminuria was associated with a more rapid decline in creatinine clearance [54].

ELDERLY
Microalbuminuria is a marker of increased mortality in the elderly [59] and of the subsequent development of coronary heart disease (CHD) especially in those with high circulating insulin levels [60].

FACTORS THAT MAY CONTRIBUTE TO CARDIOVASCULAR DISEASE IN DIABETIC AND NON-DIABETIC SUBJECTS WITH MICROALBUMINURIA
The reason for the interaction between microalbuminuria and cardiac disease is uncertain. There is an aggregation of conventional cardiovascular risk factors but this does not explain all of the excess risk [61].

Familal Predisposition
Positive family histories of hypertension or CVD in the non-diabetic parents are related to the development of albuminuria in the diabetic proband emphasising the shared predisposition to these two conditions. These associations hold true for both Type 1 and Type 2 diabetes after adjustment for age, sex and duration of diabetes [62,63]. There is

also some evidence for a familial predisposition to develop microalbuminuria in association with essential hypertension. Children with one hypertensive parent have a higher AER than children of a normotensive parent while normotensive adults with at least one hypertensive parent have elevated AER compared to normotensive adults with a negative family history for arterial hypertension [64,65].

Smoking

In both Type 1 and Type 2 diabetes smoking is an independent risk factor for the development of microalbuminuria [12,66]. The association between smoking and microalbuminuria is not strong however and it seems unlikely that smoking explains much of the excess cardiovascular risk.

Lipid Abnormalities

In both Type 1 and Type 2 diabetes, an unfavourable lipid profile is present at a very early stage of albuminuria. The concentrations of total cholesterol, VLDL cholesterol LDL cholesterol, triglycerides and fibrinogen rise with increasing AER in patients with Type 1 diabetes 11 - 14 % higher in microalbuminuria and 26 - 87% higher in macroalbuminuria [67]. In addition, there is an increase in LDL mass and atherogenic small dense LDL particles, which correlates with the plasma triglyceride concentrations. HDL levels also tend to be reduced with a disadvantageous alteration in their composition [13,68-71].

Similarly in the non -diabetic population, those with elevated UAE have increased Lipoprotein (a), LDL: HDL cholesterol ratios and lower Apolipoprotein A-1 and HDL cholesterol levels [72].

Insulin Resistance

In both non - diabetic subjects and in those with Type 1 and Type 2 diabetes, persistent microalbuminuria is associated with insulin resistance [73,74]. Thus, microalbuminuria may form part of a metabolic syndrome that predisposes to accelerated atherogenesis.

Endothelial dysfunction and haemostatic abnormalities

Levels of Von Willebrand factor (vWF), PAI1, Factor VII and fibrinogen are higher in patients with microalbuminuria as compared with controls suggesting an association with endothelial activation and a hypofibrinolytic, hypercoagulable state [45,75,76]. Recent evidence suggests that the increase in vWF may precede the onset of microalbuminuria in type 1 diabetes [77]. In addition there is a generalised increase in vascular permeability in both the non – diabetic and diabetic population indicated by an increased transcapillary escape of albumin [78-80].

INTERVENTION

Glycaemic control
The question of whether improved glycaemic control is of benefit in preventing CVD in either Type 1 Diabetes or Type 2 diabetes remains unresolved.

In the Diabetes Control and Complications Trial intensive insulin therapy lowered the risk of microalbuminuria and concomitantly reduced development of hypercholesterolaemia with a 41% reduction in the risk of macrovascular disease (combined cardiovascular and peripheral vascular). The number of outcome events was small however as the trial was carried out in relatively young Type 1 Diabetes subjects and the difference was not statistically significant [81]. The UKPDS showed that intensive glycaemic control reduced the risk of myocardial infarction by 16% over a ten-year follow up although this just failed to be statistically significant [82].

In an open, parallel trial for ~ 4 years at the STENO diabetes centre 160 patients were allocated to either standard treatment based on current guidelines or intensive treatment – a programme of behaviour modification and pharmacological therapy targeting hyperglycaemia, hypertension, dyslipidaemia, and microalbuminuria [83]. The intensively treated group had significantly lower rates of progression to nephropathy (odds ratio 0·27 [95% CI 0·10-0·75]), progression of retinopathy (0·45 [0·21-0·95]), and progression of autonomic neuropathy (0·32 [0·12-0·78]) than those in the standard group. No effect was seen on mortality or macrovascular events althought the study lacked sufficent power to look at this .

Lipid Lowering therapy
In the intensified multifactorial intervention study at the STENO lipid lowering strategies were used . AS stated above a reduction in microvascular end-points was seen but no significant effect was seen on macrovaccular events or on mortality [83].

Blood pressure reduction
In diabetes effective blood pressure treatment is able to lower AER and reduce the risk of progression to macroalbuminuria. There is also evidence for a specific benefit AER lowering effect of ACE inhibitors [84]. Studies in non – diabetic people have also shown a benefit of anti –hypertensive treatment in reducing microalbuminuria and suggested that inhibition of the renin – angiotensin system may have specific benefits in renal protection [85,86]. However again there are no specific studies with CVD mortality end points available.

The Hypertension in Diabetes study within the UKPDS showed that intensive therapy (144/82 c.f. 154/87) using primarily either an ACE inhibitor or a β-blocker resulted in significantly less strokes, heart failure and diabetes related deaths although not less myocardial infarctions [87].

The MICRO-HOPE substudy of the Heart Outcomes Prevention Evaluation Study (HOPE) has published the benefits of treatment with an ACE inhibitor in patients with type 2 diabetes and microalbuminuria. 3577 patients aged 55 years or older with a history of diabetes and at least one other cardiovascular risk factor (lipid abnormalities, hypertension, microalbuminuria or current smoking) were enrolled in the HOPE study. Urinary AER was measured at baseline, 1 year and study end (4.5 years). Microalbuminuria was defined as an early morning albumin/creatinine ratio of 2mg/mmol or higher in men and women. At baseline ~ 30% of patients had microalbuminuria 553 of whom were randomly allocated to treatment wiuth ramipril and 587 to placebo. The study was terminated by the data motiroing committee as ramipril lowered the risk of a primary combined end-point of myocardial infarction, stroke or CVD death by 25 % and total mortality by 24%. Treatment with ramipril lowered the risk of overt nephropathy in all patients with diabetes. In addition, ramipril lowered the risk of the primary combined end-point in all patients, including those with microalbuminuria [88].

This data is supported by the Appropriateness of Blood pressure Control in Diabetes trial (ABCD) compared first-line treatment with either enalapril or nisoldipine in 235 patients in each group for 5 years. Patients in the enalapril group had fewer fatal and non-fatal myocardial infrarctions (Risk ratio 7) [89]. Similar findings were also seen in the FACET trial comparing fosinopril with amlodipine in type 2 diabetes [90]. It is not believed that calcium antagonists were deleterious rather that ACE inhibitors had an additional benefit . This study however did not discriminate thus far between those with microalbuminuria and normal AER.

SUMMARY

Microalbuminuria is associated with an excess all cause and cardiovascular mortality in both diabetic and non-diabetic people. An intensive strategy of risk factor reduction may be necessary to tackle this problem and more specific studies that address the issue of risk reversibility are required.

REFERENCES

1. Keen H, Chlouverakis C, Fuller J, Jarrett RJ. The concomitants of raised blood sugar: studies in newly- detected hyperglycaemics. II. Urinary albumin excretion, blood pressure and their relation to blood sugar levels. Guys Hospital Reports 118:247-54. 1969;
2. Keen H, Chlouverakis C. An immunoassay method for urinary albumin at low concentration. Lancet 1963;ii913-4.
3. Krolewski AS, Czyzyk A, Janeczko D, Kopczynski J. Mortality from cardiovascular diseases among diabetics. Diabetologia 13:345-50. 1977;
4. Stamler J, Vaccaro O, Neaton JD, Wentworth D. Diabetes, other risk factors, and 12-yr cardiovascular mortality for men screened in the Multiple Risk Factor Intervention Trial. Diabetes Care 16:434-44. 1993;

5. Jarrett RJ, Viberti GC, Argyropoulos A, Hill RD, Mahmud U, Murrells, TJ. Microalbuminuria predicts mortality in non-insulin-dependent diabetics. Diabet Med 1:17-9. 1984;

6. Schmitz A, Vaeth M. Microalbuminuria: a major risk factor in non insulin dependent diabetes. A 10 year follow up study of 503 patients. Diabet Med 5:126-34. 1988;

7. Damsgaard EM, Froland A, Jorgensen OD, Mogensen CE. Eight to nine year mortality in known non-insulin dependent diabetics and controls. Kidney Int 41:731-5. 1992;

8. Macleod JM, Lutale J, Marshall SM. Albumin excretion and vascular deaths in NIDDM. Diabetologia 38:610-6. 1995;

9. Forsblom CM, Sane T, Groop PH, Totterman KJ, Kallio M, Saloranta C, Laasonen L, Summanen P, Lepantalo M, Laatikainen L, Matikainen E, Teppo, AM, Koskimies S, Groop L. Risk factors for mortality in Type II (non-insulin-dependent) diabetes: evidence of a role for neuropathy and a protective effect of HLA-DR4. Diabetologia 41:1253-62. 1998;

10. Neil A, Hawkins M, Potok M, Thorogood M, Cohen D, Mann J. A prospective population-based study of microalbuminuria as a predictor of mortality in NIDDM. Diabetes Care 16:996-1003. 1993;

11. Gall MA, Borch-Johnsen K, Hougaard P, Nielsen FS, Parving HH. Albuminuria and poor glycemic control predict mortality in NIDDM. Diabetes 44:1303-9. 1995;

12. Mattock MB, Barnes DJ, Viberti G, Keen H, Burt D, Hughes JM, Fitzgerald, AP, Sandhu B, Jackson PG. Microalbuminuria and coronary heart disease in NIDDM: an incidence study. Diabetes 47:1786-92. 1998;

13. Uusitupa MI, Niskanen LK, Siitonen O, Voutilainen E, Pyorala K. Ten-year cardiovascular mortality in relation to risk factors and abnormalities in lipoprotein composition in type 2 (non-insulin-dependent) diabetic and non-diabetic subjects. Diabetologia 36:1175-84. 1993;

14. Mather HM, Chaturvedi N, Kehely AM. Comparison of prevalence and risk factors for microalbuminuria in South Asians and Europeans with type 2 diabetes mellitus. Diabet Med 15:672-7. 1998;

15. Tindall H, Martin P, Nagi D, Pinnock S, Stickland M, Davies JA. Higher levels of microproteinuria in Asian compared with European patients with diabetes mellitus and their relationship to dietary protein intake and diabetic complications. Diabet Med 11:37-41. 1994;

16. Abuaisha B, Kumar S, Malik R, Boulton AJ. Relationship of elevated urinary albumin excretion to components of the metabolic syndrome in non-insulin-dependent diabetes mellitus. Diabetes Research & Clinical Practice 39:93-9. 1998;

17. Araki S, Haneda M, Togawa M, Sugimoto T, Shikano T, Nakagawa T, Isono, M, Hidaka H, Kikkawa R. Microalbuminuria is not associated with cardiovascular death in Japanese NIDDM. Diabetes Research & Clinical Practice 35:35-40. 1997;

18. Araki S, Kikkawa R, Haneda M, Koya D, Togawa M, Liang PM, Shigeta Y. Microalbuminuria cannot predict cardiovascular death in Japanese subjects with non-insulin-dependent diabetes mellitus. Journal of Diabetes & its Complications 9:323-5. 1995;

19, Dineen SF, Gerstein HC. The Association of Microalbuminuria and Mortality in Non-Insulin Dependent Diabetes Mellitus. Arch Intern Med 1997;1571413-8.

20. Viberti GC, Hill RD, Jarrett RJ, Argyropoulos A, Mahmud U, Keen H. Microalbuminuria as a predictor of clinical nephropathy in insulin-dependent diabetes mellitus. Lancet 1:1430-2. 1982;

21. Messent JW, Elliott TG, Hill RD, Jarrett RJ, Keen H, Viberti GC. Prognostic significance of microalbuminuria in insulin-dependent diabetes mellitus: a twenty-three year follow-up study. Kidney Int 41:836-9. 1992;

22. Rossing P, Hougaard P, Borch-Johnsen K, Parving HH. Predictors of mortality in insulin dependent diabetes: 10 year observational follow up study. BMJ 313:779-84. 1996;

23. Jensen T, Richter EA, Feldt-Rasmussen B, Kelbaek H, Deckert T. Impaired aerobic work capacity in insulin dependent diabetics with increased urinary albumin excretion. British Medical Journal Clinical Research Ed . 296:1352-4. 1988;

24. Earle KA, Mishra M, Morocutti A, Barnes D, Stephens E, Chambers J, Viberti GC. Microalbuminuria as a marker of silent myocardial ischaemia in IDDM patients. Diabetologia 39:854-6. 1996;

25. Sato A, Tarnow L, Parving HH. Prevalence of left ventricular hypertrophy in Type 1 diabetic patients with diabetic nephropathy. Diabetologia 1999;42(1):76-80.

26. Spring MW, Raptis AE, Chambers J, Viberti G.C. Left ventricular structure and function are associated with microalbuminuria independently of blood pressure in type 2 diabetes. [Abstract] Diabetes 1997;46:(109)AO426

27. Jensen JS, Feldt-Rasmussen B, Borch-Johnsen K, Clausen P, Appleyard M, Jensen G. Microalbuminuria and its relation to cardiovascular disease and risk factors. A population-based study of 1254 hypertensive individuals. Journal of Human Hypertension 11:727-32. 1997;

28. Jensen JS, Borch-Johnsen K, Feldt-Rasmussen B, Appleyard M, Jensen G. Urinary albumin excretion and history of acute myocardial infarction in a cross-sectional population study of 2,613 individuals. Journal of Cardiovascular Risk 4:121-5. 1997;

29. Yudkin JS, Forrest RD, Jackson CA. Microalbuminuria as predictor of vascular disease in non-diabetic subjects. Islington Diabetes Survey. Lancet 2:530-3. 1988;

30. Winocour PH, Harland JO, Millar JP, Laker MF, Alberti KG. Microalbuminuria and associated cardiovascular risk factors in the community. Atherosclerosis 93:71-81. 1992;

31. Haffner SM, Stern MP, Gruber MK, Hazuda HP, Mitchell BD, Patterson JK. Microalbuminuria. Potential marker for increased cardiovascular risk factors in nondiabetic subjects? Arteriosclerosis 10:727-31. 1990;

32. Parving HH, Mogensen CE, Jensen HA, Evrin PE. Increased urinary albumin-excretion rate in benign essential hypertension. Lancet 1:1190-2. 1974;

33. Ljungman S. Microalbuminuria in essential hypertension. Am J Hypertens 3:956-60. 1990;

34. Gerber LM, Shmukler C, Alderman MH. Differences in urinary albumin excretion rate between normotensive and hypertensive, white and nonwhite subjects. Arch Intern Med 152:373-7. 1992;

35. Bigazzi R, Bianchi S, Campese VM, Baldari G. Prevalence of microalbuminuria in a large population of patients with mild to moderate essential hypertension. Nephron 61:94-7. 1992;

36. Hishiki S, Tochikubo O, Miyajima E, Ishii M. Circadian variation of urinary microalbumin excretion and ambulatory blood pressure in patients with essential hypertension. J Hypertens 16:2101-8. 1998;

37.   Bigazzi R, Bianchi S, Baldari D, Sgherri G, Baldari G, Campese VM. Microalbuminuria in salt-sensitive patients. A marker for renal and cardiovascular risk factors. Hypertension 23:195-9. 1994;

38.   Bigazzi R, Bianchi S, Baldari G, Campese VM. Clustering of cardiovascular risk factors in salt-sensitive patients with essential hypertension: role of insulin. Am J Hypertens 9:24-32. 1996;

39.   Morimoto A, Uzu T, Fujii T, Nishimura M, Kuroda S, Nakamura S, Inenaga, T, Kimura G. Sodium sensitivity and cardiovascular events in patients with essential hypertension. Lancet 350:1734-7. 1997;

40.   Bianchi S, Bigazzi R, Baldari G, Sgherri G, Campese VM. Diurnal variations of blood pressure and microalbuminuria in essential hypertension. Am J Hypertens 7:23-9. 1994;

41.   Bigazzi R, Bianchi S. Microalbuminuria as a marker of cardiovascular and renal disease in essential hypertension. Nephrology, Dialysis, Transplantation 10 Suppl 6:10-4. 1995;

42.   Pontremoli R, Sofia A, Ravera M, Nicolella C, Viazzi F, Tirotta A, Ruello N, Tomolillo C, Castello C, Grillo G, Sacchi G, Deferrari G. Prevalence and clinical correlates of microalbuminuria in essential hypertension: the MAGIC Study. Microalbuminuria: A Genoa Investigation on Complications. Hypertension 30:1135-43. 1997;

43.   Cirillo M, Senigalliesi L, Laurenzi M, Alfieri R, Stamler J, Stamler R, Panarelli W, De Santo NG. Microalbuminuria in nondiabetic adults: relation of blood pressure, body mass index, plasma cholesterol levels, and smoking: The Gubbio Population Study. Arch Intern Med 158:1933-9. 1998;

44.   Mykkanen L, Zaccaro DJ, Wagenknecht LE, Robbins DC, Gabriel M, Haffner, SM. Microalbuminuria is associated with insulin resistance in nondiabetic subjects: the insulin resistance atherosclerosis study. Diabetes 47:793-800. 1998;

45.   Pedrinelli R, Giampietro O, Carmassi F, Melillo E, Dell'Omo G, Catapano G, Matteucci E, Talarico L, Morale M, De Negri F, et al. Microalbuminuria and endothelial dysfunction in essential hypertension. Lancet 344:14-8. 1994;

46.   Agewall S, Fagerberg B, Attvall S, Ljungman S, Urbanavicius V, Tengborn, L, Wikstrand J. Microalbuminuria, insulin sensitivity and haemostatic factors in non-diabetic treated hypertensive men. Risk Factor Intervention Study Group. J Intern Med 237:195-203. 1995;

47.   Agewall S, Persson B, Samuelsson O, Ljungman S, Herlitz H, Fagerberg B. Microalbuminuria in treated hypertensive men at high risk of coronary disease. The Risk Factor Intervention Study Group. J Hypertens 11:461-9. 1993;

48.   Bigazzi R, Bianchi S, Nenci R, Baldari D, Baldari G, Campese VM. Increased thickness of the carotid artery in patients with essential hypertension and microalbuminuria. Journal of Human Hypertension 9:827-33. 1995;

49.   Ruilope LM, Campo C, Rodriguez-Artalejo F, Lahera V, Garcia-Robles R, Rodicio JL. Blood pressure and renal function: therapeutic implications. J Hypertens 14:1259-63. 1996;

50.   Tomura S, Kawada K, Saito K, Lin YL, Endou K, Hirano C, Yanagi H, Tsuchiya S, Shiba K. Prevalence of microalbuminuria and relationship to the risk of cardiovascular disease in the Japanese population. Am J Nephrol 19:13-20. 1999;

51.   Nilsson T, Svensson A, Lapidus L, Lindstedt G, Nystrom E, Eggertsen R. The relations of microalbuminuria to ambulatory blood pressure and myocardial wall thickness in a population. J Intern Med 244:55-9. 1998;

52. Agrawal B, Berger A, Wolf K, Luft FC. Microalbuminuria screening by reagent strip predicts cardiovascular risk in hypertension. J Hypertens 14:223-8. 1996;

53. Mykkanen L, Zaccaro DJ, O'Leary DH, Howard G, Robbins DC, Haffner SM. Microalbuminuria and carotid artery intima-media thickness in nondiabetic and NIDDM subjects. The Insulin Resistance Atherosclerosis Study (IRAS). Stroke 28:1710-6. 1997;

54. Bigazzi R, Bianchi S, Baldari D, Campese VM. Microalbuminuria predicts cardiovascular events and renal insufficiency in patients with essential hypertension. J Hypertens 16:1325-33. 1998;

55. Agewall S, Wikstrand J, Ljungman S, Fagerberg B. Usefulness of microalbuminuria in predicting cardiovascular mortality in treated hypertensive men with and without diabetes mellitus. Risk Factor Intervention Study Group. Am J Cardiol 80:164-9. 1997;

56. Agrawal B, Wolf K, Berger A, Luft FC. Effect of antihypertensive treatment on qualitative estimates of microalbuminuria. Journal of Human Hypertension 10:551-5. 1996;

57. Erley CM, Risler T. Microalbuminuria in primary hypertension: is it a marker of glomerular damage? Nephrology, Dialysis, Transplantation 9:1713-5. 1994;

58. Titov VN, Tarasov AV, Sokolova RI, Volkova EI, Arabidze, GG. [A comparison of selective microproteinuria with histomorphology of the kidneys in patients with arterial hypertension]. [Russian]. Laboratornoe Delo :43-8. 1989;

59. Damsgaard EM, Froland A, Jorgensen OD, Mogensen CE. Microalbuminuria as predictor of increased mortality in elderly people. BMJ 300:297-300. 1990;

60. Kuusisto J, Mykkanen L, Pyorala K, Laakso M. Hyperinsulinemic microalbuminuria. A new risk indicator for coronary heart disease. Circulation 91:831-7. 1995;

61. Mattock MB, Morrish NJ, Viberti GC, Keen H, Fitzgerald AP, Jackson G. Prospective study of microalbuminuria as predictor of mortality in NIDDM. Diabetes 41:736-41. 1992;

62. Earle K, Viberti GC. Familial, hemodynamic and metabolic factors in the predisposition to diabetic kidney disease. Kidney Int 45:434-7. 1994;

63. Earle KA, Walker J, Hill C, Viberti GC. Familial clustering of cardiovascular disease in patients with insulin-dependent diabetes and nephropathy. N Engl J Med 326:673-7. 1992;

64. Grunfeld B, Perelstein E, Simsolo R, Gimenez M, Romero, JC. Renal functional reserve and microalbuminuria in offspring of hypertensive parents. Hypertension 15:257-61. 1990;

65. Fauvel JP, Hadj-Aissa A, Laville M, Fadat G, Labeeuw M, Zech P, Pozet N. Microalbuminuria in normotensives with genetic risk of hypertension [letter]. Nephron 57:375-6. 1991;

66. The Microalbuminuria Collaborative Study Group United Kingdom. Predictors of development of microalbuminuria in patients with type 1 diabetes: a seven year prospective study. Diabet Med 1999;16(11):918-25.

67. Jensen T, Stender S, Deckert T. Abnormalities in plasmas concentrations of lipoproteins and fibrinogen in type 1 (insulin-dependent) diabetic patients with increased urinary albumin excretion. Diabetologia 31:142-5. 1988;

68. Groop PH, Elliott T, Ekstrand A, Franssila-Kallunki A, Friedman R, Viberti GC, Taskinen MR. Multiple lipoprotein abnormalities in type I diabetic patients with renal disease. Diabetes 45:974-9. 1996;

69.   Groop PH, Viberti GC, Elliott TG, Friedman R, Mackie A, Ehnholm C, Jauhiainen M, Taskinen MR. Lipoprotein(a) in type 1 diabetic patients with renal disease. Diabet Med 11:961-7. 1994;

70.   Jones SL, Close CF, Mattock MB, Jarrett RJ, Keen H, Viberti GC. Plasma lipid and coagulation factor concentrations in insulin dependent diabetics with microalbuminuria. BMJ 298:487-90. 1989;

71.   Lahdenpera S, Groop PH, Tilly-Kiesi M, Kuusi T, Elliott TG, Viberti GC, GC, Taskinen MR. LDL subclasses in IDDM patients: relation to diabetic nephropathy. Diabetologia 37:681-8. 1994;

72.   Campese VM, Bianchi S, Bigazzi R. Hypertension, hyperlipidemia and microalbuminuria. Contrib Nephrol 120:11-21. 1997;

73.   Yip J, Mattock MB, Morocutti A, Sethi M, Trevisan R, Viberti G. Insulin resistance in insulin-dependent diabetic patients with microalbuminuria. Lancet 342:883-7. 1993;

74.   Bianchi S, Bigazzi R, Quinones Galvan A, Muscelli E, Baldari G, Pecori, N, Ciociaro D, Ferrannini E, Natali A. Insulin resistance in microalbuminuric hypertension. Sites and mechanisms. Hypertension 26:789-95. 1995;

75.   Gruden G, Pagano G, Romagnoli R, Frezet D, Olivetti C, Cavallo-Perin P. Thrombomodulin levels in insulin-dependent diabetic patients with microalbuminuria. Diabet Med 12:258-60. 1995;

76.   Gruden G, Cavallo-Perin P, Bazzan M, Stella S, Vuolo A, Pagano G. PAI-1 and factor VII activity are higher in IDDM patients with microalbuminuria. Diabetes 43:426-9. 1994;

77.   Stehouwer CD, Fischer HR, van Kuijk AW, Polak BC, Donker AJ. Endothelial dysfunction precedes development of microalbuminuria in IDDM. Diabetes 44:561-4. 1995;

78.   Feldt-Rasmussen B. Increased Transcapillary Escape of albumin in Type 1 (insulin-dependent) diabetic patients with microalbuminuria. Diabetologia 29:282-6. 1986;

79.   Nannipieri M, Rizzo L, Rapuano A, Pilo A, Penno G, Navalesi R. Increased transcapillary escape rate of albumin in microalbuminuric type II diabetic patients. Diabetes Care 18:1-9. 1995;

80.   Jensen JS, Borch-Johnsen K, Jensen G, Feldt-Rasmussen B. Microalbuminuria reflects a generalized transvascular albumin leakiness in clinically healthy subjects. Clin Sci (Colch) 88:629-33. 1995;

81.   The Diabetes Control and Complications Trial Research Group. The effect of intensive treatment of diabetes on the development and progression of long-term complications in insulin-dependent diabetes mellitus. The Diabetes Control and Complications Trial Research Group. N Engl J Med 329:977-86. 1993;

82.   UKPDS Prospective Diabetes Study (UKPDS) Group. Intensive blood-glucose control with sulphonylureas or insulin compared with conventional treatment and risk of complications in patients with type 2 diabetes (UKPDS 33). UK Prospective Diabetes Study (UKPDS) Group. Lancet 352:837-53. 1998;

83.   Gaede P, Vedel P, Parving HH, Pedersen O. Intensified multifactorial intervention in patients with type 2 diabetes mellitus and microalbuminuria: the Steno type 2 randomised study. Lancet 353:617-22. 1999;

84.   Weidmann P, Schneider M, Bohlen L. Therapeutic efficacy of different antihypertensive drugs in human diabetic nephropathy: an updated meta-analysis. Nephrology, Dialysis, Transplantation 10 Suppl 9:39-45. 1995;

85. Bianchi S, Bigazzi R, Baldari G, Campese VM. Microalbuminuria in patients with essential hypertension. Effects of an angiotensin converting enzyme inhibitor and of a calcium channel blocker. Am J Hypertens 4:291-6. 1991;

86. Ruilope LM, Alcazar JM, Hernandez E, Praga M, Lahera V, Rodicio JL. Long-term influences of antihypertensive therapy on microalbuminuria in essential hypertension. Kidney International - Supplement 45:S171-3. 1994;

87. UKPDS Prospective Diabetes Study (UKPDS) Group. Tight blood pressure control and risk of macrovascular and microvascular complications in type 2 diabetes: UKPDS 38. UK Prospective Diabetes Study Group. BMJ 317:703-13. 1998;

88. Heart Outcomes Prevention Evaluation (HOPE) Study Investigators. Effects of Ramipril on csardiovascular and microvascular outcomes in people with diabetes mellitus: results of the HOPE study and MICRO-HOPE substudy. Lancet 2000;355253-9.

89. Estacio RO, Jeffers BW, Hiatt WR, Biggerstaff SL, Gifford N, Schrier RW. The effect of nisoldipine as compared with enalapril on cardiovascular outcomes in patients with non-insulin-dependent diabetes and hypertension. N Engl J Med 338:645-52. 1998;

90. Tatti P, Pahor M, Byington RP, Di Mauro P, Guarisco R, Strollo G, Strollo F. Outcome results of the Fosinopril Versus Amlodipine Cardiovascular Events Randomized Trial (FACET) in patients with hypertension and NIDDM [see comments]. Diabetes Care 21:597-603. 1998;

5.   THE HEART IN DIABETES: RESULTS OF TRIALS

Giulio Zuanetti*, Roberto Latini* and Aldo P Maggioni*°
* Istituto Mario Negri, Milano, Italy, ° Centro Studi ANMCO, Firenze, Italy

It has been known for many years that diabetes has profound consequences on the cardiovascular system leading to increased morbidity and mortality in diabetic patients [1]. In the last years, the completion of several large trials allowed to gather critical information on the efficacy and safety of different drugs in patients with a variety of cardiovascular diseases. In most of these trials diabetic patients, generally identified on the basis of clinical history and with no distinction between type 1 and type 2 diabetes, represented an important proportion of the randomised population, ranging between 10 and 25 %. In this brief review, we will summarise how these trials helped in widening our knowledge of the pathophysiology, prognosis and pharmacological treatment of diabetic patients with cardiovascular disease. Table 5-1 shows the meaning of the acronyms of the trials quoted in this review, where three specific settings will be discussed: acute myocardial infarction (MI); congestive heart failure (CHF) and treatment of myocardial ischemia with coronary angioplasty (PTCA).

ACUTE MYOCARDIAL INFARCTION IN DIABETICS IN THE FIBRINOLYTIC ERA

The widespread use of fibrinolytic agents and aspirin led to a marked improvement in the prognosis of acute MI patients. This notwithstanding, the difference in post-MI survival between diabetic and non-diabetic patients, documented by several studies performed before the introduction of fibrinolysis [2,3] remains mostly unaffected. Data from the GISSI-2 [4], GUSTO-1 [5] and TIMI-2 [6] trials, in which all patients received fibrinolytic agents, show a 30 to 100% higher in-hospital mortality in diabetic patients of both genders compared to non-diabetics.

Although concomitant risk factors such as hypertension, hyperlipidemia and increased body mass index may all contribute to a decreased survival post-MI, diabetes *per se* exerts an independent negative role, as consistently documented in all studies.

Mogensen C.E. (ed.), THE KIDNEY AND HYPERTENSION IN DIABETES MELLITUS.
Copyright© 2000 by Kluwer Academic Publishers, Boston ● Dordrecht ● London. All rights reserved.

Efficacy of pharmacological treatment

So far, only one prospective study, the DIGAMI trial [7,8], evaluated specifically the effect of pharmacological treatment on prognosis of diabetic patients after acute MI. In this study, diabetic patients were randomized to receive either standard treatment or an intensive treatment with insulin-glucose infusion targeted to achieve a tight control of blood glucose. The insulin treatment was then continued long-term. Data showed that this "intensive" hypoglycemic treatment was associated with a lower 1 year morbidity and mortality and that the beneficial effect was even more evident during long-term follow-up. Subsequent analysis have shown that blood glucose at entry was a strong predictors of mortality in control but not in treated patients [9].

Table 5-1 Significance of acronyms of trials quoted

AIRE =	The Acute Infarction Ramipril Efficacy
ASSENT-2=	Assessment of the Safety and Efficacy of a New Thrombolytic
CARE =	Cholesterol and Recurrent Events
CCS-1 =	Chinese Cardiac Study Collaborative Groups 1
CONSENSUS-2 =	Cooperative New Scandinavian Enalapril Survival Study 2
DIGAMI =	Diabetes Mellitus Insulin-Glucose Infusion in Acute Myocardial Infarction
GISSI =	Gruppo Italiano per lo Studio della Sopravvivenza nell'Infarto miocardico
GUSTO =	Global Utilization of Streptokinase and Tissue Plasminogen Activator for Occluded Coronary Arteries
HOPE	Heart Outcomes Prevention Evaluation
ISIS-2 =	International Study of Infarct Survival 2
MERIT-HF	Metoprolol CR/XL Randomised Intervention Trial in Congestive Heart Failure
MOCHA =	Multicentric Oral Carvedilol Heart Failure Assessment
PURSUIT =	Platelet IIb/IIIa in Unstable angina: Receptor SUppression Using Integrilin Therapy
PRISM=	Platelet Receptor Inhibition in Ischemic Syndrome Management
SAVE =	Survival and Ventricular Enlargement
SOLVD =	Studies of Left Ventricular Dysfunction
TAMI =	Thrombolysis and Angioplasty in Myocardial Infarction
TIMI-2 =	Thrombolysis in Myocardial Infarction 2
TRACE =	Trandolapril Cardiac Evaluation

Most of the information on the effect of commonly used cardiovascular drugs in diabetics with MI has been obtained only from retrospective subgroup analyses of some large trials or as non-randomized comparisons between control and drug-treated patients. The evidence for several classes of drugs, summarised in Table 5-2, will be discussed below.

FIBRINOLYTIC AGENTS

Based on their tendency toward a more thrombogenic, less profibrinolytic state, it may be expected that thrombolytic treatment would be less effective in diabetic patients. However, the relative decrease in mortality of diabetics with fibrinolytic treatment has been at least similar to that observed in non diabetics. The overview of fibrinolytic trials in acute MI [10] found that fibrinolytic treatment was associated with a 35 days mortality of 13.6% vs 17.3% in diabetics (-21.7%, or 37 lives saved per 1000 treated patients) and 8.7% vs 10.2% in non diabetics (-14.3% or 15 lives saved per 1000 treated patients). One of the major concerns in administering thrombolytic treatment to diabetics was the possibility of a higher incidence of adverse effects, particularly stroke and retinal hemorrage. The incidence of stroke in diabetics (1.9% in fibrinolytic treated patients vs 1.3% in control) is higher than in non-diabetics (1.0% vs 0.6% respectively); however, this increased risk is by far outweighted by the beneficial effect on mortality. Also, no retinal hemorrages in diabetics treated with fibrinolysis were observed in the TAMI trial [11], despite presence of documented retinopathy in several patients, thus diabetes can not be considered a contraindication to fibrinolytic treatment.

The relative efficacy of newer fibrinolytic treatment regimens has been determined in several trials, such as GUSTO-IV, ASSENT-2 and other, all showing that there was no specific clinical advantage of newer fibrinolytics such as reteplase or tecneteplase, over standard thrombolytic treatment.

Table 5.2 Pharmacological agents in diabetic patients and acute MI

	Prevention of MI in high-risk patients	Treatment of MI In-hospital	Treatment of MI Post-discharge
Fibrinolytics	NA	++	NA
Aspirin	++	+	++
ACE-inhibitors	+++	+++	++*
Beta-blockers	++	+++	+++
Statins	?	NA	++
Nitrates	NA	+?	NA
Calcium antagonists	?	?	?

*   efficacy evaluated only in patients with left ventricular dysfunction
+++   efficacy higher than that in non-diabetics
++   efficacy similar to that in non-diabetics
+   efficacy lower than that in non-diabetics
NA   not applicable
?   data for diabetics not available or controversial

ASPIRIN AND OTHER ANTIPLATELET AGENTS

The role of aspirin as first-line therapy in the treatment of patients with acute MI has been firmly established [12]. However, the optimal dosage in the diabetic population remains unclear, since these patients have a higher platelet aggregability. Interestingly, in ISIS-2 [12] there was no reduction in mortality among diabetic patients receiving aspirin 160 mg daily compared with a 20% reduction in non-diabetic patients. On the other hand aspirin 325 mg in GISSI-3 trial (a non-randomized treatment) was associated to an independent beneficial effect on 6-week mortality [unpublished data]. Finally, the antiplatelet trialists collaboration overview [13] on patients with unstable angina, acute MI, prior MI, stroke or transient ischemic attack indicate a similar benefit (38 vs 36 vascular events saved /1000 treated patients) in diabetics vs non-diabetics. Taken together, these data would suggest that the beneficial effect of aspirin is maintained in diabetics, but the optimal dosage remains undefined.

Attention has recently shifted toward selective antiplatelet agents, such as the glycoprotein IIb/IIIa antagonists, particularly in patients with unstable angina and/or non-Q myocardial infarction. Preliminary data from subgroup analysis of the several trials recently completed, such as PURSUIT with eptifibatide and PRISM with tirofiban appear to suggest that these agents are as effective in diabetic as in non diabetic patients.

BETA-BLOCKERS

Beta-blockers are able to reduce mortality post-MI in diabetic patients, with an absolute and relative beneficial effect in most cases larger than that observed in non-diabetics. However, current evidence is based on subgroup analysis of several trials performed during the eighties and on non-randomized studies [14]. Further, in these trials the population of patients with diabetes was scarcely represented. However, the pooled data indicate a 37% mortality reduction during the acute phase (13% in non diabetics) and a 48% mortality reduction post-discharge (33% in non-diabetics). Since all these studies have been performed before the advent of fibrinolytic therapy, the question remains whether this marked beneficial effect is still present in more "updated" populations. Data from a subgroup analysis of DIGAMI study [15], where beta-blockers were not randomized, suggest that this is the case, and a very recent retrospective evaluation of the National Cooperative Cardiovascular Project on diabetic patients not receiving insulin indicates a HR of 0.77, 95% Cl 0.67-0.89 [16].

ACE-INHIBITORS

Several recent trials used ACE-inhibitors as a new therapeutic strategy in the attempt to reduce mortality and morbidity after acute MI. The studies in which ACE-inhibitors have been started within 24 to 36 hrs after the onset of symptoms showed an overall reduction of about 5 deaths for 1000 treated patients. In the GISSI 3 study [17] information on diabetic status was available for 18,294 patients (97% of total population); 2.7% of patients had a type 1(n=496) and 12.5 % had a type 2 (n=2294). In this study, treatment with lisinopril was associated with a decreased 6-week mortality in both type1 (11.8% vs 21.1%, p<0.05) and type 2 (8.0% vs 10.6%, p<0.05) patients corresponding to a 44.1 and 24.5% reduction respectively [18]. The treatment was associated with an increased incidence of persistent hypotension and renal dysfunction, an effect similar to that observed in the general population. The metaanalysis by the "ACE-inhibitor in MI Collaborative Group" [19], including data from GISSI-3, CCS-1 and CONSENSUS 2, confirmed that the subgroup of diabetic patients experienced a 30 days lower mortality (10.3 vs 12.0 %, or 17.3 lives saved per 1000 patients) when treated early with an ACE-inhibitor. Impressive data on the preventive effect of ACE-inhibitors in diabetics at risk of an ischemic event have been obtained in the HOPE study [20], where after four years of treatment with ramipril in patients with diabetes there was a 24% reduction in the RR of developing MI, stroke or cardiovascular death, with a significant reduction in RR for each of the three components of the primary outcome: 21% reduction in MI, 32% reduction in stroke, 25% RR reduction in total mortality.

CALCIUM ANTAGONISTS

Calcium antagonists have been always considered as a rather homogeneous class, despite the well known pharmacodynamic and pharmacokinetic differences, particularly between non-dihydropiridines and dihydropiridines [21]. These differences are most apparent in terms of the relative action of these agents at myocardial vs vascular level, but may include effects also at renal level that can be important particularly for the diabetic patient. Several trials have been performed with calcium antagonists in acute MI and, in general, non dihydropiridine ("heart rate lowering") calcium antagonists proved to be neutral or effective in patients recovering from acute MI, short-acting dihydropiridines were detrimental in the acute MI setting and long-acting dihydropiridines were neutral in patients with congestive heart failure. Data in the diabetic subpopulation seem to mirror those obtained in non-diabetics.

Some intriguing findings on a possible detrimental effect of dihydropiridine CCB in the *prevention* of MI and other CV complications in diabetic hypertensive patients have been shown in the ABCD trial [22] and in the FACET [23] trials. The design and interpretation of the results of the two studies has been challenged; however, in both studies, a higher incidence of CV complications was observed with dihydropiridines as compared with ACE-inhibitors.

STATINS

Three recent studies, the 4S [24], CARE [25] and LIPID trials, evaluated the effect of statins in reducing morbidity and mortality in patients with an history of ischemic heart disease (mainly previous MI). The main difference among these trials lies in the cut-off of cholesterol level for enrolment, that were much tighter for 4S than for CARE or LIPID. In all trials diabetics had a worsened outcome compared to non diabetics; also, in all trials, the reduction in mortality was proportionally at least similar to that observed in non diabetics. Despite the obvious limitations of this post-hoc analyses, these data suggest that statins confer long-term protection from cardiovascular events in diabetic patients recovering from MI at least to the same extent as in non-diabetics.

CONGESTIVE HEART FAILURE

The interest toward this clinical condition has grown recently mainly due to the increasing prevalence of this disease as a consequence of chronic ischemic heart disease, to the better understanding of pathophysiological mechanisms responsible for its evolution and to the availability of drugs that appear to markedly improve prognosis.

Again, data obtained in diabetic patients with CHF have been gathered mainly through the post-hoc analysis of clinical trials in patients with overt or silent CHF. There is strong evidence indicating that ischemic heart disease in diabetics, particularly the post-MI setting, is associated with an increased incidence of CHF. This has been documented even in the fibrinolytic era by data from the GISSI -2 [4] as well as other studies.

Also, analysis of crude mortality and morbidity rates in diabetics vs non-diabetics with CHF again indicates that diabetics have a worse outcome. For example, the metaanalysis of the major trials in this setting, including about 13,000 patients from SAVE [26], AIRE[27], TRACE [28] and a subpopulation of SOLVD trials [29] showed mortality of 36.4% in diabetics and 24.7% in non diabetics [unpublished data]. The relative role of concomitant risk factors in this setting remains undefined

Efficacy of pharmacological treatment

Together with diuretics, two classes of drugs appear as critical in the management of patients with heart failure: ACE-inhibitors, which are now indicated in all classes of CHF patients, and beta-blockers, whose efficacy in reducing morbidity and mortality has rapidly emerged from the latest trials.

ACE-INHIBITORS

The landmark studies in the evaluation of the efficacy of ACE-inhibitors have been performed in the eighties and early nineties, when the CONSENSUS, SOLVD treatment [29] and SOLVD prevention trials were completed. A subanalysis of the SOLVD trial showed that ACE-inhibitors are as effective in diabetics as in non diabetics in reducing mortality and hospitalisation rates [30]. More recently, the attention of researchers shifted toward patients with overt CHF and/or with left ventricular dysfunction resulting from acute MI. All the "long-term" studies enrolling patients with left ventricular dysfunction some time after MI have shown a significant benefit of ACE-inhibitor therapy, with a risk reduction in mortality of 19 to 27% over a 2.5-4 years follow-up. The metaanalysis of the major trials in this setting mentioned earlier indicate that the beneficial effect of ACE-inhibitors documented in the overall population is present also when limiting the analysis to patients with a history of diabetes. More in detail, the benefit per 1000 patients was 36 in the 10501 non diabetics and 48 in the 2282 diabetics [unpublished data].

BETA-BLOCKERS

For many years beta-blockers have been contraindicated in CHF patients, and even more so in diabetic patients, where the accentuation of altered lipid levels induced by these drugs and the fear of masking hypoglycemic episodes have been considered strong contraindications to their use; however, the pionering work performed in the seventies and the eighties particularly by Scandinavian groups [31] led the way to their targeted use in patients with asymptomatic or overt CHF [32]. A retrospective analysis performed by Kjeskhus et al [33] showed that diabetic patients with CHF post-MI benefited even more than those with preserved left ventricular function. Recently, the investigators of the MOCHA trial [34] reported that the effect of treatment with carvedilol was associated to a dramatic decrease in mortality, that was most evident in diabetic patients, with a 6.1% mortality after a median of 6 months, compared to a 30% mortality in the control group. At variance with these data, in the MERIT-HF study [35], the proportional effect of the betablocker metoprolol was similar in diabetics as in non-diabetics.

CORONARY ANGIOPLASTY (PTCA)

A history of diabetes is associated with a higher incidence of complications during PTCA and to increased morbidity and mortality during follow-up. The mechanisms responsible for an increased incidence of restenosis are several, as well reviewed by Aronson et al [36]. Interestingly, in the BARI trial [37] in patients with multivessel disease, diabetic patients treated with PTCA had a higher incidence of mortality (35 vs 19%, p<0.02) as compared with coronary bypass surgery (CABG), whereas no difference was observed in non diabetic patients using the two different approaches. Also, older data derived from the TIMI-2 trial showed that primary angioplasty in patients with acute MI (a rapidly emerging new treatment of acute MI patients) was associated with a higher mortality than in patients treated with a more conservative strategy (6). A prospective reassessment of the use of PTCA in diabetic patients with newer techniques is therefore warranted. Specifically the role of stenting implantation after direct PTCA is not yet completely defined either in non-diabetic or in diabetic patients, despite the large use in clinical practice.

Efficacy of pharmacological treatment
So far, no conclusive data are available to indicate the best pharmacological treatment to prevent restenosis in this setting. Patients are usually treated with aspirin as a standard treatment with or without ticlopidine. Studies with ACE-inhibitors, calcium antagonists or statins usually failed to show any consistent effect of these agents in reducing the incidence of restenosis or morbility during long-term follow-up. On the other hand data obtained with antithrombotic agents suggest that drugs such as abciximab [38] are effective in the general population. Due to the rapid evolution in the technique used for this intervention, including the use of stents and other devices, targeted to achieve a more stable vessel lumen after angioplasty, it is extremely difficult to quantify the value of results obtained and published even very recently. Overall, there has been a lack of

focus of the researchers on diabetic patients as a relevant subgroup to study in this setting and thus data on diabetic patients are scanty. Available unpublished data do suggest that the efficacy (or lack of efficacy) of different agents is similar irrespective of the diabetic status of patients. Thus, currently the treatment of diabetic patients undergoing PTCA mirrors that of non-diabetic patients. In particular, no data are available to indicate whether a careful control of blood glucose during the peri-intervention period would decrease morbidity and mortality after PTCA.

IMPLICATIONS FOR CLINICAL PRACTICE

The continuous progresses in the management of patients with cardiovascular diseases have radically changed their prognosis. This is particularly true for diabetic patients, whose rate of morbidity and mortality has been shown to be beneficially affected by a variety of interventions, as summarized in this review. Several issues however should be underlined. First, most of these data have been obtained as post-hoc subgroup analysis of trials performed in a general population of patients with cardiovascular disease. This would imply the need to confirm these findings in appropriate prospective studies; although some ongoing studies with ACE-inhibitors target diabetic patients as a predefined subgroup where drug efficacy will be assessed, no further studies are ongoing or planned with most of the agents reviewed in this article, indicating that the evidence so far gathered will be the one to rely upon. Second, the application of these research findings in clinical practice remains a major challenge, since drugs consistently documented to be effective in specific patients population are often underused in clinical practice. Finally, the burden of morbidity and mortality of diabetic patients with cardiovascular disease remains high and deserves testing novel therapeutic approaches targeting the several pathophysiological alterations present in diabetic patients with cardiovascular diseases.

REFERENCES

1   Jacoby RM, Nesto RW. Acute myocardial infarction in the diabetic patient: pathophysiology, clinical course and prognosis. J Am Coll Cardiol 1992; 20:736-44.
2   Smith JW, Marcus FI, Serokman R, Multicenter Postinfarction Research Group. Prognosis of patients with diabetes mellitus after acute myocardial infarction. Am J Cardiol 1984; 54:718-21.
3   Stone PH, Muller JE, Hartwell T, et al. The effect of diabetes mellitus on prognosis and serial left ventricular function after acute myocardial infarction: contribution of both coronary disease and diastolic left ventricular dysfunction to the adverse prognosis. J Am Coll Cardiol 1989; 14:49-57.
4   Zuanetti G, Latini R, Maggioni AP, Santoro L, Franzosi MG, GISSI-2 Investigators. Influence of diabetes on mortality in acute myocardial infarction: data from the GISSI-2 study. J Am Coll Cardiol 1993; 22:1788-94.

5   Lee KL, Woodlief LH, Topol EJ, Weaver D, Betriu A, Col J, Simoons M, Aylward P, Van de Werf F, Califf RM, for the GUSTO-I Investigators. Predictors of 30-day mortality in the era of reperfusion for acute myocardial infarction. Results from an international trial of 41 021 patients. Circulation 1995; 91:1659-68.

6   Mueller HS, Cohen LS, Braunwald E, Forman S, Feit F, Ross A, Schweiger M, Cabin H, Davison R, Miller D, Solomon R, Knatterud GL, for the TIMI Investigators. Predictors of early morbidity and mortality after thrombolytic therapy of acute myocardial infarction. Analyses of patient subgroups in the thrombolysis in myocardial infarction (TIMI) trial, phase II. Circulation 1992; 85:1254-64.

7   Malmberg K, Rydén L, Efendic S, Herlitz J, Nicol P, Waldenström A, Wedel H, Welin L, on behalf of the DIGAMI Study Group. Randomized trial of insulin-glucose infusion followed by subcutaneous insulin treatment in diabetic patients with acute myocardial infarction (DIGAMI Study): effects on mortality at 1 year. J Am Coll Cardiol 1995; 26:57-65.

8   Malmberg K for the DIGAMI (Diabetes Mellitus Insulin Glucose Infusion in Acute Myocardial Infarction) Study Group. Prospective randomised study of intensive insulin treatment on long term survival after acute myocardial infarction in patients with diabetes mellitus. BMJ 1997; 314:1512-5.

9.   Malmberg K; Norhammar A; Wedel H; Rydén L Glycometabolic state at admission: important risk marker of mortality in conventionally treated patients with diabetes mellitus and acute myocardial infarction: long-term results from the Diabetes and Insulin-Glucose Infusion in Acute Myocardial Infarction (DIGAMI) study. Circulation, 1999, 99:, 2626-32

10   Fibrinolytic Therapy Trialists' (FTT) Collaborative Group. Indications for fibrinolytic therapy in suspected acute myocardial infarction: collaborative overview of early mortality and major morbidity results from all randomised trials of more than 1000 patients. Lancet 1994; 343:311-22.

11   Granger CB, Califf RM, Young S, Candela R, Samaha J, Worley S, Kereiakes DJ, Topol EJ, and the Thrombolysis and Angioplasty in Myocardial Infarction (TAMI) Study Group. Outcome of patients with diabetes mellitus and acute myocardial infarction treated with thrombolytic agents. J Am Coll Cardiol 1993; 21:920-5.

12   ISIS-2 Collaborative Group. Randomized trial of intravenous streptokinase, oral aspirin, both or neither among 17187 cases of suspected acute myocardial infarction: ISIS 2 Lancet 1988; ii:349-60.

13   Antiplatelet Trialists' Collaboration. Collaborative overview of randomised trials of antiplatelet therapy—I: prevention of death, myocardial infarction, and stroke by prolonged antiplatelet therapy in various categories of patients. Br Med J 1994; 308:81-106.

14   Kendall MJ, Lynch KP, Hjalmarson Å, Kjekshus J. ß-Blockers and sudden cardiac death. Ann Intern Med 1995; 123:358-67.

15   Malmberg K, Rydén L. Intense metabolic control decreases long-term mortality in diabetics with acute myocardial infarction: predictors of one year mortality. J Am Coll Cardiol 1996; 27 Suppl. A , 82A.

16   Chen J, Marciniak TA, Radford MJ, Wang Y, Krumholz HM. Beta-blocker therapy for secondary prevention of myocardial infarction in elderly diabetic patients. Results from the National Cooperative Cardiovascular Project. J Am Coll Cardiol,1999; 34: 1388-94,

17   Gruppo Italiano per lo Studio della Sopravvivenza nell'Infarto Miocardico. GISSI-3: effects of lisinopril and transdermal glyceryl trinitrate singly and together on 6-week mortality and ventricular function after acute myocardial infarction. Lancet 1994; 343:1115-22.

18   Zuanetti G, Latini R, Maggioni AP, Franzosi MG, Santoro L, Tognoni G, on behalf of GISSI-3 Investigators. Effect of the ACE-inhibitor lisinopril on mortality in diabetic patients with acute myocardial infarction: the data from the GISSI-3 study. Circulation 1997, 96: 4239-4245

19.   Zuanetti G Cardiovascular Disease and Diabetes in New Concept in Diabetes and its treatment, Basel Karger 2000, vol 133, in press

20.   The Heart Outcomes Prevention Evaluation Study Investigators. Effects of an angiotensin converting-enzyme inhibitor, ramipril on cardiovascular events in high-risk patients. N Engl J Med, 2000; 302:145-53.

21   Abernethy DR, Schwartz JB: Drug Therapy: Calcium Antagonists N Engl J Med 1999; 341, 1447-1457

22   Estacio RO, Jeffers BW, Hiatt WR, Biggerstaff SL, Gifford N, Schrier RW. The effect of nisoldipine as compared to enalapril on cardiovascular outcomes in patients with non-insulin dependent diabetes and hypertension N Engl J Med 1998; 338: 645-52

23   Tatti P, Pahor M, Byington RP et al Outcome reuslts of the Fosinopril versus Amlodpine cardiovascular events randomized trial (FACET) in patients with hypertension and NIDDM Diabetes Care 1998; 21: 597-603

24   Pyorala K, Pedersen TR, Kjekshus J, Faergeman O, Olsson AG, Thorgeirsson G, The Scandinavian Simvastatin Survival Study (4S) Group. Cholesterol lowering with simvastatin improves prognosis of diabetic patients with coronary heart disease. A subgroup analysis of the Scandinavian Simvastatin Survival Study (4S). Diabetes Care 1997; 20:614-20.

25   Sacks FM, Pfeffer MA, Moye LA, Rouleau JL, Rutherford JD, Cole TG, Brown L, Warnica JW, Arnold JMO, Wun C-C, Davis BR, Braunwald E, for the Cholesterol and Recurrent Events Trial Investigators. The effect of pravastatin on coronary events after myocardial infarction in patients with average cholesterol levels. N Engl J Med 1996; 335:1001-9.

26   Moyé LA, Pfeffer MA, Wun CC, Davis BR, Geltman E, Hayes D, Farnham DJ, Randall OS ,Dinh H, Arnold JMO, Kupersmith J, Hager D, Glasser SP, Biddle T, Hawkins CM, Braunwald E, for the SAVE Investigators. Uniformity of captopril benefit in the SAVE study: subgroup analysis. Eur Heart J 1994; 15:2-8.

27.   The Acute Infarction Ramipril Efficacy (AIRE) Study Investigators. Effect of ramipril on mortality and morbidity of survivors of acute myocardial infarction with clinical evidence of heart failure. Lancet 1993; 342:821-28.

28   Torp-Pedersen C, Kober L, Carlsen J, on behalf of the TRACE Study Group. Angiotensin-converting enzyme inhibition after myocardial infarction: the Trandolapril Cardiac Evaluation Study. Am Heart J 1996; 132:235-43.

29   The SOLVD Investigators. Effect of enalapril on survival in patients with reduced left ventricular ejection fractions and congestive heart failure. N Engl J Med 1991; 325:293-302.

30   Shindler DM, Kostis JB, Yusuf S, Quinones MA, Pitt B, Stewart D, Pinkett T, Ghali JK, Wilson AC, for the SOLVD Investigators. Diabetes mellitus, a predictor of morbidity and mortality in the studies of left ventricular dysfunction (SOLVD) trials and registry. Am J Cardiol 1996; 77:1017-20.

31.   Waagstein F, Hjalmarson A, Varnauskas E, Wallentin J. Effect of chronic betaadrenergic receptor blockade in congestive cardiomyopathy. Br Heart J 1975; 37:1022-36.

32.   Packer M, Bristow MR, Cohn JN. The effect of carvedilol on morbidity and mortality in patients with chronic heart failure. N Engl J Med 1996;334:1349-55

33   Kjeskhus J, Gilpin E, Cali G, Blackey AR, Henning H, Ross J Jr. Diabetic patients and betablockers after acute myocardial infarction. Eur Heart J 1990; 11:43-50.

34   Bristow MR, Gilbert EM, Abraham WT, Adams KF, Fowler MB, Hershberger R, Kybo SH, Narahara KA, Robertson AD, Krueger S, for the MOCHA Investigators. Effect of carvedilol on left ventricular function and mortality in diabetic versus non-diabetic patients with ischaemic or non-ischaemic dilated cardiomyopathy. Eur Heart J 1996; 17(Suppl.):78.

35.   MERIT-HF Study Group. Effect of metoprolol CR/XL in chronic heart failure: Metoprolol CR/XL Randomised Intervention Trial in Congestive Heart Failure (MERIT-HF).Lancet 1999; 353: 2001-2007

36.   Aronson D, Bloomgarden Z, Rayfield EJ. Potential mechanisms promoting restenosis in diabetic patients. J Am Coll Cardiol 1996; 27:528-35.

37   The Bypass Angioplasty Revascularization Investigation (BARI) Investigators. Comparison of coronary bypass surgery with angioplasty in patients with multivessel disease. N Engl J Med 1996; 335:217-25.

38   Topol EJ, et al. Long-term protection from myocardial ischemic events in a randomized trial of brief integrin ß3 blockade with percutaneous coronary intervention. JAMA 1997; 278:479-84.

6. ALBUMINURIA IN NON-INSULIN-DEPENDENT DIABETES – RENAL OR "EXTRA" RENAL DISEASE ?

Anita Schmitz
Medical Department, Horsens Sygehus, Horsens, Denmark

Microalbuminuria and overt proteinuria in IDDM have been decisively established as indicators of various stages in diabetic renal disease. Persistent microalbuminuria defines the stage of 'incipient nephropathy', that is the stage that heralds progression to overt nephropathy in more than 80 percent of cases within a decade, with proteinuria and relentless decline in kidney function, unless intervention is undertaken. Subsequent research concerning patients with NIDDM has clearly demonstrated, that the course of complications and the implication of albuminuria differ in several respects between the two types of diabetes [1-3].

Microalbuminuria and proteinuria are frequent in NIDDM amounting to 20-40% and 5-15% [4-8] respectively. This pertain also to newly or recently diagnosed patients [4,8-13], though at that point elevated albuminuria is reversible to some degree [12,14,15]. As an apparent paradox the incidence of renal impairment is of a low order of magnitude, 3-8% (in Caucasian NIDDM patients) [3,4,16]. Because of the large and increasing number of patients with NIDDM, however, renal failure constitutes an important health care problem [17-19], yet the poorer prognosis in NIDDM is due mainly to cardiovascular disease. As an additional ambiguity microalbuminuria has been brought into focus as a marker of cardiovascular disease and probably also increased mortality among non-diabetic subjects. Furthermore microalbuminuria may precede or even predict the onset of NIDDM [20].

The first reports that microalbuminuria is associated with an increased mortality in NIDDM appeared in 1984 [21,22].

MICROALBUMINURIA - A MAJOR RISK MARKER.

We investigated the prognostic influence of microalbuminuria, also in relation to other potential risk factors in a 10-year follow-up study [5] of 416 Caucasian non-insulin-

Mogensen C.E. (ed.), THE KIDNEY AND HYPERTENSION IN DIABETES MELLITUS.

dependent patients with urinary albumin concentration (UAC) ≤ 200µg/ml [23]. UAC was measured in first morning urine samples at each outpatient attendance during one year. Inclusion criteria were: age 50-75 years, age at diagnosis ≥ 45 years, and treatment managed without insulin for a period of at least 2 years. Clinical data are presented in table 6-1; 15 µg/ml was chosen as the upper limit of a normal UAC, and the patients were divided into three categories accordingly. Weight recorded during all visits, was related to "ideal" and treatment modality was recorded as the most "severe" (insulin > tablets > diet) during the 10-year period, since treatment modality often changes over time.

Table 6-1. Clinical data.

	Urinary albumin concentration (µg/ml)			
	≤15 n = 290	>15-≤40 n = 72	>40-≤200 n = 54	
Age (years)	65.6 ±6.5 50-75	66.9±5.7 50-75	67.2±5.0 54-75	NS[e]
Age at diagnosis (years)	59.4±7.2 45-75	59.8±6.6 47-74	59.8±6.9 46-71	NS
Known diabetes duration (years)	6.2±4.9 0-23	7.1±5.4 0-22	7.5±5.2 1-21	NS
Systolic blood Pressure (mmHg)	159±23 113-250	162±23 108-210	166±26 110-231	NS
Diastolic blood pressure (mmHg)	91±12 60-130	92±14 60-134	94±12 70-128	NS
Fasting plasma glucose (mmol/liter)	8.8±2.1 4.6-15.8	9.5±2.6 4.4-15.8	9.6±2.5 6.1-17.6	P=0.005
Fasting plasma glucose (all visits) (mmol/liter)	8.7±1.6 5.3-14.1	9.3±1.9 6.4-13.6	9.3±1.8 5.8-16.3	P=0.002
Relative weight (all visits) (%)	111±18 73-207	114±22 76-231	111±16 82-163	NS
Serum creatinine (mg%)[a]	0.9 x/÷1.2 0.6-2.8	1.0x/÷1.3 0.6-3.1	1.1x/÷1.4 0.7-3.3	P=0.000
Sex (M/F)[b]	126/164	35/37	23/31	NS
Retinopathy (N/B/P)[c]	238/42/0	51/16/0	43/10/0	NS
Treatment (D/T/I)[d]	33/201/56	8/44/20	5/34/15	NS

[a]Geometric mean x/÷ tolerance factor
[b]M/F, male/female
[c]N/B/P, normal/background/proliferative
[d]D/T/I, diet/tablet/insulin
[e]NS, not significant

It appears that the only significant differences between the groups were higher level of plasma glucose (r = 0.17, p < 0.001) and serum creatinine (r = 0.26, p < 0.001) in patients with elevated UAC. Blood pressures (BP) were comparable and hypertensive (BP > 160 mmHg systolic or > 95 mmHg diastolic, n= 255) and normotensive (n=161) patients had mean UAC values of 11.0 µg/ml x/÷ 2.8 and 9.3 µg/ml x/÷ 2.8 respectively. Frequency of retinopathy tended to be higher in the groups with microalbuminuria.

After 10 years 219 patients had died. The prognostic influence of the variables listed in table 6-1 was first evaluated separately using a log rank test, and subsequently by Cox regression analyses. The significant independent prognostic variables and hazard ratios are given in Table 6-2. By these analyses, the remaining variables had no significant influence on survival.

Table 6-2 Significant prognostic variables and the way they were presented in the Cox regression analyses.

Risk factor		Regression coefficient	p-value	Relative risk
Age in years		0.070	0.0000	1.07
Diabetes duration >10		0.385	0.015	1.47
Serum creatinine >1.3		0.463	0.043	1.59
UAC	>15	0.503	0.003	1.65
UAC	>40	0.382	0.078	1.46
			(0.000002)	(2.41)

The hazard ratios in the groups with elevated UAC relative to those with UAC≤15µg/ml were 1.65 (p=0.003) and 2.41 (p=0.000002) respectively.

Figure 6-1 presents the survival curves for the three UAC categories after correction for the influence of the other independent prognostic variables. From this it is clear, that even a minor increase in albuminuria , i.e. UAC 16-40 µg/ml, predicts a significantly reduced survival probability. A further increase in albuminuria i.e. 41-200µg/ml, is associated with a worse prognosis. No additional increase in mortality was detected in patients with UAC > 200 µg/ml [5], but the latter were few (n = 25). Fifty-six per cent died from acute myocardial infarction, cardiac insufficiency, or stroke, whereas no more than 2.3% died from or with uraemia. These cases tended however to be increasingly frequent through the three albuminuria groups (0.8, 2.1 and 7.5 %).The major predictive power of microalbuminuria for mortality has later been further documented [24-26] and a very similar relative risk was found in a population based study in patients with NIDDM [27]. That study and also more recent reports confirm that renal disease mortality is rare in white NIDDM patients [28-29].

Considering the results in two prospective outpatient cohort studies, attention is called to high *normo*albuminuria carrying a risk. In the study by Gall et al. [29] among patients with normal urinary albumin excretion (AER <30 mg/24h), those with values above the median AER of 8 mg/24 h had a relative mortality risk of 2.7 during five years of observation, compared to the remainder. MacLeod et al.[28] defined a group of "borderline microalbuminuria": AER 10.6-29.9 µg/min with significant excess of deaths over an eight year period.

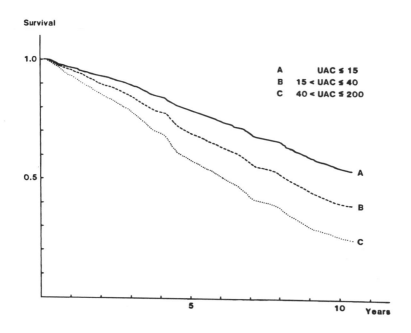

Figure 6-1. Survival curves for the three UAC groups, after correction for the other independent significant prognostic variables, age, known diabetes duration and serum creatinine. N=407, (subjects with missing value(s) excluded.

A further challenge to the understanding and definition of microalbuminuria is the findings of increased prevalence of cardiovascular risk factors [30] and reduced life expectancy [25,31] in non-diabetic persons with raised albuminuria. In one study [25] among 216 elderly non-diabetics 8-9 year mortality was increased in those with an UAE above the median of 7.52 µg/min. These observations raises questions as regards the cut-off level of abnormal albuminuria in NIDDM, including the limit for a normal albumin excretion in healthy people (not to mention the problem of defining healthiness). Originally the values defining microalbuminuria in NIDDM were adapted from IDDM. Any solid explanation for the association between elevated urinary albumin excretion and cardiovascular disease and death has so far not emerged. Albuminuria in non-insulin-dependent patients is predominantly of glomerular origin [32], but the exact mechanism behind the increased escape of albumin is not known in either type of diabetes [33-35]. Elevated albumin excretion is associated with both coronary heart disease, cardiac failure (even minor degrees of left ventricular dysfunction), ischemic stroke as well as peripheral vascular disease [3,10,36-40]. A number of cardiovascular risk factors have been linked also with albuminuria, such as lipoprotein abnormalities, hyperinsulinemia and markers of endothelial dysfunction as well as hypertension. It is predominantly systolic BP (also isolated systolic hypertension), that carries the risk [3,35,41-47]. None of these factors, however either alone or in combination have been able to "explain" the increased cardiovascular mortality in diabetic patients with microalbuminuria [3,35,41]. Consequently new risk factors are suggested [48].

ALBUMINURIA AND GLOMERULAR STRUCTURE

Diabetic glomerulopathy definitely does develop in non-insulin-dependent diabetes leading in some cases to renal impairment [49,50]. Information concerning the relationship between quantitative glomerular morphology and clinical renal parameters is however scarce in NIDDM.

In order to study the possible relation between urinary albumin excretion and glomerular structure [51] autopsy kidney tissue was sampled from 19 NIDDM patients, without other known renal disease, who had died within 18 months, mean 9 months, after UAC had been measured. They were aged 76 years (59-89),(mean, (range)), with known diabetes duration of 11 years (2-24), and UAC 29.7 µg/ml x/÷ 5.5 (1.4-710). Autopsy kidney tissue from 19 consecutive comparable non-diabetics was sampled for control.

A quantitative light-microscopic examination was performed on periodic-acid-Schiff- (P.A.S.) stained sections. The classic diabetic glomerulopathy is characterized by increased amounts of basement membrane and mesangial matrix (P.A.S.-positive) in the glomerular tuft (Chapter 17). The volume of P.A.S.-positive material as percent of tuft volume (defined as the minimal convex circumscribed polygon), estimated by point counting, was significantly increased in the group of diabetics. In this series there was no correlation between the quantitative structural parameters obtained and UAC, figure 6-2. Notably, a high UAC was not necessarily associated with more advanced glomerulopathy. In a later light- and electron microscopic study of biopsies from 20 NIDDM patients with proteinuria [52], the degree of glomerulopathy was estimated by measurement of basement membrane thickness, mesangial and matrix volume fractions (i.e volume per glomerular volume), and frequency of glomerular occlusion. Patients were aged 55 years (37-67), known diabetes duration was 8 years (1-19), urinary albumin excretion (UAE) 1.5 g/24h (0.3-8.7) and glomerular filtration rate (GFR) 90 ml/min/1.73 m^2 (24-146). Data were compared with previous data on 22 IDDM patients aged 35 years (24-47), diabetes duration 20 years (12-31), UAE 1.4 g/24h (0.3-7.9) and GFR 57 ml/min/1.73m^2 (16-104). Also, reference was made to 13 (age 51 years (21-68)) non-diabetic living renal transplant donors. There was a striking variation in the severity of glomeru-lopathy among NIDDM patients, and some proteinuric patients presented   structural parameters within the normal range, figures 6-3 and 6-4. When retinopathy was taken into account, patients with this complication all showed a glomerulopathy index (index is a calculated expression of the sum of changes in peripheral basement membrane and mesangium) above normal. In those without retinopathy approximately half had a *nor-mal* glomerular structure. Notably, GFR was rather well preserved in NIDDM compared with the younger IDDM patients, with the same degree of proteinuria.

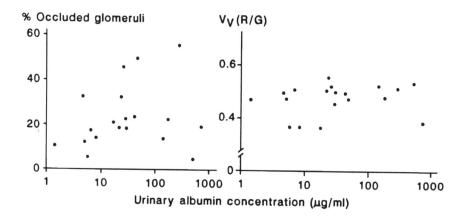

Figure 6-2. Relationship between urinary albumin concentration (μg/ml) and frequency of glo-merular occlusion (left panel) and volume fraction of P.A.S. positive material in the glomerular tuft (Vv(R/G)) in 19 NIDDM patients. Data obtained from light-microscopic studies on autopsy kidneys. Reproduced with permission from the American Diabetes Association, Inc.

In accordance with our findings Fioretto in a biopsy study on NIDDM patients with microalbuminuria found approximately 30% with a normal or near normal glomerular structure (see chapter 19). In our study kidney function was certainly associated with the structure, as an inverse correlation obtained between severity of glomerulopathy (index) and current glomerular filtration rate. Also the structural index correlated with the ensu-ing rate of decline in GFR (r = 0.84).

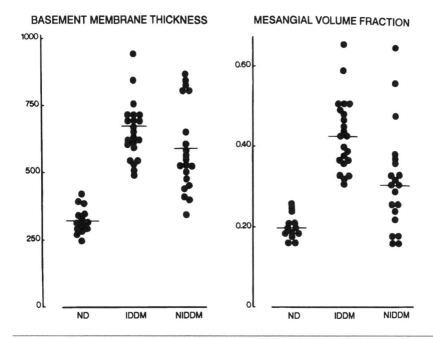

BASEMENT MEMBRANE THICKNESS   MESANGIAL VOLUME FRACTION

Figure 6-3 Basement membrane thickness in non-diabetic kidney transplant donors (ND) and IDDM and NIDDM patients with proteinuria. Data obtained from electron microscopic studies on kidney biopsies.

Figure 6-4. Mesangial volume per glomerulus (defined as the minimal convex polygon). See legend to figure 6-3.

No clear association between the structural quantities and albuminuria was however seen. Interestingly in three different studies around 60 percent of NIDDM patients with proteinuria had no retinopathy [5-7].

These observations underline the rather poor relation between albuminuria and microvascular complications compared to conditions in IDDM, and thus imply, that albuminuria has also causes other than diabetic glomerulopathy. Renal diseases unrelated to diabetic nephropathy may contribute, and has been reported to be present in as much as 30% [53, 54], though others did not confirm this high frequency [55,56] but rather around 12%. As commented above, abnormalities in albumin excretion may reflect cardiovascular disorders and essential hypertension.

Noticeable in this context, is the relation between systolic blood pressure and albumin excretion, which is demonstrated in several studies [3,5,6,9,27,44,57], whereas the relation to diastolic pressure is modest. Systolic hypertension expresses reduced vascular compliance, rather than "real" hypertension. Both systolic BP and albuminuria are related to coronary heart disease [3,58] in NIDDM as well as in non-diabetic subjects.

Albuminuria may thus express widespread vascular disease [3,35]. To elucidate why an increased urinary albumin excretion reflects non-renal complications, several hypotheses have been suggested. One recent remarkable clue for explaining this relation between albuminuria and atherosclerosis, was the finding of an increased transcapillary escape rate of albumin in otherwise clinically healthy subjects with elevated albuminuria [59]. Thus, NIDDM patients and non-diabetic persons share a relation between abnormal albuminuria and cardiovascular risk factors and disease. Transcapillary escape rate of albumin was increased in one study in NIDDM patients with microalbuminuria [60] but we were not able to confirm this [61]. Further research is needed to explain these matters.

ALBUMINURIA AND FUTURE RENAL FUNCTIONAL DETERIORATION
As in IDDM, microalbuminuria in NIDDM obviously also progresses to overt proteinuria, but overall does so to a less extent, around 20 % over a decade [62]. Also, the cumulative risk for renal failure 10 years after the appearance of proteinuria, was reported to be 11% in a population based study, [63] far more rare than in IDDM. Either the rate of progression to renal failure is misjudged as many patients are selected out by death from other causes, or raised albuminuria has "non-glomerulopathy" causes. Finally, the development of diabetic glomerulopathy may indeed be a slower process in NIDDM, perhaps with a better potential for compensation [52]. The implication of microalbuminuria in a single individual is thus difficult to decide disabling the notion "incipient nephropathy" [64] in NIDDM . (For further on the clinical course of renal function see Chapter 7).

PROGRESSION OF ALBUMINURIA
Although important for the evaluation of intervention measures, the knowledge of the rate of progression of albuminuria and factors with influence on this progression is modest. We followed of cohort of 278 NIDDM patients [65] during 6 years and estimated the average relative rate of increase to 17% per year, but with considerable interindividual variation. Systolic blood pressure and level of albuminuria were with significant influence on the rate of progression, but only a modest fraction of the variation between subjects could be explained by these factors. Progressors were then defined as those who both changed category of albuminuria (e.g. normo → micro) and increased more than 20%. These patients were characterised by elevated systolic blood pressure (165 vs 156 mmHg) a higher level of albuminuria as well as a more poor glycemic control (HbA$_{1C}$ 8.2 vs 7.7%) as compared to their non-progressing counterparts. It should be noted though that a few progressors had a very low initial level of albuminuria (1μg/ml)

stressing that serial measurements are imperative. In a more recent study [66] rather analogous differences were seen at baseline, only blood pressure did not appear as an independent predictor of progression of albuminuria.

Overall however, it is plausible from these and few other data [67], that progression of albuminuria is on average associated with a higher level of albumin excretion, more poor glycemic control and a higher blood pressure, especially the systolic. These factors are items for intervention.

CONCLUSIONS AND CONTROVERSIES

Microalbuminuria in NIDDM is a major independent risk marker for early cardiovascular mortality, but intervention is possible [68]. NIDDM patients and non-diabetic persons share a relation between raised albuminuria and atherosclerosis and its risk factors.

Elevated albumin excretion may reflect diabetic glomerulopathy, but other renal diseases or complications as well as macrovascular disease are common causes. A normal glomerular structure is seen in many patients with both microalbuminuria and proteinuria. Microalbuminuria is thus not synonymous to "incipient nephropathy" in NIDDM. As high "normoalbuminuria" carries a risk the limits for abnormal albuminuria may need reconsideration [69].

REFERENCES

1   Mogensen CE, Schmitz O. The diabetic kidney: From hyperfiltration and microalbuminuria to endstage renal failure. Med Clin North Am 1988; 72:1465-1492.

2   Mogensen CE, Damsgaard EM, Frøland A, Nielsen S, de Fine Olivarius N, Schmitz A. Microalbuminuria in non-insulin-dependent diabetes. Clin. Nephrol 1992; 38: s28-s39.

3   Schmitz A. The kidney in non-insulin-dependent diabetes. Studies in glomerular structure and function and the relationship between microalbuminuria and mortality. Acta Diabetol 1992; 29: 47-69.

4   Fabre J, Balant LP, Dayer PG, Fox HM, Vernet AT. The kindney in maturity onset diabetes mellitus: A clinical study of 510 patients. Kidney Int. 1982; 21:730-738.

5   Schmitz A, Væth M. Microalbuminuria: A major risk factor in non-insulin-dependent diabetes. A 10-year follow-up study of 503 patients. Diabetic Med 1988; 5:126-134.

6   Gall M-A, Rossing P, Skøtt P, Damsbo P, Vaag A, Bech K, Dejgaard A, Lauritzen M, Lauritzen E, Hougaard P, Beck-Nielsen H, Parving H-H. Prevalence of micro- and macro-albuminiuria, arterial hypertension, retinopathy and large vessel disease in European Type 2 (non-insulin-dependent) diabetic patients. Diabetologia 1991; 34: 655-661.

7   Marshall SM, Alberti KGMM. Comparison of the prevalence and associated features of abnormal albumin excretion in insulin-dependent and non-insulin-dependent diabetes. Q J Med 1989; 70: 61-71.

8   Damsgaard EM. »Prevalence and incidence of microalbuminuria in non-insulin-dependent diabetes: Relations to other vascular lesions.« In *The Kidney and Hypertension in Diabetes Mellitus, 1. ed.*, C.E. Mogensen, ed. Boston: Martinus Nijhoff Publishing, 1988; pp 59-63.

9   Olivarius N de F, Andreasen AH, Keiding N, Mogensen CE. Epidemiology of renal involvement in newly-diagnosed middle-aged and elderly diabetic patients. Cross-sectional data from the population-based study " Diabetes care in Generel Practice", Denmark. Diabetologia 1993; 36: 1007-1016.

10   Standl E, Stiegler H. Microalbuminuria in a random cohort of recently diagnosed Type 2 (non-insulin-dependent) diabetic patients living in the Greater Munich area. Diabetologia 1993; 36: 1017-1020.

11   Ballard DJ, Humphrey LL, Melton LJ III, Frohnert PP, Chu C-P, O'Fallon WM, Palumbo PJ.
     Epidemiology of persistent proteinuria in type II diabetes mellitus. Population-based study in Rochester, Minnesota. Diabetes 1988; 37: 405-412.

12   Schmitz A, Hvid Hansen H, Christensen T. Kidney function in newly diagnosed Type 2 (non-insulin-dependent) diabetic patients, before and during treatment. Diabetologia 1989; 32: 434-439.

13   Uusitupa M, Siitonen O, Penttilä I, Aro A, Pyörälä K. Proteinuria in newly diagnosed type II diabetic patients. Diabetes Care 1987; 10: 191-194.

14   Martin P, Hampton KK, Walton C, Tindall H, Daview JA. Microproteinuria in Type 2 diabetes mellitus from diagnosis. Diabetic Med 1990; 7:315-318.

15   Patrick AW, Leslie PJ, Clarke BF, Frier BM. The natural history and associations of microalbuminuria in type 2 diabetes during the first year after diagnosis. Diabetic Med 1990; 7: 902-908.

16   Tung P, Levin SR. Nephropathy in non-insulin-dependent diabetes mellitus. Am J Med 1988; 85: Suppl 5A: 131-136.

17   Mauer SM, Chavers BM. »A Comparison of kidney disease in Type 1 and Type II diabetes.« In *Comparison of Type 1 and Type II Diabetes. Similarities and dissimilarities in etiology, pathogenesis, and complications*, M. Vranic, C.H. Hollenberg, G. Steiner, eds. New York, London: Plenum Press, 1985; pp 299-303.

18   Rosansky SJ, Eggers PW. Trends in the US end-stage renal disease population: 1973-1983. Am J Kidney Dis. 1987; 9: 91-97.

19   Brunner FP, Brynger H, Challah S, Fassbinder W, Geerlings W, Selwood NH, Tufveson G, Wing AJ. Renal replacement therapy in patients with diabetic nephropathy, 1980-1985. Report from the European Dialysis and Transplant Association Registry. Nephrol Dial Transplant 1988; 3: 585-595.

20   Mykkänen L, Haffner SM, Kuusisto J, Pyorälä K, Laakso M. Microalbuminuria precedes the development of NIDDM. Diabetes 1994 ;43: 552-557.

21   Jarrett RJ, Viberti GC, Argyropoulos A, Hill RD, Mahmud U, Murrells TJ. Microalbuminuria predicts mortality in non-insulin-dependent diabetes. Diabetic Med 1984; 1: 17-19.

22   Mogensen CE. Microalbuminuria predicts clinical proteinuria and early mortality in maturity-onset diabetes. N Engl J Med 1984; 310: 356-360.

23   Mogensen CE, Chachati A, Christensen CK, Close CF, Deckert T, Hommel E, Kastrup J, Lefebvre P, Mathiesen ER, Feldt-Rasmussen B, Schmitz A, Viberti GC. Microalbuminuria: an early marker of renal involvement in diabetes. Uremia Invest 1985-86; 9: 85-95.

24   Mattock MB, Morrish Nj, Viberti GC, Keen H, Fitzgerald AP, Jackson G. Prospective study of microalbuminuria as predictor of mortality in NIDDM. Diabetes 1992; 41: 736-741.

25   Damsgaard EM, Frøland A, Jørgensen OD, Mogensen CE. Eight to nine year mortality in known non-insulin dependent diabetics and controls. Kidney Int 1992; 41: 731-735.

26   Dinneen SF, Gerstein HC. The association of microalbuminuria and mortality in Non-insulin-dependent diabetes mellitus. Arch Intern Med; 157: 1413-1418.

27   Neil A, Hawkins M, Potok M, Thorogood M, Cohen D, Mann J. A Prospective population-based study of microalbuminuria as a predictor of mortality in NIDDM. Diabetes Care 1993; 16: 996-1004.

28   MacLeod JM, Lutale J,Marshall SM. Albumin excretion and vascular deaths in NIDDM. Diabetologia 1995; 38: 610-616.

29   Gall M-A, Borch-Johnsen K, Hougaard P, Nielsen FS, Parving HH. Albuminuria and poor glycemic control predict mortality in NIDDM. Diabetes 1995; 44: 1303-1309.

30   Jensen JS, Borch-Johnsen K, Jensen G, Feldt-Rasmussen B. Atherosclerotic risk factors are increased in clinically healthy subjects with microalbuminuria. Atherosclerosis 1995; 112: 245-252.

31   Yudkin JS, Forrest RD, Jackson CA. Microalbuminuria as predictor of vascular disease in non-diabetic subjects. Islington diabetes survey. Lancet 1988; 2: 530-3.

32   Damsgaard EM, Mogensen CE, Microalbuminuria in elderly hyperglycaemic patients and controls. Diabetic Med 1986; 3: 430-435.

33   Hostetter TH, Rennke HG, Brenner BM. The case for intrarenal hypertension in the initiation and progression of diabetic and other glomerulopathies. Am J Med 1982; 72: 375-380.

34   Schmitz A. Increased urinary haemoglobin in diabetics with microalbuminuria – measured by an ELISA. Scand J Clin Lab Invest 1990; 50: 303-308.

35   Deckert T, Feldt-Rasmussen B, Borch-Johnsen K, Jensen T, Kofoed-Enevoldsen A. Albuminuria reflects widespread vascular damage. The Steno hypothesis. Diabetologia 1989; 32: 219-226.

36   Mattock MB, Keen H, Viberti GC, El-Gohari MR, Murrells TJ, Scott GS, Wing JR, Jackson PG. Coronary heart disease and urinary albumin excretion rate in type 2 (non-insulin-dependent) diabetic patients. Diabetologia 1988; 31: 82-87.

37   Eiskjær H, Bagger JP, Mogensen CE, Schmitz A, Pedersen EB. Enhanced urinary excretion of albumin in congestive heart failure: effect of ACE-inhibition. Scand J Clin Lab Invest 1992; 52: 193-199.

38   Kelbæk H, Jensen T, Feldt-Rasmussen B, Christensen NJ, Richter EA, Deckert T, Nielsen SL. Impaired left-ventricular function in insulin-dependent diabetic patients with increased urinary albumin excretion. Scand J Clin Lab Invest 1991; 51: 467-473.

39   Beamer NB, Coull BM, Clark WM, Wynn M (1999). Microalbuminuria in ischemic stroke. Arch Neurol, 56: 699-702.

40   Keen H. »Macrovascular disease in diabetes mellitus.« In *Diabetic Complications: Early Diagnosis and Treatment*, D. Andreani, G. Crepaldi, U. Di Mario, G. Pozza, eds. John Wiley & Sons Ltd., 1987; pp 3-12.

40   Jensen T *Albuminuria – a marker of renal and generalized vascular disease in insulin-dependent diabetes mellitus* (thesis). Copenhagen: København: Lægeforeningens Forlag, 1991.

42   Winocour PH, Durrington PN, Ishola M, Anderson DC, Cohen H. Influence of proteinuria on
vascular disease, blood pressure, and lipoproteins in insulin dependent diabetes mellitus. BMJ 1987; 294: 1648-1651.

43   Niskanen L, Uusitupa M, Sarlund H, Siitonen O, Voutilainen E, Penttilä I, Pyörälä K. Microalbuminuria predicts the development of serum lipoprotein abnormalities favouring atherogenesis in newly diagnosed Type 2 (non-insulin-dependent) diabetic patients. Diabetologia 1990; 33: 237-243.

44   Strandl E, Stiegler H, Janka HU, Mehnert H. Risk profile of macrovascular disease in diabetes mellitus. Diabete Metab (Paris) 1988; 14: 505-511.

45   Schmitz A, Ingerslev J. Haemostatic measures in Type 2 diabetic patients with microalbuminuria.Diabetic Med 1990; 7: 521-525.

46   Stehouwer CDA, Nauta JJP, Zeldenrust GC, Hackeng WHL, Donker AJM, den Ottolander GJH.
Urinary albumin excretion, cardiovascular disease and endothelial dysfunction in non-insulin-dependent diabetes mellitus. Lancet 1992; 340: 319-323.

47   Jensen T, Bjerre-Knudsen J, Feldt-Rasmussen B, Deckert T. Features of endothelial dysfunction in early diabetic nephropathy. Lancet 1989; i: 461-463.

48   Yudkin JS. Coronary heart disease in diabetes mellitus : three new risk factors and a unifying hypothesis. J Intern Med 1995; 238: 21-30.

49   Gellman DD, Pirani CL, Soothill JP, Muehrcke RC, Kark RM. Diabetic nephropathy, a clinical and pathologic study based on renal biopsies. Medicine 1959; 38: 321-367.

50   Thomsen AC. The Kidney in Diabetes Mellitus (thesis). Copenhagen: Munksgaard, 1965.

51   Schmitz A, Gundersen HJG, Østerby R. Glomerular morpology by light microscopy in non-insulin-dependent mellitus. Lack of glomerular hypertrophy. Diabetes 1988; 37: 38-43.

52   Østerby R, Gall M-A, Schmitz A, Nielsen FS, Nyberg G, Parving H-H. Glomerular structure and function in proteinuric Type 2 (non-insulin-dependent) diabetic patients. Diabetologia 1993; 36: 1064-1070.

53   Parving H-H, Gall M-A, Skøtt P, Jørgensen HE, Løkkegaard H, Jørgensen F, Nielsen B, Larsen S. Prevalence and causes of albuminuria in non-insulin-dependent diabetic patients. Kidney Int 1992; 41: 758-762.

54   Taft JL, Billson VR, Nankervis A, Kincaid-Smith P, Martin FIR. A clinical-histological study of individuals with diabetes mellitus and proteinuria. Diabetic Med 1990; 7: 215-221.

55   Olsen S, Mogensen CE. Non-diabetic renal disease in NIDDM proteinuric patients may be rare in biopsies from clinical practice (Abstract). JASN 1995; 6: 454.

56   Waldherr R, Ilkenhans C, Ritz E. How frequent is glomerulonephritis in diabetes mellitus type II ? Clin Nephrol 1992; 37: 271-273.

57   Keen H, Chlouverakis C, Fuller J, Jarrett RJ. The concomitants of raised blood sugar: studies in newly-detected hyperglycaemics II: Urinary albumin excretion, blood pressure and their relation to blood sugar levels. Guys Hosp Rep 1969; 118: 247-254.

58   Ibsen H, Hilden T. New views on the relationship between coronary heart disease and hypertension. J Intern Med 1990; 227: 77-79.

59   Jensen JS, Borch-Johnsen K, Jensen G, Feldt-Rasmussen B. Microalbuminuria reflects a generalized transvascular albumin leakiness in clinically healthy subjects. Clinical Science 1995; 88: 629-633.

60   Nannipieri M, Rizzo L, Rapuano A, Pilo A, Penno G, Navalesi R. Increased transcapillary escape rate of albumin in microalbuminuric Type II diabetic patients. Diabetes Care 1995; 18: 1-9.

61   Nielsen S, Schmitz A, Bacher T, Rehling M, Ingerslev J, Mogensen CE.Transcapillary escape rate and albuminuria in type 2 diabetes. Effects of short-term treatment with low molecular weight heparin, Diabetologia, 1999; 42: 60-67.

62   Mogensen CE. Microalbuminuria as a predictor of clinical diabetic nephropathy. Kidney Int 1987; 31: 673-689.

63   Humphrey LL, Ballard DJ, Frohnert PP, Chu C-P, O'Fallon WM, Palumbo PJ. Chronic renal failure in non-insulin-dependent diabetes mellitus. A population based study in Rochester, Minnesota. Ann Intern Med 1989; 111: 788-796.

64   Schmitz A. Renal function changes in middle-aged and elderly Caucasian Type 1 (non-insulin-dependent) diabetic patients – a review. Diabetologia 1993; 36: 985-992.

65   Schmitz A, Væth M, Mogensen CE. Systolic blood pressure relates to the rate of progression of albuminuria in NIDDM. Diabetologia 1994; 37: 1251-1258.

66   Gall MA, Hougaard P, Borch-Johnsen K, Parving HH. Risk factors for development of incipient and overt diabetic nephropathy in patients with non-insulin dependent diabetes mellitus: prospective,observational study. BMJ 1997; 314: 783-788.

67   Kikkawa R, Haneda M. »Risk factor for progression of microalbumiuria in relatively young NIDDM-patients.« In *Kidney and Hypertension in Diabetes Mellitus, 2. ed.,* C.E. Mogensen, ed. Boston, Dordrecht, London: Kluwer Academic Publishers, 1994; pp 103-109.

68   The Heart Outcomes Prevention Evaluation (HOPE) Study Investigators. Effects of an angiotensin-converting-enzyme inhibitor, ramipril, on cardiovascular events in high-risk patients. New Engl J Med, 2000; 342: 145-53.

69   Schmitz A (1997). Microalbuminuria, blood pressure, metabolic control and renal involvement. Longitudinal studies in white non-insulin-dependent diabetic patients. Am J Hypertension, 10: 189S-197S.

7. THE CLINICAL COURSE OF RENAL DISEASE IN CAUCASIAN NIDDM PATIENTS.

Søren Nielsen and Anita Schmitz
Medical Department M, Aarhus Kommunehospital, Aarhus, Denmark

Diabetic nephropathy is now the most prevalent cause of end-stage renal disease (ESRD) in the western world [1], accounting for approximately 30% of all patients entering end-stage renal failure programs [2]. Albeit diabetes is the single most important cause of ESRD in the United States [3], the percentage of patients with diabetes requiring renal replacement therapy in the European population is somewhat lower [4], about 13%, leaving glomerulonephritis and renal vascular disease due to hypertension as the most frequent causes of ESRD [5]. Approximately one-half of the diabetes related ESRD occur in NIDDM patients [6,7].

Clinical monitoring of diabetic nephropathy includes consecutive determinations of glomerular filtration rate (GFR) and measurements of the urinary albumin excretion rate (UAE) in 24 hour or in overnight collections [8]. In addition to indicating the degree of renal involvement UAE also serves as a cardiovascular risk marker. Even a minor abnormality, microalbuminuria, with UAE in the range of 20-200 µg/min (i.e. dipstick-negative albuminuria), predicts an increased incidence of overt diabetic nephropathy as characterized by proteinuria (i.e. UAE>200 µg/min) and of cardiovascular mortality [9-11]. Moreover, studies in both Caucasian subjects and the Pima Indians have shown that proteinuria is associated with a poor prognosis in terms of survival [12,13].

Measurement of the plasma clearance of an intravenously injected, single-dose of ^{51}Cr-EDTA is considered a reliable and reproducible method for routine determination of GFR, and superior to assessment of the endogenous creatinine clearance [14,15]. The coefficient of variation (CV) in an unselected group of patients with various renal disorders has been reported to be 4.1% in patients with GFR 30 ml/min and 11.6% in patients with a GFR<30 ml/min [15]. The reproducibility of GFR determinations in diabetic patients was recently evaluated and showed a CV of the single-shot ^{51}Cr -EDTA procedure similar to that of the aforementioned patients and similar to the constant ^{125}I-iothalamate infusion technique [16]. The plasma clearance technique offers an advantage in a diabetic population since it does not rely on timed urine sampling.

NEWLY DIAGNOSED NIDDM
In *newly diagnosed* Caucasian NIDDM subjects abnormal renal hemodynamics, increased kidney volume, and elevated albuminuria has been found. Thus, Vora et al. found that as many as 45% of the patients had a GFR above 120 ml/min/1.73 m^2 (i.e. the mean +2SD of an age matched control group) [17]. Other studies of newly diagnosed Caucasian subjects have shown that GFR is elevated by 10-20%[18-20] and in some reports renal plasma flow (RPF) and kidney volume have been found to be increased as well. Frank hyperfiltration (GFR>140 ml/min/1.73 m^2) was not observed by Schmitz et al. [18] in contrast to the 16% of the patients reported by Vora et al. [17]. In a population based study [21] one hour creatinine clearance was not increased in 81 subjects with fasting hyperglycaemia (i.e. previously undiagnosed diabetes) as compared to healthy sex and age matched control subjects.

IMPACT OF INITIAL METABOLIC TREATMENT
Schmitz et al first demonstrated that correction of glycaemic control over 3 months in 10 newly diagnosed NIDDM patients (mean (SD) age 59 (5) years) was associated with a reduction in both GFR and kidney volume to normal values as well as a decline in UAE which correlated with the fall rate of GFR [18]. Recently, Vora et al. [22] examined renal hemodynamics before and after 6 months of antidiabetic treatment in 76 newly diagnosed NIDDM patients (age 54 (10) years). GFR and albuminuria declined significantly during treatment, whereas mean values of RPF and filtration fraction were unchanged. The fall rate in GFR was significantly, but not very precisely, correlated with reductions of HBA_{1c} and RPF, but not with changes in UAE, blood pressure or lipids. The decline in GFR was more pronounced in younger patients with GFR levels above 120 ml/min/1.73 m^2 before treatment. Despite the reduction after 6 months, GFR remained greater than 120 ml/min/1.73 m^2 in a considerable number (32%) of patients as compared to pretreatment level of 45%. In a recent study Wirta et al. [20] also observed significantly higher GFR levels in 149 NIDDM patients with a disease duration of less than one year as compared with 150 healthy control subjects (117 (27) vs 103 (24) ml/min/1.73 m^2).

ESTABLISHED NIDDM
In *established* NIDDM cross sectional studies have shown that GFR is well preserved in patients with uncomplicated diabetes [23] as well as in patients with microalbuminuria [23-27]}(Table 7-1). Glomerular hyperfiltration has not been a consistent finding [21,23,24,27-29] although some studies have described high levels of GFR in some

patients [30-32]. Wirta et al. found that the glomerular hyperfiltration observed during the first year of diabetes persisted after 6 years [26]. In addition, measurements of kidney volume suggested a relationship with increased kidney size [30]. Recently, significantly higher GFR levels were reported in NIDDM patients with microalbuminuria as compared with normoalbuminuric patients and healthy subjects [33]. The prevalence of glomerular hyperfiltration among the microalbuminuric patients was 37%. Moreover, the GFR of the microalbuminuric patients was positively related to age, diabetes duration, glycaemic control, and urinary sodium excretion. On the other hand, significantly lower GFR levels have been found in NIDDM patients with arterial hypertension as compared with normotensive patients [34,35]. If indeed glomerular hyperfiltration is associated with microalbuminuria then increased GFR may be considered a risk marker for diabetic nephropathy [33]. On the other hand, the presence of arterial hypertension is associated with significantly lower GFR levels in NIDDM patients without overt nephropathy as compared to normotensive NIDDM patients [34,35]. However, it is also clear that GFR is related to a number of factors that by themselves modulate the levels of GFR and UAE. The prognostic significance of glomerular hyperfiltration in NIDDM is, however, still not known.

Table 7-1
Glycemic control, risk factors and kidney function in normo- and microalbuminuric NIDDM-patients

	Normoalbuminuria	Microalbuminuria
Sex (male/female)	14/5	14/5
Age (years)	64±4.5	64.5±4.2
Diabetes duration	7.3±5.6	8.4±6.8
Body mass index (kg m^{-2})	27.1±3.2	28.2±3.7
Fasting p-glucose (mmol. l^{-1})	8.5±2.5	9.1±2.7
HbA1c (%)	7.7±1.5	7.1±1.3
UAE (µg.min^{-1})	7.0x/÷1.6	61.7x/÷2.3
GFR (ml.min^{-1} 1.73 m^{-2})	94±13	91±20
Kidney volume (ml. 1.73^{-2})	220±45	260±54*
Systolic blood pressure (mmHg)	154±17	164±22
Diastolic blood pressure (mmHg)	81±11	86±11
Retinopathy (N/B/P)	16/3/0	9/8/2*
Antidiabetic treatment (diet/oha)	6/13	4/15
Antihypertensive treatment (%)	21	37
Smokers/non-smokers	7/12	12/7

LONGITUDINAL STUDIES
Only a few studies have evaluated the rate of decline in kidney function using the insulin clearance or isotopic techniques in NIDDM patients with different levels of albuminuria [36-38]. These studies describe the clinical course of renal function, not the natural history of diabetic nephropathy, since any drug therapy (e.g. antihypertensive therapy),

which may influence renal function and albuminuria was continued and adjusted during the studies.

NORMO- AND MICROALBUMINURIA

Longitudinal studies have shown, that NIDDM patients with normo- and microalbuminuria have preserved renal function. In a 3.4 year follow-up study of 37 patients (age 63 (5) years, known diabetes duration 7 (5) years) Nielsen et al. [36] found, that the average rate of decline in GFR in both normo- and microalbuminuric patients was similar to that reported in healthy, non-diabetic individuals (-1.0 ml/min/1.73 m^2) [39]. However, the change in GFR varied considerably between individuals: from -13.5 to +4.3 ml/min/1.73 m^2 per year (patients with normoalbuminuria) and from -7.0 to +4.2 ml/min/1.73 m^2 per year (patients with microalbuminuria). Both univariate and multiple regression analysis revealed that the fall rate of GFR was significantly related to the systolic blood pressure at baseline (Figure 7-1), as well as the mean systolic blood pressure during the study. This relationship was also found when the analysis was confined to the patients (73%) without antihypertensive treatment. The fall rate of GFR was not related to the level of albuminuria, metabolic parameters, or baseline GFR [36]. Thirty-one patients from the same study population were further followed for a mean of 5.5 (range: 3.3-7.5) years. The average fall rate of GFR did not differ from the abovementioned rate [40]. However, other relationships emerged during the prolonged follow-up period. Low baseline GFR was found to predict the decline of GFR. Moreover, poorer glycaemic control and higher level of albuminuria were independently associated with a higher fall rate of GFR in patients without antihypertensive treatment (Table 7-1). Conversely, the previously reported relationship with systolic blood pressure was not reproduced. This can probably be explained by relatively good blood pressure control for that age group (patients on antihypertensive treatment: 163/86 mm Hg; patients with no antihypertensive treatment: 148/79 mm Hg). In a recent short-term study of hypertensive NIDDM patients microalbuminuria predicted a drop in GFR whereas no increase was found in normoalbuminuric patients [27]. Many of the patients were on antihypertensive treatment and the achieved blood pressures were normal in the group of normoalbuminuric patients (137/77 mm Hg) and moderately, but significantly higher the microalbuminuric group (152/88 mm Hg). Moreover, the higher fall rate in the microalbuminuric patients was associated with a further increase in diastolic blood pressure. On the other hand a relationship between the decline in renal function and mean blood pressure was found in an Israeli study of somewhat younger (age 42 (2) years, known diabetes duration<2 years), normotensive (blood pressure <150/95 mm Hg) patients followed for 14 years [41]. Although patients who developed proteinuria and/or hypertension during the study were excluded from the analysis timed urine collection was not employed and renal function was estimated from the reciprocal plasma creatinine concentration. In a Brazilian study of normoalbuminuric NIDDM patients (age 53 ±7 (mean ±SD) years, diabetes duration 7 ±5 years) followed for 5 years blood pressure did not determine the fall rate of GFR [37]. Among these patients only 6 of the 32 patients studied were characterized by hypertension at baseline. The study also provides some evidence that glomerular hyperfiltration (baseline GFR > mean+2 SD of normal control values) may be associated with an increased rate of decline of GFR although regression to the mean should be kept in mind. In another prospective study serum prorenin, the inactive precursor of renin, was not related to microalbuminuria, nor did prorenin predict the rate of decline of GFR or progression rate of albuminuria [42]. Thus, it can be concluded from these studies that a normal (or fairly treated) blood pressure is not a primary determinant of renal function changes in this patient group. However, by studying such patients other factors, operating beyond blood pressure, may be disclosed.

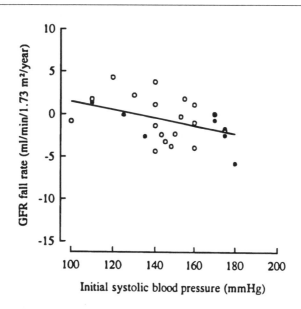

Figure 7-1

DIABETIC NEPHROPATHY

The clinical course of renal function in NIDDM patients with proteinuria was evaluated by Gall et al. in a prospective study of 26 patients (age 52 (SE 2) years, known diabetes duration 9 (1) years) followed for 5.2 (range: 1.0-7.0) years and in whom a kidney biopsy had shown diabetic glomerulosclerosis [38]. An average of 7 (range: 3-10) GFR measurements were performed in each patient. GFR decreased from 83 (24-146) to 58 (2-145) ml/min/1.73 m^2, with a mean reduction of 5.7 ml/min/1.73 m^2 per year. Again, considerable interindividual variation was found, ranging from a decrease of 22.0 to an increase of 3.5 ml/min/1.73 m^2 per year. Concomitantly, albuminuria increased from 1.2 (0.3-7.2) (geometric mean (range)) to 2.3 (0.4-8.0) g/24 h (p<0.001). Systolic blood pressure, mean blood pressure and baseline GFR correlated significantly with the rate of decline in GFR in a univariate analysis whereas no correlations were found between the fall rate of GFR and dietary protein intake, total cholesterol, HDL-cholesterol or HbA_{1c} concentrations during the follow-up period. Multiple regression analysis revealed that the systolic blood pressure during the study was the only factor significantly determining the rate of decline in GFR. Although blood pressure was unchanged throughout the study (162/93 at entry versus 161/89 mm Hg at exit) the prevalence of arterial hypertension was quite high as judged from the substantial number of patients requiring antihypertensive medication (62% at entry versus 81% at exit). The overall mortality was 27%. Three patients died from uremia and 4 patients from cardiovascular diseases. Two patients needed renal replacement therapy at the end of the study.

Other studies have indicated that systolic blood pressure has a major impact on the progression renal function deterioration. Stornello et al. reported that normotensive NIDDM patients with persistent proteinuria treated with placebo for 12 months had stable GFR [43]. Finally, studies of Biesenbach et al. [44] and Pugh et al. [45] found comparable fall rates of GFR (creatinine clearance) in proteinuric IDDM and NIDDM patients with normal GFR at baseline. Although these were studies of the most severely affected patients, namely the subgroup that eventually progressed to ESRD, the association between the fall rate of GFR and blood pressure was clearly demonstrated [44].

Thus, elevated systolic blood pressure is an important factor associated with a progressive decline in GFR in NIDDM patients. However, it is also clear, that the decline in renal function is negligible in normo- and microalbuminuric patients with a systolic blood pressure below 150 mm Hg [36] or a mean blood pressure around 95 mm Hg in younger subjects [46]. Even in patients with systolic blood pressures above 150 mm Hg the decline in GFR is quite low, and ESRD does not affect the long-term prognosis of the majority of these patients. In patients with overt proteinuria, however, deterioration in kidney function is accelerated in some patients and related to the systolic blood pressure [38].

INTERVENTION STUDIES

The list of abnormalities reported to be associated with NIDDM and abnormal albuminuria (e.g. obesity, sedentary lifestyle, hypertension, dyslipidemia, hemostatic abnormalities and insulin resistance) opens a wide spectrum of options for intervention studies focusing on the rate of progression of diabetic nephropathy. So far there have been no reports of the effect of optimized *metabolic control* on renal function in Caucasian patients with long standing NIDDM. Moreover, the influence of *non-*

pharmacological intervention, such as diet, exercise, and weight loss on renal function in Caucasian NIDDM patients have not been reported.

Studies evaluating the renal effects of different pharmacological treatments are sparse, mainly short-term, uncontrolled, and inconsistent in terms of the methods used for estimation of GFR.

ANTIHYPERTENSIVE THERAPY

Only a few randomized long-term trials have evaluated the effects of antihypertensive treatment on the progressive decline in GFR. Many studies have shown that ACE-inhibitors are superior to other antihypertensive drugs in terms of reducing albuminuria[47]. A similar advantage with respect to preventing deterioration of renal function has, however, not been documented [48,49]. Thus, blood pressure reduction is more important than the type of antihypertensive drug used.

Microalbuminuria was significantly reduced during treatment with an ACE-inhibitor or a calcium channel antagonist in a study [50] of a mixed group of diabetic patients (62% NIDDM). This effect was predominantly seen in hypertensive patients, who also exhibited the greatest blood pressure reduction. Patients with GFR above 135 ml/min/1.73 m^2 at baseline showed a significant decrease in GFR (from 186 to 161 ml/min/1.73 m^2), while patients with lower baseline levels displayed stable GFR values (from 96 to 92 ml/min/1.73 m^2). In an uncontrolled, long-term (36 months) study of 10 hypertensive NIDDM patients with microalbuminuria, using the single shot ^{51}Cr-EDTA procedure, treatment with Indapamide significantly reduced blood pressure from 180/100 to 140/85 mm Hg and albuminuria from (81.5 (SE 1) mg/24 h to 29.0 (4.5) mg/24 h, whereas GFR was unaffected during treatment, 95 ml/min/1.73 m^2 [51]. Similar results have been described by Lacourciére et al. [52]. Ravid et al. [46] conducted a randomized, double-blind, placebo controlled trial, in which they demonstrated, that treatment of normotensive, microalbuminuric NIDDM patients (mean age 45 years, diabetes duration 7 years) with an ACE-inhibitor (Enalapril 10 mg per day) (n=49) for five years exerted a stabilizing effect on albuminuria and kidney function (estimated by the reciprocal creatinine level), while a progression was observed in the placebo group (n=45). A concomitant significant rise in mean blood pressure was noted only in the placebo treated patients, stressing the importance of blood pressure in the progression of renal disease in NIDDM. These results have now been confirmed in a further 2 year unblinded extension of the study [53]. In a recent Italian study of hypertensive normo- and microalbuminuric NIDDM patients aggressive treatment of blood pressure (<140/85 mm Hg) with cilazapril and amlodipin for 3 years was associated with an average annual fall rate of GFR of 2-2.5 ml/min/1.73 m^2 [54]. In contrast, another Italian study observed increased GFR levels in a small group of microalbuminuric hypertesive patients with biopsy proven diabetic glomerulopathy treated with enalapril or nitrendipin for 27 months [55,56].

Published studies in Caucasian NIDDM patients with proteinuria are sparse and mostly short-term (6-12 months or less). In two studies of 6 months treatment with captopril a beneficial effects on GFR was observed by Stornello et al. [43], whereas a decline in GFR from 57 to 51 ml/min/1.73 m^2 was found by Valvo et al. [57]. However, both studies were uncontrolled and included only 9 and 12 patients, respectively. More convincing results were reported by Nielsen et al. in a study comparing the effects of 12 months treatment with lisinopril (n=21) and atenolol (n=22) in hypertensive NIDDM patients with proteinuria [58]. Although blood pressure was markedly reduced by both treatments (from 162/85 to 136/72 mm Hg (lisinopril) and from 161/91 to 145/81 mm Hg (atenolol)) only lisinopril lowered albumin excretion rate. However, no evidence of a stabilizing effects on GFR could be demonstrated since the annual decline in GFR was (12 (SE 2) ml/min/1.73 m^2 (lisinopril) and 11 (1) ml/min/1.73 m^2 (atenolol). It is to be noticed, however, that the blood pressure levels refer to 24 hour ambulatory measurements and that auscultatory clinical blood pressure values attained after 12 months treatment were rather high (158/81 mm Hg (lisinopril) and 160/83 mm Hg (atenolol). Recently, results from a 37 months follow-up of the same patients (open label treatment after the first 12 months) were published showing that the rate of decline of GFR was similar during both treatments, but that a slower progression rate (7-8 ml/min/1.73 m^2) was found after the first 6 months of treatment [59] (a pattern also described in IDDM). Taft et al. also found similar rate of decline in creatinine clearance (3-4 ml/min/year) between patients treated with or without ACE-inhibitors [60]. Conversely, in normotensive patients with persistent proteinuria, low dose administration of ß-blockers or ACE-inhibitors for 6-12 months reduce albuminuria in the absence of any effect on systemic blood pressure or GFR [43,61].

LIPIDE LOWERING AGENTS

Lipoprotein metabolism is frequently found abnormal in NIDDM. In particular, high triglycerides, low HDL-cholesterol and small dense LDL particles are common in combination with decreased insulin sensitivity. Dyslipidemia has been described to be more common in subjects with abnormal albuminuria [24,25,62-64]. Moreover, dyslipidemia has been proposed to promote chronic progressive renal disease [65-67] and worsen insulin resistance. Hypercholesterolaemia is not a prominent finding in NIDDM although high levels have been described [68]. However, dyslipidemia [69] and hypercholesterolaemia [70], enhances the risk of cardiovascular mortality in NIDDM. Moreover, cholesterol lowering therapy with simvastatin reduces the risk [70]. A number of animal studies have shown that experimental and physiological dyslipidemia, particularly hypercholesterolaemia, promotes renal damage and that lipid lowering therapy protects against changes in renal histology and function [67]. In humans, however, fewer and less consistent results of the prognostic significance of dyslipidemia on renal function are available. Thus, some studies have shown a positive relationship between cholesterol or triglycerides concentrations and the decline in renal function or rise in UAE [71-76] while other studies have failed to show a relationship [68,77]. Studies in Chinese and Japanese NIDDM subjects have suggested a beneficial effect of statin treatment on GFR [78] and UAE [79]. Simvastatin reduces hepatic cholesterol synthesis and increases synthesis of hepatic LDL receptors resulting in increased LDL and VLDL remnant clearance and reduced triglycerides, LDL- and VLDL-cholesterol concentrations [80,81]. In an uncontrolled study of simvastatin a significant reduction in proteinuria was observed in patients with nephrotic syndrome [82]. In another study 12 weeks treatment with simvastatin did no change proteinuria in IDDM patients with overt nephropathy and mild hypercholesterolaemia [83]. In Caucasians, the effect of lipid lowering therapy on kidney function in NIDDM has only been sparsely studied.

Nielsen et al. [84] examined the effects of pharmacological lipid lowering therapy with simvastatin on renal function in NIDDM patients with microalbuminuria and moderate hypercholesterolaemia (serum cholesterol ≥5.5 mmol/l). In a double blind, randomized design 18 patients were treated with either simvastatin 10 mg daily or placebo. The dose was adjusted in order to achieve a serum cholesterol level below 5.2 mmol/l. After 18 weeks the placebo treatment was discontinued whereas patients on simvastatin continued treatment in an unblinded design for another 18 weeks. Simvastatin treatment significantly reduced the dyslipidemia whereas no change in GFR or UAE was observed. Thus, these results are not in favor of the hypothesis that improvement of dyslipidemia has a beneficial effect on renal function in NIDDM. Recently, a reduction in microalbuminuria was reported in an Italian study of NIDDM subjects treated with simvastatin for one year [85]. The reason why some studies show an improvement in GFR and/or UAE during simvastatin as opposed to other studies showing no effect is not clear. The study period may have been too short to pick up an effect on renal function. Moreover, effects on GFR may be more difficult to detect than effects on UAE due to the low average rate of decline of GFR in microalbuminuric NIDDM. Finally, the simvastatin dose may have been too small.

Presently, studies evaluating the renal effects of intervention against hemostatic parameters and insulin resistance are not available, but in progress. General aspects of diabetic renal disease in NIDDM patients have recently been reviewed in depth [86].

REFERENCES

1. FitzSimmons, SC, Agodoa, L, Striker, L, Conti, F, Striker, G. Kidney disease of diabetes mellitus: NIDDK initiatives for the comprehensive study of its natural history, pathogenesis, and prevention. Am J Kidney Dis 1989; 8: 7-10.
2. Eggers, PW. Effect of transplantation on the medicare end-stage renal disease program. N Engl J Med 1993; 381: 223-229.
3. Walker, WG. Hypertension-related renal injury: a major contributor to end- stage renal disease. Am J Kidney Dis 1993; 22: 164-173.
4. Raine, AEG. Epidemiology, development and treatment of end-stage renal failure in Type 2 (non-insulin-dependent) diabetic patients in Europe. Diabetologia 1993; 36: 1099-1104.

5.   Brunner, FP and Selwood, NH. Profile of patients on RRT in Europe and death rates due to major causes of death groups. Kidney Int 1992; 42 Suppl 38: S4-S15.
6.   Rettig, B and Teutsch, SM. The incidence of end-stage renal disease in type I and type II diabetes mellitus. Diabetic Nephropathy 1984; 3: 26-27.
7.   Grenfell, A, Bewick, M, Parsons, V, Snowden, S, Taube, D, Watkins, PJ. Non-insulin-dependent diabetes and renal replacement therapy. Diabetic Med 1988; 5: 172-176.
8.   Mogensen, CE, Damsgaard, EM, Frøland, A, Nielsen, S, Fine Olivarius, Nd, Schmitz, A. Microalbuminuria in non-insulin-dependent diabetes. Clin Nephrol 1992; 38 Suppl 1: S28-S38.
9.   Mogensen, CE. Microalbuminuria predicts clinical proteinuria and early mortality in maturity-onset diabetes. N Engl J Med 1984; 310: 356-360.
10.   Jarrett, RJ, Viberti, GC, Argyropoulos, A, Hill, RD, Mahmud, U, Murrells, TJ. Microalbuminuria predicts mortality in non-insulin-dependent diabetics. Diabetic Med 1984; 1: 17-19.
11.   Schmitz, A and Vaeth, M. Microalbuminuria: a major risk factor in non-insulin-dependent diabetes. A 10-year follow-up study of 503 patients. Diabetic Med 1988; 5: 126-134.
12.   Stephenson, JM, Kenny, S, Stevens, LK, Fuller, JH, Lee, E. Proteinuria and mortality in diabetes: the WHO multinational study of vascular disease in diabetes. Diabetic Med 1995; 12: 149-155.
13.   Nelson, RG, Pettitt, DJ, Carraher, MJ, Baird, HR, Knowler, WC. Effect of proteinuria on mortality in NIDDM. Diabetes 1988; 37: 1499-1504.
14.   Bröchner-Mortensen J. A simple method for the determination of glomerular filtration rate. Scand J Clin Lab Invest 1972; 30: 271-274.
15.   Bröchner-Mortensen, J and Rødbro, P. Selection of routine method for determination of glomerular filtration rate in adult patients. Scand J Clin Lab Invest 1976; 36: 35-43.
16.   Mogensen, CE, Hansen, KW, Nielsen, S, Mau Pedersen, M, Rehling, M, Schmitz, A. Monitoring diabetic nephropathy: Glomerular filtration rate and abnormal albuminuria in diabetic renal disease - reproducibility, progression, and efficacy of antihypertensive intervention. Am J Kidney Dis 1993; 22: 174-187.
17.   Vora, JP, Dolben, J, Dean, JD, Thomas, D, Williams, JD, Owens, DR, Peters, JR. Renal hemodynamics in newly presenting non-insulin dependent diabetes mellitus. Kidney Int 1992; 41: 829-835.
18.   Schmitz, A, Hansen, HH, Christensen, T. Kidney function in newly diagnosed type 2 (non-insulin- dependent) diabetic patients, before and during treatment. Diabetologia 1989; 32: 434-439.
19.   Keller, CK, Bergis, KH, Fliser, D, Ritz, E. Renal findings in patients with short-term type 2 diabetes. J Am Soc Nephrol 1996; 7: 2627-2635.
20.   Wirta, O, Pasternack, A, Mustonen, J, Oksa, H, Koivula, T, Helin, H. Albumin excretion rate and its relation to kidney disease in non- insulin-dependent diabetes mellitus. J Intern Med 1995; 237: 367-373.
21.   Damsgaard, EM and Mogensen, CE. Microalbuminuria in elderly hyperglycaemic patients and controls. Diabetic Med 1986; 3: 430-435.
22.   Vora, JP, Dolben, J, Williams, JD, Peters, JR, Owens, DR. Impact of initial treatment on renal function in newly-diagnosed Type 2 (non-insulin-dependent) diabetes mellitus. Diabetologia 1993; 36: 734-740.

23. Schmitz, A, Christensen, T, Jensen, FT. Glomerular filtration rate and kidney volume in normoalbuminuric non-insulin-dependent diabetics - lack of glomerular hyperfiltration and renal hypertrophy in uncomplicated NIDDM. Scand J Clin Lab Invest 1989; 48: 103-108.

24. Schmitz, A, Christensen, T, Møller, A, Mogensen, CE. Kidney function and cardiovascular risk factors in non-insulin- dependent diabetics (NIDDM) with microalbuminuria. J Intern Med 1990; 228: 347-352.

25. Savage, S, Nagel, NJ, Estacio, RO, Lukken, N, Schrier, RW. Clinical factors associated with urinary albumin excretion in type II diabetes. Am J Kidney Dis 1995; 25: 836-844.

26. Wirta, O, Pasternack, A, Laippala, P, Turjanmaa, V. Glomerular filtration rate and kidney size after six years disease duration in non-insulin-dependent diabetic subjects. Clin Nephrol 1996; 45: 10-17.

27. Berrut, G, Bouhanick, B, Fabbri, P, Guilloteau, G, Bled, F, Le Jeune, JJ, Fressinaud, P, Marre, M. Microalbuminuria as a predictor of a drop in glomerular filtration rate in subjects with non-insulin-dependent diabetes mellitus and hypertension. Clin Nephrol 1997; 48: 92-97.

28. Fabre, J, Balant, LP, Dayer, PG, Fox, HM, Vernet, AT. The kidney in maturity onset diabetes mellitus: A clinical study of 510 patients. Kidney Int 1982; 21: 730-738.

29. Gragnoli, G, Signorini, AM, Tanganelli, I, Fondelli, C, Borgogni, P, Borgogni, L, Vattimo, A, Ferrari, F, Guercia, M. Prevalence of glomerular hyperfiltration and nephromegaly in normo- and microalbuminuric type 2 diabetic patients. Nephron 1993; 65: 206-211.

30. Wirta, OR and Pasternack, AI. Glomerular filtration rate and kidney size in type 2 (non-insulin-dependent) diabetes mellitus. Clin Nephrol 1995; 44: 1-7.

31. Silveiro, SP, Friedman, R, Gross, JL. Glomerular hyperfiltration in NIDDMpatients without overt proteinuria. Diabetes Care 1993; 16: 115-119.

32. Nowack, R, Raum, E, Blum, W, Ritz, E. Renal hemodynamics in recent-onset type II diabetes. Am J Kidney Dis 1992; 20: 342-347.

33. Vedel, P, Obel, J, Nielsen, FS, Bang, LE, Svendsen, TL, Pedersen, OB, Parving, HH. Glomerular hyperfiltration in microalbuminuric NIDDM patients. Diabetologia 1996; 39: 1584-1589.

34. Rius, F, Pizarro, E, Castells, I, Salinas, I, Sanmarti, A, Romero, R. Renal function changes in hypertensive patients with non-insulin- dependent diabetes mellitus. Kidney Int Suppl. 1996; 55: S88-90.

35. Rius, F, Pizaro, E, Salinas, I, Lucas, A, Sanmarti, A, Romero, R. Age as a determinant of glomerular filtration rate in non- insulin-dependent diabetes mellitus. Nephrol Dial Transplant 1995; 10: 1644-1647.

36. Nielsen, S, Schmitz, A, Rehling, M, Mogensen, CE. Systolic blood pressure relates to the rate of decline of glomerular filtration rate in Type 2 diabetes mellitus. Diabetes Care 1993; 16: 1427-1432.

37. Silveiro, SP, Friedman, R, De Azevedo, MJ, Canani, LH, Gross, JL. Five-year prospective study of glomerular filtration rate and albumin excretion rate in normofiltering and hyperfiltering normoalbuminuric NIDDM patients. Diabetes Care 1996; 19: 171-174.

38. Gall, M-A, Nielsen, FS, Smidt, UM, Parving, H-H. The course of kidney function in Type 2 (non-insulin-dependent) diabetic patients with diabetic nephropathy. Diabetologia 1993; 36: 1071-1078.

39.   Rowe, JW, Andres, R, Tobin, JD, Norris, AH, Shock, NW. The effect of age on creatinine clearance in men: A cross- sectional and longitudinal study. J Gerontology 1976; 31: 155-163.

40.   Nielsen, S, Schmitz, A, Rehling, M, Mogensen, CE. The clinical course of renal function in NIDDM patients with normo- and microalbuminuria. J Intern Med 1997; 241: 133-141.

41.   Ravid, M, Savin, H, Lang, R, Jutrin, I, Shoshana, L, Lishner, M. Proteinuria, renal impairment, metabolic control, and blood pressure in type 2 diabetes mellitus. Arch Intern Med 1992; 152: 1225-1229.

42.   Nielsen, S, Schmitz, A, Derkx, FHM, Mogensen, CE. Prorenin and renal function in NIDDM patients with normo- and microalbuminuria. J Intern Med 1995; 238: 499-505.

43.   Stornello, M, Valvo, EV, Scapellato, L. Angiotensin converting enzyme inhibition in normotensive type II diabetics with persistent mild proteinuria. J Hypertens 1989; 7 Suppl 6: 314-315.

44.   Biesenbach, G, Janko, O, Zazgornik, J. Similar rate of progression in the predialysis phase in type I and type II diabetes mellitus. Nephrol Dial Transplant1994; 9: 1097-1102.

45.   Pugh, JA, Medina, R, Ramirez, M. Comparison of the course to end-stage renal disease of type 1 (insulin-dependent) and type 2 (non-insulin-dependent) diabetic nephropathy. Diabetologia 1993; 36: 1094-1098.

46.   Ravid, M, Savin, H, Jutrin, I, Bental, T, Katz, B, Lishner, M. Long-term stabilizing effect of angiotensin-converting enzyme inhibition on plasma creatinine and on proteinuria in normotensive type II diabetic patients. Ann Intern Med 1993; 118: 577-581.

47.   Kasiske, BL, Kalil, RS, Ma, JZ, Liao, M, Keane, WF. Effect of antihypertensive therapy on the kidney in patients with diabetes: a meta-regression analysis. Ann Intern Med 1993; 118: 129-138.

48.   Ritz, E and Orth, SR. Nephropathy in patients with type 2 diabetes mellitus. N Engl J Med 1999; 341: 1127-1133.

49.   Parving, H-H and Rossing, P. The use of antihypertensive agents in prevention and treatment of diabetic nephropathy. Current Opinion Nephrol Hypertens 1994; 3: 292-300.

50.   Melbourne Diabetic Nephropathy Study Group. Comparison between perindopril and nifedipine in hypertensive and normotensive diabetic patients with microalbuminuria. BMJ 1991; 302: 210-216.

51.   Gambardella, S, Frontoni, S, Lala, A, Felici, MG, Spallone, V, Scoppola, A, Jacoangeli, F, Menzinger, G. Regression of microalbuminuria in type II diabetic hypertensive patients after long-term indapamide treatment. Am Heart J 1991; 122: 1232-1238.

52.   Lacourcière, Y, Nadeau, A, Poirier, L, Tancrède, G. Captopril or conventional therapy in hypertensive type II diabetics.Three-year analysis. Hypertension 1993; 21: 786-794.

53.   Ravid, M, Lang, R, Rachmani, R, Lishner, M. Long-term renoprotective effect of angiotensin-converting enzyme inhibition in non-insulin-dependent diabetes mellitus. A 7-year follow-up study. Arch Intern Med 1996; 156: 286-289.

54.   Velussi, M, Brocco, E, Frigato, F, Zolli, M, Muollo, B, Maioli, M, Carraro, A, Tonolo, G, Fresu, P, Cernigoi, AM, Fioretto, P, Nosadini, R. Effects of cilazapril and amlodipine on kidney function in hypertensive NIDDM patients. Diabetes 1996; 45: 216-222.

55.   Ruggenenti, P, Mosconi, L, Bianchi, L, Cortesi, L, Campana, M, Pagani, G, Mecca, G, Remuzzi, G. Long-term treatment with either enalapril or nitrendipine stabilizes albuminuria and increases glomerular filtration rate in non-insulin-dependent diabetic patients. Am J Kidney Dis 1994; 24: 753-761.

56. Mosconi, L, Ruggenenti, P, Perna, A, Mecca, G, Remuzzi, G. Nitrendipine and enalapril improve albuminuria and glomerular filtration rate in non-insulin dependent diabetes. Kidney Int 1996 Suppl; 55: S91-93.

57. Valvo, E, Bedogna, V, Casagrande, P, Antiga, L, Zamboni, M, Bommartini, F, Oldrizzi, L, Rugiu, C, Maschio, G. Captopril in patients with type II diabetes and renal insufficiency: Systemic and renal hemodynamic alterations. Am J Med 1988; 85: 344-348.

58. Nielsen, FS, Rossing, P, Gall, M-A, Skøtt, P, Smidt, UM, Parving, H-H. Impact of lisinopril and atenolol on kidney function in hypertensive NIDDM subjects with diabetic nephropathy. Diabetes 1994; 43: 1108-1113.

59. Nielsen, FS, Rossing, P, Gall, MA, Skøtt, P, Smidt, UM, Parving, HH. Long-term effect of lisinopril and atenolol on kidney function in hypertensive NIDDM subjects with diabetic nephropathy. Diabetes 1997; 46: 1182-1188.

60- Taft, JL, Nolan, CJ, Yeung, SP, Hewitson, TD, MartinI, IR. Clinical and histological correlations of decline in renal function in diabetic patients with proteinuria. Diabetes 1994; 43: 1046-1051.

61. Stornello, M, Valvo, EV, Scapellato, L. Persistent albuminuria in normotensive non-insulin-dependent (type II) diabetic patients: comparative effects of angiotensin-converting enzyme inhibitors and β-adrenoceptor blockers. Clin Sci 1992; 82: 19-23.

62. Jensen, JS, Borch-Johnsen, K, Jensen, G, Feldt-Rasmussen, B. Atherosclerotic risk factors are increased in clinically healthy subjects with microalbuminuria. Atherosclerosis 1995; 112: 245-252.

63. Zambon, S, Manzato, E, Solini, A, Sambataro, M, Brocco, E, Sartore, G, Crepaldi, G, Nosadini, R. Lipoprotein abnormalities in non-insulin-dependent diabetic patients with impaired extrahepatic insulin sensitivity, hypertension, and microalbuminuria. Arterioscler Thromb 1994; 14: 911-916.

64. Haffner, SM, Stern, MP, Gruber, MKK, Hazuda, HP, Mitchell, BD, Patterson, JK. Microalbuminuria. Potential marker for increased cardiovascular risk factors in nondiabetic subjects? Arteriosclerosis 1990; 10: 727-731.

65. Moorhead, JF, Chan, MK, El-Nahas, M, Varghese, Z. Lipid nephrotoxicity in chronic progressive glomerular and tubulo-interstitial disease. Lancet 1982; 1309-1311.

66. Schmitz, PG, Kasiske, BL, O'Donnell, MP, Keane, WF. Lipids and progressive renal injury. Seminars Nephrol 1989; 9, No 4: 354-369.

67. Kasiske, BL, O'Donnell, MP, Cowardin, W, Keane, WF. Lipids and the kidney. Hypertension 1990; 15: 443-450.

68. Walker, WG. Relation of lipid abnormalities to progression of renal damage in essential hypertension, insulin-dependent and non insulin-dependent diabetes mellitus. Miner Electrolyte Metab 1993; 19: 137-143.

69. Laakso, M, Lehto, S, Penttilä, I, Pyörälä, K. Lipids and lipoproteins predicting coronary heart disease mortality and morbidity in patients with non-insulin-dependent diabetes. Circulation 1993; 88: 1421-1430.

70. Pyörälä, K, Pedersen, TR, Kjekshus, J, Faergeman, O, Olsson, AG, Thorgeirsson, G. Cholesterol lowering with simvastatin improves prognosis of diabetic patients with coronary heart disease. A subgroup analysis of the Scandinavian Simvastatin Survival Study (4S). Diabetes Care 1998; 20: 614-620.

71. Mulec, H, Johnson, SA, Björck, S. Relation between serum cholesterol and diabetic nephropathy. Lancet 1990; 335: 1537-1538.

72. Hasslacher, C, Bostedt Kiesel, A, Kempe, HP, Wahl, P. Effect of metabolic factors and blood pressure on kidney function in proteinuric type 2 (non-insulin-dependent) diabetic patients. Diabetologia 1993; 36: 1051-1056.

73. Niskanen, L, Uusitupa, M, Sarlund, H, Siitonen, O, Voutilainen, E, Penttilä, I, Pyörälä, K. Microalbuminuria predicts the development of serum lipoprotein abnormalities favouring atherogenesis in newly diagnosed type 2 (non-insulin-dependent) diabetic patients. Diabetologia 1990; 33: 237-43.

74. Smulders, YM, Rakic, M, Stehouwer, CD, Weijers, BNM, Slaats, EH, Silberbusch, J. Determinants of progression of microalbuminuria in patients with NIDDM. Diabetes Care 1997; 20: 999-1005.

75. Ravid, M, Brosh, D, Ravid-Safran, D, Levy, Z, Rachmani, R. Main risk factors for nephropathy in type 2 diabetes mellitus are plasma cholesterol levels, mean blood pressure, and hyperglycemia. Arch Intern Med 1998; 158: 998-1004.

76. Gall, M-A, Hougaard, P, Borch-Johnsen, K, Parving, H-H. Risk factors for development of incipient and overt diabetic nephropathy in patients with non-insulin dependent diabetes mellitus: Prospective, observational study. BMJ 1997; 314: 783-788.

77. Forsblom, C, Groop, PH, Ekstrand, A, Totterman, KJ, Sane, T, Saloranta, C, Groop, L. Predictors of progression from normoalbuminuria to microalbuminuria in NIDDM. Diabetes Care 1998; 21: 1932-1938.

78. Lam, KSL, Cheng, IKP, Janus, ED, Pang, RWC. Cholesterol-lowering therapy may retard the progression of diabetic nephropathy. Diabetologia 1995; 38: 604-609.

79. Sasaki, T, Kurata, H, Nomura, K, Utsunomiya, K, Ikeda, Y. Amelioration of proteinuria with pravastatin in hypercholesterolemic patients with diabetes mellitus. Jpn J Med 1990; 29(2): 156-163.

80. Grundy, SM. HMG-CoA reductase inhibitors for treatment of hypercholesterolaemia. N Engl J Med 1988; 319: 24-33.

81. Garg, A and Grundy, SM. Lovastatin for lowering cholesterol levels in non-insulin-dependent diabetes mellitus. N Engl J Med 1988; 318: 81-86.

82. Rabelink, AJ, Hené, RJ, Erkelens, DW, Joles, JA, Koomans, HA. Partial remission of nephrotic syndrome in patients on long term simvastatin. Lancet 1990; 335: 1045-1046.

83. Hommel, E, Andersen, P, Gall, M-A, Nielsen, F, Jensen, B, Rossing, P, Dyerberg, J, Parving, H-H. Plasma lipoproteins and renal function during simvastatin treatment in diabetic nephropathy. Diabetologia 1992; 35: 447-451.

84. Nielsen, S, Schmitz, O, Møller, N, Pørksen, N, Klausen, IC, Alberti, KGMM, Mogensen, CE. Renal function and insulin sensitivity during simvastatin treatment in Type 2 (non-insulin-dependent) diabetic patients with microalbuminuria. Diabetologia 1993; 36: 1079-1086.

85. Tonolo, G, Ciccarese, M, Brizzi, P, Puddu, L, Secchi, G, Calvia, P, Atzeni, MM, Melis, MG, Maioli, M. Reduction of albumin excretion rate in normotensive microalbuminuric Type 2 diabetic patients during long-term simvastatin treatment. Diabetes Care 1997; 20: 1891-1895.

86. Ritz, E and Stefanski, A. Diabetic nephropathy in type II diabetes. Am J Kidney Dis 1996; 27: 167-194.

8. SERUM CREATININE AND OTHER MEASURES OF GFR IN DIABETES

Peter Rossing MD
Steno Diabetes Center, 2820 Gentofte, Denmark

The measurement of renal function or the glomerular filtration rate (GFR) in diabetes can be used 1) to estimate the renal clearance of drugs to guide dosing or to identify patients at increased risk for radiocontrast-induced acute renal failure, 2) for confirming the need for treatment of end stage renal disease, or 3) to measure progression of chronic renal disease i.e. diabetic nephropathy. The evaluation of progression in renal disease is important in the clinical setting for the monitoring of development of renal insufficiency and evaluation of the effectiveness of treatment in the individual, as well as in research to evaluate the importance of putative progression promoters in observational studies or to assess and compare the rate of progression in experimental groups in clinical trials. In order to obtain a valid assessment of the rate of decline in GFR it is necessary with regular measurements of GFR over a period of at least (2)-3 years applying a method with high precision and accuracy [1]. This is due to the usually rather slow rate of decline in GFR in diabetic nephropathy. The ideal method for assessing GFR does not exist and the available methods differ regarding precision and accuracy, cost, inconvenience and safety. In general the more precise methods are being more expensive and inconvenient. Thus one has to select a method according to the clinical situation.

SERUM CREATININE AS A MEASURE OF GFR
The level of serum creatinine is the most widely used measure of renal function in clinical practice. Serum creatinine can be assessed at a low cost and with little inconvenience for the patient. The reciprocal relationship between serum creatinine and the creatinine clearance allows a simple estimation of renal function (Figure 8-1). When progression in renal disease is evaluated the slope of either 1/serum creatinine or log (serum creatinine) is used. This is particularly useful when serum creatinine exceeds 200 µmol/l [2].

There are however several problems related to the use of serum creatinine as a marker of renal function as reviewed by Levey [3]. Firstly there are technical difficulties with interfering substances (glucose, ketones) which can be solved by the use of a reaction kinetic principle, high performance liquid chromatography (HPLC) or gas chromatography with mass spectrometry (GC-MS) [4]. Secondly the level of serum creatinine is not only dependent on the GFR: the generation of creatinine is influenced by changes in muscle mass and dietary intake of protein. In particular the ingestion of cooked meat may lead to a fast increase in serum creatinine [5]. Furthermore creatinine does not behave like an ideal filtration marker, there is tubular secretion leading to an overestimation of GFR by a factor of at least 1.2, and the proportion of tubular secretion to glomerular filtration changes with variation in the level of GFR [6], and it is affected by several drugs (e.g. cimetidine, salicylates and trimethoprim). In addition there is extra-renal elimination particularly in patients with low GFR. These conditions make it difficult to use serum creatinine to correctly estimate the level of renal function.

Problems related to differences in creatinine production affecting serum creatinine as well as the influence of extra-renal creatinine elimination, can be avoided by measuring creatinine clearance which in addition to the blood sample requires a 24 hour urine collection. However this adds the problem with accuracy of timed urine collections. The problems with tubular secretion can be avoided if the tubular secretion is blocked, for instance with the use of cimetidine [4,7], but this further adds to the complexity of the measurement.

Because of the difficulties with urine collections, it has been attempted to solve the problems due to sex and age related changes in muscle mass with formulas like that of Cockroft and Gault [8] using serum creatinine to estimate creatinine clearance (Cl_{crea}) taking sex, age and body weight into account: Cl_{crea}=(140-Age)*K*body weight*(1/p-creatinine), (K=1.23 for men, 1.05 for women, p-creatinine in μmol/l, weight in kg and age in years). Cross-sectional data suggest that the formula gives an accurate estimate of glomerular filtration rate in diabetic nephropathy in some [9] but not all studies [10,11]. In a study evaluating the formula in type 2 diabetic patients with normal renal function the formula significantly underestimated GFR [12]. It has been suggested that very accurate results are obtained from the formula, if the methods for the measurement of creatinine are improved by the use of HPLC or enzymatic assays in combination with blockade of tubular creatinine secretion by administration of cimetidine over 24 hours [13]. Only few studies have evaluated if the formulas for estimation of GFR can be used to predict the decline in renal function. In a cohort of type 1 diabetic patients with nephropathy and long follow-up, the mean decline of the cohort could be predicted using the Cockroft – Gault formula, but it was not accurate in the individual patient [11] and similarly poor results were found in a study of normoalbuminuric type 2 diabetic patients, in particular when the decline in GFR was small [13].

Recently Levey et al. suggested a more accurate prediction equation to estimate GFR, rather than Cl_{Crea}, based on data from 1628 patients in the MDRD study, using age, sex, race, serum creatinine, urea nitrogen and albumin concentration [12].

In patients with declining renal function there is an increase in fractional tubular secretion and extrarenal elimination [6]. Usually there is a lowering in muscle mass and often a restriction in protein intake. All of which will tend to preserve the level of serum creatinine despite declining GFR. Accordingly Shemes et al. [6] found that patients with a GFR as low as ~30 ml/min/1.73m² may have normal serum creatinine, and in their follow up study [6] reductions in GFR of 50% were not associated with increases in serum creatinine of the expected magnitude, and even a lack of increase in some patients, thus when evaluating progression in renal disease, an increase in serum creatinine is not a very sensitive measurement of a decrease in renal function. This is in particular the case in patients with normal renal function due to the reciprocal relationship between serum creatinine and GFR, large variations in GFR are only associated with small changes in serum creatinine. On the other hand an elevation in serum creatinine is very specific for a decline in GFR. Thus an elevated serum creatinine or a doubling of the baseline serum creatinine have been used as endpoints in clinical trials [13], but this is only valid if changes in serum creatinine are not due to changes in therapy, muscle mass or diet. Illustrating this problem the Modification of Diet in Renal Disease study [14] concluded, that while a significant beneficial effect of low protein diet could not be demonstrated when using a true marker of GFR (^{125}I-iothalamate), such an effect would erroneously have been found if creatinine data had been used [15].

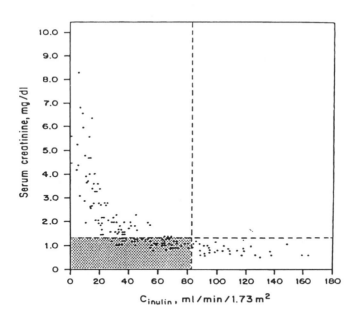

Fig. 8-1. Simultaneous measurement of serum creatinine and insulin clearance in 171 patients with glomerular disease. Vertical dashed line correspond to the lower limit of insulin clearance (82 ml/min/1.73m²), the horizontal line corresponds to the upper limit for serum creatinine (1.4 mg/dl). The shaded area include values for patients in whom insulin clearance is reduced but serum creatinine is normal. (from Shemesh et al [4]).

Other endogenous markers of GFR have been evaluated including ß$_2$-microglobulin which seems to be a more reliable method for evaluation of GFR than serum creatinine in cross sectional as well as longitudinal studies [16,17], but determination of ß$_2$-microglobulin is expensive and not a routine method at most laboratories. In addition very high levels are found in serum in patients with certain malignant disorders or immunological diseases.

GLOMERULAR FILTRATION RATE

An ideal marker for determination of glomerular filtration rate should fulfil the following requirements: it should be freely filtered at the glomerulus, no tubular secretion or reabsorption, it should not be metabolized, and it should be physiologically inert without affecting renal function, distribute instantaneously and freely in the extracellular volume, and should be easily measured [18]. Such a marker does not exist. However the renal clearance of inulin during constant infusion has been considered the gold standard for determination of GFR. The clearance is corrected for body surface area and normalised to 1.73 m^2 to take into account the relationship between kidney and body size and permit comparisons between patients. The renal clearance (Cl) during constant infusion is calculated from the plasma inulin level (P), urinary inulin concentration (U) and urine flow rate (V) as Cl=UV/P. The clearance is measured in three to five 30-minute periods during an oral water load. If during a constant infusion both distribution volume and plasma inulin concentration are constant the rate of infusion equals the rate of excretion. Then inulin clearance can be calculated from inulin infusion rate and plasma inulin concentration. However it is difficult to obtain constant inulin concentrations thus this technique is rarely used. The cumbersome procedures, difficulties with measuring inulin and its limited availability and cost has encouraged the search for alternative filtration markers.

The radioisotope-labelled markers ^{125}I-Iothalamate, ^{99m}Tc-DTPA and ^{51}Cr-EDTA have been found to give accurate and precise estimates of GFR [19] when used with constant infusion renal clearance techniques. To avoid problems with incomplete urine collections, a frequent phenomenon in diabetic patients due to cystopathy [20], plasma clearance techniques can be applied. The radioactive markers have particularly been used with such techniques. With these methods the GFR is determined without urine sampling as total plasma clearance from the declining plasma concentration followed as a function of time after injection of a bolus of the marker [21]. The clearance is calculated as the ratio of the injected amount of marker (Q) and the area under the plasma curve (A) (Cl=Q/A). Determination of the entire area under the plasma curve requires the drawing of many blood samples (10 to 20) during a time period of several hours depending on the level of renal function (three to five hours in normal to moderately decreased renal function, but up to 24 hours is recommended if GFR is below 15 ml/min). The final elimination follows a monoexponential curve which is extrapolated to infinity. Simplified methods have been developed using the final slope only, determined by two to seven blood samples, the calculated area can be mathematically corrected to the total area under the curve preserving very high precision and accuracy which is necessary in longitudinal studies [22-25]. The simplified single injection technique has frequently been used in clinical studies or as a routine method for determination of GFR [21,26].

^{51}Cr-EDTA (ethylenediaminetetraacetic acid) has been extensively used for plasma clearance studies and has been found to have a renal clearance ~10% lower than clearance of inulin [27], the difference has not been explained but could be due to plasma protein binding, tubular reabsorption or dissociation of the radionuclide from EDTA. The plasma clearance is slightly higher than the renal clearance due to extrarenal elimination (~4 ml/min) [23]. The half life of the isotope is 27 days. ^{125}I-Iothalamate can be administered as subcutaneous or intravenous injection. Due to a half life of radioactive ^{125}I of 60 days, samples can be stored before radioisotope counting, which makes it useful for multicenter studies with a central laboratory as demonstrated in the MDRD study [14]. ^{99m}Tc-DTPA (diethylenetriaminepenta-acetic acid) is also used for renal scans, and it is inexpensive compared to the rather expensive ^{125}I-Iothalamate. Protein binding is potentially of concern and radiochemical instability varies among DTPA kits making quality control critical [28]. The radiolabelling of DTPA has to be carried out immediately before use due to instability. The half life of ^{99m}Tc is only 6 hours thus samples must be counted soon after the procedure.

Plasma clearance can be measured without drawing plasma samples at all, with the use of a gamma camera measuring renal elimination of a radioactive marker such as ^{99m}Tc-DTPA [29]. This technique is not as accurate as when plasma samples are collected, but it is possible to determine the contribution from each kidney, which is particularly useful when reno-vascular disease or unilateral nephrectomy is considered.

The use of radioactive markers exposes the patients to radiation, but the radiation dose is very small and for one measurement of GFR with ^{51}Cr-EDTA it is comparable to the daily background radiation dose (Effective dose equivalent <0.01 mSv.). But even if the radiation doses are small, the use of radioactive isotopes is usually avoided in children and pregnant women. As a non-radioactive alternative the radiocontrast agents such as iohexol have been suggested [30,31], it has also been possible to measure small concentrations of inulin with HPLC methods making plasma clearance of inulin after a single injection a possibility [32].

SUMMARY

The selection of method for assessment of GFR depends on the situation. In many clinical situations the use of serum creatinine or estimated creatinine clearance based on formulas or nomograms is sufficient if the limitations are recalled. In clinical studies a more accurate and precise method is warranted. In case of severe oedema, ascites or if the renal haemodynamics are changing within hours, renal clearance methods has to be used. Apart from these special situations the simplified single injection plasma clearance methods yield sufficiently accurate and precise assessments of GFR with a minimum of inconvenience, particularly useful in long term follow-up studies.

REFERENCES:

1.   Levey AS, Gassman J, Hall PM, Walker WG. Assessing the progression of renal disease in clinical studies: effects of duration of follow-up and regression to the mean. J Am Soc Nephrol. 1991;1:1087-94.

2.   Mitch WE, Walser M, Buffington GA, Lemann J. A simple method of estimating progression of chronic renal failure. Lancet. 1976;ii:1326-8.

3.   Levey AS, Perrone RD, Madias NE. Serum creatinine and renal function. Ann Rev Med. 1988;39:465-90.

4.   Kemperman FAW, Silberbusch J, Slaats EH, et al. Glomerular filtration rate estimation from plasma creatinine after inhibition of tubular secretion: relevance of the creatinine assay. Nephrol Dial Transplant. 1999;14:1247-51.

5.   Jacobsen FK, Christensen CK, Mogensen CE, Andreasen F, Hejlskov NSC. Pronounced increase in serum dreatinine concentration after eating cooked meat. Br Med J. 1979;1049-50.

6.   Shemesh O, Golbetz HV, Kriss JP, Myers BD. Limitations of creatinine as a filtration marker in glomerulopathic patients. Kidney Int. 1985;28:830-8.

7.   van Acker BAC, Koome GCM, Koopman MG, de Waart DR, Arisz L. Creatinine clearance during cimetidine administration for measurement of glomerular filtration rate. Lancet. 1992;340:1326-9.

8.   Cockcroft DW, Gault MH. Prediction of creatinine clearance from serum creatinine. Nephron. 1976;16:31-41.

9.   Sampson MJ, Drury PL. Accurate estimation of glomerular filtration rate in diabetic nephropathy from age, body weight, and serum creatinine. Diabetes Care. 1992;15:609-12.

10. Waz WR, Qattrin T, Feld LG. Serum creatinine, height, and weight do not predict glomerular filtration rate in children with IDDM. Diabetes Care. 1993;16:1067-70.

11. Rossing P, Astrup A-S, Smidt UM, Parving H-H. Monitoring kidney function in diabetic nephropathy. Diabetologia. 1994;37:708-12.

12. Nielsen S, Rehling M, Schmitz A, Mogensen CE. Validity of rapid estimation of glomerular filtration rate in type 2 diabetic patients with normal renal function. Nephrol Dial Transplant, 1999; 14:615-9.

13. Kemperman FAW, Krediet RT, Arisz L. Validity of rapid estimation of glomerular filtration rate in type 2 diabetic patients with normal renal function (letter). Nephrol Dial Transplant, 1999; 14: 2964.

14. Levey AS, Bosch JP, Breyer JA et al. A more accurate method to estimate glomerular filtration rate from serum creatinine: a new prediction equation. Ann Intern Med, 1999; 130:461-

15. Walser M, Drew HH, Guldan JL. Prediction of glomerular filtration rate from serum creatinine concentration in advanced chronic renal failure. Kidney Int, 1993; 44:1145-8.

16. Lewis E, Hunsicker L, Bain R, Rhode R. The effect of angiotensin-converting-enzyme inhibition on diabetic nephropathy. N Engl J Med, 1993; 329: 1456-62.

17. Klahr S, Levey AS, Beck GJ, et al. The effects of dietary protein restriction and blood-pressure control on the progression of chronic renal disease. N Engl J Med. 1994;330:877-84.

18. Levey AS, Bosch JP, Coggins CH et al. Effects of diet and antihypertensive therapy on creatinine clearance and serum creatinine concentration in the modification of diet in renal disease study. J Am Soc Nephrol, 1996; 7:556-65.

19. Parving H-H, Andersen AR, Smidt UM. Monitoring progression of diabetic nephropathy. Upsala J Med Sci. 1985;90:15-23.

20. Viberti GC, Bilous RW, Mackintosh D, Keen H. Monitoring glomerular function in diabetic nephropathy. Am J Med. 1983;74:256-64.

21. Kasiske BL, Keane WF. Laboratory assessment of renal disease: clearance, urinalysis and renal biopsy. In: Brenner BM, ed.The Kidney. 5th ed. Philadelphia: Saunders, 1997:1137-74.

22. Levey AS. Assessing the effectiveness of therapy to prevent the progression of renal disease. Am J Kidney Dis. 1993;22:207-14.

23. Frimondt-Møller C. Diabetic cystopathy. Dan Med Bull. 1978;25:49-60.

24. Bröchner-Mortensen J. Current status on assessment and measurement of glomerular filtration rate. Clin Physiol. 1985;5:1-17.

25. Bröchner-Mortensen J. Routine methods and their reliability for assessment of glomerular filtration rate in adults with special reference to total $[^{51}Cr]$EDTA plasma clearance. Dan Med Bull. 1978;25:181-202.

26. Bröchner-Mortensen J, Rödbro P. Selection of routine method for determination of glomerular filtration rate in adult patients. Scand J Clin Lab Invest. 1976;36:35-45.

27. Bröchner-Mortensen J. A simple method for the determination of glomerular filtration rate. Scand J Clin Lab Invest. 1972;30:271-4.

28. Sambataro M, Tomaseth K, Pacini G, et al. Plasma clearance rate of 51 Cr-EDTA provides a precise and convenient technique for measurement of glomerular filtration rate in diabetic humans. J Am Soc Nephrol. 1996;7:118-27.

29. Parving H-H, Smidt UM, Hommel E, et al. Effective Antihypertensive Treatment Postpones Renal Insufficiency in Diabetic Nephropathy. Am J Kidney Dis. 1993;22:188-95.

30. Chantler C, Garnett ES, Parsons V, Veall N. Glomerular filtration rate measurement in man by the single injection method using ^{51}Cr-EDTA. Clin Sci. 1969;37:169-80.

31. Carlsen JE, Lehd Møller M, Lund JO, Trap-Jensen J. Comparison of four commercial Tc-99 DTPA preparations used for the measurement of glomerular filtration rate: concise communication. Journal of Nuclear Medicine. 1980;126-9.

32. Rodby RA, Ali A, Rohde RD, Lewis E. Renal scanning ^{99m}Tc diethylene-triamine pentaacetic acid glomerular filtration rate (GFR) determination compared with iothalamate clearance GFR in diabetics. Am J Kidney Dis. 1992;20:569-73.

33. Stake G, Moon E, Rootwell IT, Monclair T. The clearance of iohexol as a measure of glomerular filtration rate in children with chronic renal failure. Scand J Clin Lab Invest. 1991;51:729-34.

34. Chowdhury TA, Dyer PH, Bartlett WA, et al. Glomerular filtration rate determination in diabetic patients using iohexol clearance -comparison of single and multiple plasma sampling methods. Clinica Chimica Acta. 1998;277:153-8.

32. Jung K, Henke W, Schulze BD, Sydow K, Precht K, Klotzek S. Practical approach for determining glomerular filtration rate by single injection inulin clearance. Clin. Chem. 1992;38:403-7.

9. FAMILIAL FACTORS IN DIABETIC NEPHROPATHY

Giuseppina Imperatore[1], David J. Pettitt[2], Robert L. Hanson[1], William C. Knowler[1] and Robert G. Nelson[1]
[1]*Phoenix Epidemiology and Clinical Research Branch, NIDDK, Phoenix, Arizona, USA*
[2]*Sansum Medical Research Institute, Santa Barbara, California, USA*

Reports of nephropathy developing in some patients with apparently well controlled diabetes and not developing in some patients even after years of severe hyperglycemia lead to the conclusion, expressed by several researchers [1-5], that some, but not all, individuals are predisposed to the development of diabetic renal disease. This chapter reviews some of the data that indicate that there are familial differences in the predisposition to diabetic renal disease. If this familial predisposition is genetic, there must be an interaction between the genes and the environment, and it is often difficult to differentiate between genetic inheritance and the effect of a common environment shared by family members.

RACIAL DIFFERENCES IN PREVALENCE

Some familial clustering of diabetic nephropathy may be accounted for by racial background, as diabetic nephropathy occurs at different rates in different racial groups. Several inter-racial comparisons have been made [6-10]. Rostand et al. [6] and Cowie et al. [9] both reported higher rates of end-stage renal disease in American Blacks than Whites, and Pugh et al. [7] reported higher rates in Mexican Americans than in Non-Hispanic Whites. Diabetes duration, which is a strong risk factor for end-stage renal disease, may account for some of the racial differences in these studies. However, with diabetes duration accounted for, Haffner et al. [8] found higher rates of proteinuria among Mexican Americans, and there are several reports of very high rates of renal disease among the Pima Indians [11-14], a population that has high rates of type 2 diabetes [15,16]. The incidence of end-stage renal disease in Pima Indians was similar to that in subjects with type 1 diabetes in Boston, Massachusetts [11], but almost four times as high as in Caucasians with type 2 diabetes in Rochester, Minnesota [14].

The reasons for inter-population differences in rates of renal disease are unclear. Rostand [10] has argued that barriers to medical care for Black and Mexican Americans

Mogensen C.E. (ed.), THE KIDNEY AND HYPERTENSION IN DIABETES MELLITUS.

may impede early detection, and therefore, control of microalbuminuria and hypertension with a consequent adverse effect on the prevalence of renal disease. However, the cost, one of the major barriers to medical care, is not a factor for the Pima Indians, who have access to free medical care by providers who are well aware of the high risk of diabetic renal disease in this population. Thus, cost of medical care cannot be the only reason for racial differences. However, other aspects of access to medical care, such as transportation or cultural barriers, could be important.

Genes predisposing to renal disease might well exist at different rates in different races resulting in differences in susceptibility. Thus, if renal disease is genetic its prevalence would be expected to differ by race. However, finding different rates in different races is consistent not only with genetic inheritance but also with differing environmental exposures or with differences in competing causes of death.

SIBLINGS OF AFFECTED INDIVIDUALS

Diabetic siblings of individuals with diabetic nephropathy are at higher risk for nephropathy than are diabetic siblings of diabetic individuals without nephropathy. This familial aggregation has been found in diverse populations with both type 1 and type 2 diabetes. Seaquist et al. [17] reported familial clustering of nephropathy among diabetic siblings of diabetic probands recruited from either the University of Minnesota kidney transplant registry or from a family diabetes study. Nephropathy was found among 83% of the diabetic siblings of diabetic probands with nephropathy but among only 17% of siblings of probands without nephropathy (figure 9-1).

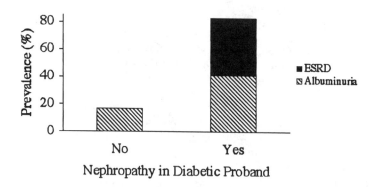

Figure 9-1. Prevalence of albuminuria and end-stage renal disease (ESRD) in diabetic siblings of diabetic probands with or without nephropathy. Adapted from Seaquist et al [17].

Furthermore, 41% of the siblings of probands with nephropathy had end-stage renal disease. Clustering of diabetic nephropathy among siblings was confirmed by Borch-Johnsen et al. [18], and higher albumin excretion was found in the nondiabetic siblings of probands with type 2 diabetes than of those without [19]. Quinn et al. [20] examined 110 probands for nephropathy status and found that the cumulative incidence of nephropathy for siblings of probands with diabetic nephropathy was 71.5% and only 25.4% for siblings of probands without nephropathy. The magnitude of the risk difference between the two groups of siblings suggests that genetic factors are very important. Similar results were observed in Brazilian subjects with type 2 diabetes [21]. Furthermore, Fioretto et al. [22] observed strong concordance in severity and patterns of glomerual lesions among sibling pairs with type 1 diabetes, despite lack of concordance in glycemia. These data, which are consistent with the hypothesis that genetic heredity is a major determinant of diabetic nephropathy, are also consistent with the hypothesis that an environmental factor or factors shared by siblings is responsible for the development of nephropathy in some families.

OFFSPRING OF AFFECTED INDIVIDUALS

Proteinuria and elevated serum creatinine concentrations were studied in Pima Indian families with diabetes in two generations [23]. Proteinuria occurred among 14% of the diabetic offspring of diabetic parents if neither parent had proteinuria, 23% if one parent had proteinuria, and 46% if both parents had diabetes with proteinuria (figure 9-2). The familial occurrence of an elevated creatinine was limited to male offspring, among whom 11.7% had a high creatinine if the parent had a high creatinine but only 1.5% did so if the diabetic parent had a normal creatinine. These data demonstrate that proteinuria and elevated creatinine aggregate in Pima families and suggest that the susceptibility to renal disease is inherited independently of the diabetes. As with the sibling concordance described above, the inheritance could be a shared environment, but since the environments of parents and of their children are very likely to differ more than those of siblings, a genetic inheritance is a strong possibility. A useful approach for discriminating between environmental and genetic factors is performing segregation analysis. This statistical method allows testing of the hypothesis that familial aggregation of diabetic nephropathy is due to the major effect of a single gene. In Pima Indians with type 2 diabetes, this analysis supported a major gene effect on the prevalence of nephropathy when duration of diabetes was accounted for. The model suggests that individuals homozygous or heterozygous for the putative high risk disease allele have a high risk for diabetic nephropathy, particularly after many years of diabetes while those homozygous for the low risk allele have very little nephropathy, regardless of duration of diabetes [24]. Similarly, segregation analysis of albumin excretion rate conducted in Caucasians with type 2 diabetes was consistent with the effect of a single gene [25]. Other data from the Pima Indians indicate that diabetic nephropathy in parents is a risk factor for diabetes in the offspring [26]. The prevalence of diabetes at 25 to 34 years of age was 46% among the offspring of two diabetic parents if one had proteinuria and only 18% if neither had proteinuria. Corresponding rates among subjects with one diabetic and one nondiabetic parent were 29% if the diabetic parent had proteinuria and 11% if not. Thus, multiple loci or homozygosity at a single locus may determine susceptibility to both diabetes and renal disease. In other words, parents with diabetes and renal disease may have a higher genetic load which increases the risk of diabetes in the offspring as well as increasing the risk of nephropathy once the diabetes develops.

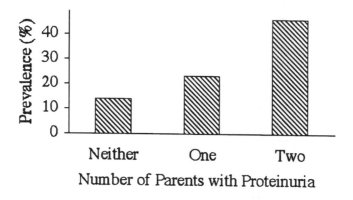

Figure 9-2. Prevalence of proteinuria by number of parents with proteinuria adjusted for age, sex blood pressure, diabetes duration and glucose concentration. Adapted from Pettitt et al. [23].

FAMILIAL HYPERTENSION AND RENAL DISEASE

The frequent association of renal disease with hypertension has led to the examination of blood pressure in nondiabetic family members of persons with diabetes and in individuals thought to be at high risk of developing diabetes in the future. Viberti et al. found that both systolic and diastolic blood pressures were significantly higher in the parents of diabetic subjects with proteinuria than in the parents of diabetic subjects without proteinuria [27]. The difference between the mean blood pressures averaged 15 mm Hg. Similarly, Krolewski et al. [28] reported that the risk of nephropathy among subjects with type 1 diabetes was three times as high in those having a parent with a history of hypertension as in those whose parents had no such history, and Takeda et al. [29] found evidence suggesting that paternal hypertension might be related to the development of nephropathy in patients with type 2 diabetes. Beatty et al. [30] found more insulin resistance as well as higher blood pressures in the offspring of hypertensive than of normotensive parents. These offspring, therefore, are presumably at increased risk of developing diabetes. Since they already have significantly higher blood pressures, they may be at particular risk of renal disease if they do develop diabetes.

Among diabetic Pima Indians whose parents did not have proteinuria, those with hypertensive parents had a higher prevalence of proteinuria than those with normotensive parents [31]. This finding was observed even among those with nondiabetic parents (figure 9-3).

Sodium-lithium countertransport activity in red cells, a genetically transmitted trait, is reported in some studies to be abnormal in subjects at risk of essential hypertension [32-35]. Rates of countertransport activity are higher in diabetic subjects with renal disease than in those with diabetes alone [28, 36]. Higher sodium-lithium activity has also been reported in parents of patients with type 1 diabetes and persistent proteinuria than in parents of patients with normoalbuminuria [37]. Kelleher et al. [38] reported more hypertension among the siblings of hypertensive than of normotensive subjects with type 1 diabetes. However, hypertension among siblings of subjects with type diabetes was more prevalent than among siblings of subjects with type 1 diabetes and was not related to hypertension in the diabetic proband. Given the association between hypertension and nephropathy, it is reasonable to assume that these hypertensive diabetic patients may be at risk for developing nephropathy, or may already have some nephropathy, and the hypertensive siblings might be at risk themselves if they were to develop diabetes.

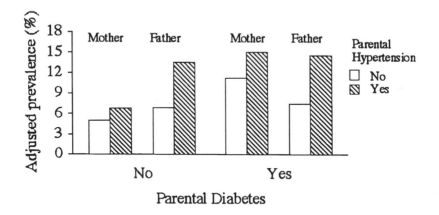

Figure 9-3. Prevalence of proteinuria according to parental hypertension and diabetes, adjusted for age, sex, diabetes duration and post-load plasma glucose Adapted from Nelson et al. [31].

Among Pima Indians, higher mean blood pressure measured at least one year prior to the onset of diabetes predicted an abnormal urinary excretion of albumin determined after the diagnosis of diabetes [39]. Thus, the hypertension so often associated with diabetic nephropathy cross-sectionally does not appear to be entirely a result of the renal disease. This hypertension, which appears to be familial in several studies, may precede and contribute to the renal disease seen after several years of diabetes in some subjects.

GENETIC MARKERS

This subject is reviewed more extensively elsewhere in this publication. The possibility of genetic causes for diabetic microvascular complications has stimulated the search for a disease gene or for linkage between the disease and a genetic marker. The data for type 1 diabetes have been reviewed extensively [40]. Several reports of associations between markers and retinopathy are encouraging [41,42], but the findings of associations with renal disease are mixed [41,43,44]. Among patients with type 1 diabetes, Barbosa [41] found similar frequencies of HLA-A and HLA-B antigens, but Christy et al. [43] found a different distribution of HLA/DR markers in those with and in those without nephropathy. Walton et al. [44], in a very small sample, also found no evidence of an HLA association with nephropathy. Similarly, in a large cohort of patients with type 1 diabetes Chowdhury et al. [45] found no association between HLA loci and diabetic nephropathy. Mijovic's [46] findings suggest that microangiopathy (not limited to renal disease) was influenced by genes in linkage disequilibrium with both the major histocompatibility complex and the Gm loci. A number of association studies for diabetic nephropathy have been conducted with candidate genes selected by their possible role in the pathogenesis of this condition. The most widely studied variant has been the insertion/deletion polymorphism in the angiotensin-I converting enzyme gene on chromosome 17. While several studies have shown that individuals homozygous for the deletion genotype are at increased risk for diabetic nephropathy [47,48], others studies have shown no effect [49-52]. Doria et al. [53] reported that, among subjects with type 1 diabetes, an uncommon DNA sequence for the angiotensin I converting enzyme was more common in those with nephropathy than in those without. A meta-analysis of 18 studies showed a modest association of the deletion allele with diabetic nephropathy (odds ratio 1.32), but there appeared to be publication bias [54]. Moczulski et al [55] conducted a linkage study on a candidate region containing the angiotensin-II type 1 receptor on chromosome 3 in a small number of sibling pairs with type 1 diabetes and found evidence for linkage in this region. However, they did not identify any disease-associated polymorphisms in the angiotensin-II type 1 receptor gene. Among Pima Indians with type 2 diabetes, Imperatore et al. [56] found suggestive linkage for nephropathy on chromosome 7. These findings were confirmed in Caucasians with type 2 diabetes [57]. This chromosomal region contains three potential candidate genes: the aldose reductase (*ALDR1*), endothelial nitric oxide synthase-3 (*NOS3*) and the T-cell receptor b-chain (*TCRBC*). Studies of a dinucleotide-repeat polymorphism in the *ALDR*1 gene are equivocal [58, 59]. In patients with type 1 diabetes, the a-deletion allele of the *NOS3* gene was associated with an increased risk of advanced nephropathy [60].

MODIFICATION OF DISEASE

Environmental factors, most of which probably remain unknown, that influence the development or progression of renal disease in subjects with diabetes are likely to be shared with other family members resulting in concordance of renal disease. Therapeutic manipulations of several factors alter the course of diabetic renal disease in individuals, but it will take family studies to see if the response to therapies is also genetic or influenced by other environmental factors.

Various treatments, which will be discussed in detail in subsequent chapters, may alter the familial aggregation of renal disease. Reichard et al. [61] showed that intensive insulin therapy in type 1 diabetes can reduce the development of microvascular complications including diabetic kidney disease. Similar results were reported by the Diabetes Control and Complications Trial [62]. The results of the United Kingdom Prospective Diabetes Study, also, showed that intensive blood glucose control decreases the risk of microvascular complications, in patients with type 2 diabetes [63].

Dietary protein may induce glomerular hyperfiltration [64], and beneficial effects of dietary protein restriction have been described [65-68]. As the renal effects differ with different types of protein [69], familial aggregation of renal disease may be due to a common diet rather than to genetics. Likewise, the beneficial effects of protein restriction may differ in different families depending, not only on genetic differences, but also on the type and the amount of protein consumed before the intervention.

Treatment of hypertension in subjects with diabetic nephropathy retards the progression of the renal disease [70], especially with the use of drugs that inhibit angiotensin converting enzyme [71]. Recently, in several randomized trials, angiotensin converting enzyme inhibitors were shown to slow the progression of renal disease and reduce mortality in subjects with proteinuria, regardless of hypertension [72-76]. It is of interest to note that there is evidence suggesting that ACE insertion/deletion polymorphism may be involved in the responsiveness to the ACE inhibitors [77,78].

In summary, much of the intriguing information regarding the familial occurrence of diabetic renal disease suggests a genetic component for this disorder but is also consistent with environmental effects. The epidemiology of renal disease is complicated by the fact that several forms of therapy currently employed to treat hyperglycemia, proteinuria and hypertension can alter the progression of renal disease and may, in some cases, even prevent its development. Selective prevention of renal disease will likely alter the familial aggregation of the disease. If there are important genes providing susceptibility to renal disease or influencing the response to treatment, even if the contribution is small, their identification could increase the clinician's knowledge about the risk for a given patient and help identify those for whom intensive therapy may be most beneficial.

REFERENCES

1.   Deckert T, Poulsen JE: Diabetic nephropathy: fault or destiny? Diabetologia 21:178-183, 1981.
2.   Moloney A, Tunbridge WMG, Ireland JT, Watkins PJ: Mortality from diabetic nephropathy in the United Kingdom. Diabetologia 25:26-30, 1983.
3.   Krolewski AS, Warram JH, Christlieb AR, Busick EJ, Kahn CR: The changing natural history of nephropathy in type I diabetes. Am J Med 78:785-794, 1985.
4.   Seaquist ER, Goetz FC, Povey S: Diabetic nephropathy: an hypothesis regarding genetic susceptibility for the disorder. Minnesota Med 69:457-459, 1986.
5.   What causes diabetic renal failure? [Editorial] Lancet 1:1433-1434, 1988.
6.   Rostand SG, Kirk KA, Rutsky EA, Pate BA: Racial differences in the incidence of treatment for end-stage renal disease. N Engl J Med 306:1276-1279, 1982.
7.   Pugh JA, Stern MP, Haffner SM, Eifler CW, Zapata M: Excess incidence of treatment of end-stage renal disease in Mexican Americans. Am J Epidemiol 127:135-144, 1988.
8.   Haffner SM, Mitchell BD, Pugh JA, Stern MP, Kozlowski MK, Hazuda HP, Patterson JK, Klein R: Proteinuria in Mexican Americans and non-Hispanic Whites with NIDDM. Diabetes Care 12:530-536, 1989.
9.   Cowie CC, Port FK, Wolfe RA, Savage PJ, Moll PP, Hawthorne VM: Disparities in incidence of diabetic end-stage renal disease according to race and type of diabetes. N Engl J Med 321:1074-1079, 1989.
10.   Rostand SG: Diabetic renal disease in blacks? inevitable or preventable? [Editorial] N Engl J Med 321:1121-1122, 1989.
11.   Nelson RG, Newman JM, Knowler WC, Sievers ML, Kunzelman CL, Pettitt DJ, Moffett CD, Teutch SM, Bennett PH: Incidence of end-stage renal disease in type 2 (non-insulin-dependent) diabetes mellitus in Pima Indians. Diabetologia 31:730-736, 1988.
12.   Kunzelman CL, Knowler WC, Pettitt DJ, Bennett PH: Incidence of proteinuria in type 2 diabetes mellitus in the Pima Indians. Kidney Int 35:681-687, 1989.
13.   Nelson RG, Knowler WC, Pettitt DJ, Saad MF, Bennett PH: Diabetic kidney disease in Pima Indians. Diabetes Care [Suppl 1] 16:335-341, 1993.
14.   Nelson RG, Knowler WC, McCance DR, Sievers ML, Pettitt DJ, Charles MA, Hanson RL, Liu QZ, Bennett PH: Determinants of end-stage renal disease in Pima Indians with Type 2 (non-insulin-dependent) diabetes mellitus and proteinuria. Diabetologia 36:1087-1093, 1993.
15.   Bennett PH, Burch TA, Miller M. Diabetes mellitus in American (Pima) Indians. Lancet 2:125-128, 1971.
16.   Knowler WC, Pettitt DJ, Saad MF, Bennett PH: Diabetes mellitus in the Pima Indians: incidence, risk factors and pathogenesis. Diabetes Metab Rev 6:1-27, 1990.
17.   Seaquist ER, Goetz FC, Rich S, Barbosa J: Familial clustering of diabetic kidney disease: evidence for genetic susceptibility to diabetic nephropathy. N Engl J Med 320:1161-1165, 1989.
18.   Borch-Johnsen K, Nørgaard, Hommel E, Mathiesen ER, Jensen JS, Deckert T, Parving H-H: Is diabetic nephropathy an inherited complication? Kidney Int 41:719-722, 1992.
19.   Faronato PP, Maioli M, Tonolo G, Brocco E, Noventa E, Piarulli F, Abaterusso C, Modena F, de Bigontina G, Velussi M, Inchiostro S, Santeusanio F, Bueti kA, Nosadini R. Clustering of albumin excretion rate abnormalities in Caucasian patients with NIDDM. Diabetologia 40:816-823, 1997.
20.   Quinn M, Angelico MC, Warram JH, Krolewski AS: Familial factors determine the development of diabetic nephropathy in patients with IDDM. Diabetologia 39:940-945, 1996.

21. Canani LH, Gerchman F, Gross JL: Familial clustering of diabetic nephropathy in Brazilian type 2 diabetic patients. Diabetes 48:909-913, 1999.

22. Fioretto P, Steffes MW, Barbosa J, Rich SS, Miller ME, Mauer M: Is diabetic nephropathy inherited? Studies of glomerular structure in type 1 diabetic sibling pairs. Diabetes 48:865-869, 1999.

23. Pettitt DJ, Saad MF, Bennett PH, Nelson RG, Knowler WC: Familial predisposition to renal disease in two generations of Pima Indians with type 2 (non-insulin-dependent) diabetes mellitus. Diabetologia 33:438-443, 1990.

24. Imperatore G, Hanson RL, Pettitt DJ, Kobes S, Bennett PH, Knowler WC: Segregation and linkage analyses of diabetic nephropathy in Pima Indians. (Abstract) AJHG 61 (Suppl):A280, 1997.

25. Fogarty DG, Rich SS, Wantman M, Warram JH, Krolewski AS: Albumin excretion in families with NIDDM is strongly influenced by a major gene: results of a segregation analysis. (Abstract) Diabetes 47 (Suppl 1):A12, 1998

26. McCance DR, Hanson RL, Pettitt DJ, Jacobsson LTH, Bennett PH, Bishop DT, Knowler WC. Diabetic nephropathy: a risk factor for diabetes mellitus in offspring. Diabetologia 38:221-226, 1995.

27. Viberti GC, Keen H, Wiseman MJ: Raised arterial pressure in parents of proteinuric insulin dependent diabetics. Br Med J 295:515-517, 1987.

28. Krolewski AS, Canessa M, Warram JH, Laffel LMB, Christlieb AR, Knowler WC, Rand LI: Predisposition to hypertension and susceptibility to renal disease in insulin-dependent diabetes mellitus. N Engl J Med 318:140-145, 1988.

29. Takeda H, Ohta K, Hagiwara M, Hori K, Watanabe K, Suzuki D, Tanaka K, Machimura H, Ya-Game M, Kaneshige H, Sakai H. Genetic predisposing factors in non-insulin-dependent diabetes with persistent albuminuria. Tokai J Exp Clin Med 17:199-203, 1992.

30. Beatty OL, Harper R, Sheridan B, Atkinson AB, Bell PM: Insulin resistance in offspring of hypertensive parents. Br Med J 307:92-96, 1993.

31. Nelson RG, Pettitt DJ, de Courten MP, Hanson RL, Knowler WC, Bennett PH: Parental hypertension and proteinuria in Pima Indians with NIDDM. Diabetologia 39:433-438, 1996.

32. Canessa M, Adragna N, Solomon HS, Connolly TM, Tosteson DC: Increased sodium-lithium countertransport in red cells of patients with essential hypertension. N Engl J Med 302:772-776, 1980.

33. Woods JW, Falk RJ, Pittman AW, Klemmer PJ, Watson BS, Namboodiri K: Increased red-cell sodium-lithium countertransport in normotensive sons of hypertensive parents. N Engl J Med 306:593-595, 1982.

34. Clegg G, Morgan DB, Davidson C: The heterogeneity of essential hypertension: relation between lithium efflux and sodium content of erythrocytes and a family history of hypertension. Lancet 2:891-894, 1982.

35. Cooper R, LeGrady D, Nanas S, Trevisan M, Mansour M, Histand P, Ostrow D, Stamler J: Increased sodium-lithium countertransport in college students with elevated blood pressure. JAMA 249:1030-1034, 1983.

36. Mangili R, Bending JJ, Scott G, Li LK, Gupta A, Viberti GC: Increased sodium-lithium countertransport activity in red cells of patients with insulin-dependent diabetes and nephropathy. N Engl J Med 318:146-150, 1988.

37. Walker JD, Tariq T, Viberti G Sodium-lithium countertransport activity in red cells of patients with insulin dependent diabetes and nephropathy and their parents. Br Med J 301:635-638, 1990.

38.   Kelleher C, Kingston SM, Barry DG, Cole MM, Ferriss JB, Grealy G, Joyce C, O'Sullivan DJ: Hypertension in diabetic clinic patients and their siblings. Diabetologia 31:76-81, 1988.

39.   Nelson RG, Pettitt DJ, Baird HR, Charles MA, Liu QZ, Bennett PH, Knowler WC: Pre-diabetic blood pressure predicts urinary albumin excretion after the onset of type 2 (non-insulin-dependent) diabetes mellitus in Pima Indians. Diabetologia 36:998-1001, 1993.

40.   Doria A, Warram JH, Krolewski AS. Genetic susceptibility to nephropathy in insulin-dependent diabetes: from epidemiology to molecular genetics. Diabetes/Metab Rev 11:287-314, 1995.

41.   Barbosa J: Is diabetic microangiopathy genetically heterogeneous? HLA and diabetic nephropathy. Horm Metab Res Suppl 11:77-80, 1981.

42.   Scaldaferri E, Devidè A: Microangiopatia diabetica: esiste una suscettibilità genetica HLA-correlata? Minerva Endocrinol 10:115-124, 1985.

43.   Christy M, Anderson AR, Nerup J, Platz P, Ryder L, Thomsen M, Morling M, Svejgaard A: HLA/DR in longstanding IDDM with and without nephropathy? evidence for heterogeneity? [abstr] Diabetologia 21:259, 1981.

44.   Walton C, Dyer PA, Davidson JA, Harris R, Mallick NP, Oleesky S: HLA antigens and risk factors for nephropathy in type 1 (insulin-dependent) diabetes mellitus. Diabetologia 27:3-7, 1984.

45.   Chowdhury TA, Dyer PH, Barnett AH, Bain SC: HLA and insulin (INS) genes in Caucasians with type 1 diabetes and nephropathy. (Abstract) Diabetologia 41 (Suppl 1)A296, 1998.

46.   Mijovic C, Fletcher JA, Bradwell AR, Barnett AH: Phenotypes of the heavy chains of immunoglobulins in patients with diabetic microangiopathy: evidence for an immunogenetic predisposition. Br Med J 292:433-435, 1986.

47.   Marre M, Bernadet P, Gallois Y, Savagner F, Guyene TT, Hallab M, Cambien F, Passa P, Alhenc-Gelas F Relationships between angiotensin I converting enzyme gene polymorphism, plasma levels, and diabetic retinal and renal complications. Diabetes 43:384-388, 1994.

48.   Jeffers BW, Estacio RO, Raynolds MV, Schrier RW: Angiotensin-converting enzyme gene polymorphism in non-insulin dependent diabetes mellitus and its relationship with diabetic nephropathy. Kidney Int 52:473-477, 1997.

49.   Schmidt S, Schone N, Ritz E: Association of ACE gene polymorphism and diabetic nephropathy? The Diabetic Nephropathy Study Group. Kidney Int 47:1176-1181, 1995.

50.   Tarnow L, Cambien F, Rossing P, Nielsen FS, Hansen BV, Lecerf L, Poirier O, Danilov S, Parving HH: Lack of relationship between an insertion/deletion polymorphism in the angiotensin I-converting enzyme gene and diabetic nephropathy and proliferative retinopathy in IDDM patients. Diabetes 44:489-494, 1995.

51.   Chowdhury TA, Dronsfield MJ, Kumar S, Gough SL, Gibson SP, Khatoon A, MacDonald F, Rowe BR, Dunger DB, Dean JD, Davies SJ, Webber J, Smith PR, Mackin P, Marshall SM, Adu D, Morris PJ, Todd JA, Barnett AH, Boulton AJ, Bain SC: Examination of two genetic polymorphisms within the renin-angiotensin system: no evidence for an association with nephropathy in IDDM. Diabetologia 39:1108-1114, 1996.

52.   Grzeszczak W, Zychma MJ, Lacka B, Zukowska-Szczechowska E: Angiotensin I-converting enzyme gene polymorphisms: relationship to nephropathy in patients with non-insulin dependent diabetes mellitus. J Am Soc Nephrol 9:1664-1669, 1998.

53.   Doria A, Warram JH, Krolewski AS: Genetic predisposition to diabetic nephropathy: evidence for a role of the angiotensin I-converting enzyme gene. Diabetes 43:690-695, 1994.

54. Fujisawa T, Ikegami H, Kawaguchi Y, Hamada Y, Ueda H, Shintani M, Fukuda M, Ogihara T: Meta-analysis of association of insertion/deletion polymorphism of angiotensin I-converting enzyme gene with diabetic nephropathy and retinopathy. Diabetologia 41:47-53, 1998

55. Moczulski DK, Rogus JJ, Antonellis A, Warram JH, Krolewski AS: Major susceptibility locus for nephropathy in type 1 diabetes on chromosome 3q: results of novel discordant sib-pair analysis. Diabetes 47:1164-1169, 1998.

56. Imperatore G, Hanson RL, Pettitt DJ, Kobes S, Bennett PH, Knowler WC, the Pima Diabetes Genes Group: Sib-pair linkage analysis for susceptibility genes for microvascular complications among Pima Indians with type 2 diabetes. Diabetes 47:821-830, 1998.

57. Fogarty DG, Moczulski DK, Makita Y, Araki S, Rogus JJ, Krolewski AS: Evidence for a susceptibility locus for diabetic nephropathy on chromosome 7q in Caucasian families with type 2 diabetes. (Abstract). Diabetes 48 (Suppl 1):A47, 1999.

58. Heesom AE, Hibberd ML, Millward A, Demaine AG: Polymorphism in the 5'-end of the aldose reductase gene is strongly associated with the development of diabetic nephropathy in type I diabetes. Diabetes 46:287-291, 1997.

59. Moczulski DK, Burak W, Doria A, Zychma M, Zukowska-Szczechowska E, Warram JH, Grzeszczak W: The role of aldose reductase gene in the susceptibility to diabetic nephropathy in Type II (non-insulin-dependent) diabetes mellitus. Diabetologia 42:94-97, 1999.

60. Zanchi A, Wantman M, Moczulski DK, Warram JH: Genetic susceptibility to diabetic nephropathy in IDDM is related to polymorphism in the endothelial nitric oxide synthase (eNOS) gene. (Abstract). Diabetes 47 (Suppl 1)A52, 1998.

61. Reichard P, Nilsson B-Y, Rosenqvist U: The effect of long-term intensified insulin treatment on the development of microvascular complications of diabetes mellitus. N Engl J Med 329:304-309, 1993.

62. The Diabetes Control and Complications Trial Research Group: The effect of intensive treatment of diabetes on the development and progression of long-term complications in insulin-dependent diabetes mellitus. N Engl J Med 329:977-986, 1993.

63. UK Prospective Diabetes Study (UKPDS) Group: Intensive blood-glucose control with sulphonylureas or insulin compared with conventional treatment and risk of complications in patients with type 2 diabetes (UKPDS 33). Lancet 352:837-853, 1998.

64. Krishna GP, Newell G, Miller E, Heeger P, Smith R, Polansky M, Kapoor S, Hoeldtke R: Protein-induced glomerular hyperfiltration: role of hormonal factors. Kidney Int 33:578-583, 1988.

65. Wiseman MJ, Dodds R, Bending JJ, Viberti GC: Dietary protein and the diabetic kidney. Diabetic Med 4:144-146, 1987.

66. Walker JD, Dodds RA, Murrells TJ, Bending JJ, Mattock MB, Keen H, Viberti GC: Restriction of dietary protein and progression of renal failure in diabetic nephropathy. Lancet 2:1411-1415, 1989.

67. Mitch WE: Dietary protein restriction in chronic renal failure: nutritional efficacy, compliance, and progression of renal insufficiency. J Am Soc Nephrol 2:823-831, 1991.

68. Zeller K, Whittaker E, Sullivan L, Raskin P, Jacobson HR: Effect of restricting dietary protein on the progression of renal failure in patients with insulin-dependent diabetes mellitus. N Engl J Med 324:78-84, 1991.

69. Nakamura H, Ito S, Ebe N, Shibata A: Renal effects of different types of protein in healthy volunteer subjects and diabetic patients. Diabetes Care 16:1071-1075, 1993.

70. Mogensen CE: Long-term antihypertensive treatment inhibiting progression of diabetic nephropathy. Br Med J 285:685-688, 1982.

71.   Parving H-H, Hommel E, Smidt UM: Protection of kidney function and decrease in albuminuria by captopril in insulin dependent diabetics with nephropathy. Br Med J 297:1086-1091, 1988.

72.   Marre M, Chatellier G, Leblanc H, Guyene TT, Menard J, Passa P: Prevention of diabetic nephropathy with enalapril in normotensive diabetics with microalbuminuria. Br Med J 297:1092-1095, 1988.

73.   Mathiesen ER, Hommel E, Giese J, Parving H-H: Efficacy of captopril in postponing nephropathy in normotensive insulin dependent diabetic patients with microalbuminuria. Br Med J 303:81-87, 1991.

74.   Ravid M, Savin H, Jutrin I, Bental T, Katz B, Lishner M: Long-term stabilizing effect of angiotensin-converting enzyme inhibition on plasma creatinine and on proteinuria in normotensive type II diabetic patients. Ann Int Med 118, 577-581, 1993.

75.   Lewis EJ, Hunsicker LG, Bain RP, Rohde RD. The effect of angiotensin-converting-enzyme inhibition on diabetic nephropathy. N Engl J Med 329:1456-1462, 1993

76.   The Microalbuminuria Captopril Study: Captopril reduces the risk of nephropathy in IDDM patients with microalbuminuria. Diabetologia 39:587-593, 1996.

77.   van Essen GG, Rensma PL, de Zeeuw D, Sluiter WJ, Scheffer H, Apperloo AJ, de Jong PE: Association between angiotensin-converting-enzyme gene polymorphism and failure of renoprotective therapy. Lancet 347:94-95, 1996.

78.   Penno G, Chaturvedi N, Talmud PJ, Cotroneo P, Manto A, Nannipieri M, Luong LA, Fuller JH: Effect of angiotensin-converting enzyme (ACE) gene polymorphism on progression of renal disease and the influence of ACE inhibition in IDDM patients: findings from the EUCLID Randomized Controlled Trial. EURODIAB Controlled Trial of Lisinopril in IDDM. Diabetes 47: 1507-11, 1998.

10.   GENETICS AND DIABETIC NEPHROPATHY

Michel Marre[+], Samy Hadjadj[++], Béatrice Bouhanick[+++]
Diabetes Departments, [+]Hôpital Bichat, Paris; [++]Centre Hospitalier Universitaire, Poitiers; [+++]Centre Hospitalier Universitaire, Angers, France

INTRODUCTION

Both genetic determinants and environmental conditions can affect enzyme activity. As all type 1 diabetes complications are secondary to long lasting hyperglycemia, the search for a genetic basis to diabetic nephropathy represents a typical example of search for gene-environment interaction. Furthermore, gene-gene interactions must be expected, as determinants for type 1 diabetes complications are multifactorial. Lastly, the level of evidence for one given gene polymorphism is currently low to account for diabetic nephropathy. Thus, practical implications for this type of investigation in patient care are currently premature.

EPIDEMIOLOGICAL EVIDENCES FOR A GENETIC BASIS TO DIABETIC NEPHROPATHY

One study published by SIPERSTEIN et al in 1968 suggested that capillary basement membrane enlargement (a typical sign for diabetic microangiopathy) preceded diabetes, and consequently that type 1 diabetes complications could be genetically determined independently of glycemic level [1]. However, large amounts of experimental and clinical data have accumulated to contradict this possibility, which established that anatomical and functional signs of diabetic nephropathy are acquired and secondary to hyperglycemia and its consequent disorders [2, 3]. In diabetic patients, Jean PIRART produced a large, 25-yr, prospective, follow-up study, establishing that the development of diabetic complications (including diabetic nephropathy) was proportional to the duration of diabetes and to diabetes control (as assessed by the amount of glycosuria and by random blood glucose measurements) [4]. Last, but not the least, intervention studies in type 1 diabetes (the DCCT trial [5] being the most important quantitatively) or in type 2 diabetes [6] indicated that reduction of hyperglycemia reduced the risk of diabetic nephropathy, as assessed by the incidence of microalbuminuria and proteinuria. However, prospective, follow-up studies suggest that long-term, uncontrolled type 1 diabetes is a necessary, but not sufficient conditional for diabetic nephropathy to develop. For instance, Jean PIRART [4] noticed that concordance was not perfect between onset of each of the 3 specific complications (retinopathy, neuropathy, and nephropathy), as illustrated in Figure 10-1: hardly one fourth of the patients developing retinopathy, or neuropathy, displayed nephropathy. Diabetic nephropathy occurs in hardly half of type 1 diabetes patients, and presents with a peak of onset between the 10th and 25th year of type 1 diabetes duration, as documented by follow-up studies in the Joslin Clinic in Boston and in the Steno Memorial Hospital in Copenhagen [7-9].

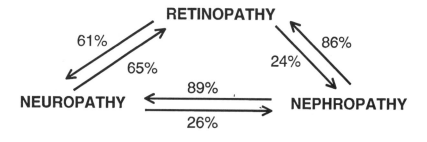

Fig. 10-1. Concordance between diabetic complications in the follow-up study by Jean Pirart [4]. For each new case of one given complication, the probability to display another complication is indicated by the percentage attached to the arrow directed to this complication (e.g. among new cases of retinopathy, 61% already had neuropathy, and 24% nephropathy.

The concept of a genetic basis for diabetic nephropathy is also supported by familial aggregation of this complication within families with several members affected by type 1 diabetes [10-12]. Moreover, phenotypes attached to diabetic nephropathy like high blood pressure seem to segregate with diabetic nephropathy in families of type 1 diabetes patients [13]. The major drawback of family studies is that members of families can share the same environmental conditions, in addition to the same genes, and this remark was applied to the study of families with several type 1 diabetes patients [14]. However, studies in Pima Indians are of importance in this respect, because families share similar environmental conditions. The fact that familial aggregation for proteinuria was found among diabetic siblings of this ethnic group is an important argument for a genetic basis to diabetic nephropathy, eventhough these patients are mostly type 2 diabetes [15]. This result was also confirmed in Caucasian type 2 diabetes patients. As in type 1 diabetes patients [12], the risk for diabetic nephropathy is three to four fold higher for type 2 diabetes siblings when the diabetic probounds display proteinuria [16]. The heritability of urinary albumin excretion and of risk for diabetic nephropathy has been established very recently [17-20]

CANDIDATE GENE VERSUS WHOLE GENOME SCREENING APPROACH
The whole genome screening approach is a promising strategy currently applied to monogenic diseases. In multifactorial diseases, this strategy may be less effective, but it was already used to study the determinants of blood pressure, a variable tightly linked to glomerular disease. For instance, an original methodological approach indicated recently that a genetic region at or near the lipoprotein lipase gene locus was related to blood pressure in humans [21]. Also, the techniques of reverse genetics lead to the discovery of a link between severe, familial hypertension, and angiotensinogen gene polymorphisms, and then angiotensinogen plasma levels [22].

The strategy of whole genome scanning was applied to search for determinants of microvascular disease related to diabetes. In type 2 diabetes, linkage analysis evidenced 2 regions in chromosome 7 and 20 that could determine susceptibility to nephropathy in Pima Indians [23]. These regions contain possible candidate genes such as NO synthase or aldose reductase. In type 1 diabetes patients, using discordant sib pairs for diabetic nephropathy, a susceptibility locus was found on chromosome 3q – Candidate genes in this region involved angiotensin II sub-type 1 receptor (AT1R), but the role for AT1R gene itself was not evidenced using known polymorphisms in this gene [24]. However, the candidate-gene approach has been the most fruitful approach in the domain of cardiovascular risk to date [25-27] and this strategy has been widely applied to diabetic nephropathy.

WHICH CANDIDATE GENES TO BE TESTED FOR DIABETIC NEPHROPATHY?
Target tissues/organs susceptible to diabetic complications are those for which insulin is not required for glucose to be trapped and/or metabolized, i.e., nerves, lens, kidneys, blood cells, epithelial and endothelial cells. Glucose metabolism is altered in these tissues/organs through a few biochemical pathways, e.g., polyol pathway or non-enzymatic glycation of proteins. On the other hand, the vascular (and especially the renal) complications encountered in type 1 diabetes can be explained by hemodynamic factors [28]: increased arteriolar vasodilatation due to high glucose [3] creates high hydraustatic capillary pressure [29] resulting into arteriosclerosis and glomerulosclerosis [30, 31]. In this context, search for candidate genes able to modulate the risk of renal complications due to long-term hyperglycemia can be divided into two avenues: first, to search gene polymorphism of enzymes driving glucose metabolism in tissue/target organs; second, to test gene polymorphism affecting background vascular risk in general population. Using the first strategy, a dinucleotide repeat polymorphism was found at the 5'end of the aldose reductase gene to be associated with early onset of retinopathy in Chinese, type 2 diabetes patients [32]. Later on, another group found this polymorphism

to be associated with diabetic nephropathy in Caucasian type 1 diabetes patients, although the interaction with presence or absence of retinopathy was not clearly delineated [33]. This positive result was rechallenged by some [34] but not all authors [35]. Thus, it is possible that aldose reductase, an enzyme able to affect glucose metabolism within target tissues/organs of diabetic microangiopathy, may affect vascular prognosis of type 1 diabetes patients, including nephropathy through variable, genetically determined, levels of its activity.

A second strategy consists in applying candidate genes for cardiovascular risk (especially those for alterations in microcirculation) to the risk for diabetic nephropathy. The working hypothesis relies on the assumption that global capillary vasodilatation provoked by hyperglycemia and/or insulinopenia in type 1 diabetes [3, 29] also affects renal circulation, and that glomerular capillary hypertension (a universal cause for progression towards glomerulosclerosis and renal failure [36]) is due to an imbalance between hyperglycemia-induced afferent glomerular vasodilatation and constitutive, efferent, glomerular relative vasoconstriction (Figure 10-2).

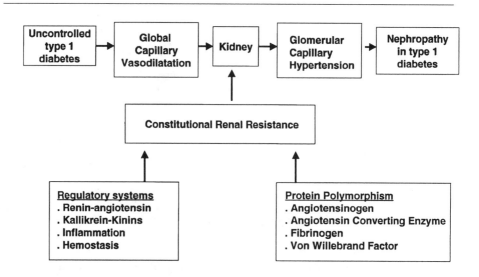

Fig. 10-2. Working hypothesis to study susceptibility to nephropathy in IDDM. Glomerular capillary hypertension, a universal cause for glomerulosclerosis and renal failure, is due to an imbalance between pre-glomerular vasodilatation produced by IDDM, and constitutional renal assistance. Renal resistances result from several regulatory systems, among them several proteins can display polymorphisms affecting the activity of the considered systems.

There are a serie of regulatory systems able to affect glomerular hemodynamics. Within each of these systems, enhanced or reduced activity of one of its components can lead to high/low glomerular hydraulic pressure. Indeed, pharmacological alterations in these systems can affect glomerular hemodynamics, as indicated by changes in albuminuria. For instance, angiotensin I converting enzyme inhibitors can block the renin-angiotensin and kallikrein-kinins systems and reduce micro- or macroalbuminuria [37, 38]. However, reduction in urinary albumin can also be obtained through blockade of prostanoïds with indomethacin [39], or alterations of hemostasis and proteoglycans with heparin [40]. Thus, new polymorphisms within each component of these various regulatory systems are worth being tested for their roles in the development of type 1 diabetes complications, especially diabetic nephropathy [41, 42]. This is especially true, if gene polymorphisms are associated with variable levels of expression of the concerned protein.

WORKING HYPOTHESIS : POLYMORPHISM OF THE RENIN-ANGIOTENSIN SYSTEM AND RISK FOR DIABETIC NEPHROPATHY

Background hypothesis
As depicted in Figure 10-3, angiotensin II (AII) generation is consequent to a serie of enzymatic reactions, and AII interacts with a well-defined membrane receptor, of which the sub-type 1 AII receptor (AT1R) is of interest. Several of these components displayed genetic polymorphisms, but only two of them displayed polymorphisms related to variable expressions of the protein: the renin substrate angiotensinogen (AGT) through the M235T and T174M polymorphisms [22], and the Angiotensin I Converting Enzyme (ACE) through an Insertion/Deletion (I/D) polymorphism located in intron 16 of the gene [43]. The effect of diabetes on glomerular circulation ressembles that of AII [44, 45]. Furthermore, ACE inhibition prevents diabetic nephropathy [46], or halts its progression [47]. If we accept the ancient hypothesis proposed by VANE that the ACE availability can limit transformation of angiotensin I into AII within the glomerular circulation [48], it was tempting to test the hypothesis of a role for ACE I/D polymorphism in the risk of diabetic nephropathy for type 1 diabetes patients. Also, genetically determined AGT levels could affect AII, in that the amount of substrate for renin (an enzyme without relevant genetic polymorphism) may limit angiotensin I production [22], although the proportion of the inter-subject variance of AGT due to genetic factors is relatively low (10-15 %), compared to that of ACE accounted for by genetic factors (~ 75 %), of which the I/D polymorphism makes ~ 50 % minimally [27]. Finally, a A1166C AT1R polymorphism was described in relation to essential hypertension [49], but no study has demonstrated to date, that it affects AII sensitivity.

Case-control studies on Diabetic Nephropathy and ACE I/D polymorphism in type 1 diabetes patients
Using the hypothesis depicted in Figure 10-2, we produced a case-control study indicating that type 1 diabetes subjects homozygotes for the ACE I allele seemed

protected against diabetic nephropathy through low circulating ACE levels [50]. In this study, controls of nephropathy were carefully matched with cases for short-and long-term glycemic control (as assessed by HbA1c and the severity of retinopathy), and not only for age, sex, and type 1 diabetes duration. This result was challenged by some other, apparently negative, case-control studies, although bia due to a better glycemic control of controls than of cases was observable in these studies [51-54].

Proteln	Polymorphism	Association with	References
Angiotensinogen	M235T, T174M	Essential Hypertension	(18)
↓ ◄—— Renin			
Angiotensin I			
↓ ◄—— ACE*	I/D	Myocardial Infarction Renal Failure	(20) (20)
Angiotensin II			
↓			
AT1R	A 1166C	Essential Hypertension	(40)

Fig. 10-3. Schematic diagram of the renin-angiotensin system. Only two proteins (angiotensinogen, ACE) display variable levels of protein expression according to genetic polymorphisms. Numbers between parantheses indicate reference numbers*, ACE: angiotensin converting enzyme.

In order to reduce the uncertainty due to the variable type 1 diabetes control and duration on the role for one given protein polymorphism in the kidney prognosis of type 1 diabetes patients, we organized a multi-center, cross-sectional study of type 1 diabetes patients having expressed their risk of kidney disease due to type 1 diabetes: those who developed proliferative retinopathy, a clear hallmark for uncontrolled type 1 diabetes [55]. Then, we found that the severity of renal involvement was dependent of ACE I/D polymorphism with a dominant effect of ACE D allele [adjusted odds ratio for renal involvement attributable to the D allele 1.889 (95 % CI 1.209-2.952)]. There was no independent effect of AGT, or AT1R polymorphisms on the risk for diabetic nephropathy, but a significant interaction between ACE I/D and AGT M235T polymorphisms, suggesting that genetically determined AGT levels can affect risk for diabetic nephropathy through angiotensin I generation, if angiotensin I transformation into AII is not restrained by ACE availability (i.e., the patients with the ACE II genotype) [55]. A family-based study showed that the T allele of the M235 T polymorphism of AGT was preferentially transmitted to make type 1 diabetes patients with nephropathy [56]. Other cross-sectional studies have produced discordant results on the role of AT1R on diabetic nephropathy. Some authors evidenced an interaction between the A1166C polymorphism of the AT1R gene and poor glycaemic control [57], but other groups failed to reproduce this result [58] or did not evidence any effect ot this genotype on diabetic nephropathy [59, 60].

Finally, some meta-analysis of all currently available studies on ACE I/D polymorphism and diabetic nephropathy support that the II genotype may confer a relative protection against diabetic nephropathy [61-63].

Clinical investigations on renal haemodynamics and ACE I/D polymorphism
Recently, J. MILLER et al reported that type 1 diabetes patients with the II genotype displayed higher glomerular filtration rate and effective renal plasma flow during normoglycemia than type 1 diabetes patients within the ID or DD genotypes [64]. These results are consistent with the effect of ACE inhibition on renal hemodynamics reported in normoalbuminuric [65] and microalbuminuric [38] subjects and consistent with a global, systemic vasodilatation due to low circulating AII levels. These alterations make protection against diabetic nephropathy [46]. Conversely, we studied recently the effect of acute hyperglycaemia in normotensive normoalbuminuric type 1 diabetes patients, and found that those with the ID or DD genotypes displayed alterations in glomerular haemodynamics consistent with a rise in glomerular capillary hydraulic pressure, while this was not observed in the patients with the II genotype [66]. Thus, these investigations are arguments to support that ACE I/D polymorphism and related ACE levels can affect constitution and progression of diabetic nephropathy.

Follow-up studies and intervention studies according to ACE I/D genotypes
One follow-up study in Austria indicated that ACE I/D polymorphism can affect the course of kidney disease in type 1 diabetes patients [67]. Thus, prospective follow-up of kidney function must be organized according to ACE genotypes and other possibly important polymorphisms. We have also confirmed in a prospective follow-up study of a cohort of 310 type 1 diabetes patients that the D allele is significantly and independently associated with the risk of development and progression of diabetic nephropathy [68]. Also, Parving et al reported that ACE I/D polymorphism can affect the course of glomerular filtration rate, once diabetic nephropathy is established [69]. Moreover, these authors [69] suggested that ACE inhibition was less effective to prevent the evolution towards renal failure, if the type 1 diabetes patients displayed the DD genotype, than if they did not [69]. Conversely, studying normo-or-microalbuminuric type 1 diabetes patients, Penno et al failed to show a substantial interaction between ACE inhibition and ACE I/D polymorphism [70]. However, these studies must be cautiously examined, because of the possible survival bia and other unidentified, hidden bias. Intervention

studies (especially with ACE inhibitors) must be designed according to ACE I/D polymorphism with an appropriate method, probably using surrogate end-point like urinary albumin excretion as main outcome in a first step.

ACE I/D polymorphism and diabetic nephropathy in type 2 diabetes patients
ACE I/D polymorphism was reported to be associated with risk for coronary heart disease in type 2 diabetes [71]. As microalbuminuria or proteinuria predicts or is associated with coronary heart disease in type 2 diabetes [72-74], it was worth looking for an association between urinary albumin and ACE I/D polymorphism in type 2 diabetes. This association was reported to be positive in the UKPDS study [75]. Also, positive studies on the association between ACE I/D polymorphism and diabetic nephropathy were reported in Japanese type 2 diabetes patients by most [76-78], if not all studies [79]. Some cross-sectional studies have been reported in Caucasians with discordant results. Pooled in a meta-analysis, the effect of the ACE I/D polymorphism is statistically significant in Japanese but not in Caucasian type 2 diabetes patients [63]. However, in a longitudinal study of type 2 diabetes Caucasian patients, the decline of GFR during the follow-up period was least in those patients with the II genotype [80]. Thus, the issue of an association between ACE I/D polymorphism remains debatable, because microalbuminuria or proteinuria is attributable to diabetic nephropathy in only a portion of cases with type 2 diabetes [81] and because the interaction between elevated urinary albumin, coronary heart disease and ACE I/D polymorphism must be clarified. Lastly, the frequency of ACE II genotype is higher among Asian (~ 40-45%) than among Caucasian (~ 20-25%) subjects, and the clinical characteristics and age at onset of type 2 diabetes are not similar in Japanese and Caucasian patients. Thus, the portion of the risk for (or of protection against) diabetic nephropathy / coronary heart disease may be different among Asian and Caucasian type 2 diabetes patients.

ACKNOWLEDGMENT
The authors thank Mrs Line GODIVEAU and Isabelle GOULEAU for their excellent secretarial assistance.

REFERENCES
1   Siperstein MD., Unger RH., Madison LL. Studies of muscle   capillary basement membranes in normal subjects, diabetic and prediabetic patients. J. Clin. Invest., 1968, 47: 1973-1999
2   Mauer S., Steffes M.W., Sutherland D.E.R., Najarian   J.S., Michael A.F., BrownD M. Studies of the rate of regression of the glomerular lesions in diabetic rats treated with pancreatic islet transplantation. Diabetes, 1975, 24: 250-255
3   Williamson JR., Chang K, Frangos M., Hasan KS., Ido Y., Kawamura F., Nyengaard RD J.R., Van Den Enden M., Kilo C., Tilton RG. Hyperglycemic pseudohypoxia and diabetic complications. Diabetes, 1993, 42: 801-813

4   Pirart J. Diabète et complications dégénératives. Présentation d'une étude prospective portant sur 4400 cas observés entre 1947 et 1973. Diabete Metab., 1977, 3: 97-107, 3: 173-182, 3: 243-256

5   The Diabetes Control and Complications Trial Research Group.The effect of intensive treatment of diabetes on the development and progression of long-term complications in insulin-dependent diabetes mellitus. N. Engl. J. Med., 1993, 329: 977-986

6   UK Prospective Diabetes Study (UKPDS) Group. Intensive blood-glucose control with sulphonylureas or insulin compared with conventional treatment and risk of complications in patients with type 2 diabetes. (UKPDS, 33). Lancet, 1998, 352: 837-853

7   Krolewski AJ., Warram JH., Rand LI., Kahn CR. Epidemiologic approach to the etiology of type I diabetes mellitus and its Complications. N. Engl. J. Med, 1987, 317: 1390-1398

8   Andersen AR., Christiansen JS., Andersen JK., Kreiner S., Deckert T. Diabetic nephropathy in type 1 (insulin-dependent) diabetes: an epidemiological Study. Diabetologia, 1983, 2: 496-501.

9   Borch-Johnsen K., Andersen P.K., Deckert T. The effect of proteinuria on relative mortality in type 1 (insulin-dependent) diabetes mellitus. Diabetologia, 1985, 28: 590-596

10   Seaquist ER., Goetz FC., Rich HS., Barbosa J. Familial clustering ofdiabetic kidney disease : evidence for genetic susceptibility to diabetic nephropathy. N. Engl. J. Med, 1989, 320: 1161-1165

11   Earle K., Walker J., Hill C., Viberti GC. Familial clustering of cardiovascular disease in patients with insulin-dependent diabetes and nephropathy. N. Engl. J. Med, 1992, 326: 673-677

12   Quinn M., Angelico MC., Warram JH., Krolewski A.S. Familial factors determine the development of diabetic nephropathy in patients with IDDM. Diabetologia, 1996, 39: 940-945

13   Viberti GC., Keen H., Wiseman MJ. Raised arterial pressure in parents of proteinuric insulin-dependent diabetics. B.M.J, 1987, 295: 515-517

14   Borch-Johnsen K., Norgaard K., Hommel E., Mathiesen ER., Jensen JS., Deckert T, Parving H-H. Is diabetic nephropathy an inherited complication? Kidney Int, 1992, 41: 719-722

15   Pettit D.J., Saad MF., Bennett PH., Nelson RG., Knowler WC. Familial predisposition to renal disease in two generations of Pima Indians with 2 (non-insulin-dependent) diabetes mellitus. Diabetologia, 1990, 33: 438-443

16   Canani LH., Gerchman F., and Gross J.L. Familial clustering of diabetic nephropathy in Brazilian type 2 diabetic patients. Diabetes, 1999, 48: 909-913

17   Gruden G., Cavallo-Perin P, Olivetti C., Repetti E., Sivieri R., Bruno A., Pagano G. Albumin excretion rate levels in non-diabetic offspring of NIDDM patients with and without nephropathy. Diabetologia, 1995, 38: 1218-1222

18   Forsblom CM., Kanninen T., Lehtovirta M., Saloranta C., Groop LC. Heritability of albumin excretion rate in families of patients with Type II diabetes. Diabetologia, 1999, 42: 1359-1366

19   Solini A., Giacchetti G., Sfriso A., Fioretto P., Sardu C., Saller A., Tonolo G., Maioli M., Mantero F., and Nosadini R. Polymorphisms of angiotensin-converting enzyme and angiotensinogen genes in type 2 diabetic sibships in relation to albumin excretion rate. Am. J. Kidney Dis, 1999, 34: 1002-1009

20   Faronato PP., Maioli M., Tonolo G., Brocco E., Noventa E., Piarulli F., Abaterusso C., Modema F., Bigontina G de, Velussi M., Inchiostro S., Santeusanio F., Bueti A., Nosadini R., on behalf of the Italian NIDDM Nephropathy Study Group. Clustering of albumin excretion rate abnormalities in Caucasian patients with NIDDM. Diabetologia, 1997, 40: 816-823

21   Wu DA., Bu X., Harden CH., Shen DDC., Jeng CY., Sheu WHH., Fuh MMT., Katsuya T., Dzau VJ., Reaven GM., Lusis AJ., Rotter JI, Chen DI. Quantitative trait locus mapping of human blood pressure to a genetic region at or near the Lipoprotein lipase gene locus on chromosome 8p22.J. Clin. Invest, 1996, 97: 2111-2118

22   Jeunemaitre X., Soubrier F., Kotelevtsev Y., Lifton R., Williams C., Charru A., HUNT S., Hopkins P., Williams R., Lalouel JM., Corvol P. Molecular basis of human hypertension: role of angiotensinogen. Cell, 1992, 71: 169-180

23   Imperatore G., Hanson RL., Pettitt DJ., Kobes S., Bennett PH., Knowler WC, and the Pima Diabetes Genes Group. Sib-Pair linkage analysis for susceptibility genes for microvascular complications among Pima Indians with type 2 diabetes. Diabetes, 1998, 47: 821-830

24   Moczulski DK., Rogus JJ., Antonellis A., Warram JH., and Krolewski AS. Major susceptibility locus for nephropathy in type 1 diabetes on chromosome 3q. Results of novel discordnt sib-pair analysis. Diabetes, 1998, 47: 1164-1169

25   Cambien F., Alhenc-Gelas F., Herberth B., Andre JL., Rakotovao R., Gonzales MF., Allegrini J., Bloch C. Familial ressemblance of plasma angiotensin converting enzyme level: the Nancy study. Am. J. Hum. Genet, 1988, 43: 774-780

26   Cambien F., Poirier O., Lecerf L., Evans A., Cambou JP., Arveiler D., Luc G., Bard JM., Bara L., Ricards S., Tiret L., Amouyel Ph., Alhenc-Gelas S F., Soubrier F. Deletion polymorphism in the gene for angiotensin converting enzyme is a potent risk factor for myocardial infarction. Nature, 1992, 359: 641-644

27   Cambien F., Costerousse O., Tiret L., Poirier O., Lecerf L., Gonzales MF., Evans A., Arveiler D., Cambou JP., Luc G., Rakotovao R., Ducimetiere P., Soubrier F., Alhenc-Gelas F. Plasma level and gene polymorphism of angiotensin concerting enzyme in relation to myocardial infarction. Circulation, 1994, 90: 669-676

28   Parving H-H., Viberti GC., Keen H., Christiansen JS., Lassen .NA. Hemodynamic factors in the genesis of diabetic microangiopathy. Metabolism, 1983, 32: 943-949

29   Tooke JE. Microvascular function in human diabetes. A physiological perspective. Diabetes, 1995, 44: 721-726

30   Zatz R., Dunn BR., Meyer TW., Anderson S., Rennke H.G., Brenner BM. Prevention of diabetic glomerulopathy by pharmacological of glomerular capillary hypertension. J. Clin. Invest, 1986, 77: 1925–1930

31   Deckert T., Feldt-Rasmussen B., Borch-Johnsen K., Jensen T., Kofoed-Enevoldsen A. Albuminuria reflects widespread vascular damage: the Steno hypothesis. Diabetologia, 1989, 32: 219-226

32   Ko BCB., Lam KSL., Wat NMS., Chung SSM. An (A-C)n dinucleotide repeat polymorphic marker at the 5' end of the aldose reductase gene is associated with early-onset diabetic retinopathy in NIDDM patients. Diabetes, 1995, 44: 727-732

33   Heesom AE., Hibberd ML., Millward A., Demaine A.G. Polymorphism in the 5'-end of the aldose reductase gene is strongly associated with the development of diabetic nephropathy in type I diabetes. Diabetes, 1997, 46 : 287-291

34   Ichikawa F., Yamada K., Ishiyama-Shigemoto S., Yuan X. and Nonoka K. Association of an (A-C)n dinucleotide repeat polymorphic marker at the 5'-region of the aldose reductase gene with retinopathy but not with nephropathy or neuropathy in Japanese patients with type 2 diabetes mellitus. Diabetic Medicine, 1999, 16: 744-748

35   Shah VO., ScaviniI M., Nikolic J., Sun Y., Vai S., Griffith JK., Dorin RI., Stidley C., Yacoub M., Vander Jagt DL., Philip Eaton R. and Zager PG. Z-2 Microsatellite allele is linked to increased expression of the aldose reductase gene in diabetic nephropathy. J Clin Endocrinol Metab, 1998, 83: 2886-2891

36   Brenner BM. Hemodynamicaly mediated glomerular injury and the progressive nature of kidney disease. Kidney Intern, 1983, 23: 617-655.,

37   Taguma Y., Kitamoto Y., Futaki G., Ueda H., Monma H., Ishizaki M., Takahashi H., Sekino H., Sasaky Y. Effect of Captopril on heavy proteinuria in azotemic diabetics. N. Engl. J. Med, 1985, 313: 1617-1620

38   Marre M., Leblanch H., Suarez L., Guyenne TT., Menard J., Passa P. Converting enzyme inhibition and kidney function in normotensive diabetic patients with persistent microalbuminuria. B.M.J, 1987, 294: 1448-1452

39   Hommel E., Mathiesen E., Olsen U.B., Parving H-H. Effects of indomethacin on kidney function in type 1 (insulin-dependent) diabetic patients with nephropathy. Diabetologia, 1987, 30: 78-81

40   Myrup B., Hansen PM., Jensen J., Kofoed-Enevoldsen A., Feldt-Rasmussen B., Gram J., Kluft C., Jespersen J., Deckert T. Effect of low-dose heparin on urinary albumin excretion in insulin-dependent diabetes mellitus. Lancet, 1995, 345: 421-422

41   Torremocha F, Marechaud R, Marre M., Passa Ph., Rodier M., Alhenc-Gelas F., Jeunemaître X. for the GENEDIAB group Lack of relation between renal kallidrein gene polymorphism and diabetic nephropathy. Diabetologia, 1997, 40, A520 (abstract)

42   Lacquemant C., Gaucher C., Delorme C., Chatellier G., Gallois Y., Rodier M., Passa Ph., Balkau B., Mazurier C., Marre M., Froguel P., and the GENEDIAB study group and the DESIR Study group. Association between high von Willebrand factor levels and the Thr 789Ala vWF gene polymorphism but not with nephropathy in type 1 diabetes. Kidney Int., 2000 (in press)

43   Rigat B., Hubert C., Alhenc-Gelas F., Cambien F., Corvol P., Soubrier F. An insertion deletion polymorphism in angiotensin I convertion enzyme gene accounting for half of the variance of serum enzyme levels. J. Clin. Invest, 1990, 86: 1343-1346

44   Hostetter TH., Troy JL., Brenner BM. Glomerular hemodynamics in experimental diabetes mellitus. Kidney Int., 1981, 19: 410-415

45   Hall JE., Guyton AC., Jackson TE., Coleman TG., Lohmeier TE., Tripodo NC. Control of glomerular filtration rate by renin-angiotensin system. Am. J. Physiol., 1977, 233: F366-F372

46   Marre M., Chatellier G., Leblanc H., Guyenne TT, Menard J., Passa P. Prevention of diabetic nephropathy with enalapril in normotensive diabetics with microalbuminuria. B.M.J., 1988, 297: 1092-1095

47   Lewis EJ., Hunsicker LG., Bain RP., Rohde RD., for the Collaborative Study Group. The effect of angiotensin-converting-enzyme inhibition on diabetic nephropathy. N. Engl. J. Med., 1993, 329: 1456-1462

48.   Vane JR. Sites of conversion of angiotensin I. In Hypertension. GENEST J., KOINE E., eds Berlin, Springer Verlag, 1972, p 523-532

49   Bonnardeaux A., Davies E., Jeunemaître X., Fery I., Charru A., Clauser E., Tiret L., Cambien F., Corvol P., Soubrier F. Angiotensin II type 1 receptor gene polymorphisms in human essential hypertension. Hypertension, 1994, 24: 63-69

50   Marre M., Bernadet P., Gallois Y., Savagner F., Guyene TT., Hallab M., Cambien F., Passa Ph., Alhenc-Gelas F. Relationships between angiotensin I converting enzyme gene polymorphism, plasma levels, and diabetic retinal and renal complications. Diabetes, 1994, 43: 384-388

51   Tarnow L., Cambien F., Rossing P., Nielsen FS., Hansen BV., Lecerf L., Poirier O., Danilov S., Parving H-H. Lack of relationship between an insertion / deletion polymorphism in the I-converting enzyme gene and diabetic nephropathy and proliferative retinopathy in IDDM patients. Diabetes, 1995, 44: 489-494

52   Schmidt S., Schone N., Ritz E., and the Diabetic Nephropathy Study Group: Association of ACE gene polymorphism and diabetic nephropathy ? Kidney Int., 1995, 47: 1176-1181

53   Powrie JK., Watts GF., Ingham JN., Taub NA., Talmud PJ., Shaw KM. Role of glycæmic control in development of microalbuminuria in patients with insulin-dependent diabetes. B.M.J., 1994, 309: 1608-1612

54   Chowdhury TA., Dronsfield MJ., Kumar S., Gough SLC., Gibson SP., Khatoon A., MacDonald F., Rowe BR., Dunger DB., Dean JD., Davies SJ., Webber J., Smith PR., Macrin P., Marshall SM., Adu D., Morris PJM., Todd JA., Barnett AH., Boulton AJM., Bain SC. Examination of two genetic polymorphisms within the renin-angiotensin system: no evidence for an association with nephropathy in IDDM. Diabetologia, 1996, 39: 1108-1114

55   Marre M., Jeunemaître X., Gallois Y., Rodier M., Chatellier G., Sert C., Dusselier L., Kahal Z., Chaillous L., Halimi S., Muller A., Sackmann H., Bauduceau B., Bled F., Passa Ph., Alhenc-Gelas F. Contribution of Genetic polymorphism in the Renin-Angiotensin System to the development of renal complications in insulin-dependent diabetes. J. Clin. Invest., 1997, 99, 1585-1595

56   Rogus JJ., Moczulski D., Freire MB., Yang Y., Warram JH., Krolewski AS. Diabetic nephropathy is associated with AGT polymorphism T235: results of a family-based study. Hypertension, 1998, 31: 627-631

57   Doria A., Onuma T., Warram JH, Krolewski AS. Synergistic effect of angiotensin II type 1 receptor genotype and poor glycaemic control on risk of nephropathy in IDDM. Diabetologia, 1997, 40: 1293-1299

58   Savage DA., Feeney SA., Fogarty DG., Maxwell AP. Risk of developing diabetic nephropathy is not associated with synergism between the angiotensin II (type 1) receptor C1166 allele and poor glycaemic control. Nephrol Dial Transplant, 1999, 14: 891-894

59   Tarnow L., Cambien F., Rossing P., Nielsen FS., Hansen V., Ricard S., Poirier O., Parving H-H. Angiotensin –II type 1 receptor gene polymorphism and diabetic microangiopathy. Nephrol Dial Transplant, 1996, 11: 1019-1023

60   Chowdhury TA., Dyer PH., Kumar S., Gough SC., Gibson SP., Rowe BR., Smith PR., Dronsfield MJ., Marshall SM., Mackin P., Dean JD., Morris PJ., Davies S., Dunger DB., Boulton AJ., Barnett AH., Bain SC. Lack of association of angiotensin II type 1 receptor gene polymorphism with diabetic nephropathy in insulin-dependent diabetes mellitus. Diabet Med, 1997, 14: 837-840

61   Staessen JA., Wang JG., Ginocchio G., Petrov., Saavedra AP., Soubrier F., Vlietinck R., Fagard R. The deletion/insertion polymorphism of the angiotensin converting enzyme gene and cardiovascular renal risk. J. Hypertension, 1997, 15: 1575-1592

62   Fusisawa T., Ikegami H., Kawaguchi Y., Hanada Y., Ueda H., Shintani M., Fukuda M., Ogihara T. Meta-analysis of association of insertion/deletion polymorphism of angiotensin I-converting enzyme gene with diabetic nephropathy and retinopathy. Diabetologia, 1998, 41: 47-53

63   Tarnow L., Gluud C., and Parving H-H. Diabetic nephropathy and the insertion/deletion polymorphism of the angiotensin-converting enzyme gene. Nephrol Dial Transplant, 1998, 13: 1125-1130

64   Miller JA., Scholey JW., Thai K., Pei YPC. Angiotensin converting enzyme gene polymorphism and renal hemodynamic function in early diabetes. Kidney International, 1997, 51: 119-124

65   Mau-Pedersen M., Schmitz A., Pedersen EB., Danielsen H., Christiansen JS. Acute and long-term renal effects of angiotensin converting enzyme inhibition in normotensive, normoalbuminuric insulin-dependent diabetic patients. Diabetic Med, 1988, 5: 562-569

66   Marre M., Bouhanick B., Berrut G., Gallois Y., LeJeune JJ., Chatellier G., Menard J., Alhenc-Gelas F. Renal Changes on hyperglycemia and angiotensin-converting enzyme in type 1 diabetes. Hypertension, 1999, 33: 775-780

67   Barnas U., Schmidt A., Illievich A., Kiener HP., Rabensteiner D., Kaider A., Prager R., Abrahamian H., Irsigler K., Mayer G. Evaluation of risk factors for the development of nephropathy in patients with IDDM: insertion/deletion angiotensin converting enzyme gene polymorphism, hypertension and metabolic control. Diabetologia, 1997, 40: 327-331

68   Hadjadj S., Belloum R., Gallois Y., Bouhanick B., Berrut G., Weekes L., Marre M. Contribution of Angiotensin I Converting Enzyme I/D Polymorphism ot the development and progression of diabetic nephropathy in type I diabetes: a 6-year follow-up study. Diabetes, 1999, 48 (suppl. 1) A36

69   Parving H-H., Jacobsen P., Tarnow L., Rossing P., Lecerf L., Poirier O., Cambien F. Effect of deletion polymorphism of angiotensin enzyme gene on progression of diabetic nephropathy during inhibition of angiotensin converting enzyme, observational follow-up study. B.M.J., 1996, 313: 591-594

70   Penno G., Chaturvedi N., Talmud PJ., Cotroneo P., Manto A., Nannipieri M., Luong LA., Fuller JH., and the EUCLID Study Group. Effect of Angiotensin-Converting Enzyme (ACE) gene polymorphism on progression of renal disease and the influence of ACE inhibition in IDDM patients. Diabetes, 1998, 47: 1507-1511

71   Ruiz J., Blanche H., Cohen N., Velho G., Cambien F., Cohen D., Passa Ph., Froguel Ph.Insertion / Deletion polymorphism of the angiotensin converting enzyme gene is strongly associated with coronary heart disease in non-insulin-dependent diabetes mellitus Proc. Natl. Acad. Sci. USA, 1994, 91: 3662-3665

72   Mogensen C.E. Microalbuminuria predicts clinical proteinuria and early mortality in maturity-onset diabetes. N. Engl. J. Med., 1984, 310: 356-360

73   Jarrett R.J., Viberti GC., Argyropoulos A., Hill RD., Mahmud U., Murrels TJ. Microalbuminuria predicts mortality in non insulin-dependent diabetics. Diabetic Med., 1984, 1: 17-19

74   Mattock MB., Morrish NJ., Viberti GC., Keen H., Fitzgerald AP., Jackson G. Prospective study of microalbuminuria as predictor of mortality in NIDDM. Diabetes 1992, 41: 736-741

75   Dubley CRK., Keavney B., Stratton IM., Turner RC., Ratcliffe PJ. U.K. prospective diabetes study XV: relationship of renin-angiotensin system gene polymorphisms with microalbuminuria in NIDDM.Kidney Int., 1995, 48: 1907-1911

76   Mizuiril S., Hemmi H., Inoue A., Yoshikawa H., Tanegashima M., Fushimi T., Ishigami M., Amagasaki Y., Ohara T., Shimatake H., Hasegawa A. Angiotensin-converting-enzyme polymorphism and development of diabetic nephropathy in non-insulin-dependent diabetes mellitus. Nephron., 1995, 70: 455-459

77   Doi Y., Yoshizumi H., Lino K., Yamamoto M., Ichikawa K., Iwase M., Fujishima M. Association between a polymorphism in the angiotensin-converting-enzyme gene and microavascular complications in Japanese patients with NIDDM. Diabetologia, 1996, 39: 97-102

78   Ohno T., Kawazu S., Tomono S. Association analyse of the polymorphisms of angiotensin-converting enzyme and angiotensinogen genes with diabetic nephropathy in Japanese non-insulin-dependent diabetics. Metabolism, 1996, 45: 218-222

79   Fujisawa T., Ikegami H., Shen GQ., Yamato E., Takekawa K., Nakagawa Y., Hamada Y.,Ueda H., Rakugi H., Higaki J., Ohishi M., Fujii K., Fukuda M., Ogihara T. Angiotensin I converting enzyme gene polymorphism is associated with myocardial infarction, but not with retinopathy or nephropathy, in NIDDM. Diabetes Care, 1995, 18: July

80   Huang XH., Rantalaiho V., Wirta O., Pasternack A., Hiltunen TP., Koivula T., Malminiemi K., NikkarlT., Lehtimaki T. Angiotensin-Converting Enzyme insertion/deletion polymorphism and diabetic albuminuria in patients with NIDDM followed up for 9 years. Nephron, 1998, 80: 17-24

81   Gambara V., Mecca G., Remuzzi G., Bertani T. Heterogeneous nature of renal lesions in type II diabetes. J. Am. Soc. Nephrol., 1993, 3: 1458-1466

11.   BIRTH, BARKER AND BRENNER: THE CONCEPT OF LOW BIRTH WEIGHT AND RENAL DISEASE

Susan Jones and Jens Randel Nyengaard
Department of Medicine, The Medical School, Newcastle upon Tyne, UK and Stereological Research Laboratory, University of Aarhus, Denmark

The concept that intra-uterine environment may influence the development of chronic disease in adulthood such as hypertension, ischaemic heart disease, impaired glucose tolerance and diabetes mellitus was proposed by Barker et al [1,2] . It is hypothesised in the event of intra-uterine malnutrition the foetus 'reserves' nutrition for the developing brain, at the expense of other less important organs such as the pancreas and kidney. These organs may subsequently suffer from diseases in adulthood as a result of deprived nutrition at a crucial stage of their development.

Brenner et al [3] proposed that essential hypertension may be the result of an inborn reduction in glomerular number resulting in a reduction in total glomerular filtration surface area. The embryological development of the kidney is very tightly controlled [4] and in vitro studies have shown that manipulation of the matrix during glomerular morphogenesis may generate less developed nephrons [5]. In vivo studies have shown that administration of gentamicin [6,7] or protein restriction [8,9] in pregnant rats results in offspring with a reduced number of glomeruli.

BARKER HYPOTHESIS
The result of malnutrition in early pregnancy may be symmetrically small babies with low birth weight. In mid-pregnancy, the placenta grows faster than the fetus and mild malnutrition in this period of time may result in a baby with low birth weight and a small or hypertrophied placenta. Late in pregnancy, malnutrition may result in thin babies, as the fetus may loose weight [10]. Retarded fetal growth can be characterised by low birth weight, low birth weight relative to placental weight or low ponderal index (birth weight / length^3) [10].

Barker and Osmond observed that the geographical distribution of mortality rates from cardiovascular disease in England and Wales were similar to the pattern of neonatal and maternal mortality rates in the early twentieth century [11,12]. In a retrospective study among 5,654 men born in Hertfordshire, UK between 1911 and 1930 they demonstrated an association between those of lowest weight at birth, or at age 1 year, and deaths from ischaemic heart disease, suggesting a link between intrauterine environment and cardiovascular disease [10]. Barker and colleagues also calculated the ponderal index as a marker of intra-uterine malnutrition. A low ponderal index (abnormal thinness) was associated with cardiovascular disease in adulthood. The observation that the geographical differences in the incidence of cardiovascular disease correlated with differences in mean blood pressure of men and women [13] prompted further study by Barker and colleagues.

A cohort of 449 men and women born between 1935 and 1942 in Preston, Lancashire, UK who still lived in the area were studied since extremely detailed maternity records had been kept for this group. Systolic and diastolic blood pressure were strongly associated with placental weight at birth in both men and women [14]. An association between the development of both impaired glucose tolerance and Type 2 diabetes mellitus and low birth weight was also found [15].

This association between LBW and chronic disease in adulthood was most noticeable in those individuals who subsequently became obese adults. These observations formed the basis of the Barker or 'fetal origins' hypothesis that intra-uterine environment could influence the development of chronic disease in adulthood and that birth weight or abnormal thinness at birth were markers of intra-uterine malnutrition.

Changes in fetal life [16], primarily focusing upon changes in maternal glucocorticoids [17,18], have attempted to explain the association between low birth weight and hypertension. Persistent changes in the secretion of fetal hormones and the altered sensitivity of different kinds of tissue to the maternal glucocorticoids may result in the development of hypertension. Dysfunction of the placental glucocorticoid barrier may result in increased maternal glucocorticoids in the fetus, resulting in impaired fetal growth. The maternal glucocorticoids, which are exposed to the fetus may effect the development of fetal vessels, thus increasing the risk of developing hypertension in adult life [17].

THE DUTCH HUNGER WINTER AND THE LENINGRAD SIEGE STUDIES

The direct effects of severe intra-uterine malnutrition have been tested in animal models and by using epidemiological studies of offspring of mothers exposed to malnutrition whilst pregnant. Examples of the latter include the Dutch Hunger Winter [19] and the Leningrad Siege [20] studies.

The Dutch Hunger Winter cohort study initially sought to examine the effects of intra-uterine malnutrition on birth weight, adulthood anthropomorphic measurements and psychiatric illness [21]. Individuals born in Amsterdam between 1944 and 1946 during a wartime famine were exposed to intra-uterine malnutrition at different stages of gestation. First trimester exposure to intra-uterine malnutrition had no effect on birth weight but was associated with increased waist-hip ratio in adulthood. In contrast, third trimester exposure was associated with a reduction in both birth weight and adulthood adiposity.

Lumey and Stein [19] subsequently examined the birth weights in offspring of mothers from the initial cohort born between 1944 and 1946. The analysis included 437 families with two siblings and 107 families with three siblings born between 1960 and 1985. Infants whose mothers had been exposed to first trimester intra-uterine malnutrition during the Dutch Hunger Winter did not show the expected increase in birth weight with increasing birth order and weighed less than their firstborn siblings. This apparent effect observed in a selected group of offspring suggests that there may be long-term biological effects that are independent of maternal birth weight and influence the subsequent generation.

During World War II, St Petersburg (formally known as Leningrad) was besieged from 1941 to 1944. In a cross sectional study Stanner et al [20] compared two groups: those born during the siege (n=169; intra-uterine group), those born before the siege (n=192; infant group). Those individuals in the intra-uterine group were exposed to significant malnutrition in utero and in early infancy. A third group not exposed to the siege, derived from those born outside the city during the siege (n=188; unexposed group), was also studied.

In contrast to Barker's studies there was no difference between the intra-uterine and infant groups with respect to the following: glucose intolerance, insulin concentration, blood pressure, lipid levels or coagulation factors. The intra-uterine group had higher levels of von Willebrand's factor, a marker of endothelial dysfunction, compared to the infant group. The intra-uterine group also exhibited a stronger association between adulthood obesity and both diastolic and systolic blood pressure but this was not statistically significant. Despite the problems of the lack of accurate birth weight data and low case ascertainment rate (only 44% of eligible subjects were screened), the Leningrad Siege Study suggests that intra-uterine malnutrition does not have a major role in the pathogenesis of adulthood glucose intolerance and hypertension.

OTHER EPIDEMIOLOGICAL STUDIES

Extreme malnutrition may have little relevance to the general population and a number of studies have retrospectively examined the effect of birth weight on the rates of chronic disease in adulthood using 'normal' subjects. In the Health Professionals Follow-up Study, including 22,846 US men, self-reported low birth weight was associated with a higher frequency of hypertension and diabetes and high birth weight was associated with adult obesity [22]. Similar associations were seen in the Nurses' Health Study [23] in 92,940 women using self-reported birth weight.

Leon et al [24] reported a large cohort study of 13,282 singleton babies born in Uppsala, Sweden between 1915 to 1929 which survived beyond the first year of life. Using linkage and census data, the group was able to trace 97% of subjects and determine cardiovascular death rates. Although low birth weight was associated with increased cardiovascular death rates this trend was only seen in males. Leon proposed that reduced fetal growth rates rather than absolute birth weight was associated with cardiovascular mortality.

Forsén et al [25] were unable to demonstrate a statistically significant association between absolute birth weight and cardiovascular mortality in adulthood within a cohort of 3,302 men born in Helsinki, Finland between 1924 and 1933. Low ponderal index and cardiovascular mortality in adulthood were, however, significantly associated. This supported the Barker hypothesis that abnormal thinness at birth is associated with increased risk of cardiovascular disease in adulthood. Forsén also observed that men, whose mothers had low body mass index in pregnancy ($\leq$ 24 kgm^{-2}), exhibited a higher rate of cardiovascular disease compared to those born to mothers with a higher body mass index. This study suggests that if intra-uterine environment is important in the pathogenesis of cardiovascular disease then birth weight per se is a poor marker of intra-uterine nutrition.

ARGUMENTS AGAINST THE BARKER HYPOTHESIS

Birth weight alone may not be an important risk factor for the development of cardiovascular disease, impaired glucose tolerance and diabetes. Firstly, despite the large numbers of women studied in the Nurses' Health Study low birth weight was only associated with 2% of non-fatal cardiovascular disease [26]. Secondly, Carlsson et al [27] recently demonstrated, in a cross-sectional study of 2,237 men born in 1938-1957, that the association with low birth weight and diabetes or impaired glucose tolerance was most marked in those individuals of low birth weight with a strong family history of diabetes. Thirdly, Barker and colleagues adjust birth weight for current body mass index [28] and thus the positive effect of birth weight on current body mass index [21] is cancelled out. Current body mass index is a better predictor of insulin concentrations than birth weight [29] and this is in direct contradiction with the Barker hypothesis. Fourthly, one would expect that growth retardation in twins would lead to an increased risk of developing cardiovascular death, according to the Barker hypothesis, because twins have greatly restricted growth in the third trimester. Apparently, the mortality of twins after the age of 6 does not differ from the background population [30]. Fifthly, in Great Britain, the initial and current place of residence contribute equally to the risk of coronary heart disease and migrants seem to acquire the mortality risk from stroke of the area to which they move [31]. Sixthly, the Barker hypothesis predicts a link between a high ratio of placental weight to fetal weight and adult hypertension, but a recent study including 2,507 pregnant women concluded that the ratio of placental weight to birth weight is an inaccurate marker of fetal growth [32]. Other factors than birth weight may carry greater importance: these factors are maternal obesity [33], maternal smoking [34], maternal diabetes [35], and gestational age [36]. Seventhly, both maternal smoking and social class are well recognised as having a significant impact on birth weight in many other studies [28]. Barker and colleagues have never taken maternal smoking into account and the social class of the mothers did not associate with birth weight in their studies. Finally in 33,545 and 10,883 subjects from Israel, low birth weight and other factors associated with poor intrauterine nutrition were poorly or not associated with higher blood pressure in late adolescence [37,38] as shown in other studies [31-39].

To date no study has conclusively demonstrated that intra-uterine environment alone is an important determinant of chronic disease in adulthood and studies showing an inverse relationship between birth weight and blood pressure present a quite weak correlation.

BRENNER HYPOTHESIS

Glomerular number shows a wide biological variability in both humans (400,000 – 1,200,000) [40,41] and rats (20,000 – 35,000) [9-42]. Brenner et al, proposed that individuals with a mean glomerular number at the lower end of or below the physiological range are at increased risk of developing hypertension [3], due to a reduction in total filtration surface area. During the growth phase of a human being, hypertension may result in glomerular capillary hypertension and later on in glomerular sclerosis, which will further reduce the total glomerular filtration surface area, thus perpetuating a vicious cycle [43]. Intra-uterine growth retardation has been associated with a 35% reduction in glomerular number in humans [44]. Estimation of glomerular number in infants who died from non-renal causes in a neonatal intensive care unit [45] suggested that infants with a birth weight below the 10th percentile had 30% fewer nephrons, compared to infants that weighed above the 10th percentile. Retrospective autopsy studies in adults with a less marked reduction in birth weight have failed to demonstrate a clear association between low birth weight and reduced glomerular number [46].

The mechanism by which glomerular number is reduced is uncertain but exogenous factors acting on the fetus may be important. Vitamin A deficiency in rats is associated with renal abnormalities [47] and, in vitro, both retinol and retinoic acid have been shown to stimulate nephrogenesis [48]. Mild vitamin A deficiency in rats results in a 50% reduction in glomerular number in fetal kidneys [49]. Low circulating levels of Vitamin A occur in women who smoke, abuse alcohol or adopt extreme weight reducing diets in pregnancy [50,51]. It is uncertain whether this reduction in circulating levels of Vitamin A produces a clinically significant reduction in glomerular number in the offspring of humans. Animal studies have demonstrated a reduction in glomerular number with gentamicin [6,7,52] but this has not been confirmed in humans.

Surgical reduction in glomerular number by unilateral nephrectomy in childhood [53] and unilateral renal agenesis [54] are associated with increased risk of hypertension. In contrast the prevalence of hypertension following unilateral nephrectomy in adulthood is low [53]. These findings suggest that the early reduction in glomerular number may be important in the pathogenesis of hypertension but the majority of patients with hypertension have not undergone nephrectomy and do not have renal agenesis.

BARKER, BRENNER AND BABIES

The variation in expression of renal disease among, for example, diabetic patients could be explained by the large variation in glomerular number and size within these patients [55,56]. Those individuals born with a greater total glomerular filtration surface area would be less prone to develop diabetic nephropathy than those with a small total glomerular filtration surface area, due to a reduced haemodynamic burden on individual glomeruli. Thus, in diabetic subjects it is possible to unify the Barker and Brenner hypotheses: Intrauterine compromise, caused by any kind of mechanism, generates babies with a low birth weight. These smaller babies have smaller kidneys with fewer and/or smaller glomeruli. Fewer and/or smaller glomeruli result in decreased total glomerular filtration surface area, giving rise to individual glomerular hypertension due to a reduced renal functional reserve. The diabetic patients with the least and/or smallest glomeruli will then be more prone to develop irreversible renal failure when exposed to a renal insult in later life.

Unification of the Barker and Brenner hypothesis with respect to diabetic nephropathy is disputed. Only one study demonstrates a direct association between birth weight and proteinuria in diabetic subjects: In 45 patients with Type 1 diabetes of greater than 20 years duration, those patients without proteinuira had a greater birth weight than those with microalbuminuria or proteinuria [57]. Short stature in adulthood, which may reflect birth weight, has also been linked to the development of diabetic nephropathy [58].

Table 11-1. The sex, age, kidney weight, glomerular number and size, and birth weight on 19 normal persons and 26 Type 2 diabetic patients (from ref 46). Data are expressed as mean ± SD and (range) unless otherwise stated.

	Controls	Type 2 Diabetes
Sex (m = males f = females)	8m / 11f	14m / 12f
Age (years)	59 ± 16 (34 – 87)	63 ± 11 (35 – 85)
Kidney Weight (grams)	137 ± 36 (91 – 206)	150 ± 38 (82 – 228)
Glomerular number (10^3)	670 ± 176 (393 – 1056)	673 ± 200 (379 – 1124)
Mean glom. volume (10^6 μm^3)	6.25 ± 1.48 (3.95 – 8.97)	5.71 ± 1.74 (2.81 – 9.18)
Birth weight (grams)	3 577 ± 400 (2 900 – 4 250)	3 489 ± 429 (2 750 – 4 500)

Three other studies in non diabetic adult subjects support the unification of the hypothesis: 1) 23 young women with scarred kidneys but stable renal function weighed more at birth than 17 similar patients with progressive renal failure [59]. 2) Birth weights correlated with the gradients of reciprocal serum creatinine regression lines in 12 patients with idiopathic membranous glomerulonephropathy [60]. 3) Amongst the Aboriginal community, which has an extremely high rate of renal failure [61], multivariant analysis suggested that increasing body mass index and blood pressure and low birth weight act together to increase urine albumin excretion with age [62]. The latter study was, however, limited by incomplete ascertainment of birth weight amongst older subjects, the high rate of post-streptococcal glomerulonephritis in the population and the use of an albumin creatinine ratio from a single random urine sample to define abnormal urine albumin excretion.

Four recent studies challenge the unification of the hypothesis: 1) there was no difference in birth weight between 25 Type 1 diabetic patients without diabetic nephropathy and 22 patients with diabetic nephropathy [63]. 2) There was no correlation between low birth weight, few and/or small glomeruli or low kidney weight and there was no difference between the four parameters in 19 control subjects and 26 Type 2 diabetic patients. (See figures 11-1+2 and table 11-1) [46]. 3) In an epidemiological study of 620 Caucasian non-diabetic subjects there was no correlation between birth weight and blood pressure or between birth weight and urinary albumin excretion rate [64] .4) Eleven non-diabetic subjects exposed to intra-uterine starvation did not have higher urinary albumin excretion than controls [65].

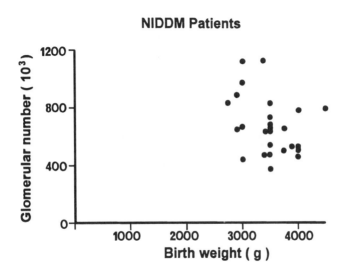

NIDDM Patients

Fig 11-1 There is no significant correlation (r = -0.33, p = 0.10) between birth weight and total glomerular number in 26 Type 2 diabetic subjects (from ref 46 with permission)

CONCLUSION
The unification of Brenner and Barker's hypothesis is deduced from observations suggesting that: low birth weight results in high blood pressure and impaired glucose tolerance in adult life; that low birth weight results in a low nephron number; and that low nephron number results in high blood pressure. In our opinion, it is likely that infants of very low birth weight (<2750g) at term may have fewer and/or smaller glomeruli. Recent data suggests that in normal persons and in Type 2 diabetes patients,

this association is of very limited importance, where many other factors may carry a far greater importance in a population where so few people have a very low birth weight.

Thus the hypothesis that low birth weight in a population of human beings should have a significant effect on the development of type 2 diabetes and smaller kidneys with few and/or small glomeruli seems relatively unimportant. It is therefore difficult to support the unification of the Brenner and Barker hypothesis with regard to diabetic kidney disease at this point in time.

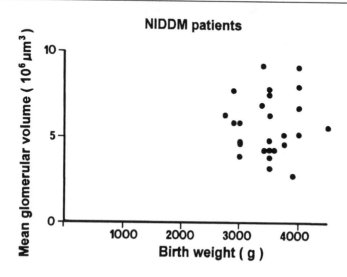

Fig 11.2 There is no significant correlation ($r = 0.06$, $p = 0.78$) between birth weight and mean glomerular volume in 26 Type 2 diabetic subjects (from ref 46 with permission)

ACKNOWLEDGEMENTS

The authors have been supported by The Danish Heart Foundation, Leo Nielsen's Foundation, The Foundation for Advancement of Medical Research, and Northern and Yorkshire NHS Executive Research Training Fellowship.

REFERENCES

1.   Barker D. Fetal and infant orgins of adult disease. London, 1992.
2.   Barker D. Mothers, babies and disease in later life. London, 1994.
3.   Brenner B, Garcia D, Anderson S. Glomeruli and blood pressure: less of one and more of the other? 1988;1:335-347.
4.   Bard J, Wolf A. Nephrogenesis and the development of renal disease. Nephrol Dial Transplant 1992;7:563-572.

5. Bard J. Traction and the formation of mesenchymal condensations in vitro. BioEssays 1990;12:389-393.

6. Gilbert T, Lelièvre-Pérgorier M, Merlet-Bénichou C. Immediate and long-term renal effects of fetal exposure to gentamicin. Pediat Nephrol 1990;8:175-180.

7. Gilbert T, Lelièvre-Pégorier M, Merlet-Bénichou C. Long-term effects of mild oligonephronia induced in utero by gentamicin in the rat. Pediat Res 1991;30:450-456.

8. Zeman F. Effects of maternal protein restriction on the kidneys of newborn young of rats. J Nutrition 1968;94:111-116.

9. Merlet-Bénichou C, Gilbert T, Muffat-Joly M, Lelièrvre-Pérgorier M, Leroy B. Intrauterine growth retardation leads to a permanent nephron deficit in the rat. Pediat Nephrol 1994;8:175-180.

10. Barker D, Osmond C, Winter P, Margetts B, Simmonds S. Weight in infancy and death from ischaemic heart disease. Lancet 1989:577-580.

11. Barker D, Osmond C. Diet and coronary heart disease in England and Wales during and after the second world war. J Epidemiol Comm Health 1986;40(1):37-44.

12. Barker D, Osmond C. Death rates from stroke in England and Wales predicted from past maternal mortality. Br Med J 1987;295:83-86.

13. Shaper A, Pocock S, Walker M, Cohen N, Wade C, Thomson A. British regional heart study: cardiovascular risk factors in middle-aged men in 24 towns. Br Med J 1981;283:179-186.

14. Barker D, Bull A, Osmond C, Simmonds S. Fetal and placental size and risk of hypertension in adult life. Br Med J 1990;302:259-262.

15. Barker D, Hales C, Fall C, Osmond C, Phipps K, Clark P. Type 2 (non-insulin dependent) diabetes mellitus, hypertension and hyperlipidaemia (syndrome X): relation to reduced fetal growth. Diabetologia 1993;36:62-67.

16. Edwards C, Benediktsson R, Lindsay R, Seckle J. Dysfunction of placental glucocorticoid barrier: link between fetal environment and adult hypertension? Lancet 1993;341:355-357.

17. Garrett P, Bass P, Sanderman D. Barker and babies - early environment and renal disease in adulthood. J Pathol 1994;173:299-300.

18. Benediktsson R, Lindsay R, Noble J, Seckle J, Edwards C. Glucocorticoid exposure in utero: new model for adult hypertension. Lancet 1993;341:339-341.

19. Lumey L, Stein A. Offspring birth weights after maternal intrauterine undernutrition: a comparison within sibships. Am J Epidemiol 1997;146:801-809.

20. Stanner S, Bulmer K, Andres C, Lantseva O, Borodina V, Poteen V, Yudkin J. Does malnutrition in utero determine diabetes and coronary heart disease in adulthood? Results from the Leningrad siege, a cross sectional study. Br Med J 1997;315:1342-1348.

21. Jackson A, Langley-Evan S, McCarthy H. Nutritional influences in early life upon obesity and other body proportions. Ciba Foundation Symposium 1996;201:118-129.

22. Curhan G, Willett W, Rimm E, Spiegelman D, Ascherio A, Stampfer M. Birth weight and adult hypertension,diabetes mellitus and obesity in US men. Circulation 1996;94:1310-1315.

23. Curhan G, Chetow G, Willett W, Spiegelman D, Colditz G, Manson J, Spiezer F, Stampfer M. Birth weight and adult hypertension, and obesity in US women. Circulation 1996;94:1310-1315.

24. Leon D, Lithell H, Vagero D, Koupilova I, Mohsen R, Berglund L, Lithell U-B, McKeigue P. Reduced fetal growth rate and increased risk of death from ischaemic heart disease: cohort study of 15 000 Swedish men and women born 1915-29. Br Med J 1998;317:241-245.

25.   Forsén T, Eriksson J, Tuomielehto J, Teramo K, Osmond C, Barker D. Mother's weight in pregnancy and coronary heart disease in a cohort of Finnish men: follow up study. Br Med J 1997;315:837 - 840.

26.   Rich-Edwards J, Stampfer M, Manson J, Rosner B, Hankinson S, Colditz G, Willett W, Hennekens C. Birth weight and risk of cardiovascular disease in a cohort of women followed up since 1976. Br Med J 1997;315:396-400.

27.   Carlsson S, Persson P-G, Alvarsson M, Efendic S, Norman A, Svanström L, Östenson C-G, Grill V. Low birth weight, family history of diabetes, and glucose intolerance in Swedish middle-aged men. Diabetes Care 1999;22(7):1043-1047.

28.   Paneth N, Susser M. Early origins of coronary heart disese ("the Barker Hypothesis"). Br Med J 1995;310:411-412.

29.   Fall C, Osmond C, Barker D, Clark P, Hales C, Stirling Y, Meade T. Fetal and infant growth and cardiovascular risk factors in women. Br Med J 1995;310:428-432.

30.   Christensen K, Vaupel J, Holm N, Yashin A. Mortality among twins after age 6: fetal origins hypothesis vs twin method. Br Med J 1995;310:432-427.

31.   Strachan D, Leon D, Dodgeon B. Mortality from cardiovascular disease among interregional migrants in England and Wales. Br Med J 1995;310:423-436.

32.   Williams L, Evans S, Newham J. Prospective cohort study of the factors influencing the relative weights of the placenta and the newborn infant. Br Med J 1997;314:1864-1868.

33.   Perry I, Beevers D, Whincup P, Beresford D. Predictors of ratio of placental weight to fetal weight in a multiethnic community. Br Med J 1995;310:436-439.

34.   Beaulac-Baillargeon L, Desrosiers C. Caffeine-cigarette interaction on fetal growth. Am J Obstet Gynae 1987;157:1236-1240.

35.   Clarson C, Tevaarweek G, Harding P, Chance G, Haust M. Placental weight in diabetic pregnancies. Placenta 1989;10:275-281.

36.   Dombrowski M, Berry S, Johnson M, Saleh A, Sokol R. Birth weight-length ratios, ponderal indexes, placental weights and birth weight-placenta ratios in a large population. Arch Pediat Adoles Med 1994;148:508-512.

37.   Seidman D, Laor A, Galc R, Stevenson D, Mashiach S, Danon Y. Birth weight, current body weight and blood pressure in late adolescence. Br Med J 1991;302:1235-1237.

38.   Laor A, Stevenson DK, Sherner J, Gale R, Seidman D. Size at birth, maternal nutritional status in pregnancy and blood pressure at age 17: population based analysis. Br Med J 1997;315:449-453.

39.   Macintyre S, Watt G, West P, Ecob R. Correlates of blood pressure in 15 year olds in the west of Scotland. J Epidemiol Community Health 1991;45:143-147.

40.   Moore R. The total number of glomeruli in the normal human kidney. Anat Rec 1931;48:153-68.

41.   Tischer C, Madsen K. Anatomy of the kidney. In: Brenner B, Rector FJ, editors. The Kidney. 3rd ed. Philadelphia: W B Saunders, 1986:3-60.

42.   Larsson L, Aperia A, Wilton P. Effect of normal development on compensatory renal growth. Kidney Int 1980;18:29-35.

43.   Brenner B, Chertow G. Congentital oligonephropathy and the etiology of adult hypertension and progressive renal injury. Am J Kidney Dis 1994;23:171-175.

44.   Hinchcliffe S, Lynch M, Sargent P, Howard C, van Velzen D. The effect of intra-uterine growth retardation on the development of nephrons. Br J Obstet Gynaecol 1992;99:296-301.

45.   Leroy B, Josset P, Morgan G, Costill J, Merlet-Bénichou C. Intrauterine growth retardation (IUGR) an nephron deficit: Preliminary study in man. Pediatric Nephrol 1992;6:3.

46. Nyengaard J, Bendtsen T, Mogensen C. Low birth weight - is it associated with few and small glomeruli in normal subjects and NIDDM patients? Diabetologia 1996;39:1634-1637.

47. Wilson J, Warkney J. Malformations in the genito-urinary tract induced by maternal vitamin A deficiency in the rat. Am J Anat 1948;83:357-407.

48. Vilar J, Gilbert T, Moreau E, Merlet-Bénichou C. Metanephros organogenesis is highly stimulated by vitamin A derivatives in organ culture. Kidney Int 1996;49:1478 - 1487.

49. Lelièvre-Pégorier M, Villar J, Ferrier M, Moreau E, Freund N, Gilbert T, Merlet-Bénichou C. Mild Vitamin A deficiency leads to inborn nephron deficit in the rat. Kidney Int 1998;54:1455-1462.

50. Gerster H. Vitamin A: Functions, dietary requirements and safety in humans. In J Vitam Nutr Res 1997; 67:71-90.

51. Bonjour J. Vitamins and alcoholism IX. Vitamin A. Int J Vitam Nutr Res 1981;51:166-177.

52. Gilbert T, Lelièvre- Pérgorier M, Maliénou R, Meulemans A, Merlet-Bénichou C. Effects of prenatal and post natal exposure to gentamicin on renal differentiation in the rat. Toxicology 1987;43:301-313.

53. Hakim R, Goldszer R, Brenner B. Hypertension and proteinuria: Long-term sequelae of unilateral nephrectomy. Kidney Int 1984;25:930-936.

54. Argueso L, Ritchley M, Boyle E, Milliner D, Bergstralh E, Kramer S. Prognosis of patients with unilateral agenesis. Pediatr Nephrol 1992;6:412-416.

55. Nyengaard J, Bendtsen T. Glomerular number and size in relation to age, kidney weight and body surface in normal man. Anat Rec 1992;232:194-201.

56. Bendtsen T, Nyengaard J. The number of glomeruli in Type 1 (insulin dependent) and Type 2 (non-insulin dependent) diabetic patients. Diabetologia 1992;35:844-850.

57. Sanderman D, Reza M, Phillips D, Barker D, Osmond C, Leatherdale B. Why do some type 1 diabetics develop nephropathy? A possible role of birthweight. Diabetic Med 1992;9(Suppl.1):36A.

58. Rossing P, Tarnow L, Neilsen F, Boelskiftes S, Brenner B, Parving H-H. Short stature and diabetic nephropathy. Br Med J 1995;310:296-297.

59. Garrett P, Sandeman D, Reza M, Rogerson M, Bass P, Dunca R, Dathan J. Weight at birth and renal disease in adulthood. Nephrol. Dial. Transplant 1993;8:920.

60. Duncan R, Bass P, Garrett P, Dathan J. Weight at birth and other factors influencing progression of idiopathic membranous nephropathy. Nephrol. Dial. Transplant 1994;9:871-880.

61. Hoy W, Mathews J, Pugsley D, Hayhurst B, Rees M, Kile E, Walker K, Wang Z. The multidimensional nature of renal disease: Rates and associations of albuminuria in an Australian Aboriginal community. Kidney Int 1998;54:1296-1304.

62. Hoy W, Rees M, Kile E, Mathews J, Wang Z. A new dimension to the Barker hypothesis: Low birth weight and susceptibility to renal disease. Kidney Int 1999;56:1072-1077.

63. Eshøj O, Vaag A, Feldt-Rasmussen B, Borch-Johnsen K, Beck-Nielsen H. No evidence of low birth weight as a risk factor for diabetic nephropathy in type 1 diabetic patients. Diabetologia 1995;38(Suppl 1):A 222.

64. Vestbo E, Damsgaard E, Frøland A, Mogensen CE. Birth weight and cardiovascular factors in an epidemiological study. Diabetologia 1996;39:1598-1602.

65. Yudkin J, Philips D, Stanner S. Proteinuria and progressive renal disease: birth weight and microalbuminuria. Nephrol Dial Trans 1997;12(Suppl 2):10 - 13.

12. EFFECTS OF INSULIN ON THE KIDNEY AND THE CARDIOVASCULAR SYSTEM

Ele Ferrannini, MD and Monica Nannipieri, MD
Department of Internal Medicine and Metabolism Unit, C N R Institute of Clinical Physiology at the University of Pisa School of Medicine, Pisa, Italy

THE CARDIOVASCULAR SYSTEM

The concept that exogenous insulin administration may be associated with haemodynamic changes has appeared in the literature soon after the purified hormone became available for use in humans (eg [1]). Subsequently, however, these changes have mostly been ascribed to the counter-regulatory hormone response to insulin-induced hypoglycaemia. It has not been until the introduction of the glucose clamp technique, by which hyperinsulinaemia can be uncoupled from hypoglycaemia, that the existence of specific vascular actions of the hormone has been recognised. Interest has initially focussed on insulin-induced vasodilatation [2]; more recently, a wider range of haemodynamic effects of insulin has been characterised, and their possible physiological significance is beginning to be appreciated.

BLOOD FLOW

Against a background of mostly negative reports, the careful studies of Baron and his co-workers [3] have established that insulin infusion with maintenance of glycaemia is followed by an increase in leg blood flow in healthy, young volunteers. Typically in these studies [3,4], following a few hours of euglycaemic hyperinsulinaemia (in the range of 300-700 pmol/l) leg blood flow, as measured by thermodilution, rose approximately 2-fold above baseline values in resting subjects under controlled experimental conditions.

As this effect was found to be blunted in patients with insulin resistance of glucose uptake (obese [3], hypertensive [5] or diabetic [6,7]), Baron [8] pioneered the interpretation that insulin-induced vasodilatation, by increasing substrate and hormone delivery to target tissues such as skeletal muscle, is a physiological determinant of insulin action on glucose uptake. Both the basic observation and its interpretation have been challenged, and still are a subject of controversy. Discrepancies have been imputed to the technique for measuring blood flow (indicator dilution, thermodilution, venous occlusion plethysmography, Doppler ultrasound, positron-emitting tomography [PET]), the limb tested (forearm vs calf), the dose and duration of insulin administration, and the selection of study subjects. As recently reviewed [9], insulin exposure (ie dose x time) and limb muscularity appear to be more important factors than the anatomical site or the experimental technique in contributing to the variability of insulin-induced vasodilatation.

By compiling a vast amount of data in the literature, the relationship between insulin exposure (with the hormone infused locally - through the brachial or femoral artery - or systemically through a forearm vein) and changes in blood flow (forearm or calf) can be schematised as depicted in Fig. 12-1: within the physiological range of insulin exposure (the darker shade), limb blood flow may rise up to 30% of its baseline value, with a rather wide scatter of the results depending on the experimental circumstances.

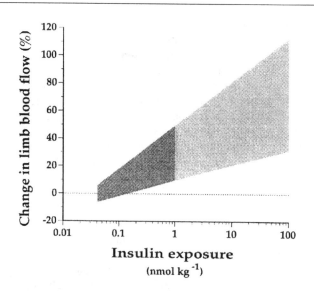

Fig. 12-1 Relationship between insulin exposure (expressed as total amount infused per kilogram of body weight or per 10 kg of forearm muscle, for systemic intravenous and local intra-arterial administration, respectively) and percent change in limb blood flow (re-calculated from ref. 8).

Thus, insulin does have intrinsic, if weak, vasoactive properties. The physiological impact of insulin-induced vasodilatation on glucose metabolism is, however, marginal on several accounts. Firstly, resting skeletal muscle has a low extraction coefficient for glucose, and is therefore little sensitive to changes in blood flow. Recent PET studies [10] have demonstrated that leg muscle blood flow is distributed in a heterogeneous pattern, and that glucose uptake co-localises with higher perfusion rates in response to strong insulin stimulation. These findings, however, may simply reflect regional differences in muscle fibre composition, as oxidative type I fibres are both more sensitive to insulin and more richly capillarised [11]. By itself, co-localisation of flow and metabolism does not prove that insulin actually recruits previously unperfused or underperfused areas, thereby exposing more tissue to its metabolic action. In addition, relative to the time-course of insulin action on glucose extraction, insulin vasodilatation is a late phenomenon [12,13]. Finally, in the forearm of insulin resistant subjects, insulin-mediated extraction of glucose is impaired but the exchange of other substrates (lactate, pyruvate, and lipid substrates) is not appreciably different from that of insulin sensitive individuals [14]. This observation argues against significant flow-limitation of glucose uptake during insulin stimulation. In keeping with this, insulin vasodilatation has been reported to be unaltered in native states of insulin resistance (type 1 diabetes [15], type 2 diabetes [10,16], essential hypertension [7], and familial hypertension [18]). Moreover, in insulin resistant patients with essential hypertension the intra-arterial infusion of an endogenous vasodilator, adenosine [19], or of a direct nitric oxide donor, sodium nitroprusside [20], fails to overcome the insulin resistance. On the other hand, local co-infusion of high doses of vitamin C - which oppose endogenous peroxidation - induces an increase in forearm blood flow that is not accompanied by an enhanced uptake of arterial glucose [21]. Collectively, these observations indicate that exposure to acute insulinisation is followed by some increase in limb blood flow, but this haemodynamic effect is of limited consequence for insulin stimulation of glucose uptake within the physiological range of insulin concentrations in humans.

The mechanism by which insulin increases blood flow is interesting. Neither adrenergic nor cholinergic blockade abolishes insulin-induced stimulation of calf blood flow [22], whilst both NG-monomethyl-L-arginine (L-NMMA), a competitive inhibitor of nitric oxide (NO) synthase [23,24], and ouabain, which blocks the insulin-stimulatable sodium potassium pump, have been shown to antagonise insulin-induced vasodilatation [25,26].

Furthermore, in both normal subjects and patients with essential hypertension local insulin infusion in physiological amounts potentiates acetylcholine-induced vasodilatation [27]. The exact site of this action of insulin, whether endothelial or smooth muscle cells, is not known. Both cell types carry insulin receptors as well as Na^+-K^+-ATPase activity in their plasma membrane [28,29], and can synthesise and release NO. In cultured smooth muscle [30], insulin attenuates agonist-induced increases in intracellular calcium concentrations, thereby causing relaxation. This effect may be due to antagonism of inositol-triphosphate-sensitive calcium release from intracellular stores. As L-NMMA blocks the insulin-induced decrease in cytosolic calcium in smooth muscle cells, NO-mediated increases in cyclic nucleotides (both cAMP and cGMP) appear to be involved [31]. In turn, NO can activate Na^+-K^+-ATPase in a cGMP-independent fashion [32]. In endothelial cells, on the other hand, activation of Na^+-K^+-ATPase leads to a rise in intracellular calcium, which would stimulate synthesis and release of NO [33]. Thus, insulin impacts on a regulatory system involving at least two tissues - the endothelium and the underlying smooth muscle -and two effectors - NO and Na^+-K^+-ATPase - which interact in a complex fashion to elicit vasodilatation.

Clearly, additional investigation is needed to understand the cellular basis of insulin-induced vasodilatation. While the weight of evidence indicates that insulin-mediated vasodilatation is endothelium-dependent, endothelial dysfunction per se does not appear to segregate either with insulin resistance of glucose metabolism or with insulin resistance of vasodilatation. Thus, both in normotensive subjects [34] and hypertensive patients [35], acetylcholine-induced vasodilatation is similar in very insulin-resistant and insulin sensitive individuals; conversely, insulin-mediated vasodilatation is intact in obese individuals in whom bradykinin-mediated vasodilatation is impaired [36].

BLOOD VOLUME
Recent studies [37] have shown that administration of insulin in physiological amounts under euglycaemic conditions leads to a 3% rise in haematocrit and a 7% reduction in blood volume, ie haemoconcentration. This effect, if small in size, is consistent, and is closely related to the concomitant change in diastolic blood pressure levels (Fig. 12-2).

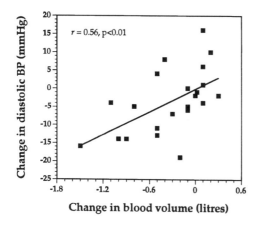

Fig. 12-2 Direct relationship between concomitant changes in blood volume and diastolic blood pressure induced by physiological hyperinsulinaemia (~600 pmol/l) under euglycaemic conditions. Note that the regression line predicts a 1 mmHg fall in blood pressure for each 0.1 litre decrease in blood volume.

Loss of intravascular water to the extravascular space could be due to redistribution of blood flow to capillary beds with higher hydrostatic or lower oncotic pressure. Alternatively, insulin could vasoconstrict post-capillary venules, thereby leading to a generalised increase of the hydrostatic pressure in the capillary bed. The latter explanation is compatible with insulin-induced activation of the adrenergic nervous system (see below).

CARDIAC OUTPUT AND BLOOD PRESSURE

During systemic insulin administration at physiological doses, cardiac output increases by 10-15% as a result of a slight but consistent acceleration of heart rate (2 bpm on average) coupled with an increase in stroke volume [38]. These haemodynamic responses are mediated by adrenergic activation, as documented by a dose-dependent rise in circulating noradrenaline concentrations [39], an enhanced firing rate in the sympathetic fibres of the peroneal nerve, as measured by microneurography [4], and an upward shift in the sympathetic/vagal activity ratio, as measured by spectral analysis of heart rate variability [38]. The overall effect of simultaneous changes in cardiac output, blood volume, and peripheral vascular resistance in response to euglycaemic hyperinsulinaemia is maintenance of mean arterial blood pressure [38].

This, however, is a compound of opposite changes in systolic and diastolic blood pressure. The former, in fact, tends to increase as cardiac dynamics are excited by enhanced adrenergic discharge, while the latter decreases due to the drop in peripheral vascular resistances (Table 12-1). It is interesting to note that the effects of insulin on the cardiovascular system are mediated by both peripheral reflexes and direct central neural influences.

Table 12-1. Haemodynamic effects of insulin under euglycaemic conditions

Effect	Change	Mechanism
Stroke volume	↑	Adrenergic stimulation
Heart rate	↑	Adrenergic stimulation
Blood volume	↓	Haemoconcentration
Peripheral vascular resistance	↓	Vasodilatation
Systolic blood pressure	↑	Adrenergic stimulation
Diastolic blood pressure	↓	Vasodilatation
Mean blood pressure	⇔	

Thus, direct relaxation of resistance arteries by insulin evokes tachycardia through the unloading of arterial baroreceptors, a reflex arch that involves central relays. In addition, insulin appears to directly desensitise the sinoatrial node to the baroreflex control of heart rate [38]. Mounting evidence [40], however, indicates that insulin, by trespassing (by transcytosis) the blood-brain barrier in the periventricular area, binds to neurons in the arcuate and paraventricular nuclei, which then send inhibitory impulses to the vagus and excitatory impulses to the sympathetic nuclei. This reaction is completed by the release of corticotropin releasing hormone (CRH), which orchestrates a response including stimulation of cortisol and prolactin release and depression of growth hormone and thyroid stimulating hormone [38,41]. Overall, even in the absence of hypoglycaemia the cardiovascular system responds to acute insulin administration with a moderate, specific stress reaction. The full physiological significance and the possible pathophysiological implications of this response in states of chronic hyperinsulinaemia and insulin resistance - such as obesity and early stages of human diabetes - remain to be established; collectively, they appear to enhance cardiovascular risk.

THE KIDNEY

Insulin and glomerular function

With regard to the effect of insulin on glomerular filtration rate (GFR), observations in the isolated kidney, in experimental animals, and in humans have yielded contradictory results, as decreased, increased or unchanged GFRs have all been reported (reviewed in [42]). In healthy subjects under conditions of forced water diuresis - when changes in plasma volume are prevented - euglycaemic hyperinsulinaemia did not affect GFR [43]. Likewise, in a dose-response study in type 1 diabetic patients under fasting conditions, insulin was without significant effect on GFR [44]. Neither renal plasma flow (as measured with ^{131}I-hippuran) nor renal vascular resistances are affected by acute insulin administration. The role of plasma glucose concentration itself in the induction and/or maintenance of hyperfiltration has been controversial. During oral glucose loading, if large fluid volumes are co-administered, plasma volume and, in turn, GFR will increase.

On the other hand, a large glucose delivery to the proximal tubule could increase hydrostatic pressure in the tubular lumen, thereby leading to decreased GFR. Collectively, it appears that hyperglycaemia may be associated with small changes in GFR in either direction depending on factors such as duration of hyperglycaemia, hydration, and urine flow. An important question is whether insulin affects glomerular permeability to albumin and other proteins.

We recently examined the acute effect of insulin on the systemic transcapillary escape rate (as measured by the ^{131}I-labelled albumin technique) and the urinary excretion of albumin under time-controlled, steady-state conditions of glucose concentrations, urine output, blood pressure, and creatinine clearance [38]. While producing no significant change in albumin exit from the vascular compartment, physiological hyperinsulinaemia increased urinary albumin excretion by 50% in normoalbuminuric patients with type 2 diabetes but not in healthy subjects. In these patients, this effect was accompanied by an enhanced excretion of N-acetyl-β-D-glucosaminidase and retinol-binding protein - which are released and reabsorbed in the proximal tubule, respectively -, whereas the excretion of two proteins handled by the distal tubule (Tamm-Horsfall protein and epidermal growth factor) was unaffected (Fig. 12-3). These findings lend support to the notion that even modest increments in the glomerular permeability of albumin decrease the reabsorptive capacity of the proximal tubules, thereby leading to leakage of other tubular proteins. Moreover, this tubular albumin overload is intrinsically toxic to the interstitium, where it leads to the over-expression of inflammatory and vasoactive molecules [45,46]. Thus, perturbation of the glomerulo-tubular feed-back, rather than solely an increase in glomerular permeability, may be the trigger for nephropathy. In this context, the interaction between insulin and hyperglycaemia on glomerulo-tubular function deserves further investigation as it may be an early sign of renal involvement in diabetes.

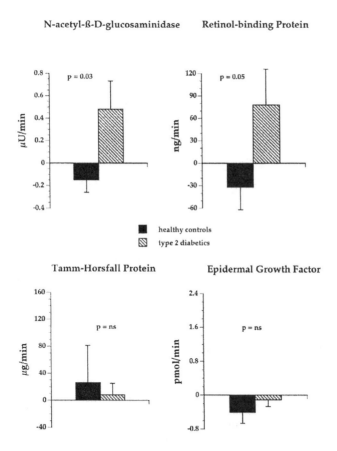

Fig. 12-3. Renal excretion of tubular proteins in response to isoglycaemic hyperinsulinaemia in healthy subjects and patients with type 2 diabetes. Bars are mean (±1 SE) changes in excretion between normoinsulinaemia and hyperinsulinaemia under steady-state conditions (redrawn from reference 37).

INSULIN AND TUBULAR FUNCTION

Specific binding of insulin is greatest in the thick ascending limb and distal convoluted tubules [47]. Insulin has been found to stimulate sodium transport in proximal tubules in the rabbit [48], and to increase chloride reabsorption by the loop segment in the rat [49]. Human studies, however, have indicated that the anti-natriuretic action of insulin takes place in the distal tubule [50,51]. Whether insulin affects sodium absorption by a direct effect on the renal tubules or through modulation of local or systemic factors that control sodium chloride reabsorption is still uncertain. Friedberg et al. [52], for example, reported that the anti-natriuretic effect of insulin could no longer be observed when insulin-induced hypokalaemia was prevented by a simultaneous potassium administration. To test this hypothesis, we performed oral glucose tolerance tests with or without potassium replacement in a group of healthy subjects [53].

Moreover, to determine whether the anti-natriuretic effect of insulin is preserved in patients with impaired insulin action on glucose metabolism, a group of non-diabetic patients with essential hypertension was also studied. We found that healthy individuals and hypertensive patients exhibited similar insulin anti-natriuresis whether or not exogenous potassium was given to clamp serum potassium at basal levels.

Also, insulin anti-natriuresis was independent of the presence of metabolic (= glucose metabolism) insulin resistance. The discordance with the results of Friedberg et al. [52] may depend on the differences between their experimental conditions (forced water diuresis, euglycaemic hyperinsulinaemia) and ours (maintenance of basal urine output, hyperglycaemic hyperinsulinaemia). In fact, in vitro studies have shown that glucose increases anti-natriuresis due to enhanced glucose-sodium co-transport at the level of the convoluted proximal tubule [48]. In vivo studies using lithium clearance have demostrated that proximal sodium reabsorption is stimulated by hyperglycaemia in rats [54]; in patients with type 1 diabetes, sodium excretion is lower under hyperglycaemic than euglycaemic conditions [55]. At least in part, the effect of hyperglycaemia can be ascribed to the brush-border sodium co-transport, where the glucose:sodium stoichiometry is 1:2 [56]. In a series of elegant studies, Nosadini et al. [57] found that patients with type 2 diabetes and metabolic insulin resistance retained more sodium than non-diabetic subjects at similar plasma glucose concentrations and filtered glucose.

Moreover, at comparable degrees of hyperglycaemia the more insulin resistant patients exhibited more sodium retention, suggesting that metabolic insulin resistance may be coupled with an intrinsic renal abnormality.

In summary, both insulin alone and hyperglycaemia restrain renal sodium excretion; the most probable sites of action are the proximal tubule for hyperglycaemia, the distal portions of the nephron for insulin (though the latter is still somewhat uncertain). These two actions are combined in the physiological response to feeding [53]. Most importantly, in individuals with insulin resistance of glucose metabolism - ie diabetic [57], hypertensive [58], or obese [59] patients - insulin anti-natriuresis is preserved.

Thus, the compensatory hyperinsulinaemia of insulin resistant subjects imposes a chronic anti-natriuretic pressure on the kidney. This may play a role in the development or maintenance of high blood pressure. Insulin has a major role in potassium homeostasis. In dose-response studies in humans [60], euglycaemic hyperinsulinaemia stimulated potassium uptake by both liver and peripheral tissues. Insulin-induced hypokalaemia is accompanied by a reduction in urinary potassium excretion. Insulin does not appear to have a direct effect on renal potassium handling, however. Thus, in our own studies [53] the anti-kaliuretic response to oral glucose was abolished when insulin-induced hypokalaemia was prevented. Importantly, when plasma potassium concentrations were clamped at their basal levels, glucose-induced insulin secretion was significantly heightened [53]. Thus, insulin modulates renal potassium excretion and its own release by the β-cell through the same signal, ie hypokalaemia. This constitutes a dual feedback loop, or glucose-potassium cycle, which serves the function of storing glucose and potassium in cells while limiting the risk of hypoglycaemia. Sodium and uric acid excretion parallel one another under many physiological conditions [61,62]. During euglycaemic hyperinsulinaemia, serum uric acid levels and creatinine clearance do not change, whereas the clearance rate and fractional excretion of uric acid decrease by 30%. The change in uric acid excretion is significantly related to the concomitant fall in urinary sodium excretion [63]. In patients with essential hypertension [58] and in obese subjects (unpublished observations), we have found that the anti-uricosuric effect of insulin is maintained, and thus is independent of metabolic insulin resistance. The finding that uric acid and sodium urinary excretion are both restrained by physiological hyperinsulinaemia provides an explanation for the clustering of hyperuricaemia with insulin resistant states such as hypertension, obesity, and diabetes mellitus [64,65].

REFERENCES

1.   Zierler KL. Theory of the use of arteriovenous concentration differences for measuring metabolism in steady state and non-steady states. J Clin Invest 1961; 40:2111-2125

2.   Steinberg HO, Chaker H, Leaming R, Johnson A, Brechtel G, Baron AD. Obesity/insulin resistance is associated with endothelial dysfunction. Implications for the syndrome of insulin resistance. J Clin Invest 1996; 97:2601-2610

3.   Laakso M, Edelman SV, Brechtel G, Baron AD. Decreased effect of insulin to stimulate skeletal muscle blood flow in obese man. J Clin Invest 1990; 85:1844-1852

4.   Anderson EA, Hoffman RP, Balon TW, Sinkey CA, Mark AL. Hyperinsulinemia produces both sympathetic neural activation and vasodilatation in normal humans. J Clin Invest 1991; 87:2246-2252

5.   Baron AD, Brechtel-Hook G, Johnson A, Hardin D. Skeletal muscle blood flow. A possible link between insulin resistance and blood pressure. Hypertension 1993; 21:129-135

6.   Baron AD, Laakso M, Brechtel G, Edelman SV. Mechanism of insulin resistance in insulin-dependent diabetes mellitus: a major role for reduced skeletal muscle blood flow. J Clin Endocrinol Metab 1991; 73:637-643

7.   Laakso M, Edelman SV, Brechtel G, Baron AD. Impaired insulin-mediated skeletal muscle blood flow in patients with NIDDM. Diabetes 1992;41: 1076-1083

8.   Baron AD, Steinberg HO, Chaker H, Leaming R, Johnson A, Brechtel G. Insulin-mediated skeletal muscle vasodilatation contributes to both insulin sensitivity and responsiveness in lean humans. J Clin Invest 1995; 96:786-792

9.   Yki-Järvinen H, Utriainen T. Insulin-induced vasodilatation: physiology or pharmacology? Diabetologia 1998; 41:369-379

10. Utriainen T, Nuutila P, Takala T, Vicini P, Ruotsalainen U, Rönnemaa T, Tolvanen T, Raitakari M, Haaparanta M, Kirvelä O, Cobelli C, Yki-Järvinen H. Intact insulin stimulation of skeletal muscle blood flow, its heterogeneity and redistribution but not of glucose uptake in non-insulin-dependent diabetes mellitus. J Clin Invest 1997; 100:777-785

11. Utriainen T, Holmäng A, Björntorp P, Mäkimattila S, Sovijärvi A, Lindholm H, Yki-Järvinen H. Physical fitness, muscle morphology and insulin-stimulated limb blood flow in normal subjects. Am J Physiol 1996; 270:E905-E911

12. Utriainen T, Malmström R, Mäkimattila S, Yki-Järvinen H. Methodological aspects, dose-response characteristics and causes of inter-individual variation in insulin stimulation of limb blood flow in normal subjects. Diabetologia 1995; 38:555-564

13. Tack CJJ, Schefman AEP, Willems JL, Thien T, Lutterman JA, Smits P. Direct vasodilator effects of physiological hyperinsulinaemia in human skeletal muscle. Eur J Clin Invest 1996; 26:772-778

14. Natali A, Santoro D, Palombo C, Cerri M, Ghione S, Ferrannini E. Impaired insulin action on skeletal muscle metabolism in essential hypertension. Hypertension 1991; 17:170-178

15. Mättimakila S, Virtamäki A, Malmström R, Utriainen T, Yki-Järvinen H. Insulin resistance in type I diabetes mellitus: a major role for reduced glucose extraction. J Clin Endocrinol Metab 1996; 81:707-712

16. Tack CJJ, Smits P, Willemsen JJ, Lenders JWM, Thien T, Lutterman JA. Effects of insulin on vascular tone and sympathetic nervous system in NIDDM. Diabetes 1996; 45:15-22

17. Hunter SJ, Harper R, Ennis CN, Sheridan B, Atkinson AB, Bell PM. Skeletal muscle blood flow is not a determinant of insulin resistance in essential hypertension. J Hypertens 1997; 15:73-77

18. Hulten UL, Endre T, Mattiasson I, Berglund G. Insulin and forearm vasodilatation in hypertension-prone men. Hypertension 1995; 25:214-218

19. Natali A, Bonadonna R, Santoro D, Quiñones Galvan A, Baldi S, Frascerra S, Palombo C, Ghione S, Ferrannini E. Insulin resistance and vasodilatation in essential hypertension. Studies with adenosine. J Clin Invest 1994; 94:1570-1576

20. Natali A, Quiñones Galvan A, Toschi E, Pecori N, Sanna G, Ferrannini E. Vasodilation with sodium nitroprusside does not improve insulin action in essential hypertension. Hypertension 1998; 31:632-636

21. Natali A, Sironi AM, Toschi E, Camastra S, Sanna G, Perissinotto A, Taddei S, and Ferrannini E. Effect of vitamin C on forearm blood flow and glucose metabolism in essential hypertension. (in press)

22. Randin D, Vollenweider P, Tappy L, Jequier E, Nicod P, Scherrer U. Effects of adrenergic and cholinergic blockade on insulin-induced stimulation of calf blood flow in humans. Am J Physiol 1994; 266:R809-R816

23. Steinberg HO, Brechtel G, Johson A, Fireberg N, Baron AD. Insulin-mediated skeletal muscle vasodilatation is nitric oxide dependent. A novel action of insulin to increase nitric oxide release. J Clin Invest 1994; 94:1172-1179

24. Scherrer U, Randin D, Vollenweider P, Vollenweider L, Nicod P. Nitric oxide release accounts for insulin's vascular effects in humans. J Clin Invest 1994; 94:2511-2615

25. Ferrannini E, Taddei S, Santoro D, Natali A, Boni C, Del Chiaro D, Buzzigoli G. Independent stimulation of glucose metabolism and Na^+-K^+ exchange by insulin in the human forearm. Am J Physiol 1988; 266:E953-E958

26.   Tack CJJ, Lutterman JA, Vervoot G, Thien T, Smits P. Activation of the sodium-potassium pump contributes to insulin-induced vasodilatation in humans. Hypertension 1996; 28:426-432

27.   Taddei S, Virdis A, Mattei P, Natali A, Ferrannini E, Salvetti A. Effect of insulin on acetylcholine-induced vasodilatation in normotensive subjects and patients with essential hypertension. Circulation 1995; 92:2911-2918

28.   Meharg JV, McGowan-Jordan J, Charles A, Parmelee JT, Cutaia MV, Rounds S. Hydrogen peroxide stimulates sodium-potassium pump activity in cultured pulmonary arterial endothelial cells. Am J Physiol 1993; 265:L613-L621

29.   Tirupattur PR, Ram JL, Tandley PR, Sowers JR. Regulation of Na^+-K^+-ATPase gene expression by insulin in vascular smooth muscle cells. Am J Hypertens 1993; 6:626-629

30.   Kahn AM, Seidel CL, Allen JC, O'Neil G, Shelat H, Song T. Insulin reduces contraction and intracellular calcium concentration in vascular smooth muscle. Hypertension 1993; 22:735-742

31.   Trovati M, Anfossi G. Insulin, insulin resistance and platelet function: similarities with the insulin effects on cultured smooth muscle cells. Diabetologia 1998; 41:609-622

32.   Gupta S, McArthur C, Grady C, Ruderman NB. Stimulation of vascular Na^+-K^+-ATPase activity by nitric oxide: a cGMP-independent effect. Am J Physiol 1994; 266:H2146-2151

33.   Moncada S, Palmer RMJ. The L-arginine-nitric oxide pathway in the vessel wall. In: Moncada S, Higgs B, eds. Nitric Oxide from L-arginine: a Bioregulatory System. Amsterdam, Elsevier, 1990, pp 19-33

34.   Utriainen T, Mäkimattila S, Virkamäki A, Bergholm R, Yki-Järvinen H. Dissociation between insulin sensitivity of glucose uptake and endothelial function in normal subjects. Diabetologia 1996; 39:1477-1482

35.   Natali A, Taddei S, Quiñones Galvan A, Camastra S, Baldi S, Frascerra S, Virdis A, Sudano I, Salvetti A, Ferrannini E. Insulin sensitivity, vascular reactivity, and clamp-induced vasodilatation in essential hypertension. Circulation 1997; 96:849-855

36.   Laine H, Yki-Järvinen H, Kirvela O, Tolvanen T, Raitakari M, Solin O, Haaparanta M, Knuuti J, Nuutila P. Insulin resistance of glucose uptake in skeletal muscle cannot be ameliorated by enhancing endothelium-dependent blood flow in obesity. J Clin Invest 1998; 101:1156-1162

37.   Catalano C, Muscelli E, Quiñones Galvan A, Baldi S, Masoni A, Gibb I, Torffvit O, Seghieri G, Ferrannini E. Effect of insulin on systemic and renal handling of albumin in nondiabetic and NIDDM subjects. Diabetes 1997; 46:868-875

38.   Muscelli E, Emdin M, Natali A, Pratali L, Camastra S, Baldi S, Buzzigoli G, Carpeggiani C, Ferrannini E. Autonomic and hemodynamic responses to insulin in lean and obese humans. J Clin Endocrinol Metab 1998; 83:2084-2090

39.   Rowe JW, Young JB, Minaker KL, Stevens AL, Pallotta J, Landsberg L. Effect of insulin and glucose infusions on sympathetic nervous system activity in normal man. Diabetes 1981; 30:219-225.

40.   Davis SN, Colburn C, Robbins R, Nadeau S, Neal D, Williams P, Cherrington AD. Evidence that the brain of the conscious dog is insulin sensitive. J Clin Invest 1995; 95:593-602

41.   Schwartz MW, Figlewicz DP, Baskin DB, Woods SC, Porte D, Jr. Insulin in the brain: a hormonal regulator of energy balance. Endocr Rev 1992; 13:81-113

42.   Quiñones-Galvan A, Ferrannini E. Renal effects of insulin in man. J Nephrol 1997; 10:188-191

43.   DeFronzo RA, Cooke CR, Andres R, Faloona GR, Davis PJ. The effect of insulin on renal handling of sodium, potassium, calcium, and phosphate in man. J Clin Invest 1975; 55:845-855.

44.   Christiansen JS, Frandsen M, Parving H-H. The effect of intravenous insulin infusion on kidney function in insulin-dependent diabetes mellitus. Diabetologia 1981; 20:199-204.

45.   Tucker BJ, Rasch R, Blantz RC. Glomerular filtration and tubular reabsorption of albumin in preproteinuric and proteinuric diabetic rats. J Clin Invest 1993; 92:686-694.

46.   Benigni A, Remuzzi G. Glomerular protein trafficking and progression of renal disease to terminal uremia. Semin Nephrol 1996; 16:151-159.

47.   Butlen D, Vadrot S, Roseau S, Model F. Insulin receptors along the rat nephron: [125I] insulin binding in microdissected glomeruli and tubules. Pflugers Arch 1988; 412:604-612.

48.   Baum M. Insulin stimulates sodium transport in rabbit proximal convoluted tubule. J Clin Invest 1987; 79:1104-1109.

49.   Kirchner KA. Insulin increases loop segment chloride reabsorption in the euglycemic rat. Am J Physiol 1988; 24:F1206-F1213.

50.   DeFronzo RA, Goldberg M, Agus Z. The effects of glucose and insulin on renal electrolyte transport. J Clin Invest 1976; 58:83-90.

51.   Skott P, Vaag A, Bruun NE, Hother-Nielsen O, Gall MA, Beck-Nielsen H, Parving H-H. Effect of insulin on renal sodium handling in hyperinsulinemic Type 2 (non-insulin-dependendent) diabetic patients with peripheral insulin resistance. Diabetologia 1991; 34:275-281.

52.   Friedberg CE, Buren MW, Bijisma JA, Koomans HA. Insulin increases sodium reabsorption in diluting segments in humans: evidence for indirect mediation through hypokalemia. Kidney Int 1991; 40:251-256.

53.   Natali A, Quiñones-Galvan A, Santoro D, Pecori N, Taddei S, Salvetti A, Ferrannini E. Relationship between insulin release, antinatriuresis and hypokalemia after glucose ingestion in normal and hypertensive man. Clin Sci 1993; 85;327-335.

54.   Bank N, Anynedjan HS. Progressive increases in luminal glucose stimulate proximal tubular reabsorption in normal and diabetic rats. J Clin Invest 1990; 86:309-316.

55.   Hannedouche JP, Delgado AG, Guionshade DA, Boitard C, Lacour B, Grunfeld JP. Renal hemodynamics and segmental tubular reabsorption in early type I diabetes. Kidney Int 1989; 37:1126-1133. 56.

56.   Turner RJ, Moran A. Further studies of proximal tubular brush border membrane D-glucose heterogeneity. J Membr Biol 1982; 70:37-45.

57.   Nosadini R, Sambataro M, Tomaseth K, Pacini G, Cipollina MR, Solini A, Carraro A, Velussi M, Frigato F, Crepaldi G. Role of hyperglycemia and insulin resistance in determining sodium retention in non-insulin dependent diabetes. Kidney Int 1993; 44:139-146.

58.   Muscelli E, Natali A, Bianchi S, Bigazzi R, Quiñones-Galvan A, Sironi AM, Frascerra S, Ciociaro D, Ferrannini E. Effect of insulin on renal sodium and uric acid handling in essential hypertension. Am J Hypertens 1996; 9:746-752

59.   Rocchini AP, Katch V, Kveselis D, Moorehead C, Martin M, Lampman R, Gregory M. Insulin and renal sodium retention in obese adolescents. Hypertension 1989; 14:367-374

60.   DeFronzo RA, Felig P, Ferrannini E, Wahren J. Effect of graded doses of insulin on splanchnic and peripheral potassium metabolism in man. Am J Physiol 1980; 238:E421-E427.

61.   Cannon PJ, Svahn DS, Demartini FE. The influence of hypertonic saline infusion upon the fractional reabsorption of urate and other ions in normal and hypertensive man. Circulation 1970; 41:97-108.

62. Holmes WE, Kelley NW, Wyngaarden JB. The kidney and uric acid excretion in man. Kidney Int 1972; 2:115-118.

63. Quiñones-Galvan A, Natali A, Baldi S, Frascerra S, Sanna G, Ciociaro D, Ferrannini E. Effect of insulin on uric acid excretion in humans. Am J Physiol 1995; 268:E1-E5.

64. Cannon PJ, Stason WB, Demartini FE, Sommers SC, Laragh JH. Hyperuricemia in primary and renal hypertension. N Engl J Med 1966; 275:457-464..

65. Modan M, Halkin H, Karasik A, Lusky A. Elevated serum uric acid – a facet of hyperinsulinaemia. Diabetologia 1987; 30:713-718.

13. VALUE OF SCREENING FOR MICROALBUMINURIA IN PEOPLE WITH DIABETES AS WELL AS IN THE GENERAL POPULATION

Bo Feldt-Rasmussen, Jan Skov Jensen and Knut Borch-Johnsen
Rigshospitalet University Hospital, Department of Nephrology, Copenhagen, and Steno Diabetes Center, Gentofte, Denmark

The concept of microalbuminuria was first introduced among diabetologists [1,2]. It is diagnosed when the urinary albumin excretion rate (UAER) is slightly elevated compared with a normal reference range but lower than what is seen when the classical dipstix are positive for protein or albumin. Microalbuminuria is a marker of an increased risk of diabetic nephropathy and of cardiovascular disease in patients with insulin-dependent (IDDM) as well as with non-insulin-dependent (NIDDM) diabetes mellitus [1-18]. A high number of studies of the pathophysiology and of interventional measures in these patients have been published as reviewed in a number of dissertations and reviews since 1989 [19-27] and seven sets of recommendations on the prevention of diabetic nephropathy, with special reference to microalbuminuria have been published [28-34]. More recently microalbuminuria has been brought into a wider perspective because it has been found to be associated with cardiovascular disease also in the non-diabetic population. In fact microalbuminuria may show to be a *risk factor* of cardiovascular disease among otherwise apparently healthy persons [35-52].

DEFINING MICROALBUMINURIA
Microalbuminuria has been defined using different units of measurement. According to the Gentofte-Montecatini convention [53] microalbuminuria is present when the UAER in a 24-hour urine or a short time collected urine during daytime is in the range of 30 to 300 mg/24h (20 to 200 µg/min) equivalent to 0.46 to 4.6 µmol/24h [53,54]. The upper level is corresponding to a total urinary protein concentration of approximately 0.5 g/l which was previously considered to be the first marker of clinical diabetic nephropathy.

Mogensen, C.E. (ed.), THE KIDNEY AND HYPERTENSION IN DIABETES MELLITUS.
Copyright© 2000 by Kluwer Academic Publishers, Boston • Dordrecht • London. All rights reserved.

The lower limit predicting nephropathy was defined on the basis of the results of four prospective studies in IDDM patients [1-4] (table 13-1). As shown in the table the studies have used different sampling periods, number of urine samples, reference range and they differed with respect to the length of the follow up periods. Nevertheless an international agreement was made on a lower predictive level of 30 mg/24h (20 µg/min) in order to make it possible to compare the outcome of studies from the various international study groups [53].

In the non-diabetic population clinical cardiovascular disease is often present in subjects with an UAER in the range of 30 to 300 mg/24h [35-52] (table 13-2). Therefore the level of microalbuminuria must be lower if the measuring of UAER also should *predict* cardiovascular disease in the population. This will be discussed at the end of this chapter.

METHODOLOGICAL PROBLEMS

The concentration of albumin in the urine can be assayed using a number of immunoassays [20]. The major problem is the day to day variation of 23 to 52 %.

Table 13-1. Four prospective studies demonstrating that an increased urinary albumin excretion rate (UAER) is a predictor of nephropathy in IDDM patients.

	Gentofte (1)[*])	London (2)	Aarhus (3)	Gentofte 2 (4)
Number of patients	23	63	44	71
Method for collecting urine UAER	24 hours			24 hours
Predictive Value for nephropathy (µg/min)	30	30	15	70
Observation (years)	6	14	10	6
Number of patients with UAER above the predictive value who progressed to nephropathy	5/8	7/8	12/14	7/7
[*])the patients from this study were also included as a part of Gentofte 2.				

This variation is similar regardless of the urine collection procedure used: 24h, overnight collection, timed collection at daytime, during water diureses or by calculating an albumin/creatinine-ratio [4,20,22,54]. It is therefore recommended that presence of microalbuminuria is confirmed in at least two more urine collections [50].

The UAER is increased in the presence of urinary tract infections, menstrual bleedings, nephrological diseases other than diabetic nephropathy, severe hypertension and severe cardiac disease which all have to be excluded. It is also elevated during heavy physical exercise but not significantly affected in healthy subjects during normal daily life activities [20,22].

The UAER is elevated in diabetic patients in very poor glycaemic control with ketonuria and during episodes of ketoacidoses [20].

The collection period is also of importance. The level is similar in urines collected over 24-h and in timed daytime urine collections but reduced by 25% in urines collected overnight. Therefore the range of microalbuminuria in overnight urines should be an UAER of 23 to 230 mg/24h (15 to 150 µg/min) [20,23].

The pathophysiology of development of microalbuminuria is not yet clarified [55-60]. If a timed collection cannot be obtained, an index of albumin/creatinine (µg/µ mol) can be calculated. Microalbuminuria is present at an index >3.5 (sensitivity > 95%, specificity >65%) [34]. A close time-relationship between increase in UAER and increase in blood pressure has been demonstrated. The increase in UAER may precede the increase in blood pressure [61].

MICROALBUMINURIA AS A RISK FACTOR

Insulin-dependent diabetes mellitus (IDDM)
The prevalence of microalbuminuria is 16 to 22% [27,62]. Normally no other signs of micro- or macroangiopathy are present at the first diagnosis of microalbuminuria. Later on with higher levels of microalbuminuria retinopathy will become much more frequent, and in fact microalbuminuria is a strong risk marker of severe retinopathy [20,22,23]. The blood-pressure is usually below 160/95 mmHg, but the mean blood-pressure is increasing by 3 mmHg per year [20,22,63]. The kidney function in terms of S-creatinine and glomerular filtration rate (GFR) are normal. The loss of kidney function is observed only in patients with the highest levels of UAER in the microalbuminuric range in whom a decline rate of GFR of 3 to 4 ml/(min*year) has been described [20,22,63]. The risk of clinical diabetic nephropathy is the highest among patients with an UAER in the range of 100 to 300 mg/24h (70 to 200 µg/min) [63,64]. The classical definition of clinical diabetic nephropathy at levels of UAER above 300 mg/24h therefore seems to be historical and dictated by the low sensitivity of the older methods for determining protein in urine.

IDDM patients with classical proteinuria >0.5g/l are carrying almost the entire burden of the overmortality of diabetic patients [19]. This overmortality is only to a small extent caused by end stage renal failure. By far most of the patients are dying from cardiovascular diseases [19]. It is therefore widely accepted that microalbuminuria in the IDDM patient should be a valuable diagnostic parameter being highly predictive of excess mortality and cardiovascular morbidity [7-10]. The predictive value of microalbuminuria for cardiovascular diseases seems to be independent of conventional atherosclerotic risk factors, diabetic nephropathy, and diabetes duration and control [7].

It is important to identify all IDDM patients with microalbuminuria because the progression of their disease can be delayed. Antihypertensive treatment reduces the fall rate of GFR by 50 % from 10 to less than 5 ml/(min*year) as observed in patients with clinical nephropathy [65-68]. The effect may be even more impressive when treatment is started at the first signs of an increasing blood-pressure but before development of overt hypertension [69,70].

The effect of antihypertensive treatment is further emphasized by the important observation in Denmark of an increased patient survival following the implementation of early antihypertensive treatment [71].

Optimizing the glycaemic control has also shown to be effective in arresting the progression of diabetic renal disease in its early stages i.e. delaying development and in some cases also the progression of microalbuminuria [63,72-76].

Non-insulin-dependent mellitus (NIDDM)

The prevalence of microalbuminuria is also high in NIDDM patients : 30 to 40 % [24,25,77]. Microalbuminuria is often present at diagnosis of the diabetic state. It is primarily associated to cardiovascular disease and NIDDM patients with microalbuminuria are at an increased risk of cardiovascular death compared with NIDDM patients with a normal UAER [11-18,25].

End stage renal failure only occurs in 3 to 8 % of NIDDM patients despite the high prevalence of microalbuminuria. On the other hand microalbuminuria is a predictor of increasing levels of very low density lipoprotein cholesterol and a decrease of high density lipoprotein cholesterol [78]. Microalbuminuria therefore seems to be a *risk factor* of generalized disease to an even higher extent than in IDDM patients.

Also in NIDDM patients the causal link between microalbuminuria and generalized vascular disease is speculative. It is likely that a link should be found in alterations in the composition of the basal membranes of the capillaries and of the extracellular matrices as also hypothesized in IDDM patients. In any case presence of the well-known risk factors is not sufficient to explain the entire overmortality of patients with NIDDM: hypertension, dyslipidaemia, atherogenic changes in the haemostatic system (increased von Willebrand factor and plasma fibrinogen) [24,25]. In contrast microalbuminuria appears to be an independent risk factor as is the case in IDDM patients.

The diabetic state per se and its associated syndrome of insulin resistance is also likely to be an important risk factor.

Treating normotensive NIDDM patients with microalbuminuria with ACE inhibitors delays the progression to diabetic nephropathy [79,80].

Non-diabetics

Microalbuminuria is also present in the non-diabetic population. This has now been described in a number of studies [35-52]. Whenever mentioned, the reference range of the UAER seems to be rather low in relation to the classical definition of microalbuminuria. In table 13-3 is shown the reference range of UAER in 10 different studies. Except for one study with a higher level, the median or mean value of UAER is given from 2.6 to 8 µg/min and the upper 95% percentile in more than 50% of the studies as 15 µg/min or below [36,37,41,43,44,46,48,57,81-83]. Microalbuminuria in its classical definition therefore seems to represent a relatively high UAER among non-diabetics. In an English 4-year follow-up study microalbuminuria, however, increased the mortality rate 24 times [36]. In a Danish study UAER was measured in 216 non-diabetic subjects, 60 to 74 years of age [37]. The median UAER was 7.52 µg/min (25 and 75 percentiles were 4.77 and 14.85 µg/min). The subjects were reexamined 7 years later. Among the 107 subjects with an initial UAER above the median value 23 had died in contrast to 8 out of 107 below the median UAER (p<0.008). In both studies the predictive effect of microalbuminuria was independent of the conventional atherosclerotic risk factors [36,37] which are usually increased among non-diabetic subjects with microalbuminuria (table 13-2).

More recently two larger scaled population based studies have confirmed that a UAER above a certain level is predictive of developing ischaemic heart disease and increased mortality [47]. In a Finnisch study of Kuusisto et al, 1.069 elderly inhabitants were followed for 3-4 years. Those who at baseline had an A/C ratio above the upper quintile (>3.2 mg albumin/mmol creatinine) had a higher morbidity and mortality from ischaemic heart disease (odds ratio 2.2) [49]. In our own study of 2.181 participants of the 1st Monica Population Study, Glostrup, Copenhagen County, an A/C ratio above the upper decile (>0.65 mg albumin/mmol creatinine) was significantly associated with an increased relative risk of 2.3 for development of ischaemic heart disease [47]. Also in the two latter studies, the predictive effect of microalbuminuria was independent of the conventional atherosclerotic risk factors.

Therefore, the link between microalbuminuria and cardiovascular disease may be explained by other pathophysiologic mechanisms, e.g. an universally increased transvascular albumin leakage [84,85] as well as other signs of endothelial dysfunction [86,87].

Prospective population studies including our own are in progress aiming to further clarify the role of UAER as a predictor of premature death of cardiovascular disease in apparently healthy subjects.

Author	Haffner	Wino-cour	Woo	Metcalf	Go-uld	Dim-mitt	Beatty	Myk-känen	Jensen
Publica-tion year	1990	1992	1992	1992 & 1993	1993	1993	1993	1994	1997
Microal-buminura	U_{alb}>30 mg/l	U_{alb}>20 mg/l	U_{alb}/U_{Cre} at >90%-ile	U_{alb} continuous variable	UAER 20-200µg/min	U_{alb}>media l	UAER 20-200µg/min	U_{alb}/U_{create}>2	UAER>90%-ile
Sample size	316	447	1.333	5.349	959	474	264	1.068	2.613
Male sex					↑	↑			↑
Age					↑	↓		↑	
Blood pressure	↑	↑	↑	↑	↑			↑	↑
S-insulin	↑		↑					↑	
P-lipids	↑			↑		↑	↑	↑	
Body mass index				↑					↑
Smoking				↑					↑
Height					↓				
B-glucose					↑		↑		

↑, microalbuminuria is assoiated with increased levels of the risk factor; ↓, microalbuminuria is assoiated with increased levels of the risk factor.

U_{alb}, urinary albumin concentretion; U_{creat}, urinary creatinine concentretion; UAER, urinary albumin excretion rate.

Table 13-2. Associations between microalbuminuria and atherosclerotic risk factors.

CONCLUSIONS AND RECOMMENDATIONS

Measuring the UAER is a well documented and a well established part of monitoring *IDDM patients*. The most simple urine sampling procedures can be used as long as the UAER is not significantly elevated i.e. as long as the albumin/ creatinine index is below 3.5 µg/µmol. It should be examined at least once a year. When microalbuminuria is suspected, a method of quantitating the UAER should be used at all subsequent visits in the out-patient clinic or until it is found normal at three consecutive visits. Presence of microalbuminuria warrants intensified follow up in order to diagnose and to intervene against retinopathy, nephropathy, hypertension and, if necessary to optimize the glycaemic control [88].

In *patients with NIDDM* the UAER should be measured at diagnosis and once a year. Measuring the UAER is part of the general description of the cardiovascular risk profile of the individual patient. If the UAER is elevated the indications are that treatment with ACE inhibitors may be beneficial. Presence of microalbuminuria will

Table 13-3. Reference values of urinary excretion in non-diabetic individuals.

Study (Author, country, publication year)	Urine collection	Sample size (Numbers	Age (Years)	Sex (M/F)	Urinary albumin excretion
Marre et al, France (1987)	Timed overnight	60	40±13	28/32	4.2±4.1 µ/min[a] a
Marre et al, France (1987)	Timed daytime	60	40±13	28/32	6.6 ±7.7 µ/min[a] a
Marre et al, France (1987)	Timed 24-hours	60	40±13	28/32	8.0±8.1 µ/[a]min a
Watts et al, UK (1988)	Morning spot	127	33±12	59/68	3.9(0.9-16.2)[a] mg/l f
Watts et al, UK (1988)	Timed overnight	127	33±12	59/68	3.2(1.2-8.6) µg/[a]min f
Watts et al, UK (1988)	Timed daytime	127	33±12	59/68	4.5(1.0-9.1) µg/[a]min f
Yudkin et al, UK (1988)	Timed daytime	184	60±12	68/116	2.8(0.09-154.6) [a] µg/min c
Gosling & Beevers, UK (1989)	Timed 24-hours	199	40±11	99/100	3.7(0.1-22.9) µg[a]/min c
Damsgaard et al, Denmark (1990)	Timed daytime	223	68(64-71)	89/134	7.5(4.8-14.9) µg/[b]min b
Metcalf et al, New Zealand (1992)	Morning spot	5.670	49(40-78)	4.106/1.564	5.2(5.1-5.4) mg/l[c] g
Dimmitt et al, Australia (1993)	Morning spot	474	34(17-64)	241/233	5.3 mg/ ch
Mykkänen et al, Finland (1994)	Morning spot	826	69.0± 0.1	312/514	23.7±2.5mg/l[d] d
Gould et al, UK (1994)	Timed overnight	812	40-75	359/453	2.6(0.1-148.8)[e] µg/min c
Gould et al, UK (1994)	Timed daytime	913	40-75	411/502	4.1(0.1-165.6) µg/min c
Jensen et al, Denmark (1997)	Timed overnight	2.613	30-70	1.340/1.273	2.8(1.2-7.0)µg/[e]min i

[a]Mean±SD [b]Median (1-3. Interquartile range) [c]median (range) [d]mean± SE [e]range [f]mean (95% C.I.) [g]geometric mean (95% C.I.) [h]median [i]median(10-90 interpercentile range)

emphasize the need for intervention against any other risk factor present (hypertension, dyslipidaemia, tobacco smoking and obesity).

Among non-diabetic subjects an increased UAER is a marker of cardiovascular disease as well as a risk factor of premature death. Examining the UAER is recommended as part of the routine medical check up of the adult and to replace the less sensitive examination for protein in the urine which after all only serves to disclose diseases of the kidneys and the urinary tract. As was the case in NIDDM patients precense of increased values will reinforce the need to intervene against any other risk factor present. Values of UAER above the microalbuminuric range should obviously lead to routine examinations to exclude nephro-urological diseases. The significance of an increased UAER on development of cardiovascular disease is to some extent clarified but so far no direct clinical consequences should be drawn of microalbuminuria per se.

Among non-diabetic subjects the present indications are that UAER is significantly elevated and predictive of disease at a much lower level than in diabetic patients i.e. at a level below the classical definition of microalbuminuria.

Further research is needed for this clarification as well as for the investigation of interventional measures. Microalbuminuria is therefore at present in focus in numerous epidemiological and pathophysiological studies. Measurement is also relevant in relation races, because hypertension and diabetes seem very prevalent in several areas of the world, e.g. among Africans in Cameroon [89].

REFERENCES

1.   Parving H-H, Oxenbøll B, Svendsen PAa, Christiansen JS, Andersen AR. Early detection of patients at risk of developing diabetic nephropathy. Acta Endocrinol (Copenh) 1982; 100: 550-555.

2.   Viberti GC, Hill RD, Jarret RJ, Argyropoulos A, Mahmud U, Keen H. Microalbuminuria as a predictor of clinical nephropathy in insulin-dependent diabetes mellitus. Lancet 1982; i: 1430-1432.

3.   Mogensen CE, Christensen CK. Predicting diabetic nephropathy in insulin-dependent patients. N Engl J Med 1984; 311: 89-93.

4.   Mathiesen ER, Oxenbøll B, Johansen K, Svendsen PAa, Deckert T. Incipient nephropathy in Type 1 (insulin-dependent) diabetes. Diabetologia 1984; 26: 406-410.

5.   Mogensen CE. Microalbuminuria predicts clinical proteinuria and early mortality in maturity onset diabetes. N Engl J Med 1984; 310: 356-360.

6.   Jarrett RJ, Viberti GC, Argyropoulos A, Hill RD, Mahmud U, Murrels TJ. Microalbuminuria predicts mortality in non-insulin-dependent diabetes. Diabetic Med 1984; 1: 17-19.

7. Deckert T, Yokoyama H, Mathiesen ER, Rønn B, Jensen T, Feldt-Rasmussen B, Borch-Johnsen K, Jensen JS. Cohort study of predictive value of urinary albumin excretion for atherosclerotic vascular disease in patients with insulin dependent diabetes. BMJ 1996; 312: 871-874.

8. Messent JWC, Elliot TG, Hill RD, Jarrett RJ, Keen H, Viberti GC. Prognostic significance of microalbuminuria in insulin-dependent diabetes mellitus: A twenty-three year follow-up study. Kidney Int 1992; 41: 836-839.

9. Torffvit O, Agardh C-D. The predictive value of albuminuria for cardiovascular and renal disease. A 5-year follow-up study of 476 patients with type 1 diabetes mellitus. J Diabetic Compl 1993; 7: 49-56.

10. Jensen T, Borch-Johnsen K, Kofoed-Enevoldsen A, Deckert T. Coronary heart disease in young type 1 (insulin-depedent) diabetic patients with and without diabetic nephropathy: Incidence and risk factors. Diabetologia 1987; 30: 144-148.

11. Schmitz A, Vaeth M. Microalbuminuria: A major risk factor in non-insulin-dependent diabetes. A 10-year follow-up study of 503 patients. Diabetic Med 1988; 5: 1126-1134.

12. Mattock MB, Morrish NJ, Viberti GC, Keen H, Fitzgerald AP, Jackson G. Prospective study of microalbuminuria as predictor of mortality in NIDDM. Diabetes 1992; 41: 736-741.

13. Neil A, Hawkins M, Potok M, Thororgood M, Cohen D, Mann J. A prospective population-based study of microalbuminuria as a predictor of mortality in NIDDM. Diabetes Care 1993; 16: 996-1003.

14. Gall M-A, Borch-Johnsen K, Hougaard P, Nielsen FS, Parving H-H. Albuminuria and poor glycemic control predict mortality in NIDDM. Diabetes 1995; 44: 1303-1309.

15. Rossing P, Hougaard P, Borch-Johnsen K, Parving H-H. Predictors of mortality in insulin dependent diabetes: 10 year observational follow up study. BMJ 1996; 313: 779-784.

16. Damsgaard EM, Frøland A, Jørgensen OD, Mogensen CE. Eight to nine year mortality in known non-insulin dependent diabetics and controls. Kidney Internat 1992; 41: 731-735.

17. MacLeod JM, Lutale J, Marshall SM. Albumin excretion and vascular deaths in NIDDM. Diabetologia 1995; 38: 610-616.

18. Beilin J, Stanton KG, McCann VJ, Knuiman MW, Divitini ML. Microalbuminuria in type 2 diabetes: an independent predictor of cardiovascular mortality. Aust Nz J Med 1996; 26: 519-525.

19. Borch-Johnsen K. The prognosis of insulin-dependent diabetes - an epidemiological approach (Thesis). Dan Med Bull 1989; 36: 336-348.

20. Feldt-Rasmussen B. Microalbuminuria and clinical nephropathy in Type 1 (insulin-dependent) diabetes mellitus: Pathophysiological mechanisms and intervention studies (Thesis). Dan Med Bull 1989; 36: 405-415.

21. Jensen T. Albuminuria - a marker of renal and general vascular disease in IDDM (Thesis). Dan Med Bull 1991; 38: 134-144.

22. Christensen CK. The pre-proteinuric phase of diabetic nephropathy (Thesis). Dan Med Bull 1991; 38: 145-159.

23. Mathiesen ER. Prevention of diabetic nephropathy: Microalbuminuria and perspectives for intervention in insulin-dependent diabetes (Thesis). Dan Med Bull 1993; 40: 273-285.

24. Schmitz A. The kidney in non-insulin-dependent diabetes. Studies on glomerular structure and function and the relationship between microalbuminuria and mortality. Acta Diabetologica 1992; 29: 47-69.

25. Gall M. Albuminuria in non-insulin-dependent diabetes mellitus: prevalence, causes and consequences (Thesis). Dan Med Bull 1997: 44: 465-485.

26. Deckert T, Feldt-Rasmussen B, Borch-Johnsen K, Jensen T, Kofoed-Enevoldsen A. Albuminuria reflects widespread vascular damage. The Steno hypothesis. Diabetologia 1989; 32: 219-226.

27. Mogensen CE, Hansen KW, Sommer S et al. »Microalbuminuria: studies in diabetes, essential hypertension and renal disease as compared with the background population.« In *Advances in Nephrology*. Grunfeld JP, ed. Mosby Year Book, 1991; vol 20: 191-228.

28. Viberti GC, Mogensen CE, Passa P, Bilous R, Mangili R. »St Vincent Declaration, 1994: Guidelines for the prevention of diabetic renal failure.« In *The Kidney and Hypertension in Diabetes Mellitus*, 2nd ed. Mogensen CE, ed. Boston, Dordrecht, London: Kluwer Academic Publishers, 1994; pp 515-527.

29. Anon. Prevention of diabetes mellitus: report of a WHO study group. WHO Tech Rep Ser 844. Geneva: WHO, 1994: 55-59.

30. Jerums G, Cooper M, Gilbert R, O'Brien R, Taft J. Microalbuminuria in diabetes. Med J Aust 1994; 161: 265-268.

31. Consensus development conference on the diagnosis and management of nephropathy in patients with diabetes mellitus. Diabetes Care 1994; 17: 1357-1361.

32. Bennett PH, Haffner S, Kaiske BL, et al. Screening and management of microalbuminuria in patients with diabetes mellitus: recommendations to the scientific advisory board of the National Kidney Foundation from an ad hoc committee of the council on diabetes mellitus of the National Kidney Foundation. Am J Kidney Dis 1995; 25: 107-112.

33. Striker GE. Report on a workshop to develop management recommendations for the prevention of progression in chronic renal disease (Bethesda, April, 1994). Nephrol Dial Transplant 1995; 10: 290-292.

34. Mogensen CE, Keane WF, Bennett PH, Jerums G, Parving H-H, Passa P, Steffes MW, Striker GE, Viberti GC. Prevention of diabetic renal disease with special reference to microalbuminuria. Lancet 1995; 346: 1080-1084.

35. Jensen JS. Microalbuminuria and the risk of atherosclerosis. Dan Med Bull (in press).

36 Yudkin JS, Forrest RD, Jackson CA. Microalbuminuria as predictor of vascular disease in non-diabetic subjects: Islington diabetes survey. Lancet 1988; ii: 530-533.

37 Damsgaard EM, Frøland A, Jørgensen OD, Mogensen CE. Microalbuminuria as predictor of increased mortality in elderly people. BMJ 1990; 300: 297-300.

38. Haffner SM, Stern MP, Gruber KK, Hazuda HP, Mitchell BD, Patterson JK. Microalbuminuria. Potential marker for increased cardiovascular risk factors in non-diabetic subjects. Arteriosclerosis 1990; 10: 727-731.

39. Winocour PH, Harland JOE, Millar JP, Laker MF, Alberti KGMM. Microalbuminuria and associated cardiovascular risk factors in the community. Atherosclerosis 1992; 93: 71-81.

40. Woo J, Cockram CS, Swaminathan R, Lau E, Chan E, Cheung R. Microalbuminuria and other cardiovascular risk factors in non-diabetic subjects. Int J Cardiol 1992; 37: 345-350.

41. Metcalff P, Baker J, Scott A, Wild C, Scragg R, Dryson E. Albuminuria in people at least 40 years old: Effect of obesity, hypertension and hyperlipidemia. Clin Chem 1992; 38: 1802-1808.

42. Metcalff PA, Baker JR, Scragg RKR, Dryson E, Scott AJ, Wild CJ. Albuminuria in people at least 40 years old. Effect of alcohol consumption, regular exercise, and cigarette smoking. Clin Chem 1993; 39: 1793-1797.

43. Gould MM, Mohamed-Ali V, Goubet SA, Yudkin JS, Haines AP. Microalbuminuria: associations with height and sex in non-diabetic subjects. BMJ 1993; 306: 240-242.

44. Dimmitt SB, Lindquist TL, Mamotte CDS, Burke V, Beilin LJ. Urine albumin excretion in healthy subjects. J Human Hypertens 1993; 7: 239-243.

45. Beatty OL, Atkinson AB, Browne J, Clarke K, Sheridan B, Bell PM. Microalbuminuria does not predict cardiovascular disease in a normal general practice population. Ir J Med Sci 1993; 163: 140-142.

46. Mykkänen L, Haffner SM, Kuusisto J, Pyorälä K, Laakso M. Microalbuminuria precedes the development of NIDDM. Diabetes 1994; 43: 552-557.

47. Jensen JS, Borch-Johnsen K, Feldt-Rasmussen B, Jensen G, Feldt-Rasmussen B. Atherosclerotic risk factors are increased in clinically healthy subjects with microalbuminuria. Atherosclerosis 1995; 112: 245-252.

48. Gould MM, Mohamed-Ali V, Goubet SA, Yudkin JS, Haines AP. Associations of urinary albumin excretion rate with vascular disease in Europid nondiabetic subjects. J Diabetic Compl 1994; 8: 180-188.

49. Kuusisto J, Mykkänin L, Pyörälä K, Laakso M. Hyperinsulinemic microalbuminuria. A new risk indicator for coronary heart disease. Ciculation 1995: 91: 831-837.

50. Jensen JS, Borch-Johnsen K, Feldt-Rasmussen B, Appleyard M, Jensen G. Urinary albumin excretion and history of acute myocardial infarction in a cross-sectional population study of 2613 individuals. Journal of Cardiovascular Risk 1997; 4: 121-125.

51. Borch-Johsen K, Feldt-Rasmussen B, Strandgaard S, Schroll M, Jensen SR. Urinary albumin excretion. An independent predictor of ischemic heart disease. Aterioscler Thromb Vasc Biol 1999, 19:1992-1997.

52. Jensen JS, Feldt-Rasmussen B, Clausen P, Borch Johnsen K, Jensen G. Aterial hypertension, microalbuminuria, and the risk of ischaemic heart disease. Hypertension (in press).

53. Mogensen CE, Chachati A, Christensen CK, Close CF, Deckert T, Hommel E, Kastrup J, Lefebvre P, Mathiesen ER, Feldt-Rasmussen B, Schmitz A, Viberti GC. Microalbuminuria: an early marker of renal involvement in diabetes. Uremia Invest 1985-86; 9: 85-95.

54. Feldt-Rasmussen B, Dinesen B, Deckert M. Enzyme immuno assay. an improved determination of urinary albumin in diabetics with incipient nephropathy. Scand J Clin Lab Invest 1985; 45: 539-544.

55. Christiansen JS. Glomerular hyperfiltration in diabetes mellitus. Diabetic Med 1985; 2: 235-239.

56. Parving H-H, Mogensen CE, Jensen HÆ et al. Increased urinary albumin excretion rate in benign essential hypertension. Lancet 1974; i: 1190-1192.

57.   Gosling P, Beevers DG. Urinary albumin excretion and blood pressure in the general population. Clin Sci 1989; 76: 39-42.
58.   Hommel E, Mathiesen ER, Edsberg B, Bahnsen M, Parving H-H. Acute reduction of arterial blood pressure reduces urinary albumin excretion in type 1 (insulin-dependent) diabetic patients with incipient nephropathy. Diabetologia 1986; 29: 211-215.
59.   Deckert T, Kofoed-Enevoldsen A, Vidal P, Nørgaard K, Andreassen HB, Feldt-Rasmussen B. Size and charge selectivity of glomerular filtration in insulin-dependent diabetic patients with and without albuminuria. Diabetologia 1993; 36: 244-251.
60.   Feldt-Rasmussen B. Increased transcapillary escape rate of albumin in insulin-dependent diabetic patients with microalbuminuria. Diabetologia 1986; 29: 282-286.
61.   Mathiesen ER, Rønn B, Jensen T, Storm B, Deckert T. The relationship between blood pressure and urinary albumin excretion in the development of microalbuminuria. Diabetes 1990; 39: 245-249.
62.   Parving H-H, Hommel E, Mathiesen ER, Skøtt P, Edsberg B, Bahnsen M et al. Prevalence of microalbuminuria, arterial hypertension, retinopathy and neuropathy in patients with insulin dependent diabetes. BMJ 1988; 296: 157-160.
63.   Feldt-Rasmussen B, Mathiesen ER, Jensen T, Lauritzen T, Deckert T. Effect of improved metabolic control on loss of kidney function in insulin-dependent diabetic patients. Diabetologia 1991; 34: 164-170.
64.   Mathiesen ER, Feldt-Rasmussen B, Hommel E, Deckert T, Parving H-H. Stable glomerular filtration rate in normotensive IDDM patients with stable microalbuminuria: A 5-year prospective study. Diabetes Care 1997; 20/3: 286-289.
65.   Bjorck S, Mulec H, Johnsen SA et al. Renal protective effect of Enalapril in diabetic nephropathy. BMJ 1992; 304: 339-343.
66.   Lewis EJ, Hunsicker LG, Bain RP, Rohde RD, for the Collaborative Study Group. The effect of angiotensin-converting-enzyme inhibition on diabetic nephropathy. N Engl J Med 1993; 329: 1456-1462.
67.   Parving H-H, Andersen AR, Schmidt UM, Hommel E, Mathiesen ER, Svendsen PAa. Effect of antihypertensive treatment on kidney function in diabetic nephropathy. BMJ 1987; 294: 1443-1447.
68.   Mathiesen ER, Hommel E, Giese J, Parving H-H. Efficacy of captopril in postponing nephropathy in normotensive insulin-dependent diabetic patients with microalbuminuria. BMJ 1991; 303: 81-87.
69.   Mathiesen ER, Hommel E, Hansen HP, Smidt UM, Parving H-H. Randomised controlled trial of long term efficacy of captopril on preservation of kidney function in normotensive patients with insulin dependent diabetes and microalbuminuria. BMJ 1999; 319: 24-25.
70.   Viberti GC, Mogensen CE, Groop L, Pauls JF, for the European Microalbuminuria Captopril Study Group. Effect of captopril on progression to clinical proteinuria in patients with insulin-dependent diabetes mellitus and microalbuminuria. JAMA 1994; 271: 275-279.
71.   Parving H-H, Hommel E. Prognosis in diabetic nephropathy. BMJ 1989; 299: 230-233.
72.   Dahl-Jørgensen K, Hanssen KF, Kierulf P, Bjøro T, Sandvik L, Aagenaess Ø. Reduction of urinary albumin excretion after 4 years of continuous subcutaneous insulin infusion in insulin-dependent diabetes mellitus. Acta Endocrinol (Copenh) 1988; 117: 19-25.

73. Reichard P, Berglund B, Britz A, Cars I, Nilsson BY, Rosenqvist U. Intensified conventional insulin treatment retards the microvascular complications of insulin-dependent diabetes mellitus (IDDM). The Stockholm Diabetes Intervention Study after five years. J Intern Med 1991; 230: 101-108.

74. The Diabetes Control and Complications Trial Research Group. The effect of intensive treatment of diabetes on the development and progression of long-term complications in insulin-dependent diabetes mellitus. N Engl J Med 1993; 329: 977-986.

75. Diabetes Control and Complications (DCCT) Research Group. Effect of intensive therapy on the development and progression of diabetic nephropathy in the diabetes control and complications trial. Kidney Int 1995; 42: 1703-1720.

76. Microalbuminuria Collaborative Study Group, United Kingdom. Intensive therapy and progression to clinical albuminuria in patients with insulin dependent diabetes mellitus and microalbuminuria. BMJ 1995; 311: 973-977.

77. Gall M, Rossing P, Skøtt P, Damsbo P, Vaag A, Bech K et al. Prevalence of micro- and macro-albuminuria, arterial hypertension, retinopathy and large vessel disease in European Type 2 (non-insulin-dependent) diabetic patients. Diabetologia 1991; 34: 655-661.

78. Niskanen L, Uusitupa M, Sarlund H, Siitonen O, Voutilainen E, Penttila I et al. Microalbuminuria predicts the development of serum lipoprotein abnormalities favouring atherogenesis in newly diagnosed Type 2 (non-insulin-dependent) diabetic patients. Diabetologia 1990; 33: 237-243.

79. Ravid M, Savin H, Jutrin I, Bental T, Katz B, Lishner M. Long-term stabilizing effect of angiotensin-converting enzyme inhibition on plasma creatinine and on proteinuria in normotensive type II diabetic patients. Ann Intern Med 1993; 118: 577-581.

80. Gaede P, Vedel P, Parving H-H, Pedersen O. Intensified multifactorial intervention in patients with type 2 diabetes mellitus and microalbuminuria: The Steno type 2 randomised study. Lancet 1999; 353: 617-622.

81. Marre M, Claudel J-P, Ciret P, Luis N, Suarez L, Passa P. Laser immunonephelometry for routine quantification of urinary albumin excretion. Clin Chem 1987; 33: 209-213.

82. Watts GF, Morris RW, Khan K, Polak A. Urinary albumin excretion in healthy adult subjects: reference values and some factors affectin their interpretation. Clin Chim Acta 1988; 172: 191-198.

83. Jensen JS, Feldt-Rasmussen B, Borch-Johnsen K, Jensen G and the Copenhagen City Heart Study Group. Urinary albumin excretion in a population based sample of 1011 middle aged non-diabetic subjects. Scand J Clin Lab Invest 1993; 53: 867-872

84. Jensen JS, Borch-Johnsen K, Jensen G, Feldt-Rasmussen B. Microalbuminuria reflects a generalized transvascular albumin leakiness in clinically healthy subjects. Clin Sci 1995; 88: 629-33.

85. Jensen JS, Borch-Johnsen K, Deckert T, Deckert M, Jensen G, Feldt-Rasmussen B. Reduced glomerular size- and charge-selectivity in clinically healthy individuals with microalbuminuria. Eur J Clin Invest 1995; 25: 608-614.

86. Clausen P, Feldt-Rasmussen B, Jensen G, Jensen JS. Endothelial haemostatic factors are associated with progression of urinary albumin excretion in clinically heathy subjects: a 4-year prospective study. Clinical Science 1999; 97: 37-43.

87.   Stehouwer CDA, Lambert J, Donker AJM, van Hinsbergh VWM. Endothelial dysfunction and pathogenesis of diabetic angiopathy. Cardiovascular Research 1997; 34: 55-68.

88.   Borch-Johnsen K, Wenzel H, Viberti GC, Mogensen CE. Is screening and intervention for Microalbuminuria worthwhile in patients with insulin dependent diabetes? BMJ 1993; 306: 1722-1725.

89.   Ducorps M, Bauduceau B, Poirier JM, Cosson E, Belmejdoub G, Mayaudon H. Hypertension in black African diabetics (Abstract). Diabetologia 1996; 39: Suppl. 1: A287.

14. INCIDENCE OF NEPHROPATHY IN IDDM AS RELATED TO MORTALITY. COSTS AND BENEFITS OF EARLY INTERVENTION.

Knut Borch-Johnsen,
Steno Diabetes Centre, Gentofte Denmark

Development of persistent proteinuria - the clinical manifestation of diabetic nephropathy - is a strong prognostic marker in IDDM-patients. Not only does it precede the development of end stage renal failure, it is also associated with an increased risk of proliferative retinopathy, visual impairment and blindness, and with an increased risk of atherosclerosis leading to peripheral vascular disease and amputations, coronary artery disease, myocardial infarction, sudden death and cerebrovascular disease and stroke.

As discussed elsewhere in this book, effective antihypertensive treatment has improved the prognosis of patients with diabetic nephropathy, but in many countries diabetic nephropathy is still the most frequent condition, leading to dialysis and transplantation. Thus, the focus of this chapter is:

■ the epidemiological pattern of diabetic nephropathy
■ mortality in patients with and without nephropathy
■ mortality and microalbuminuria
■ prospects for prevention, including health economical aspects

EPIDEMIOLOGICAL PATTERN OF DIABETIC NEPHROPATHY
Clinical diabetic nephropathy (i.e. persistent proteinuria $\geq$ 0.5 g/24 h or $\geq$ 300 mg albumin/24 h) is rare in the first 10 years of diabetes duration, but thereafter the incidence increases to a maximum of 2-3 %/year after 13-20 years of duration. Thereafter, the incidence decreases and remains at a level of < 0.5 %/year. This incidence pattern has been demonstrated in several studies [1-4] and it has remained remarkably constant over time [1, 2]. The incidence of nephropathy has, however, decreased markedly during the

last 50 years, and in Denmark [1, 2] as well as in USA [3], and the life time of nephropathy decreased from 50 % to 25 %. In Sweden an even more dramatic reduction was observed in cohorts of children with IDDM, an in the youngest cohort no cases of nephropathy was observed at all [5]. These result were obtained in a paediatric clinic which has proven to be able to maintain remarkably low HbA_{1C} values in their patients. This result is encouraging and demonstrates the importance of strict metabolic control, but unfortunately the same level of HbA_{1C} has not been obtainable in other countries [6] and that may well explain why a similar decline in the incidence has not been found in other countries [7].

The reason why the life time risk of nephropathy has decreased from 50% to 25 % is only partly known. Improved metabolic regulation is likely to be the most important single factor. It is likely that the modifications in care, therapeutic strategies and introduction of the "self care" principle has lead to improved metabolic control. Furthermore, the DCCT-study has not only demonstrated a beneficial effect of good metabolic control, it also showed that the most dramatic absolute risk reduction was obtained in the high range of HbA_{1C} values. Other factors like antihypertensive treatment and dietary changes may have contributed to a lesser degree to the decrease in incidence of nephropathy by reducing the risk of progression from microalbuminuria to overt nephropathy.

Studies from different parts of the world consistently show, that IDDM-patients have an excess mortality compared with the non-diabetic population. The excess mortality varies with age and diabetes duration [1], and also shows considerable variation between countries [2]. As shown in table 14-1, the distribution of causes of death varies according to diabetes duration.

While acute, metabolic complications and infections dominates in patients with short diabetes duration, diabetic nephropathy and cardiovascular diseases account for 70-80 % of all deaths in patients with longer diabetes duration.

In 1972 Watkins et al suggested, that development of proteinuria was a strong prognostic marker in diabetes, and probably even stronger than grading of nephropathy on the basis of histo-pathological findings [11]. In our study of excess mortality in 1030 IDDM patients followed for 30 to 50 years we found [12], (figure 14-1) that the very high excess mortality of IDDM-patients was found only in patients who developed persistent proteinuria (clinical diabetic nephropathy), while patients not developing clinical nephropathy had a low and rather constant excess mortality.

MORTALITY AND PROTEINURIA

The high mortality of patients with nephropathy has been confirmed by several other studies [13, 14]. In patients with nephropathy the leading causes of death are uraemia/end stage renal failure and macrovascular disease. Myocardial infarction and stroke is 10 times more frequent in patients with than in patients without nephropathy [15] and below the age of 50 years the excess mortality from macrovascular disease is almost entirely confined to patients with diabetic nephropathy [16]. Thus, in conclusion from these studies, the most effective way of improving the prognosis of IDDM would be to prevent development of diabetic nephropathy. As already mentioned the incidence of nephropathy has decreased, and thus it is not surprising, that in a study of the relative mortality of IDDM-patients in Denmark during the period from 1930 to 1981 we found [17] that the excess mortality decreased by nearly 40 %. The study included nearly three thousand patients diagnosed before the age of 31 years, diagnosed during the period 1933 to 1972 and admitted to the Steno Memorial Hospital (Steno Diabetes Centre). All patients were followed up from their first admission to the hospital until death, emigration or January 1st 1982. The major decrease in the excess mortality took place in patients diagnosed from 1940 to 1955, but a constant and gradual decline was found over the entire period.

Table 14-1. Cause of death according to diabetes duration in a cohort of 2,900 Danish IDDM-patients diagnosed 1932-1972, before the age of 31 years [17]

Cause of death	Diabetes Duration		
	0-15 years (n=124)	16-30 years (n=513)	> 30 years (n=199)
Vascular			
Acute myocardial infarction	9%	17%	36%
Other cardiovascular	4%	3%	11%
Cerebrovascular	2%	4%	10%
Diabetic nephropathy	17%	52%	15%
Ketoacidosis	18%	2%	3%
Hypoglycaemia	6%	3%	2%
Diabetes NOD	2%	1%	1%
Infections	14%	5%	10%
Suicide	8%	3%	3%
Cancer	2%	3%	4%
Other	19%	7%	9%

MORTALITY AND MICROALBUMINURIA

Patients with microalbuminuria i.e. urinary albumin excretion rate from 30 to 300 mg/24 h have long been known as a high risk group for development of diabetic nephropathy [18-20]. Dyslipidaemia and changes in other cardiovascular risk factors including blood pressure and rheological factors are well established characteristics of patients with microalbuminuria [21, 22], and in NIDDM patient's microalbuminuria is associated with increased cardiovascular morbidity and mortality [23, 24]. Thus, the question is whether microalbuminuria predicts increased mortality - particularly from cardiovascular disease, even in IDDM patients. In non-insulin dependent diabetic patient [25, 26] as well as in non-diabetic individuals [27, 28] microalbuminuria is associated with a marked excess mortality particularly from cardiovascular disease. Very few studies have been performed in IDDM patients, and methodologically these studies are difficult to perform, as patients developing nephropathy should be excluded (censored) from the cohort at onset of nephropathy. The magnitude of this problem is illustrated in a study by Messent [30] where they followed microalbuminuric IDDM patients for more than twenty years, this group of patients had a significant excess mortality. Among the eight patients with microalbuminuria originally included in the study five died. However, all deceased patients had developed clinical nephropathy and were no longer microalbuminuric at the time of death. Among the three surviving patients, one developed renal failure while two remained microalbuminuric throughout the observation period. In a more recent study, where we combined data from several cohorts we showed [31] that microalbuminuria is associated with excess mortality even in the microalbuminuric range.

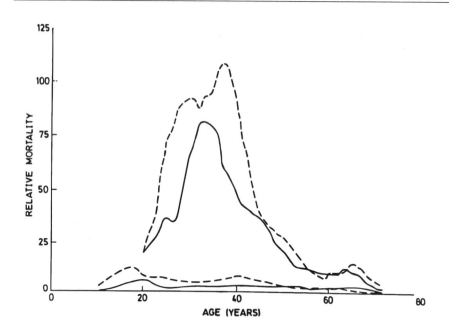

Figure 14-1 Age adjusted relative mortality of IDDM-patients with proteinuria (upper curves) and without proteinuria (lower curves) in a cohort of 1003 Danish IDDM-patients: - - - - Women, — Men. (Reproduced with permission from Diabetologia and Springer Verlag [12]).

Intervention studies have shown that strict metabolic control [8] as well as antihypertensive treatment of IDDM patients with microalbuminuria may delay or prevent progression to diabetic nephropathy, and it must therefore be assumed, that it will prevent some of these patients from developing End Stage Renal Failure and uraemia. The impact of this on all cause mortality and cardiovascular mortality in particular remains unknown, at strict metabolic control may not be able to bring mortality rates down to the same controlled clinical trials have been so small and running for so short periods of time [32-35] that an evaluation of this has been impossible so far.

PROSPECTS FOR PREVENTION

As already discussed the incidence of nephropathy has decreased markedly during the last 30-50 years, and the most likely explanation is that a gradual improvement in overall metabolic regulation has occurred during this period. Thus, primary prevention of nephropathy in IDDM patients is possible. Secondary prevention, i.e. prevention of progression from microalbuminuria to overt nephropathy is also possible by antihypertensive treatment [32-35], but other factors like smoking [36] and dietary factors [37] may also be important risk factors for progression to nephropathy. All of these factors will be dealt with in details in other chapters of this book and will not be discussed further here. The main lesson is that primary AND secondary prevention is possible. Secondary prevention is, however, possible only if patients developing microalbuminuria are identified at an early stage of the condition, where there is room for early intervention. For this reason all patients with IDDM should be screened annually for microalbuminuria. This could not only contribute to an improvement of the prognosis of the individual, but, as discussed below, even lead to considerable savings in the health care system.

SCREENING, INTERVENTION AND COST EFFECTIVENESS

As trials aiming at early intervention in the microalbuminuric stage are relatively small and few, it is difficult to estimate the cost effectiveness of different regimens for screening for and early intervention in microalbuminuria. On the other hand, treatment of end stage renal failure with dialysis or renal transplantation is so expensive (costs approximately 25 to 40.000 US $ per year) [38], that if intervention programmes are effective, then they are also likely to be cost-beneficial. Furthermore, screening for microalbuminuria is becoming increasingly simple, fast and cheap with the availability of methods described elsewhere in this book.

Two independent groups have tried to estimate the likely cost-benefit and cost effectiveness of different regimens for screening and intervention. In the study of Siegel et al [39], the authors compared the likely costs and savings related to four different programmes: 1: No screening for microalbuminuria or proteinuria, antihypertensive treatment at BP 140/90, 2: Screening for proteinuria (0.5 g/24 h) and ACE-inhibitor treatment in case of proteinuria, 3: Screening for microalbuminuria, treatment with ACE-inhibitor if UAER 100 µg/min and 4: Screening for microalbuminuria and ACE-inhibitor if UAER 20 µg/min. The authors used previously published epidemiological data regarding the natural history of diabetic nephropathy to estimate the time of progression from norm-to microalbuminuria, from microalbuminuria to proteinuria and from proteinuria to end stage renal failure. They then assumed two different potential effects of antihypertensive treatment, 50 % increase in progression time (called conservative estimate) and 75 % increased progression time (called optimistic estimate).

The second study [40], used a rather similar design including annual testing for microalbuminuria in all IDDM patients from five to 30 years of diabetes duration. Antihypertensive treatment using an ACE-inhibitor would be initiated in all patients with microalbuminuria (30 mg/24 h). The study used data from a previously published Danish epidemiological study [41] of the incidence of nephropathy and the mortality in patients with and without proteinuria to estimate mortality rates and transmission times without intervention. Based on the results from controlled clinical trials [32-35, 42] they estimated that the increase rate in UAER could be decreased by 33 or 67 per cent.

Both studies conclude, that if antihypertensive treatment can lower the annual increase rate in UAER in microalbuminuric patients, then screening- and intervention programmes will save money for the providers of the health care system. In our own study, we found [40] that even when taking discounting into consideration, a treatment effect of the antihypertensive treatment of 8 to 12 % would be sufficient to out-balance costs and savings. In patients with nephropathy, antihypertensive treatment has been shown to decrease the decline-rate in GFR and to decrease the mortality rates by 67 % [43, 44]. If this was the case also in patients with microalbuminuria, then screening and intervention for microalbuminuria would increase the median life-expectancy of IDDM patients by more than 10 years, and the life-time risk of developing end stage renal failure would decrease by more than 60 %.

The conclusions drawn in the studies by Siegel et al. [39] and Borch-Johnsen et al [40] have been disputed by Kiberd and Jindal [46]. Like the two previous studies they performed a cost-effectiveness study, but compared a scenario with screening for microalbuminuria with a scenario screening for hypertension. They concluded that screening for hypertension would be more cost effective than screening for microalbuminuria. In their paper they, however, never defined hypertension, making it difficult to take recommendations from their study. Furthermore, their analysis was based on a set of critical assumptions, including that: i) Insulin dependent diabetic patients with microalbuminuria usually develop hypertension before they develop nephropathy. Ii) A diagnosis of hypertension can be made precisely without false positive and false negative cases of hypertension and iii) prevention of nephropathy is the only reason for surveillance and intervention. The premises for assumptions i) and ii) are discussed elsewhere in this book, but it is likely that microalbuminuria and increasing blood pressure develops in parallel [46]. Furthermore, it is well known that there is a huge variability in blood pressure, particularly when measured in routine clinical settings [47]. Microalbuminuria is a marker, not only of early renal disease, but also of generalised micro-and macrovascular disease [21, 31]. Thus, it is a marker of high risk individuals that should be screened regularly for other complications, and therefore premise iii) is not valid. Finally, as discussed later in this book, antihypertensive treatment with ACE-inhibitors is indicated even in normotensive patients with microalbuminuria and thus screening for hypertension would NOT identify the target population.

CONCLUSION

Proteinuria and microalbuminuria are both not only well established risk factors for end stage renal failure but also the strongest prognostic markers ever identified in diabetic individuals. In IDDM patients, a diagnosis of proteinuria and microalbuminuria has therapeutic implications (e.g. strict metabolic control, antihypertensive treatment etc.) and they will indicate that this is a high risk patient who needs intensified care to prevent macroangiopathy (i.e. focus on the entire cardiovascular risk profile) and to prevent proliferative retinopathy and visual impairment. As neither microalbuminuria nor proteinuria causes any subjective symptoms to the patient, they reflect the large group of clinically silent but life threatening conditions that can only be detected by screening.

REFERENCES

1. Andersen AR, Christiansen JS, Andersen JK, Kreiner S & Deckert T. Diabetic nephropathy in Type 1 (insulin-dependent) diabetes: and epidemiological study. Diabetologia 1983;25:496-501.
2. Kofoed-Enevoldsen A, Borch-Johnsen K, Kreiner S, Nerup J, Deckert T. Declining incidence of persistent proteinuria in Type 1 (insulin-dependent) diabetic patients in Denmark. Diabetes 1987;36:205-209.
3. Krolewski AS, Warram JH, Christlieb ARE, Busick EJ, Kahn CR. The changing natural history of nephropathy in Type 1 diabetes. Am J Med 1985;78:785-794.
4. Tchobroutsky G. Relation of diabetic control to development of microvascular complications. Diabetologia 1978;15:143-153.
5. Bojestig M, Arnqvist HJ, Hermansson G, Karlberg BE, Ludvigsson J. Declining incidence of nephropathy in insulin-dependent diabetes mellitus. N Engl J Med 1994;330:15-18.
6. Mortensen HB, Hougaard P. Comparison of metabolic control in a cross-sectional study of 2,873 children and adolescents with IDDM from 18 countries. Diabetes Care 1997;20:714.
7. Rossing P, Rossing K, Jacobsen P, Parving HH. Unchanged incidence of diabetic nephropathy in IDDM patients. Diabetes 1995;44:739-743.

8.   The Diabetes Control and Complications Trial Research Group. The effect of intensive treatment of diabetes on the development and progression of long-term complications in insulin-dependent diabetes mellitus. N Engl J Med 1993;329:977-986.
9.   Borch-Johnsen K. The prognosis of insulin-dependent diabetes mellitus. Dan Med Bull 1989;36:336-348.
10.   Diabetes Epidemiology Research International (DERI) Mortality Study Group. Major Cross-Country differences in risk of dying for people with IDDM. Diabetes Care 1991;14:49-54.
11.   Watson PJ, Blainey JD, Brewer DB, Fitzgerald MG, Malins JM, O'Sullivan DJ, Pinto JA. The natural history of diabetic renal disease. Q J Med 1972;164:437-456.
12.   Borch-Johnsen K, Andersen PK, Deckert T. The effect of proteinuria on relative mortality in Type 1 (insulin-dependent) diabetes mellitus. Diabetologia 1985;28:590-596.
13.   Parving HH, Hommel E. Prognosis in diabetic nephropathy. BMJ 1989;299:230-233.
14.   Rossing P, Hougaard P, Borch-Johnsen K, Parving HH. Predictors of mortality in insulin dependent diabetes: 10 year observational follow up study. BMJ 1996;313:779-784.
15.   Jensen T, Borch-Johnsen K, Deckert T. Coronary heart disease in young Type 1 (insulin-dependent) diabetic patients with diabetic nephropathy: Incidence and risk factors. Diabetologia 1987;30:144-148.
16.   Borch-Johnsen K, Kreiner S. Proteinuria: value as predictor of cardio-vascular mortality in insulin-dependent diabetes mellitus. Br Med J 1987;294:1651-1654.
17.   Borch-Johnsen K, Kreiner S, Deckert T. Mortality of Type 1 (insulin-dependent) diabetes mellitus in Denmark. Diabetologia 1986;29:767-772.
18.   Viberti GC, Jarrett RJ, Mahmud U, Hill RD, Argyropoulos A, Keen H. Microalbuminuria as a predictor of clinical nephropathy in insulin dependent diabetes mellitus. Lancet 1982;i:1430-1432.
19.   Mogensen CE, Christensen CK. Predicting diabetic nephropathy in insulin-dependent patients. N Engl J Med 1984;311:89-93.
20.   Mathiesen ER, Oxenbøll B, Johansen K, Svendsen PAa, Deckert T. incipient nephropathy in Type 1 (insulin-dependent) diabetes. Diabetologia 1984;26:406-410.
21.   Jensen T. Albuminuria - a marker of renal and generalized vascular disease in insulin-dependent diabetes mellitus. Dan Med Bull 1991;38:134-144.
22.   Feldt-Rasmussen B. Microalbuminuria and clinical nephropathy in Type 1 (insulin-dependent) diabetes mellitus: pathophysiological mechanisms and intervention studies. Dan Med Bull 1989;36:405-415.
23.   Gall M-A, Borch-Johnsen K, Hougaard P, Nielsen FS, and Parving H-H. Albuminuria and poor glycemic control predict mortality in NIDDM. Diabetes 1995;44:1303-1309.
24.   Agewall S, Wikstrand J, Ljungman S, Herlitz H, and Fagerberg B. Does microalbuminuria predict cardiovascular events in nondiabetic men with treated hypertension? AJH 1995;8:337-342.
25.   Mogensen CE. Microalbuminuria predicts clinical proteinuria and early mortality in maturity onset diabetes. N Engl J Med 1984;310:356-360.
26.   Jarrett RJ, Viberti GC, Argyropoulos A, Hill RD, Mahmud U, Murrells TJ. Microalbuminuria predicts mortality in non-insulin-dependent diabetes. Diabetic Med 1984;I:17-19.

27. Yudkin JS, Forrest RD, Jackson CA. Microalbuminuria as predictor of vascular disease in non-diabetic subjects. Lancet 1988;ii:530-533.

28. Damsgaard EM, Frøland A, Jørgensen OD, Mogensen CE. Micro-albuminuria as predictor of increased mortality in elderly people. BMJ 1990;300:297-300.

29. Borch-Johnsen K, Feldt-Rasmussen B, Strandgaard S, Schroll M, Jensen JS. Microalbuminuria: a novel independent risk factor for ischemic heart disease. Submitted BMJ 1997.

30. Messent JWC, Elliott TG, Hill RD, Jarrett RJ, Keen H, Viberti GC. Prognostic significance of microalbuminuria in insulin-dependent diabetes mellitus: a twenty year follow-up study. Kidney Int 1992;41:836-839.

31. Deckert T, Yokoyama H, Mathiesen ER, Rønn B, Jansen T, Feldt-Rasmussen B, Borch-Johnsen K, Jensen JS. Cohort study of predictive value of urinary albumin excretion for atherosclerotic vascular disease in insulin dependent diabetes. BMJ 1996;312:871-874.

32. Marre M, Chatellier G, Leblanc H, Guyene TT, Menard J, Passa P. Prevention of diabetic nephropathy with enalapril in normotensive diabetics with microalbuminuria. BMJ 1988;297:1092-1095.

33. Mathiesen ER, Hommel E, Giese J, Parving H-H. Efficacy of captopril in postponing nephropathy in normotensive insulin-dependent diabetic patients with microalbuminuria. BMJ 1991;303:81-87.

34. Melbourne Diabetic nephropathy study group. Comparison between perindopril and nifedipine in hypertensive and normotensive diabetic patients with microalbuminuria. BMJ 1991;302:210-216.

35. Viberti GC, Mogensen CE, Groop L, Pauls JF for the European Microalbuminuria Captopril Study Group. Effect of captopril on progression to clinical proteinuria in patients with insulin-dependent diabetes mellitus and microalbuminuria. JAMA 1994;271:275-279.

36. Sawicki PT, Mühlhaser I, Bender R, Pethke W, Heinemann L, Berger M. Effects of smoking on blood pressure and proteinuria in patients with diabetic nephropathy. J Intern Med 1996;239:345-352.

37. Pedrini MT, Levey AS, Lau J, Chalmers TC, Wang PH. The effect of dietary protein restriction on the progression of diabetic and non-diabetic renal disease: a meta-analysis. Ann Intern Med 1996;124:627-632.

38. Eggers PW. Health Care Policies/economics of the geriatric renal population. Am J Kidney Dis 1990;16:384-391.

39. Siegel JE, Krolewski AS, Warram JH, Weinstein MC. Cost-effectiveness of screening and early treatment of nephropathy in patients with insulin-dependent diabetes mellitus. J AM Soc Nephrol 1992;3:3111-3119.

40. Borch-Johnsen K, Wenzel H, Viberti GC, Mogensen CE. Is screening and intervention for Microalbuminuria worthwhile in patients with insulin dependent diabetes? BMJ 1993;306:1722-1725.

41. Ramlau-Hansen H, Bang Jespersen NC, Andersen PK, Borch-Johnsen K, Deckert T. Life insurance for insulin-dependent diabetics. Scand Actuarial J 1987;19-36.

42. Feldt-Rasmussen B, Mathiesen ER, Jensen T, Lauritzen T, Deckert T. Effect of improved metabolic control on loss of kidney function in Type 1 (insulin-dependent) diabetic patients: an update of the Steno studies. Diabetologia 1991;34:164-170.

43. Parving H-H, Andersen ARE, Smidt UM, Svendsen PAA. Early aggressive antihypertensive treatment reduces the rate of decline in kidney function in diabetic nephropathy. Lancet 1983;i:1175-1179.

44. Mathiesen ER, Borch-Johnsen K, Jensen DV, Deckert T. Improved survival in patients with diabetic nephropathy. Diabetologia 1989;32:884-886.

45. Kiberd BA, Jindal KK. Screening to prevent renal failure in insulin dependent diabetic patients: an economical evaluation: BMJ 1995;311:595-599.

46. Microalbuminuria Collaborative Study Group, UK. Risk factors for development of microalbuminuria in insulin dependent diabetic patients: a cohort study. BMJ 1993;306:1235-1239.

47. Hansen KW, Christensen CK, Andersen PH, Mau Pedersen M, Christiansen JS, Mogensen CE. Ambulatory blood pressure in microalbuminuric type 1 diabetic patients. Kidney Int 1992;41:847-854.

15. DYSFUNCTION OF THE VASCULAR ENDOTHELIUM AND THE DEVELOPMENT OF RENAL AND VASCULAR COMPLICATIONS IN DIABETES

Coen D.A. Stehouwer
Department of Medicine, University Hospital Vrije Universiteit, Amsterdam, The Netherlands

This chapter will specifically consider whether endothelial dysfunction can explain why, both in type 1 and in type 2 diabetes, the presence of microalbuminuria or clinical proteinuria is associated with a very high risk of developing severe vascular complications, i.e. proliferative retinopathy, renal insufficiency, and cardiovascular disease, as reviewed elsewhere [1]. It will also discuss at what stage of diabetes endothelial dysfunction becomes manifest as well as its potential causes.

WHAT IS ENDOTHELIAL DYSFUNCTION?

The endothelium is an important locus of control of vascular functions. It actively regulates vascular tone, vascular permeability to leukocytes and macromolecules, the balance between coagulation and fibrinolysis, the composition of the subendothelial matrix, and the proliferation of vascular smooth muscle cells. To carry out these functions, the endothelium produces components of the extracellular matrix and a variety of regulatory mediators, such as nitric oxide (NO), prostanoids, endothelin, angiotensin-II, thrombomodulin, heparan sulphate, tissue factor pathway inhibitor, tissue-type plasminogen activator (t-PA), plasminogen activator inhibitor-1 (PAI-1), von Willebrand factor (vWf), adhesion molecules and cytokines. Normally, the endothelium actively decreases vascular tone; maintains vascular permeability within narrow bounds; inhibits platelet adhesion and aggregation; limits activation of the coagulation system; and stimulates fibrinolysis. The endothelium can adapt to temporal and local requirements. Dysfunction of the endothelium can be considered present when its properties have changed in a way that is inappropriate with regard to the preservation of organ function. For example, basement membrane synthesis may be altered, resulting in changes in cell-matrix interactions which can contribute to arterial stiffening and increased microvascular permeability; vascular tone and permeability may increase, which contributes to increased blood pressure and atherogenesis; and the endothelium may lose its antithrombotic and profibrinolytic properties and may instead acquire prothrombotic and antifibrinolytic properties. Such alterations do not necessarily occur simultaneously and may differ according to the nature of the injury and the intrinsic properties of the endothelium (e.g., venous versus arterial versus microvascular endothelium, and heart versus kidney versus skeletal muscle endothelium).

Endothelial function cannot be measured directly in humans. Estimates of different types of endothelial dysfunction may be obtained indirectly by measuring endothelium-dependent vasodilation, plasma levels of endothelium-derived regulatory proteins and, possibly, microalbuminuria. The assumptions underlying this approach and its general validity have been discussed elsewhere [1-4]. In brief, reasonable but not perfect estimates exist for assessing endothelial function in vivo in humans. The most extensive experience has been gained with three particular estimates: endothelium-dependent vasodilation, plasma vWf level and microalbuminuria. With regard to the latter, it is unlikely that the presence of microalbuminuria always and exclusively reflects a generalised increase of endothelial permeability; it may be wholly or partly a local renal haemodynamic phenomenon in at least some cases [5; see below].

ENDOTHELIAL DYSFUNCTION, (MICRO-)ALBUMINURIA AND CARDIOVASCULAR DISEASE IN DIABETES MELLITUS

Endothelial dysfunction is an event closely associated with the development of diabetic retinopathy, nephropathy and atherosclerosis, both in type 1 and type 2 diabetes (see ref. 1 for review).

In type 1 diabetes, microalbuminuria (early nephropathy) and macroalbuminuria (advanced nephropathy) are accompanied by a variety of markers of endothelial dysfunction, such as increased plasma concentrations of vWF and impaired endothelium-dependent, nitric oxide-mediated vasodilation [1]. In type 2 diabetes, microalbuminuria has also been shown to be related to elevated levels of plasma vWF and of other endothelial dysfunction markers [1]. In prospective cohort studies, the development of microalbuminuria was accompanied by an increase in vWF [6,7]. High vWF levels also have prognostic value with regard to the occurrence of diabetic neuropathy [8] and of cardiovascular events [7,9]. Endothelial dysfunction in type 1 and 2 diabetes complicated by micro- or macroalbuminuria is generalised, in that it affects many aspects of endothelial function and occurs both in the kidney and elsewhere [1]. These data, together with limited data showing that microalbuminuria is also associated with endothelial dysfunction in the absence of diabetes [10], have led to the concept that microalbuminuria itself is a marker of generalised renal and extrarenal endothelial dysfunction, specifically increased endothelial permeability to macromolecules. Another hypothesis is that the presence of microalbuminuria simply reflects more advanced atherosclerotic disease. A recent study provided some evidence against this idea [11].

Endothelial dysfunction may explain the typical association between (micro-) albuminuria and extrarenal complications [1], because it is a central feature of current models of atherogenesis [12] and because it may be important in the pathogenesis of albuminuria [13,14] both directly, by contributing to the synthesis of a leaky glomerular basement membrane, and indirectly, by influencing glomerular mesangial and epithelial cell function in a paracrine fashion.

IS THE LINK BETWEEN MICROALBUMINURIA AND ENDOTHELIAL DYSFUNCTION IN DIABETES HETEROGENEOUS?

Microalbuminuria in diabetes *in general* clusters with hypertension, severe retinopathy and atherosclerotic cardiovascular disease in both type 1 and type 2 diabetes [1]. There is some recent evidence, however, for heterogeneity among these relationships and for a role of vWF and retinopathy in distinguishing microalbuminuria with versus microalbuminuria without a tendency for severe extrarenal disease [5]. The EURODIAB IDDM Complications Study found, in a Europe-wide study of over 3000 type 1 diabetic patients, that the albumin excretion rate correlated significantly with both systolic blood pressure and the plasma vWF concentration, but only in subjects with diabetic retinopathy. Around half of the patients with microalbuminuria had no clinical evidence of retinopathy, and in this group there was no association of increasing albumin excretion with either blood pressure or endothelial dysfunction [15,16]. In type 2 diabetes, there is some evidence – although by no means undisputed – that both dipstick-positive proteinuria [17] and microalbuminuria [18] are morphologically heterogeneous. Fioretto et al. have recently shown that endothelial dysfunction, as estimated by plasma vWF, was present only in those microalbuminuric patients who, on renal biopsy, had either typical diabetic glomerulopathy or atypical patterns of injury but not in those with (near-) normal histology [18,19]. In two prospective studies in type 2 diabetes, microalbuminuria was associated with an increased risk of new cardiovascular events mainly when endothelial dysfunction was present [7,20]. Thus, both in type 1 and, perhaps even more so, in type 2 diabetes, the interrelationships among microalbuminuria, endothelial dysfunction, renal histology and diabetic retinopathy appear somewhat more heterogeneous than previously thought, but further study of this issue is clearly required.

AT WHAT STAGE OF DIABETES DOES ENDOTHELIAL DYSFUNCTION BECOME MANIFEST?

In type 1 diabetes, plasma vWF levels are increased in patients with an elevated urinary albumin excretion rate, but not in patients with early, uncomplicated and reasonably well-regulated type 1 diabetes, nor in those with early diabetic retinopathy [1]. A small prospective study showed that an increase in the plasma vWF level preceded the occurrence of microalbuminuria by about three years [21; figure 15-1]. Thus, limited prospective data on vWF in human type 1 diabetes indicate that endothelial dysfunction, as reflected by increased vWF, is not a feature of the diabetic state per se but does occur before microalbuminuria sets in. In accordance, abnormalities of large vessel function that may in part be endothelium-dependent, such as increased arterial stiffness, can be demonstrated in normoalbuminuric type 1 diabetic subjects and are worse in the microalbuminuric stage [22-25].

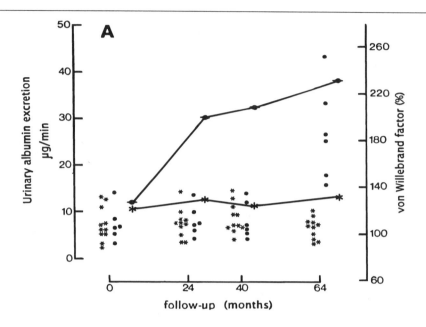

Figure 15-1 Time course of urinary albumin excretion (UAE; reference < 15 µg/min) and plasma von Willebrand factor level (vWF; reference range 50-150%) in insulin-dependent diabetes mellitus. All patients had normal UAE at the start of the follow-up (t=0). UAE remained normal in 11 patients (*); in six patients (•), microalbuminuria was present at the final follow-up (t=64). The figure shows the individual values of UAE (* and •) and the medians of the vWF levels (*-*) and (•-•). The figure illustrates that high vWF levels, indicating endothelial dysfunction, are present in patients in whom microalbuminuria develops. The increase in vWF (present at t=24) precedes the development of microalbuminuria (at t=24). Reproduced with permission [21].

It is controversial whether the bioactivity of nitric oxide, as estimated from endothelium-dependent vasodilatory responses, is impaired in otherwise uncomplicated type 1 diabetes, and whether hyperglycaemia per se is sufficient to impair nitric oxide bioactivity, both normal and impaired responses having been reported [1, 26-33]. Taken together, these data suggest that impairment of endothelium-dependent vasodilation may occur early in a subset of type 1 diabetic patients, perhaps dependent on other, environmental or genetic, factors.

The definition of "early, uncomplicated type 2 diabetes" is problematic, which complicates an analysis of the role of endothelial dysfunction in the angiopathy of type 2 diabetes. Nevertheless, endothelial dysfunction can occur in patients with normal urinary albumin excretion [1]. High levels of vWF are associated with an increased risk of cardiovascular mortality [9] and, in patients with normal urinary albumin excretion, with an increased risk of developing microalbuminuria [7]. Endothelium-dependent vasodilation appears impaired in type 2 diabetes [34-38], although some studies are difficult to interpret because both endothelium-dependent and –independent responses were found to be decreased [37,38]. Thus, there is increasing evidence for impaired endothelial function in early type 2 diabetes.

ENDOTHELIAL DYSFUNCTION AND THE INSULIN RESISTANCE SYNDROME

Insulin resistance (impaired insulin-stimulated glucose utilisation) usually precedes the development of type 2 diabetes and is often accompanied by a cluster of other risk factors, notably obesity, hypertension, high triglyceride levels, low high density lipoprotein (HDL) cholesterol levels, abnormal low density lipoprotein composition, and hyperinsulinaemia (the insulin resistance syndrome). The mechanisms underlying this clustering are still unclear, but all elements of the cluster share two important pathophysiological features, namely insulin resistance and vascular endothelial dysfunction, with most studies concentrating on endothelium-dependent vasodilation [1,39-47]. A widely accepted theory states that insulin resistance is the primary abnormality that gives rise to type 2 diabetes, hypertension and dyslipidaemia, and that endothelial dysfunction merely represents the impact of hyperglycaemia and other features of the insulin resistance syndrome. However, one needs to consider the alternative concept, i.e. that endothelial dysfunction could be a common antecedent: endothelial dysfunction in resistance vessels and metabolically important capillary beds may contribute to the development of the insulin resistance syndrome in parallel with endothelial-dysfunction-induced atherosclerosis in large arteries. There are at least two possibilities through which this may occur.

First, kinetic studies of insulin action indicate that, before insulin binds to its receptor on muscle cells, there is a rate-limiting step, which may reflect in part transendothelial insulin transport [48]. However, it is unclear whether impaired transendothelial transport is responsible for insulin resistance in subjects with type 2 diabetes or obesity, because neither the time course of transport of insulin to the interstitium nor interstitial insulin concentrations in such subjects appear to differ from those in normal subjects [49,50]. A second possible link between endothelial dysfunction and insulin resistance is through insulin's vasoactive properties. Insulin increases muscle blood flow in a time- and concentration-dependent fashion [41,42,51] through a mechanism that can be abolished by inhibiting nitric oxide synthase [52]. In insulin-resistant states, insulin's vasodilator actions are impaired and this finding has led to the concept of cross-talk between insulin's metabolic and vascular actions [41,42]. Specifically, it has been hypothesised that insulin may redirect blood flow from non-nutritive vessels to nutritive capillary beds in skeletal muscle, and thus influence glucose metabolism, even if total blood flow remains constant. Thus, an insulin-induced redistribution of capillary blood flow rather than an insulin-induced increase in total blood flow may be crucial [53-56]. Since insulin largely appears to be an endothelium-dependent vasodilator [52], the linkage between glucose metabolism and blood flow distribution may occur at an endothelial level. Most [42,57,58] but not all [59] data in humans support a relationship between insulin resistance and impaired endothelial function. Whether insulin causes capillary recruitment in humans is still unresolved [58], but muscle capillary density has been shown to be positively correlated with insulin sensitivity [60] and skin capillary recruitment is strongly related to insulin sensitivity in normal subjects [58].

Thus, the endothelium may have important roles both in the delivery of insulin and glucose, and as a target for insulin action. Reduced endothelial surface area and impaired insulin-induced, endothelium-dependent vasodilatation and microvascular (endothelium-dependent?) blood flow distribution may contribute to insulin resistance. In this way, physical integrity and normal function of the arteriolar and capillary endothelium may be prerequisites for normal insulin action. In fact, a case can be made for impaired microvascular function as a contributor to other features of the insulin resistance syndrome [1,39,40], notably hypertension [58] and dyslipidaemia [61], but much more work in this area is clearly needed.

WHAT CAUSES ENDOTHELIAL DYSFUNCTION IN DIABETES?
Human data on these issues are scarce and mostly indirect. For example, poor glycaemic control is associated with high vWF levels and other markers of endothelial dysfunction [6,62], but the relation is relatively weak. This is consistent with current thinking on the pathogenesis of nephropathy, which postulates that hyperglycaemia is necessary but not sufficient to cause severe microangiopathy [1]. Major obstacles to defining the causes of endothelial dysfunction in diabetes in humans include methodological problems with the assessment of endothelial function and the fact that assessment, in man, of the relative importance of the biochemical pathways proposed on the basis of experimental studies will require specific interventions with for example inhibitors of protein kinase C (PKC), transforming growth factor-β (TGFβ) and advanced glycation endproduct (AGE) formation, which are only just becoming available. What follows is a brief survey of the most important current hypotheses (see refs. 1 and other chapters in this book for more detailed discussions).

Hyperglycaemia.
High glucose affects endothelial function both directly, through glucose-induced impairment of normal intracellular metabolic regulation, and indirectly, through increased formation of early and advanced glycation endproducts and through affecting the function of other cells with secondary effects on the endothelium.

Endothelial cells exposed to high glucose in vitro increase the production of extracellular matrix components, such as collagen and fibronectin, and of procoagulant proteins, such as von Willebrand factor and tissue factor, and show decreased proliferation, migration and fibrinolytic potential [63], and increased programmed cell death (apoptosis; [64]) and leukocyte adhesion [65]. High glucose levels affect several interlinked pathways resulting in an increased NADH/NAD$^+$ ratio (hyperglycaemic pseudohypoxia; [66]); changes in the regulation of protein tyrosine kinases, the activity of which is influenced by the redox state of their sulphydryl groups; dysregulation of PKC, in particular the PKC-βII isotype [67,68]; and the accumulation of sorbitol [66].

One consequence of an increased NADH/NAD$^+$ ratio may be an increased sensitivity to oxidative stress [66,69]. PKC activation can potentially explain many of the vascular abnormalities observed in diabetes: in animal and in vitro models, it can affect endothelial, vascular smooth muscle and mesangial cell functions, including the regulation of permeability, contractility, blood flow and basement membrane synthesis [67,68].

Advanced glycation end products (AGEs) can affect endothelial function in at least three ways: by altering extracellular proteins, by binding to cellular receptors and by intracellular AGE formation. Thus, extracellular AGEs inhibit a normal network formation by type IV collagen; decrease heparan sulphate proteoglycan binding by vitronectin and laminin; and quench nitric oxide during its passage from endothelial to smooth muscle cells, with loss of its vasodilating and antiproliferative actions [70,71]. The binding of AGEs to their cellular receptor has been shown, in macrophages, to induce the synthesis of interleukin-1, tumour necrosis factor-α (TNF-α), and insulin-like growth factor-1; and, in endothelial cells, to increase permeability and to induce tissue factor, vascular cell adhesion molecule-1, and interleukin-6 expression. In type 1 diabetes, AGE levels are related to endothelial dysfunction [72]. Specific Amadori products may also affect endothelial function [73].

Thus, many aspects of vascular dysfunction observed in diabetes are potentially related to the effects of AGEs. AGE-induced TNFα formation may be important in inducing insulin resistance (see below), but may also activate endothelial cells and thus affect the antithrombotic properties of endothelial cells and the margination and extravasation of leukocytes.

Hyperglycaemic pseudohypoxia, glucose autooxidation and AGE formation may be important determinants of increased oxidative stress in diabetes. However, evidence that hyperglycaemia-associated oxidative stress may be linked to endothelial dysfunction in human diabetes is as yet limited [74].

Other indirect pathways by which high glucose is believed to influence endothelial cells include the synthesis of growth factors in adjacent cells, in particular TGFβ [75] and vascular endothelial growth factor (VEGF), the latter being especially important in the neovascularisation of proliferative diabetic retinopathy [76].

The insulin resistance syndrome

The endothelial dysfunction observed in subjects with the insulin resistance syndrome is likely to be multifactorial. First, once dyslipidaemia and hypertension occur (through whatever mechanisms), this will in and of itself contribute to endothelial dysfunction. Second, hyperinsulinaemia may play a role, although this is controversial [1,77]. Most evidence suggests that insulin activates vasodilator pathways in both endothelial and vascular smooth muscle cells, possibly through a phosphatidylinositol 3 (PI3)-kinase dependent pathway [52, 78,79]. On the other hand, insulin may have slow growth-promoting effects through activation of a mitogen-activated protein (MAP)-kinase-dependent pathway [80], and it is conceivable that this may cause endothelial dysfunction. Insulin may also activate certain blood-pressure-increasing mechanisms [81], although it remains unclear whether this is relevant in man [82]. A further complexity is that insulin's vascular effects may differ between men and women [78,83,84].

As alluded to above, insulin resistance/hyperinsulinaemia and impaired endothelial function are associated, but, as discussed above, this does not necessarily mean that hyperinsulinaemia *causes* endothelial dysfunction. For example, a common antecedent may, at least in part, explain the link between insulin resistance and endothelial dysfunction. An important candidate is adipose tissue. For example, increased adipose tissue and adipose-tissue-derived mediators such as TNF-α and free fatty acids, and chronic, low-grade inflammatory activity in human obesity may induce insulin resistance [1,85-89] and endothelial dysfunction [89-91]. This is an important area for further study. In addition, as discussed above, microvascular (endothelial?) dysfunction may contribute to insulin resistance. Possible causes of microvascular dysfunction, in turn, include all of the causes of endothelial dysfunction listed above, thus potentially creating several types of vicious cycle. Finally, low birth weight is associated with an increased risk of developing the insulin resistance syndrome and atherothrombotic disease. How this relates to the above discussion remains unresolved, although it is clear that there is no lack of possibilities [92,93].

CONCLUSION
There is extensive biochemical and clinical evidence that dysfunction of the vascular endothelium plays an important role in the pathogenesis of diabetic micro- and macroangiopathy. Endothelial dysfunction occurs in at least some patients without clinical evidence of angiopathy and is usually generalised by the time microalbuminuria sets in. A subset of diabetic patients with microalbuminuria may not have generalised endothelial dysfunction, and these subjects may have a relatively good prognosis. Insulin resistance is associated with endothelial dysfunction. There is evidence that insulin resistance or the metabolic defects with which it is associated cause endothelial dysfunction. In addition, microvascular endothelial dysfunction may itself contribute to insulin resistance, suggesting that endothelial dysfunction is among the earliest (and perhaps the fundamental) factors that cause vascular disease not only in type 2 diabetes, but also in subjects with the so-called insulin resistance syndrome. The proximate causes of endothelial dysfunction in diabetic man remain poorly understood but probably include direct and indirect effects of hyperglycaemia as well as adipose-tissue-derived mediators.

REFERENCES
1.   Stehouwer CDA, Lambert J, Donker AJM, van Hinsbergh VWM. Endothelial dysfunction and the pathogenesis of diabetic angiopathy. Cardiovasc Res 1997;34:55-68.
2.   Blann AD, Taberner DA. A reliable marker of endothelial dysfunction: does it exist? Br J Haematol 1995;90:244-248.
3.   Celermajer DS. Endothelial dysfunction: does it matter? Is it reversible? J Am Coll Cardiol 1997;30:325-333.
4.   Stehouwer CDA. Is measurement of endothelial dysfunction clinically useful? [editorial] Eur J Clin Invest 1999;29:459-461.

5.   Stehouwer CDA, Yudkin JS, Fioretto P, Nosadini R. How heterogeneous is microalbuminuria? The case for 'benign' and 'malignant' microalbuminuria. Nephrol Dial Transplant 1998;13:2751-2754.

6.   Stehouwer CDA, Stroes ESG, Hackeng WHL, Mulder PGH, den Ottolander GJH. von Willebrand factor and development of diabetic nephropathy in insulin-dependent diabetes mellitus. Diabetes 1991;40:971-976 [erratum, Diabetes 1991;40:1746].

7.   Stehouwer CDA, Nauta JJP, Zeldenrust GC, Hackeng WHL, Donker AJM, den Ottolander GJH. Albuminuria, cardiovascular disease, and endothelial dysfunction in non-insulin-dependent diabetes mellitus. Lancet 1992;340:319-323.

8.   Plater ME, Ford I, Dent MT, Preston FE, Ward JE. Elevated von Willebrand factor antigen predicts deterioration in diabetic periperal nerve function. Diabetologia 1996;39:336-343.

9.   Jager A, van Hinsbergh VWM, Kostense PJ, Emeis JJ, Yudkin JS, Nijpels G, Heine RJ, Bouter LM, Stehouwer CDA. Von Willebrand factor, C-reactive protein and five-year mortality in diabetic and non-diabetic subjects. The Hoorn Study. Arterioscler Tromb Vasc Biol, 1999; 19:3071-8.

10.   Clausen P, Feldt-Rasmussen B, Jensen G, Jensen JS. Endothelial haemostatic factors are associated with progression of urinary albumin excretion in clinically healthy subjects: a 4-year prospective study. Clin Sci 1999;97:37-43.

11.   Jager A, Kostense PJ, Ruhé HG, Heine RJ, Nijpels G, Dekker JM, Bouter LM, Stehouwer CDA. Microalbuminuria and peripheral arterial disease are independent predictors of cardiovascular and all-cause mortality, especially among hypertensive subjects. Five-year follow-up of the Hoorn Study. Arterioscler Thromb Vasc Biol 1999;19:617-624.

12.   Ross R. The pathogenesis of atherosclerosis: A perspective for the 1990s. Nature 1993;362:801-809.

13.   Lee LK, Neyer TW, Pollock AS, Lovett DH. Endothelial cell injury initiates glomerular sclerosis in the rat remnant kidney. J Clin Invest 1995;96:953-64.

14.   Sorensson J, Matejka GL, Ohlson, Haraldsson B. Human endothelial cells produce orosomucoid, an important component of the capillary barrier. Am J Physiol 1999;276:H530-H534.

15.   Stephenson JM, Fuller JH, Viberti G-C, Sjolie A-K, Navalesi R, the EURODIAB IDDM Complications Study Group. Blood pressure, retinopathy and urinary albumin excretion in IDDM: The EURODIAB IDDM Complications Study. Diabetologia 1995; 38:599-603.

16.   Greaves M, Malia RG, Goodfellow K, et al. Fibrinogen and von Willebrand factor in IDDM: relationships to lipid vascular risk factors, blood pressure, glycaemic control and urinary albumin excretion rate: the EURODIAB IDDM complications study. Diabetologia 1997; 40:698-705.

17.   Parving HH, Gall MA, Skott P, et al. Prevalence and causes of albuminuria in non-insulin-dependent diabetic patients. Kidney Int 1992; 41:758-762.

18.   Fioretto P, Mauer M, Brocco E, et al. Patterns of renal injury in NIDDM patients with microalbuminuria. Diabetologia 1996; 39:1569-1576.

19.   Fioretto P, Stehouwer CDA, Mauer M, Chiesura-Corona M, Brocco E, Carraro A, et al. Heterogeneous nature of microalbuminuria in non-insulin-dependent diabetes: studies of endothelial function and renal structure. Diabetologia 1998;41:233-236.

20.   Jager A, van Hinsbergh VWM, Kostense PJ, Nijpels G, Dekker JM, Heine RJ, Bouter LM, Stehouwer CDA. Prognostic implications of retinopathy and a high plasma von Willebrand factor level in NIDDM subjects with microalbuminuria. Diabetologia 1999;42(suppl.1):A259 (abstract)

21.   Stehouwer CDA, Fischer HRA, van Kuijk AWR, Polak BCP, Donker AJM. Endothelial dysfunction precedes development of microalbuminuria in insulin-dependent diabetes mellitus. Diabetes 1995;44:561-564.

22.   Kool MJF, Lambert J, Stehouwer CDA, Hoeks APG, Struijker Boudier HAJ, Van Bortel LMAB. Vessel wall properties of large arteries in uncomplicated insulin-dependent diabetes mellitus. Diabetes Care 1995;18:618-624.

23.   Lambert J, Pijpers R, van Ittersum FJ, Comans EFI, Aarsen M, Pieper EJ, Donker AJM, Stehouwer CDA. Sodium, blood pressure and arterial distensibility in insulin-dependent diabetes mellitus. Hypertension 1997;30:1162-1168.

24.   Lambert J, Smulders RA, Aarsen M, Donker AJM, Stehouwer CDA. Carotid artery stiffness is increased in microalbuminuric insulin-dependent diabetes mellitus patients. Diabetes Care 1998;21:99-103.

25.   Giannattasio C, Failla M, Piperno A, Grappiolo A, Gamba P, Paleari F, Mancia G. Early impairment of large artery structure and function in type I diabetes mellitus. Diabetologia 1999;42:987-994.

26.   Johnstone MT, Creager SJ, Scales KM, Cusco JA, Lee BK, Creager MA. Impaired endothelium-dependent vasodilation in patients with insulin-dependent diabetes mellitus. Circulation 1993;88:2510-2516.

27.   Clarkson P, Celermajer DS, Donald AE, Sampson M, Sorensen KE, Adams M et al. Impaired vascular reactivity in insulin-dependent diabetes mellitus is related to disease duration and low density lipoprotein cholesterol levels. J Am Coll Cardiol 1996;28:573-579.

28.   Lambert J, Aarsen M, Donker AJM, Stehouwer CDA. Endothelium-dependent and -independent vasodilation of large arteries in normoalbuminuric insulin-dependent diabetes mellitus. Arterioscler Thromb Vasc Biol 1996;16:705-11.

29.   Huvers FC, de Leeuw PW, Houben AJHM, de Haan CHA, Hamulyak K, Schouten H, et al. Endothelium-dependent vasodilation, plasma markers of endothelial function, and adrenergic vasoconstrictor responses in type 1 diabetes under near-normoglycemic conditions. Diabetes 1999;48:1300-1307.

30.   Vervoort G, Wetzels JF, Lutterman JA, van Doorn LG, Berden JH, Smits P. Elevated skeletal muscle blood flow in non-complicated type 1 diabetes mellitus: the role of nitric oxide and sympathetic tone. Hypertension, 1999; 34: 1080-85.

31.   Pieper GM. Enhanced, unaltered and impaired nitric oxide-mediated endothelium-dependent relaxation in experimental diabetes mellitus: importance of disease duration. Diabetologia 1999;42:204-213.

32.   Houben AJ, Schaper NC, de Haan CH, Huvers FC, Slaaf DW, de Leeuw PW, Nieuwenhuijzen Kruseman C. Local 24-h hyperglycemia does not affect endothelium-dependent or -independent vasoreactivity in humans. Am J Physiol 1996;270:H2014-H2020.

33.   Williams SB, Goldfine AB, Timimi FK, Ting HH, Roddy M, Simonson D, Creager M. Acute hyperglycemia attenuates endothelium-dependent vasodilation in humans in vivo. Circulation 1998;97:1695-1701.

34.   Goodfellow J, Ramsey MW, Luddington LA, Jones CJH, Coates PA, Dunstan F et al. Endothelium and inelastic arteries: an early marker of vascular dysfunction in non-insulin dependent diabetes. BMJ 1996;312:744-745.

35.   Yokoyama I, Ohtake T, Momomura S, Yonekura K, Woo-Soo S, Nishikawa J et al. Hyperglycemia rather than insulin resistance is related to reduced coronary flow reserve in NIDDM. Diabetes 1998;47:119-124.

36. Hogikyan RV, Galecki AT, Pitt B, Halter JB, Greene DA, Supiano MA. Specific impairment of endothelium-dependent vasodilation in subjects with type 2 diabetes independent of obesity. J Clin Endocrinol Metab 1998;83:1946-1952.

37. McVeigh GE, Brennan GM, Johnston GD, McDermott BJ, McGrath LT, Henry WR et al. Impaired endothelium-dependent and -independent vasodilation in patients with type 2 (non-insulin-dependent) diabetes mellitus. Diabetologia 1992;35:771-776.

38. Morris SJ, Shore AC, Tooke JE. Responses of the skin microcirculation to acetylcholine and sodium nitroprusside in patients with non-insulin-dependent diabetes mellitus. Diabetologia 1995;38:1337-1344.

39. Pinkney JH, Stehouwer CDA, Coppack SW, Yudkin JS. Endothelial dysfunction: cause of the insulin resistance syndrome. Diabetes 1997;46(suppl 2):S9-S13.

40. Tooke JE. The association between insulin resistance and endotheliopathy. Diabetes Obesity Metab 1999; 1(suppl. 1):S17-S22.

41. Baron AD. Cardiovascular actions of insulin in humans. Implications for insulin sensitivity and vascular tone. Bailliere's Clin Endocrinology Metab 1993;7:961-987.

42. Baron AD. The coupling of glucose metabolism and perfusion in human skeletal muscle. The potential role of endothelium-derived nitric oxide. Diabetes 1996;45(Suppl. 1):S105-S109.

43. Ferrannini E, Buzzigoli G, Bonadonna R, Giorico MA, Oleggini M, Graziadei L et al. Insulin resistance in essential hypertension. N Eng J Med 1987;317:350-357.

44. Panza JA, Quyyumi AA, Brush JE, Epstein SE. Abnormal endothelium-dependent vascular relaxation in patients with essential hypertension. N Eng J Med 1990;323:22-27.

45. Steinberg HO, Chaker H, Leaming R, Johnson A, Brechtel G, Baron AD. Obesity/insulin resistance is associated with endothelial dysfunction. Implications for the syndrome of insulin resistance. J Clin Invest 1996;97:2601-2610.

46. Kuhn FE, Mohler ER, Satler LF, Reagan K, Lu DY, Rackley CE. Effects of high-density lipoprotein on acetylcholine-induced coronary vasoreactivity. Am J Cardiol 1991; 68:1425-30.

47. Caballero AE, Arora S, Saouaf R, Lim SC, Smakowski P, Park JY, King GL, LoGerfo FW, Horton ES, Veves A. Microvascular and macrovascular reactivity is reduced in subjects at risk for type 2 diabetes. Diabetes 1999;48:1856-62.

48. Nolan JJ, Ludvik B, Baloga J, Reichart D, Olefsky JM. Mechanisms of the kinetic defect in insulin action in obesity and NIDDM. Diabetes 1997;46:994-1000.

49. Cline GW, Falk Petersen K, Krssak M, Shen J, Hundal RS, Trajanoski Z, et al. Impaired glucose transport as a cause of decreased insulin-stimulated muscle glycogen synthesis in type 2 diabetes. N Engl J Med 1999;341:240-246.

50. Castillo C, Bogardus C, Bergman R, Thuillez P, Lillioja S. Interstitial insulin concentrations determine glucose uptake rates but not insulin resistance in lean and obese men. J Clin Invest 1994;93:10-16

51. Yki-Järvinen H, Utriainen T. Insulin-induced vasodilatation: physiology or pharmacology? (Review). Diabetologia 1998:41:369-379.

52. Scherrer U, Randin D, Vollenweider P, Vollenweider L, Nicod P. Nitric oxide release accounts for insulin's vascular effects in humans. J Clin Invest 1994;94:2511-2515.

53. Bonadonna RC, Saccomani MP, Del Prato S, Bonora E, DeFronzo RA, Cobelli C. Role of tissue-specific blood flow and tissue recruitment in insulin-mediated glucose uptake of human skeletal muscle. Circulation 1998;98:234-241.

54. Clark MG, Colquhoun EQ, Rattigan S, Dora KA, Eldershaw TP, Hall JL, Ye J. Vascular and endocrine control of muscle metabolism (Review). Am J Physiol 1995;268:E797-E812.

55. Rattigan S, Clark MG, Barrett EJ. Hemodynamic actions of insulin in rat skeletal muscle. Evidence for capillary recruitment. Diabetes 1997;46:1381-1388.

56. Rattigan S, Clark MG, Barrett E. Acute vasoconstriction-induced insulin resistance in rat muscle in vivo. Diabetes 1999;48:564-569.

57. Petrie J, Ueda S, Webb DJ, Elliott HL, Connell JMC. Endothelial nitric oxide production and insulin sensitivity: a physiological link with implications for pathogenesis of cardiovascular disease. Circulation 1996;93:1331-1333.

58. Serné EH, Stehouwer CDA, ter Maaten JC, ter Wee PM, Rauwerda JA, Donker AJM, Gans ROB. Microvascular function relates to insulin sensitivity and blood pressure in normal subjects. Circulation 1999;99:896-902.

59. Utriainen TR, Makimattila S, Virkamaki A, Bergholm R, Yki-Järvinen H. Dissociation between insulin sensitivity of glucose uptake and endothelial function in normal subjects. Diabetologia 1996;39:1477-1482.

60. Lillioja S, Young AA, Culter CL, Ivy JL, Abbott WGH, Zawasski JK et al. Skeletal muscle capillary density and fiber type are possible determinants of in vivo insulin resistance in man. J Clin Invest 1987;80:415-424.

61. Kashiwazaki K, Hirano T, Yoshino G, Kurokawa M, Tajima H, Adachi M. Decreased release of lipoprotein lipase is associated with vascular endothelial damage in NIDDM patients with microalbuminuria. Diabetes Care 1998;21:2016-2020.

62. Lehmann ED, Riley WA, Clarkson P, Gosling RG. Non-invasive assessment of cardiovascular disease in diabetes mellitus. Lancet 1997; 350 (suppl I):14-19.

63. Lorenzi M. Glucose toxicity in the vascular complications of diabetes: the cellular perspective. Diab Metab Rev 1992;8:85-103.

64. Baumgartner-Parzer SM, Wagner L, Pettermann M, Grillari J, Gessl A, Waldhäusl W. High-glucose-triggered apoptosis in cultured endothelial cells. Diabetes 1995;44:1323-1327.

65. Morigi M, Angioletti S, Imberti B, Donadelli R, Micheletti G, Figliuzzi M, et al. Leukocyte-endothelial interaction is augmented by high glucose concentrations and hyperglycemia in a NF-kB-dependent fashion. J Clin Invest 1998;101:1905-1915.

66. Williamson JR, Chang K, Frangos M, Hasan KS, Ido Y, Kawamura T, et al. Hyperglycemic pseudohypoxia and diabetic complications. Diabetes 1993;42:801-813.

67. King GL, Shiba T, Oliver J, Inoguchi T, Bursell SE. Cellular and molecular abnormalities in the vascular endothelium of diabetes mellitus. Annu Rev Med 1994;45:179-188.

68. Porte D, Schwartz MW. Diabetes complications: why is glucose potentially toxic? Science 1996;272:699-670.

69. Baynes JW, Thorpe SR. Role of oxidative stress in diabetic complications: a new perspective on an old paradigm. Diabetes 1999;48:1-9.

70. Brownlee M. Glycation and diabetic complications. Diabetes 1994;43:836-841.

71. Vlassara H, Bucala R, Striker L. Pathogenic effects of advanced glycosylation: Biochemical, biologic, and clinical implications for diabetes and aging. Lab Invest 1994;70:138-151.

72. Smulders RA, Stehouwer CDA, Schalkwijk CG, Donker AJM, van Hinsbergh VWM, TeKoppele JM. Distinct associations of HbA1c and the urinary excretion of pentosidine, an advanced glycosylation end-product, with markers of endothelial function in insulin-dependent diabetes mellitus. Thromb Haemost 1998;80:52-7

73. Schalkwijk CG, Ligtvoet N, Twaalfhoven H, Jager A, Blaauwgeers HGT, Schlingemann RO, Tarnow L, Parving HH, Stehouwer CDA, van Hinsbergh VWM. Amadori-albumin in type 1 diabetic patients: correlation with markers of endothelial function, association with diabetic nephropathy and localization in retinal capillaries. Diabetes, 1999; 48: 2446-53.

74. Ting HH, Timimi FK, Boles KS, Creager SJ, Ganz P, Creager MA. Vitamin C improves endothelium-dependent vasodilation in patients with non-insulin-dependent diabetes mellitus. J Clin Invest 1996;97:22-28.

75. Wolf G, Ziyadeh FN. Molecular mechanisms of diabetic renal hypertrophy. Kidney Int 1999;56:393-405.

76. Duk E, Aiello LP. Vascular endothelial growth factor and diabetes: the agonist versus antagonist paradox. Diabetes 1999; 48: 1899-1906.

77. Catalano C, Muscelli E, Galvan AQ, Baldi S, Masoni A, Gibb I, et al. Effect of insulin on systemic and renal handling of albumin in nondiabetic and NIDDM subjects. Diabetes 1997;46:868-875.

78. Polderman KH, Stehouwer CDA, van Kamp GJ, Gooren LJG. Effects of insulin infusion on endothelium-derived vasoactive substances. Diabetologia 1996;39:1284-1292.

79. Trovati M, Anfossi G. Insulin, insulin resistance and platelet function: similarities with insulin effects on cultured vascular smooth muscle cells. Diabetologia 1998;41:609-622.

80. Begum N, Song Y, Rienzie J, Ragolia L. Vascular smooth muscle cell growth and insulin regulation of mitogen-activated protein kinase in hypertension. Am J Physiol 1998;275(1 Pt 1):C42-C49.

81. Reaven GM, Lithell H, Landsberg L. Hypertension and associated metabolic abnormalities. The role of insulin resistance and the sympathoadrenal system. N Engl J Med 1996;334:374-381.

82. Heise T, Magnusson K, Heinemann L, Sawicki PT. Insulin resistance and the effect of insulin on blood pressure in essential hypertension. Hypertension 1998;32(part2):243-248.

83. Giltay EJ, Lambert J, Elbers JMH, Gooren LJG, Asscheman H, Stehouwer CDA. Arterial compliance and distensibility are modulated by body composition in both men and women, but by insulin sensitivity only in women. Diabetologia 1999;42:214-221.

84. Giltay EJ, Lambert J, Gooren LJG, Elbers JMH, Steyn M, Stehouwer CDA. Sex steroids, insulin, and arterial stiffness in women and men. Hypertension 1999, 34: 590-97.

85. Pickup JC, Crook MA. Is Type II diabetes a disease of the innate immune system? Diabetologia 1998;41:1241-1248.

86. Perseghin G, Scifo P, De Cobelli F, Pagliato E, Battezzati A, Arcelloni C, et al. Intramyocellular triglyceride content is a determinant of in vivo insulin resistance in humans: a ^{1}H-^{13}C nuclear magnetic resonance spectroscopy assessment in offspring of type 2 diabetic parents. Diabetes 1999;48:1600-1606.

87. Schmidt MI, Duncan BB, Sharett AR, Lindberg G, Savage PJ, Offenbacher S, et al. Markers of inflammation and prediction of diabetes mellitus in adults (Atherosclerosis Risk in Communities study): a cohort study. Lancet 1999;353:1649-1652.

88. Hak AE, Stehouwer CDA, Bots ML, Polderman KH, Schalkwijk CG, Westendorp ICD, et al. Associations of C-reactive protein with measures of obesity, insulin resistance and subclinical atherosclerosis in healthy middle-aged women. Arterioscler Thromb Vasc Biol 1999;19:1986-1991.

89. Yudkin JS, Stehouwer CDA, Emeis JJ, Coppack SW. C-reactive protein in healthy subjects: associations with obesity, insulin resistance and endothelial dysfunction. A potential role for cytokines originating from adipose tissue? Arterioscler Thromb Vasc Biol 1999;19:972-978.

90. Steinberg HO, Tarshoby M, Monestel R, Hook G, Cronin J, Johnson A et al. Elevated circulating free fatty acid levels impair endothelium-dependent vasodilation. J Clin Invest 1997;100:1230-1239.

91.   Schalkwijk CG, Poland DCW, van Dijk W, Kok A, Emeis JJ, Dräger AM, van Hinsbergh VWM, Stehouwer CDA. Plasma concentration of C-reactive protein is increased in Type I diabetic patients without clinical macroangiopathy and correlates with markers of endothelial dysfunction: evidence for chronic inflammation. Diabetologia 1999;42:351-357.

92.   Barker DJP. Intrauterine programming of coronary heart disease and stroke. Acta Paediatrica 1997;423 (suppl.):178-183.

93.   Hattersley AT, Tooke JE. The fetal insulin hypothesis: an alternative explanation of the association of low birthweight with diabetes and vascular disease. Lancet 1999;353:1789-1792.

16. URINARY TRACT INFECTIONS IN PATIENTS WITH DIABETES MELLITUS

Andy I.M. Hoepelman, MD, Ph.D. & Suzanne E. Geerlings
Dept. of Medicine, Division Infectious Diseases and AIDS & Eijkman-Winkler Institute, University Medical Center, PO Box 85500, F02126, 3508 GA Utrecht, The Netherlands

URINARY TRACT INFECTIONS IN PATIENTS WITH DIABETES MELLITUS

Urinary tract infections (UTI) are second only to respiratory tract infections as problems encountered by practicing physicians. They occur most often in young healthy adult women and are easy treatable in these patients. However, in some patient groups infections occur more often, can have a complicated course, are more difficult to treat and often recur.

Many of them have easily recognizable urological abnormalities, but also more subtle conditions as age over 65 years, treatment with immunosuppressive drugs, HIV-infection with a CD-4+ count below $200/mm^3$ and last but not least diabetes mellitus lead to an enhanced susceptibility for UTI [1,2]

Diabetes mellitus (DM) is seen in about 1-2% of the population about 300.000 men and women in the Netherlands, it has been estimated that this will increase to 400-500.000 in 2010.

Besides organ complications as retinopathy, nephropathy and neuropathy, infections are common problems in these patients [3].

In a large study of bacteremic patients, it was demonstrated that two thirds of them had DM and that the urinary tract was the most prevalent infection site [4]. Since UTI complications (e.g., bacteremia, renal abscesses, and renal papillary necrosis) occur more often in diabetic patients, it is important to recognize UTI's in this patient group [3].

CLINICAL PRESENTATION

UTI's in diabetics can present themselves as asymptomatic bacteriuria (2 cultures, taken at least 24 hours apart, yielding growth, $\geq 10^5$cfu/ml of one and the same

Mogensen C.E. (ed.), THE KIDNEY AND HYPERTENSION IN DIABETES MELLITUS.

microorganism) or symptomatic UTI. Since nowadays we assume that renal infections occur through the ascending route, it is no unreasonable to assume that symptomatic infections arise from asymptomatic ones.

The presentation can be straightforward and accompanied by symptoms such as dysuria, frequency, urgency, gross hematuria, lower back and/or abdominal discomfort, and (rarely) low-grade fever; however, the same symptoms may be produced by inflammation in the urethra or by agents such as *chlamydia trachomatis*, herpes simplex or by a vaginitis (e.g. *C. albicans*). Therefore an urine specimen should be checked for pyuria (5 leukocytes/hpf or 10 leukocytes/mm^3 in unspun urine) and bacteriuria (by nitrite test or dip-slide).

Upper tract involvement is common [5,6]. Acute pyelonephritis is a clinical syndrome characterized by fever and chills, flank pain, costovertebral angle tenderness, and other symptoms, such as nausea and vomiting. There may or may not be symptoms of lower UTI, such as dysuria. Some patients only present with symptoms of lower UTI but nevertheless have upper tract involvement (subclinical pyelonephritis; see later). Very often infection leads to bacteremia. There are exceptional cases of renal abscesses, papillary necrosis and emphysematous pyelitis [7].

Renal abscess formation should be suspected in patients who do not respond to antimicrobial therapy after 72 hours. Papillary necrosis is also an important complication of diabetes. Symptoms consist of flank pain, chills, fever and renal insufficiency develops in 15% of the cases. Therefore the diagnosis should be suspected in patients poorly responding to antimicrobial therapy with developing renal insufficiency. Emphysematous pyelonephritis is a necrotizing infection characterized by gas production in and around the kidneys. The disease is seen almost exclusively in diabetics, Gram negatives are the most common isolates but multiple organisms occur. Clinical features include fever, flank pain and a palpable mass in 45% of patients. Bacteremia is a frequent complication. Diagnosis is made radiographically because plain films of the abdomen show gas in the renal fossa or preferable by CT-scanning. Survival is best with combined medial and surgical treatment.

PREVALENCE OF ASYMPTOMATIC BACTERIURIA

Several studies summarized by Zhanel & Nicolle et al have assessed the prevalence of asymptomatic bacteriuria in patients with diabetes mellitus [8]. Probably due to selection bias, not discriminating between in-and outpatients, and not selecting for severity of the underlying disease, there is a wide range in prevalence among women (0-29%; mean 20%). Previously, in a small study in our outpatient diabetic clinic we found a prevalence of 32% in our female population [9]. We recently have completed a study in 636 non-pregnant women with DM (including our University Hospital, secondary care hospitals, in-and outpatients as well as diabetics visiting their GP). The prevalence of ASB was 26% compared to 6% in the control group (p<0.001). The prevalence of ASB in the 378 women with DM type 2 was 29% (compared to 21% in those with DM type

1) [10]. Therefore, the prevalence of ASB is consistently higher in diabetic women than in non-diabetics.

In men results are more consistent, a frequency between 1-2% has been found, with no clear difference between diabetics and non-diabetics.

PATHOGENS AND SITE OF INFECTION

The bacteria causing infections are the same as in complicated UTI in non-diabetics. About 75% are caused by *Escherichia coli*, *Serratia spp.*, *Klebsiella/Enterobacter spp.* and *Streptococcus faecalis* [11,12,13] Also fungal infections with the yeast *Candida albicans* and *Torulopsis glabrata* can occur. Moreover, 80% of E. coli express type-1 fimbriae (Geerlings et al, submitted).

Localization studies have indeed shown that in about 75% of patients also the kidney is involved [5,6] This is also shown by the number of diabetics under the patients with a complicated course of their UTI (50% of the patients with papillary necrosis and 30% of the patients with perinephritic abscesses) [7].

ASSOCIATED RISK FACTORS

Factors that have been proposed constituting an enhanced risk for UTI in diabetics include: poor control, neuropathy with neurogenic bladder dysfunction and chronic urine retention, old age, previous instrumentation, recurrent vaginitis, micro-and macroangiopathy and impairment of leukocyte function [3].

Studies into the association of risk factors and asymptomatic bacteriuria yield conflicting results: on the one hand no relation with duration, type and regulation (HbA$_1$) [11,12,14,15] nor with neuropathy [14] but a positive correlation between bacteriuria and retinopathy [14,15] (although not all studies confirm this) and microangiopathy [12,15] in the kidney has been found. There also is a correlation with autonomic cardiovascular neuropathy [16] but curiously not with bladder dysfunction [13]. Many of these items seem contradictory because it is generally assumed that the longer diabetes exists the chance of microangiopathy increases. In the study mentioned above [10], the largest in its kind avoiding all the discrepancies mentioned above, risk factors for ASB in all women with DM were retinopathy, macroalbuminuria, a longer duration of the diabetes, a lower body mass index (BMI), and a symptomatic UTI in the previous year (p<0.05) [10] . Risk factors for ASB in the women with type-1 diabetes included a longer duration of the diabetes, peripheral neuropathy, and macroalbuminuria. The prevalence of ASB was 29% in women with DM type 2 [10]. Risk factors in these women included age, macroalbuminuria, a lower BMI, and a UTI in the previous year. All p-values were adjusted for age. There was no association between the diabetes regulation and the presence of a post-voiding bladder residue and the presence of ASB [10].

CONSEQUENCES OF ASYMPTOMATIC BACTERIURIA IN DIABETIC WOMEN

In a small prospective study of 58 nondiabetic women with ASB (1-year follow-up), 31% developed a symptomatic urinary tract infection (UTI) and in other studies [36,37] of nondiabetic patients it was suggested that ASB can lead to recurrent UTIs, progressive renal impairment, hypertension, and an increased mortality. It is not known, however, whether ASB leads to symptomatic UTI and/or a decline in renal function in diabetic patients [2,3]. We followed the cohort mentioned before for 18 months. Of these 589 women, 115 (20%) developed a symptomatic UTI. Antimicrobial therapy for this UTI was prescribed in the majority of them. Like other studies of ASB in non-diabetic women, we found that women with DM type 2 and ASB at baseline had an increased risk of developing UTI during the 18-month follow-up, compared to women with DM type 2 without ASB at baseline (p=0.005) [17]. There was no difference in the incidence of a symptomatic UTI between DM type 1 women with and those without ASB. Moreover, DM type 1 women with ASB had a tendency to a faster decline in renal function than those without ASB (4.6% versus 1.5%, p=0.2), which probably is the result of the ASB. To confirm this hypothesis, we will monitor these diabetic women with and without ASB for the coming 5-10 years. However, in another recent study, it was documented that 14 of the 52 (27%) diabetic women with ASB developed a pyelonefritis, moreover, while in the control group, which was kept non-bacteriuric by active treatment pyelonefritis, was only seen in 2% of diabetic women [18]. Moreover, non-treatment was associated with a significantly greater incidence of hospitalization due to pyelonefritis (RR=7.7 P=0.02). This discrepancy with our findings may have a genetic background since the group studied by Zhanel et al [18] consisted mainly of a group of aboriginals, which moved to Canada many decades ago. However, this makes our findings of a probable difference in adherence of bacteria to uroepithelial cells even more likely (see pathogenesis).

PATHOGENESIS

Studies demonstrate greater susceptibility of diabetic than of nondiabetic animals to urinary tract infection [19-22]. Suggested mechanisms are a) decreased antibacterial activity due to the "sweet urine". b) Defects in neutrophil function c) increased adherence to uroepithelial cells.

We have studied the growth rates of different *Escherichia coli* strains (three from blood cultures from urosepsis patients, two urinary isolates, two fecal isolates and one laboratory strain K12) in human urine with and without the addition of glucose and with and without a constant pH [23]. These growth rates were compared with the growth rates in Mueller Hinton broth (MHB). All isolates grew better in MHB than in urine, but with the exception of the laboratory strain, they had the same growth rate in urine. No significant difference was found between the growth rate in urine from diabetics without glucosuria and that in urine from non-diabetics. The addition of glucose (up to a concentration of 1,000 mg/dl, which is a concentration as found in poorly regulated diabetic patients) to urine and MHB enhanced the growth rate of all isolates. Therefore, it may be concluded that glucosuria enhances bacterial growth and may be one of the explanations of the increased susceptibility of diabetic patients to have bacteriuria. However, very high concentrations of glucose (up to 10,000 mg/dl) in urine and MHB caused a decrease in bacterial growth rate when urinary pH was not kept constant [23]. Moreover, diabetic rats are more susceptible to UTI caused by *S.aureus and C.albicans* [18]. The experimental settings of these animal experiments are far from ideal, however. In the "rat studies" bacteria were administered IV [19] , studying the hematogenous route of UTI instead of the more important ascending route. Also the data on impaired neutrophil function are weak. Again very unphysiological conditions in only a few patients with antique techniques were studied [24,25]; moreover, UTI's are not very prominent in other groups of patients with neutrophil defects or neutropenia [26]. And indeed we were unable to document any differences in PMN-function when comparing diabetic women with or without bacteriuria and healthy controls [9].

The experiments showing increased adherence to uroepithelium in diabetic animals are more intriguing [20].

At least two mechanisms can be responsible for this phenomenon: a) diminished anti-adherence activity of the urine and b) enhanced adherence capacity of uroepithelial cells.

It has been shown that there is a genetic predisposition in the occurrence of UTI. Patients with recurrent UTI, without a known structural abnormality, belong to certain blood group types and do not secrete blood-group antigens (non-secretor status) [27,28]. It is assumed that in non-secretors, receptors involved in adhesion are more exposed or that they express other glycosphingolipids [28,29]. Interestingly, it has not only been shown in animals but also in patients with diabetes mellitus that there is a correlation between the non-secretor status and stomatitis due to *C.albicans* [30]. A simple genetic explanation cannot be given; however, because the chromosomes involved (6 and 19) are far apart. Recently, we have documented that their is an increased adherence of type-1 fimbriated *E.coli* to uroepithelial cells from diabetic women compared to controls, while no difference was found for non-fimbriated and *E.coli* expressing P-fimbriae (unpublished information).

As said it is also possible that, the increased incidence of UTI's is due to a defective anti-adherence mechanism in urine. Known anti-adherence mechanisms in the urine are oligosaccharides and a glycoprotein called Tamm-Horsfall (THP), which covers the uroepithelium and is also excreted in the urine [31,32]. Type 1 fimbriae are important in the adherence of bacteria to buccal and vaginal cells and patients with recurrent UTI show enhanced adherence of bacteria to vaginal cells type 1 fimbriae of *E. coli*. Moreover, type-1 fimbriae (expressed by 80% of bacteria found in diabetic women) adhere to THP. It is therefore conceivable that in patients with DM and recurrent UTI, excretion and or/production of THP is deficient. Indeed it has been described that in patients with DM the glycosylation of THP is changed and that the excretion of disaggregated THP is diminished independent of the existence of nephropathy, age or control of DM [33]. However, that, a relation between diminished THP excretion and bacteriuria in diabetics does exist, remains to be shown.

Moreover, we studied the urinary IL-8 and IL-6 excretion *ex-vivo* in diabetic women with ASB and compared these cytokine concentrations with those of non-diabetic bacteriuric controls. Furthermore, we correlated these cytokine concentrations with the presence and expression of known virulence factors of *E. coli* isolated from the urine of these diabetic women. Lower urinary interleukin-8 (IL-8) and interleukin-6 (IL-6) concentrations (p=0.11 and p<0.001 respectively) and fewer known uropathogenic O: K: H-serotypes (p=0.002) were found in diabetic women than in nondiabetic controls [34]. The urinary IL-8 concentration correlated with the phenotypic expression (p=0.03) of type 1 fimbriae, the urinary IL-6 concentration with the genotypic (p=0.03) and phenotypic expression (p=0.04) of P fimbriae of *E. coli*. A lower urinary leukocyte cell count also correlated with lower urinary IL-8 and IL-6 concentrations (p<0.05) [34]. We concluded that this decreased urinary cytokine production and leukocyte count in diabetic women might explain the increased prevalence of bacteriuria in this patient group. Therefore, future research should focus on these findings.

TREATMENT

It should be clear from the previous text that UTI in diabetics should be regarded as complicated infections.

In general it can be said that complicated urinary tract infections should be treated with agents that reach high tissue levels (TMP\SMZ; Fluoroquinolones) and that treatment duration in general should be no less than 10-14 days [35] .

It is not known, however, if asymptomatic bacteriuria should be treated. Studies analyzing, the effects on renal function and the development of symptomatic infections, of keeping diabetic women non-bacteriuric are underway. Therapy makes sense if treatment of asymptomatic infections prevents the development of nephropathy and /or decline in renal function.

FUTURE RESEARCH

Answers to the following questions remain to be given: 1. Should ASB be treated (effects on the occurrence of symptoms and on renal function), 2. Do infections recur when treated and is antimicrobial prophylaxis effective? Concerning the pathogenesis, more fundamentally, 3. What is the mechanism of increased adherence of bacteria to uroepithelial cells of diabetic women and 4? Are these women hampered in their immune response (cytokine release) to LPS and whole bacteria?

REFERENCES

1. Hoepelman AIM, van Buren M, van den Broek J, Borleffs JCC. Bacteriuria in men infected with HIV-1 is related to their immune status (CD4+ cell count). Aids 1992; 6:179-184.
2. Johnson JR, Roberts PL, Stamm WE. P fimbriae and other virulence factors in *E.coli* urosepsis:association with patients' characteristics. J Infect Dis 1987; 156:225-229.
3. Wheat LJ. Infection and diabetes mellitus. Diabetes Care 1980; 3:187-197.
4. Carton JA, Maradona JA, Nuno FJ, et al: Diabetes mellitus and bacteraemia: A comparative study between diabetic and non-diabetic patients. EJM 1992; 1: 281-287
5. Forland M, Thomas V, Shelokov A. Urinary tract infections in patients with diabetes mellitus. Studies on antibody coating of bacteria. JAMA 1977; 238:1924-1926.
6. Forland M, Thomas VL. The treatment of urinary tract infections in women with diabetes mellitus. Diabetes Care 1985; 8:499-506.
7. Saiki J, Vaziri ND, Barton C. Perinephric and intranephric abscesses: a review of the literature. West J Med 1982; 136:95-102.
8. Zhanel GG, Harding GK, Nicolle LE. Asymptomatic bacteriuria in patients with diabetes mellitus. Rev Infect Dis 1991; 13:150-154.
9. Balasoiu D, Kessel v KC, Kats-Renaud v HJ, Collet TJ, Hoepelman AI: Granulocyte function in women with diabetes and asymptomatic bacteriuria. Diabetes Care 1997 20:392-395
10. Geerlings SE, Stolk RP, Camps MJL, Netten PM, Hoekstra JBL, Bouter KP, Bravenboer B, Collet TJ, Jansz AR, Hoepelman IM. Prevalence and risk factors for asymptomatic bacteriuria in women with diabetes mellitus. ICAAC, 1999, p.663, abstract 607.
11. Schmitt JK, Fawcett CJ, Gullickson G. Asymptomatic bacteriuria and hemoglobin A1. Diabetes Care 1986; 9:518-520.
12. Hansen RO. Bacteriuria in Diabetic and Non-diabetic out-patients. Acta med scand 1964; 176:721-730.
13. Joffe BI, Seftel HC, Distiller LA. Asymptomatic bacteriuria in diabetes mellitus. S Afric Med J 1974; 48:1306-1308.
14. Vejlsgaard R. Studies on urinary infection in diabetics. II. Significant bacteriuria in relation to long-term diabetic manifestations. Acta Med Scand 1966; 179:183-188.
15. Batalla MA, Balodimos MC, Bradley RF. Bacteriuria in diabetes mellitus. Diabetologia 1971; 7:297-301.
16. Sawers JS, Todd WA, Kellett HA, et al. Bacteriuria and autonomic nerve function in diabetic women. Diabetes Care 1986; 9:460-464.
17. Geerlings SE, Stolk RP, Camps MJL, Netten PM, Collet TJ, Hoepelman IM. Asymptomatic bacteriuria in diabetic females precedes symptomatic urinary tract infection. ICAAC 1999, p.662, abstract 604.
18. Zhanel GG, Nicolle LE, Harding GKM. Untreated asymptomatic bacteriuria (ABU) in women with diabetes mellitus (WWDM) is associated with high rates of pyelonefritis (P). ICAAC 1999, p. 664, abstract 609.
19. Raffel L, Pitsakis P, Levison SP, Levison ME. Experimental *Candida albicans*, Staphylococcus aureus, and Streptococcus faecalis pyelonephritis in diabetic rats. Infect Immun 1981; 34:773-779.
20. Obana Y, Nishino T. The virulence of *Enterobacter cloacae* and *Serratia marcescens* in experimental bladder infection in diabetic mice. J Med Microbiol 1989; 30:105-109.

21. Obana Y, Shibata K, Nishino T. Adherence of *Serratia marcescens* in the pathogenesis of urinary tract infections in diabetic mice. J Med Microbiol 1991; 35:93-97.

22. Levison ME, Pitsakis PG. Effect of insulin treatment on the susceptibility of the diabetic rat to *Escherichia coli*-induced pyelonephritis. J Infect Dis 1984; 150:554-560.

23. Geerlings SE, Brouwer EC, Gaastra W, Verhoef J, Hoepelman AIM. Effect of glucose and pH on uropathogenic and non-uropathogenic *Escherichia coli:* studies with urine from diabetic and non-diabetic individuals. J Med Microbiol 1999;48:535-9

24. Gargan RA, Hamilton Miller JM, Brumfitt W. Effect of pH and osmolality on in vitro phagocytosis and killing by neutrophils in urine. Infection & Immunity 1993; 61:8-12.

25. Chernew I, Braude AI. Depression of Phagocytosis by solutes in concentrations found in kidney and urine. J Clin Invest 1962; 41:1945-1953.

26. Wang QN, Qiu ZD. Infection in acute leukemia: an analysis of 433 episodes. Rev Infect Dis 1989; 11 Suppl 7:S1613-S1620.

27. Sheinfeld J, Schaeffer AJ, Cordon Cardo C, Rogatko A, Fair WR. Association of the Lewis blood-group phenotype with recurrent urinary tract infections in women. N Engl J Med 1989; 320:773-777.

28. Lomberg H, Cedergren B, Leffler H, Nilsson B, Carlstrom AS, Svanborg Eden C. Influence of blood group on the availability of receptors for attachment of uropathogenic Escherichia coli. Infect Immun 1986; 51:919-926.

29. Stapleton A, Nudelman E, Clausen H, Hakomori S, Stamm WE. Binding of uropathogenic Escherichia coli R45 to glycolipids extracted from vaginal epithelial cells is dependent on histo-blood group secretor status. J Clin Invest 1992; 90:965-972.

30. Aly FZ, Blackwell CC, Mackenzie DA, et al. Chronic atrophic oral candidiasis among patients with diabetes mellitus--role of secretor status. Epidemiol Infect 1991; 106:355-363.

31. Parkkinen J, Virkola R, Korhonen TK. Identification of factors in human urine that inhibit the binding of Escherichia coli adhesins. Infection & Immunity 1988; 56:2623-2630.

32. Reinhart HH, Spencer JR, Zaki NF, Sobel JD. Quantitation of urinary Tamm-Horsfall protein in children with urinary tract infection. Eur Urol 1992; 22:194-199.

33. Bernard AM, Ouled AA, Lauwerys RR, Lambert A, Vandeleene B. Pronounced decrease of Tamm-Horsfall proteinuria in diabetics. Clin Chem 1987; 33:1264.

34. Geerlings SE, . Cytokine Secretion Is Impaired in Women with Diabetes Mellitus. ICAAC 1999, p. 388, abstract 1609.

35. Stamm, W. E. and T. M. Hooton. Management of urinary tract infections in adults. N Engl J Med 1993;329:1328-1334.

36. Gaymans R, Haverkorn MJ, Valkenburg HA, Goslings WR. A prospective study of urinary tract infections in a Dutch general practice. Lancet, 1976; 7987: 674-77.

37. Ronald AR, Pattullo AL. The natural history of urinary tract infections in adults. Infect Dis Clin North Am, 1991: 75:299-312.

17. LIGHT MICROSCOPY OF DIABETIC GLOMERULOPATHY: THE CLASSIC LESIONS

Steen Olsen
Professor Emeritus, Department of Pathology, Herlev Hospital, DK-2730 Herlev, Denmark.

The history of our knowledge of the light microscopy of diabetic glomerulopathy began with the famous paper by Kimmelstiel and Wilson in 1936 [1]. With some justification, it can be said that it has been completed by the careful analysis of large series by Thomsen 1965 [2] and Ditscherlein 1969 [3], the first mentioned taking advantage of the introduction of percutaneous renal biopsies.

Histologic lesions of the renal glomerulus in diabetics were not totally unknown when Kimmelstiel and Wilson reported their findings, but the exact relationship of these alterations to the diabetic state was unclear. Kimmelstiel and Wilson were the first investigators to draw attention to the characteristic »intercapillary«, nodular thickening of mesangial regions and its association with a clinical syndrome consisting of severe proteinuria, edema, hypertension, and eventually a decrease in renal function.

The histology of diabetic glomerulopathy described here rests upon the cornerstones mentioned above and other important classical contributions [4-9] as well as more recent data. Arteriolar changes are included due to the close anatomic and functional connection of arterioles with the glomerulus. Some differential diagnostic problems are discussed , and a brief review of tubolointerstitial lesions is also provided since it is still not known whether they are secondary to vascular changes or have other pathogenesis.

THE DIFFUSE LESION
This consists of a uniform widening of the mesangial regions (figure 17-1). It is particularly well exhibited in sections stained by periodic acid-Schiff (PAS) or by silver methenamine that display structures often described as finger-like radiations from the glomerular hilum.

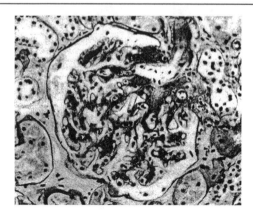

Fig. 17-1. Diabetic glomerulopathy, diffuse type. There is a slight increase of PAS-positive material in all mesangial regions, radiating from the vascular pole *(upper right)*. PAS-haematoxylin.

THE NODULAR LESION

As the volume of the mesangial matrix increases, some mesangial regions become more prominent than others and may take on a globular shape (figure 17-2). The mesangial nodule is thus created by a gradual increase of the diffuse lesion and the distinction between them is arbitrary. Several nodules may be present in each glomerulus, but usually only a few of the mesangial regions are affected in this way

The nodules are distributed in a horseshoe-shaped area corresponding to the peripheral mesangium [12]. The other mesangial regions present the diffuse lesion. Small nodules contain evenly distributed mesangial cells, but in medium-sized or large nodules, the central areas are almost always acellular. The periphery of the nodule contains one or a few layers of mesangial cells. Around the nodule, a ring of capillaries is present and they may be dilated. It has been suggested that the formation of the nodule is preceded by focal mesangiolysis [13,14].

THE FIBRINOID CAP

Insudative or exudative lesions consists of deposits of plasma proteins and lipids within renal arterioles (arteriolar hyalinosis), glomerular capillaries (fibrinoid or fibrin cap) and Bowman's capsule (capsular drop). The fibrin cap [8,9,15-17] is situated in the peripheral capillary wall and has a crescentic shape (figure 17-3).

If the basement membrane is stained by silver methenamine, the cap appears to be situated between this and the endothelium. Its structure is homogeneous although small vacuoles may be seen in which lipids can be demonstrated in frozen sections stained by oil-red.

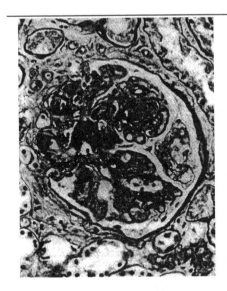

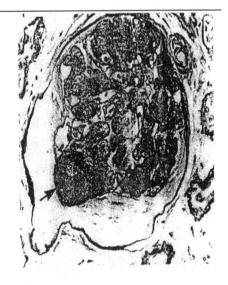

Fig. 17-2. Diabetic glomerulopathy. The diffuse component is more marked than in figure 17-1 and a nodule has been formed from a particulary voluminous region. PAS-haematoxylin.

Fig. 17-3. Fibrinoid cap in diabetic glomerulopathy. Totally obsolescent glomerulus with several fibrinoid caps, one of them indicated by an arrow. The crescent-shaped pale area to the left is subcapsular, fibrotic tissue. The PAS-positive glomerular basement membranes form a solid, retracted tuft. PAS-haematoxylin.

THE CAPSULAR DROP

This lesion [1,3] is situated on the inner side of the capsule of Bowman. It sometimes looks like a drop (figure 17-4), but it may also be more extended, as a slender, fusiform deposit. Its outer border is formed by the capsule of Bowman; its inner projects toward the urinary space.

ARTERIOLAR HYALINOSIS

In the early stage of arteriolar hyalinosis (or hyaline arteriolosclerosis), small drops of strongly eosinophilic material accumulate in the wall of the juxtaglomerular arterioles.

They may be situated in the intima or in the media. They gradually increase in size and eventually involve the whole arteriolar wall, which then appears as a strongly thickened, homogeneous structure. Arteriolar hyalinosis in diabetes involves the afferent arteriole as well as the efferent arteriole (figure 17-5).

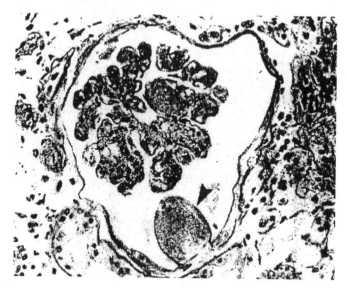

Fig. 17-4. Capsular drop in diabetic glomerulopathy. A large, drop-shaped deposit (*arrow*). PAS-haematoxylin.

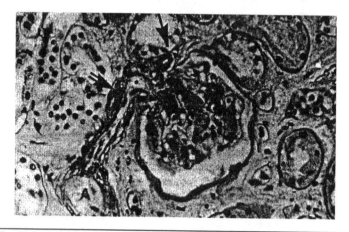

Fig. 17-5. Arteriolosclerosis in diabetes. There is moderate hyaline arteriolosclerosis in both the afferent (*double arrow*) and the efferent (*arrow*) arterioles. A, interlubular artery. PAS-haematoxylin.

STAINING CHARACTERISTICS AND HISTOCHEMISTRY

Histochemical studies have been published by several authors [10,17,18]. The most important results are presented in table 17-1. The fibrinoid cap, capsular drop, and arteriolar hyalinosis are identical in staining characteristics, which is why some authors have included them in one group.

Immunoflourescence microscopy (IF) shows often IgG in a fine linear pattern along the glomerular capillary walls [19-21]. This reaction is considered to be unspecific since albumin can also be detected in the same location and IgG cannot be eluded. The nodules are negative. Exudative lesions are postive for C3, β-lipoprotein and (weakly) for IgG [21]. Insulin or anti-insulin are not detectable by IF in the glomeruli [20,21].

Table 17-1 Staining characteristics of diabetic glomerular lesions

Stain	Diffuse	Nodular	Exudative[a]
Haematoxylineosin	+red	+red	++red
V. Gieson-Hansen	+red	+red	++yellow
Masson-trichrome	++blue	++blue	+++red
Phosphotungstic acid-haematoxylin	0	0	+++deep blue
PAS after diastase	++	++	+++
Silver-methenamine	++black	+/- black fibrils in pale matrix	0
Alcian-blue	+	0	0
Congo red, other amyloid stains	0	0	0
Neutral fat	0	(+) occasionally	+ fat vacuoles

[a]Exudative lesions are fibrinoid caps, capsular drops, and arteriolar hyalinosis

DEVELOPMENT OF THE LESIONS BY TIME

The most powerful determinant for the appearance and development of glomerular and vascular lesions in diabetes is duration of the diabetic state [2]. Diffuse glomerulopathy can be demonstrated by ultrastructural morphometry after a few years of diabetes [22], but is usually not distinct light-microscopically until 5-10 years after the onset of the disease. Nodular glomerulosclerosis demands at least 15 years of diabetes to develop. The nodules tend to disappear with marked glomerular obsolescence. Whereas the precise onset of the diabetic disease is known in insulin dependent diabetes (IDDM) this is not the case with non-insulin dependent diabetes (NIDDM) in which the disease may have been present several years before diagnosis. This is why glomerular nodules may occasionally be seen in patients with a *known* duration of diabetes of less than 15 years, and they may even occur at the time diagnosis is made. The diffuse lesion and arteriolosclerosis occur in 20% of patients before 5 years have elapsed from the apparent onset [2]. These lesions are nonspecific, and thus their presence in a patient suffering from diabetes may be unrelated to the diabetic state.

The fibrinoid cap occurs most frequently in the later stages of glomerulopathy, but, in contradistinction to all other glomerular lesions in this disease, the capsular drop is found almost as often in earlier as in later stages [2].

A peculiar and as yet unexplained fact is that about 60% of patients with long-standing diabetes do *not* develop clinical nephropathy or diabetic glomerular changes.

GLOMERULAR STRUCTURE IN THE TERMINAL PHASE

The appearance of glomeruli in advanced diabetic glomerulopathy presents a broad spectrum ranging from totally occluded to almost normal glomeruli. Glomeruli, which are still open, may be hypertrophic and often present global mesangial hypercellularity. Totally occluded glomeruli are not evenly distributed, but tend to be concentrated in radiating stripes parallel to the medullary rays [23]. There is no difference in the severity of glomerular involvement between deep and superficial cortical zones. The total number of glomeruli decreases with progression of the diabetic nephropathy, at least in IDDM [24].

It is important to realize that this terminal pattern is not exclusively due to glomerular alterations specific for diabetes. Ischemic scarring and focal glomerular sclerosis occur and may indicate that causes other than progression of diabetic glomerular lesion may be partially responsible for the development of renal failure, such as vascular constriction with glomerular ischemia and lesions due to hyperfunction of remaining glomeruli.

SPECIFICITY OF THE LESIONS

The diffuse lesion is completely nonspecific and may be present in older people without diabetes. The combination of arteriolosclerosis and the diffuse lesion often occurs in hypertension, but involvement of both the afferent arteriole and the efferent arteriole is regarded as a strong indication of diabetes [6,25,26] although even this combination is not entirely specific [15].

All insudative lesions are much more numerous and/or larger in diabetics than in controls but they are not specific. Even capsular drops and hyalinosis of efferent arterioles which have traditionally been regarded as specific lesions may be seen in small numbers in some non-diabetic controls [15].

The nodular lesion is often regarded as pathognomonic for diabetes. It is true that numerous reports of nodular lesions in non-diabetic patients have been published [for a list, see ref. 3]. Most of these reports can be criticized, however, either because of doubt as to absence of diabetes or to lack of application of precise criteria for the morphologic diagnosis. There are, however, well documented cases on record with typical nodular glomerulopathy without diabetes [27,28].

Although the *typical* nodular lesion is very strongly associated with diabetes, there exist nevertheless other conditions in which glomerular nodules may occur. Since these may present diagnostic difficulties, they will be briefly mentioned here. For a detailed report and illustrations, the reader is referred to an earlier publication [29].

In renal *amyloidosis*, abnormal homogeneous substance is deposited in the peripheral as well as mesangial parts of the glomerular capillary walls. In rare cases, the deposits may take on the shape of typical diabetic nodules with an acellular center. They can be correctly classified by the use of amyloid stains and by demonstration of typical fibrils on electron microscopy.

Some types of advanced *glomerulonephritis* (mesangial proliferative, membrano-proliferative) have a histology that resembles nodular glomerulosclerosis. In glomerulonephritis, however, there is a distinct hypercellularity and the central, acellular area that is so characteristic for diabetes is not present. Nodules in glomerulonephritis involve all mesangial areas and are of almost equal size. Immunodeposits are usually present, but are faint or absent in diabetes.

Glomerular nodules may also be present in various *dysproteinemias* (e.g. multiple myeloma and heavy-chain disease [30-35].

The clinical picture may often solve the diagnostic problem, but the occurrence of glomerular nodules in these diseases should be a reminder to the pathologist not to postulate the presence of diabetes on the prima facie detection of nodular structures in the glomeruli.

OTHER RENAL DISEASES IN DIABETES MELLITUS

Glomerulonephritis has been thought to occur more frequently in patients with diabetic renal disease than could be explained by mere coincidence [34,35]. Autopsy studies have, however, shown that complicating glomerular disease is rare and probably not exceeding prevalence in the general population [36]. In biopsy studies of patients with IDDM glomerulonephritis seems to be comparatively rare [37,38], probably around 2-3% in unselected cases with proteinuria and duration of diabetes of more than 10 years. It has recently been reported that it may be more common in NIDDM [for literature see ref 39], but data from different series are conflicting. The rates of glomulonephritis in these studies vary between 0 and 69% and those of other complicating renal diseases between 0 and 20%. Geographical differences and variable criteria for histopathological diagnosis may be partly responsible, but the main cause of the diverging results is probably selection of patients for renal biopsy. Most of the investigations are based upon biopsies from patients referred to a nephrologic clinic and in some reports it was explicitly stated that the biopsies were made due to presence of symptoms and signs considered to be caused by other diseases than diabetes. It is clear that this will favor inclusion of patients with complicating renal disease. Pinel et al [40] on the other hand, in their investigation of patients with NIDDM, have excluded all patients with clinical renal disease other than the presence of micro- or macroalbuminuria and found no complicating renal disease. Investigating a consecutive series of renal biopsies from 53 patients with NIDDM and microalbuminuria. Brocco et al did not find any with complicating glomerulonephritis [41]. Only one study, that of Parving et al., was population-based and cross sectional [42]. In this series of patients with macroalbuminuria, 23% had non diabetic glomerular disease. Half of these had, however, no glomerular lesions by light microscopy (LM) or IF and were thought to have a complicating minor change nephropathy. While most types of glomerulitis can be confidently diagnosed by proliferative or membranous glomerular changes and deposits of immunoglobulin, this is not the case with minor change disease. Albuminuria in a diabetic patient with normal glomeruli by LM and IF may be due to the still unknown factor responsible for minor change disease, to focal and segmental glomerular sclerosis missed due to sampling problems, to early diffuse diabetic glomerulopathy, not detectable by LM, or to other, hypothetical causes (vascular permeability factors? Biochemical alterations of the glomerular basement membrane?) [43]. We have at the moment no explanation of albuminuria in diabetic patients with normal glomerular structure. This group of patients should be investigated further.

Other complicating diseases. Atheroma emboli may be found in the intrarenal vessels as a complication to diabetic macroangiopathy (atherosclerosis in the aorta and renal arteries). Papillary necrosis is also a well known complication. Other renal diseases occurring in the same age as NIDDM such as amyloidosis and myeloma are probably unrelated to the diabetic state.

It is well established that long term diabetic nephropathy is associated with marked *interstitial fibrosis, tubular atrophy* and *mononuclear cell infiltration.* Formerly these changes were interpreted as evidence of complicating chronic pyelonephritis [3]. Since they were shown to be correlated to the renal microvascular alterations characteristic for long term diabetes, it was later on suggested that they were due to chronic ischemia [42,43]. Lane et al [44] found in IDDM that mesangial volume fraction, severity of arteriolar hyalinosis, percentage of globally sclerosed glomeruli, and interstitial volume fraction for total renal cortex were significantly correlated and all four structural parameters correlated with glomerular filtration rate and urinary albumin excretion. Stepwise multiple regression analysis suggested, however, that they are partially independent. Gambara et al [45] described a special subgroup of patients with diabetic renal disease in which the severe interstitial changes were not clearly correlated with glomerular or vascular lesions. Similar observations were reported by another group of investigators who analysed patients with microalbuminuria [41] and described three patterns of renal morphology. One had normal structure, another had typical diabetic glomerular changes and a third group had absent or mild glomerular changes together with disproportionately severe tubulointerstitial changes and/or arteriolar hyalinosis. Conceivably such changes may not be due to ischemia but to the diabetic metabolic abnormality, like diabetic glomerulopathy although with other pathogenesis.

REFERENCES
1.   Kimmelstiel P, Wilson C. Intercapillary lesions in the glomeruli of the kidney. Am J Pathol 1936; 12: 83-105.
2.   Thomsen AC. *The Kidney in Diabetes Mellitus* (thesis). Copenhagen: Munksgaard, 1965.
3.   Ditscherlein G. *Nierenveränderungen bei Diabetikern.* Jená: G. Fischer, 1969.

4. Allen AC. So-called intercapillary glomerulosclerosis: a lesion associated with diabetes mellitus. Arch Pathol Lab Med 1941; 32: 33-51.
5. Bell ET. Renal lesions in diabetes mellitus. Am J Pathol 1942; 18: 744-745.
6. Bell ET. Renal vascular disease in diabetes mellitus. Diabetes 1953; 2: 376-389.
7. Bell ET. *Diabetes Mellitus: A Clinical and Pathological Study of 2529 Cases*. Springfield IL: Thomas, 1960.
8. Fahr T. Über Glomerulosklerose. Virschows Arch (Pathol Anat) 1942; 309: 16-33.
9. Spühler O, Zollinger HU. Die diab. Glomerulosklerose. Dtsch Arch Klin Med 1943; 190: 321-379.
10. Muirhead EE, Montgomery POB, Booth E. The glomerular lesions of diabetes mellitus: cellular hyaline and acellular hyaline lesions of »intercapillary glomerulosclerosis« as depicted by histochemical studies. Arch Intern Med 1956; 98: 146-161.
11. Randerath E. Zur Frage der intercapillären (diabetischen) Glomerulosklerose. Virchows Arch (Pathol Anat) 1953; 323: 483-523.
12. Sandison A, Newbold KM, Howie AJ. Evidence for unique distribution of Kimmelstiel-Wilson nodules in glomeruli. Diabetes 1992; 41: 952-955.
13. Stout LC, Kumar S, Whorton EB. Focal mesangiolysis and the pathogenesis of the Kimmelstiel-Wilson nodule. Hum Pathol 1993; 24: 77-89.
14. Yafumi S, Hiroshi K, Shin-Ichi T, Mitsuhiro Y, Hitoshi Y, Yoshitaka K, Nobu H. Mesangiolysis in diabetic glomeruli: Its role in the formation of nodular lesions. Kidney Int 1988; 34: 389-396.
15. Stout LC, Kumar S, Whorton EB. Insudative lesions - their pathogenesis and association with glomerular obsolescence in diabetes: A dynamic hypothesis based on single views of advancing human diabetic nephropathy. Hum Pathol 1994; 25: 1213-1227.
16. Barrie HJ, Aszkanazy CL, Smith GW. More glomerular changes in diabetics. Can Med Assoc J 1952; 66: 428-431.
17. Koss LG. Hyaline material with staining reaction of fibrinoid in renal lesions in diabetes mellitus. Arch Pathol Lab Med 1952; 54: 528-547.
18. Rinehart JF, Farquhar MG, Jung HC, Abul-Haj SK. The normal glomerulus and its basic reactions in disease. Am J Pathol 1953; 29: 21-31.
19. Gallo GR. Elution studies in kidneys with linear deposition of immunoglobulin in glomeruli. Am J Pathol 1970; 61: 377-394.
20. Westberg NG, Michael AF. Immunohistopathology of diabetic glomerulosclerosis. Diabetes 1972; 21: 163-174.
21. Frøkjær Thomsen O. Studies of diabetic glomerulosclerosis using an immunofluorescent technique. Acta Pathol Microbiol Scand (A) 1972; 80: 193-200.
22. Østerby R, Gundersen HJG, Nyberg G, Aurell M. Advanced diabetic glomerulopathy. Quantitative structural characterization of nonoccluded glomeruli. Diabetes 1987; 36: 612-619.
23. Hørlyck A, Gundersen HJG, Østerby R. The cortical distribution pattern of diabetic glomerulopathy. Diabetologia 1986; 29: 146-150.
24. Bendtsen TF, Nyengaard JR. The number of glomeruli in Type 1 (insulin-dependent) and Type 2 (non-insulin dependent) diabetic patients. Diabetologia 1992; 35: 844-850.
25. Allen AC. *The Kidney: Medical and Surgical Diseases*, 2nd ed. London: Churchill, 1962; pp 38.
26. Heptinstall RH. *Pathology of the Kidney*, 3rd ed. Boston: Little, Brown and Company, 1983; Ch. 26.

27.   Da-Silva EC, Saldanha LB, Pestalozzi MS, Del-Bueno IJ, Barros RT, Marcondes M, Nussenzveig I. Nodular diabetic glomerulosclerosis without diabetes mellitus. Nephron 1992; 62: 289-291.

28.   Kanwar YS, Garces J, Molitch ME. Occurrence of intercapillary nodular glomerulosclerosis in the absence of glucose intolerance. Am J Kidney Dis 1990; 15: 281-283.

29.   Olsen TS. Mesangial thickening and nodular glomerular sclerosis in diabetes mellitus and other diseases. Acta Pathol Microbiol Scand (A) 1972; 80: 203-216.

30.   Sølling K, Askjær S-A. Multiple myeloma with urinary excretion of heavy chain components of IgG and nodular glomerulosclerosis. Acta Med Scand 1973; 194: 23-30.

31.   Gallo GR, Feiner HD, Katz LA, Feldman GM, Correa EB, Chuba JV Buxbaum JN. Nodular glomerulopathy associated with nonamyloidotic kappa light chain deposits and excess immunoglobulin light chain synthesis. Am J Pathol 1980; 99: 621-644.

32.   Sølling K, Sølling J, Jacobsen NO, Frøkjær Thomsen O. Nonsecretory myeloma associated with nodular glomerulosclerosis. Acta Med Scand 1980; 207: 137-143.

33.   Schubert GE, Adam A. Glomerular nodules and long-spacing collagen in kidneys of patients with multiple myeloma. J Clin Pathol 1974; 27: 800-805.

34.   Wehner H, Bohle A. The structure of the glomerular capillary basement membrane in diabetes mellitus with and without nephrotic syndrome. Virchows Arch (Pathol Anat) 1974; 364: 303-309.

35.   Yum M, Maxwell DR, Hamburger R, Kleit SA. Primary glomerulonephritis complicating diabetic nephropathy. Hum Pathol 1984; 15: 921-927.

36.   Waldherr R, Ilkenhans C, Ritz E. How frequent is glomerulonephritis in diabetes mellitus type II ? Clin Nephrol 1992; 37: 271-273.

37.   Mauer SM, Steffes MW, Ellis EN, Sutherland DER, Brown DM, Goetz FC. Structural-functional relationships in diabetic nephropathy. J Clin Invest 1984; 74: 1143-1155.

38.   Richards N, Greaves I, Lee S, Howie A, Adu D, Michael J. Increased prevalence of renal biopsy findings other than diabetic glomerulopathy in type II diabetes mellitus. Nephrol Dial Transplant 1992; 7: 397-399.

39.   Olsen S, Mogensen CE. How often is type II diabetes mellitus complicated with non-diabetic renal disease? A material of renal biopsies and an analysis of the literature. Diabetologia 1996; 39: 1638-1645.

40.   Pinel NBF, Bilous R, Corticelli P, Halimi S, Cordonnier D. Renal Biopsies in 30 Micro-and Macroalbuminuric Non-Insulin Dependent (NIDDM) Patients: Heterogeneity of Renal Lesions. Heidelberg: European Diabetic Nephropathy Study Group, 1995.

41.   Brocco E, Fioretto P, Mauer M, Saller A, Carraro A, Frigato C, Chiesura-Corona M, Bianchi L, Baggio B, Maioll M, Abaterusso C, Velussi M, Sambatoro M, Virgili F, Ossi E, Nosadini R. Renal structure and function in non-insulin dependent diabetic patients with microalbuminuria. Kidney Int. 1997; 52: Suppl. 63: S40-S44

42   Parving H-H, Gall M-A, Skøtt P,Jørgensen HE, Løkkegaard H, Jørgensen F, Nielsen B, Larsen S. Prevalence and causes of albuminuria in non-insulin-dependent diabetic patients. Kidney Int, 1992; 41: 758-762

43   Olsen S. Identification of non-diabetic glomerular disease in renal biopsies from diabetics – a dilemma. Neprol Dial Transplant 1999; 13: 1846-49.

44.   Lane PH, Steffes M, Fioretto P, Mayer SM. Renal interstitial expansion in insulin-dependent diabetes mellitus. Kidney Int 1993; 43: 661-667.

45.   Gambara V, Remuzzi G, Bertani T. Heterogenous nature of renal lesions in type II diabetes. J Am Soc Nephrol 1993; 3: 1458-1466.

18. RENAL STRUCTURAL CHANGES IN PATIENTS WITH TYPE 1 DIABETES AND MICROALBUMINURIA

Hans-Jacob Bangstad, Susanne Rudberg and Ruth Østerby
Department of Pediatrics, Aker Diabetes Research Centre, Ullevål University Hospital, Oslo, Norway,The Department of Woman and Child Health, Pediatric Unit, Karolinska Institute, Stockholm, Sweden and Laboratory for Electron Microscopy, Aarhus Kommunehospital, Aarhus, Denmark

Associations between early stages of diabetic nephropathy and structural changes is far from clarified since some reports present rather marked changes in patients in the preclinical stage whereas others found very moderate changes in the early stage of nephropathy. Hence the issue is still a challenge to further studies. This chapter concentrates on the renal morphological changes in patients with Type 1 diabetes and early nephropathy and the possibilities of influencing the progression by blood glucose control and antihypertensive treatment.

STRUCTURES IN QUESTION

Structural changes in glomeruli, termed <u>diabetic glomerulopathy</u> is the aspect that has attracted most attention. The increased thickness of the glomerular basement membrane (BM) and the mesangial expansion with accumulation of matrix are the fundamental changes [1]. The relative increase of mesangium and of mesangial matrix is expressed as volume fractions, e.g. mesangium per glomerulus, matrix per mesangium or per glomerulus. The volume fractions are relative measures, estimating the composition of glomeruli and mesangial regions. These parameters are the quantitative expressions of the characteristic appearance of diabetic glomerulopathy. The matrix star volume [2] is an estimate of the confluence and/or convexity and size of the individual branches of the matrix. An overall estimate of the glomerulopathy may be expressed by a structural index (e.g. BMT/10+Vv (matrix/glom)%). Of decisive importance for obtaining reliable data describing the earliest stages is a sufficient and unbiased sampling. In order to reduce the imprecision in the estimates of the mesangial volume fraction a method with complete

Mogensen C.E. (ed.), THE KIDNEY AND HYPERTENSION IN DIABETES MELLITUS.
Copyright© 2000 by Kluwer Academic Publishers, Boston ● Dordrecht ● London. All rights reserved.

cross-sections at 3 levels per glomerulus has been applied [2].

Another glomerular structural change of completely different nature is the glomerular hypertrophy present in the earliest phase of diabetes [3]. In advanced stages it is further expressed as a compensatory enlargement, accompanying the developing glomerulopathy [4].

Further, extra-glomerular changes may play an important role. Rather characteristic is the arteriolar hyalinosis affecting afferent and efferent arterioles. This arteriolopathy can be expressed as the volume fraction of extra-cellular material (matrix) per media. Also, expansion of the cortical interstitium is part of the whole picture. Further, measureable enlargement has been described in the juxta-glomerular apparatus and the vascular pole region.

PATIENTS WITH MICROALBUMINURIA VS. HEALTHY CONTROLS
We have studied two series of kidney biopsies from 38 normotensive young patients with Type 1 diabetes as baseline data for prospective studies [5,6]. Most of the diabetic patients had AER in the low range with a median of 31 µg/min (range 15-194). Their mean age was 19 years (14-29) and diabetes duration 11 years (6-18). The microalbuminuric (MA) patients showed a clear increment in BM thickness with a mean of 586 nm (95% confidence interval 553-619 nm) versus 350 nm (315-384) in the control group. All of the MA patients had BM thickness above the normal range. The average BM thickening during the years with diabetes was approximately 20 nm per year. This approximation was based on the assumption that the patients had a BM thickness at onset of diabetes corresponding to the mean BMT of the control group, i.e. 350 nm. A significant parallel matrix expansion in the microalbuminuric patients vs. the normal controls was observed. Matrix/glomerular volume fraction was 0.12 (0.11-0.13) vs. 0.09 (0.08-0.10) and matrix star volume 28 µm^3 (26-31) vs. 14 µm^3 (11-17) in the two groups respectively [7].

Fioretto et al. presented structural data (BMT and mesangial/glomerular volume fraction) in 33 patients with AER above 15 µg per minute. Both parameters were increased compared with those in controls and correlated with AER. Matrix parameters were not investigated. Observations different from those in our series were very high figures for mesangial volume fraction also in the low range of microalbuminuria. Furthermore, several patients had decreased creatinine clearance and hypertension [8].

It is hardly surprising that it is possible with sensitive methods to show morphological changes in Type 1 patients with clinical indications of renal impairment (microalbuminuria) when compared to healthy controls, but the extent of the changes should be emphasized.

MICROALBUMINURIA VS. NORMOALBUMINURIA
In the 60es several reports indicated that morphological changes were present at the onset of Type 1 diabetes. Later studies clearly showed that the glomeruli are normal at that time

[9] and the impact of that observation was supported by studies of identical twins discordant for Type 1 diabetes [10]. In a clinical setting the transition from normo- to microalbuminuria is of utmost importance. Walker et al. compared two groups of Type 1 diabetes patients [11]. One with normoalbuminuria (n=9, AER <20 μg/min) and one with microalbuminuria (n=6). Even though the number of patients was low, a significant increment in BM thickness, mesangial/glomerular volume fraction and also the matrix parameters was found in patients with MA compared to those with NA. The patients in the normoalbuminuric (NA) group were slightly younger and had a shorter duration of diabetes than the MA-group, although the differences were not statistically significant. The group of patients with microalbuminuria was very heterogeneous with a wide range in diabetes duration. Since the biopsies in the previously mentioned study [5] were investigated at the same laboratory as Walker et al.'s, and the MA-group in this study [5] was rather homogeneous and in fact very similar to Walker et al's normoalbuminuric patients, we compared the groups and confirmed with a greater number of patients (n=17) Walker's principal findings. These results differ from those presented by Fioretto et al. [8], who found no difference between patients with normo- and low-grade microalbuminuria (< 32 μg/min). Further, their observations in the normoalbuminuric group are remarkable as increased BMT and mesangial volume fraction are shown as well. The latter parameter (with a mean of 0.30) is in fact markedly higher than that observed in our microalbuminuric group (0.21) and expresses advanced glomerulopathy. The high prevalence of hypertension (15%) in the normoalbuminuric patients does not seem to fully explain the discrepancies between the studies. In a fairly large study of normoalbuminuric adolescents [12] also abnormal levels of basement membrane thickness and mesangial volume fraction were found in some cases, but concurrent controls were not studied, and advanced glomerulopathy was not observed.

Another recent American study reports analogous findings in children and adolescents with diabetes duration five to twelve years [13]. They found a high frequency of BM-thickening and increased mesangial volume fraction in more than fifty percent of the group, most of which (48/59) had normal AER. However, the categorization of the continuous structural variables into normal or abnormal is a rather crude way of analysing the results. Further, concurrent analysis of valid control cases was not performed and so the frequencies should be taken with some reserve. It is not surprising that some measureable changes can be observed during the normoalbuminuric period. Yet, the two reports stating occurrence of advanced lesions in cases with normal AER lead to the question whether European and American populations are really that different, or whether patient selection or quantitative methodology are part of the explanation of discrepancies.

EXTRA-GLOMERULAR CHANGES

In advanced stages of nephropathy several structural compartments in the kidney display distinct abnormalities. The hyalinosis of efferent and afferent arterioles was described a long time ago. Increase in the interstitial tissue has in fact been incriminated as a very important determinant of the late fall in renal function [14]. Some information on these structures during earlier phases of nephropathy has been obtained in recent years.

Semiquantitative studies of the hyalinosis of arterioles have dealt with a very broad clinical range. The results showed that the score of arteriolar lesions correlated with the severity of glomerulopathy and interstitial expansion and also with renal function [15]. Clearly in this composite picture with affection of all compartments it is not possible to determine which is the most important in terms of the further progression of nephropathy, in particular since abnormalities in one compartment may be very closely and causally related to that in others.

In quantitative ultrastructural studies the composition of arteriolar walls was estimated in NA and MA IDDM patients and in controls [16]. All of the patients had clinical blood pressure within the normal range. Increased matrix per media was found in afferent and efferent arterioles in the MA patients, showing that matrix abnormalities have developed in this location at the earliest stage of nephropathy. The matrix/media volume fraction of the afferent arterioles correlated with glomerular parameters, both basement membrane thickness and matrix/glomerular volume fraction. Quantitative data are now available in one follow-up study, before and after antihypertensive treatment [17]. At baseline highly significant alterations were present in afferent and efferent arterioles. Over the follow-up period a moderate progression was observed in matrix/media volume fraction in afferent arterioles, but no significant worsening in the efferent arterioles.

Another structural change has recently been demonstrated in young Type 1 patients with MA. The volume of the juxta-glomerular apparatus is increased compared with that in non-diabetic controls. Furthermore, also the size expressed relative to glomerular volume, is increased. The interrelationship with functional variables, whether causative or consequent, is not known at the present time [18].

Interstitial expansion is a companion of advanced glomerulopathy and vasculopathy. The interstitium expressed as fraction of cortical space has been shown to correlate with AER and creatinine clearance, as well as with glomerular and arteriolar changes, considering a wide range of functional impairment [15]. We estimated the interstitial volume fraction in the MA patients with low grade albuminuria, and found that it was increased compared to controls already in this early phase [5]. A positive correlation with the degree of glomerulopathy was found, indicating parallel or maybe even interactive processes.

GLOMERULOPATHY AND BLOOD GLUCOSE CONTROL

The impact of long term hyperglycaemia on the development of structural changes has been demonstrated in several animal studies [19-22]. One study in man showed that in renal allografts no significant increase in BM thickness and mesangial volume fraction was found 2-10 years after pancreas transplantation in 11 patients [23]. Specific mesangial matrix parameters were not investigated. In a prospective long term (12 years) study of renal allografts, the increment of the mesangial volume fraction, but not the BM thickening, was prevented when blood glucose control was improved [24]. Similar results have been demonstrated in patients receiving simultaneous pancreas- and kidney transplantation [25]. Those patients with a well-functioning pancreas transplant seemed to be spared the development of diabetic glomerulopathy. A recent paper presented very intrigueing data [26]. Pancreas transplanted patients with native kidneys were followed with kidney biopsies at transplantation and after five and ten years. Whereas the glomerulopathy seemed to progress from 0-5 years, less severe affection was observed after ten years, indicating that very long-term metabolic normalisation may entail reversion of established lesions. However, the patients studied after 10 years were the survivors, some patients had dropped out due to renal failure.

In our own series we studied the relationship between structural changes and preceding blood glucose control. The estimated yearly increment of BMT and matrix volume fraction from the start of diabetes correlated with mean HbA_{1c} from the year preceding the study, which probably reflects the long term blood glucose control [5]. Another study in adolescents confirmed this by finding that 5-year mean HbA1c in addition to diabetes duration and GFR, was a variable with an independent influence on the glomerulopathy index [6].

The prospective study dealing with metabolic control has been concluded after 2 and a half years period [27]. The patients were randomized to either intensive insulin treatment by continuous subcutaneous insulin infusion (CSII) or conventional treatment (CT,- mostly multiple injections). It should be noticed that the mean HbA_{1c}-values in the two groups were rather high, and that the difference between the groups was modest, although significant, 8.7% and 9.9% respectively (normal range 4.3-6.1%),. The AER was for most of the patients in the low microalbuminuric range throughout the study. In fact, 38 % of the patients had AER <15 µg/min at the end of the study and thus by definition had no longer microalbuminuria. The main finding of the study was that in the CSII-group none of the matrix-parameters increased, whereas they all increased (not significantly for matrix/glomerular volume fraction) in the CT-group. The BM thickness increased in both groups,- but the increment during the study period was significantly larger in the CT-group [140 nm (50-230) vs. 56 nm (27-86)]. The association between blood glucose control and structure was confirmed when all the patients were considered together. A strong correlation was found between mean HbA_{1c} during the study and increase in BM thickness and matrix/glomerular volume fraction (figure 18-1). We thus showed that the progression of morphological changes in the glomerulus can be identified within a short period of only 2-3 years. Furthermore, we observed that reduced mean blood glucose levels clearly retarded the progression of morphological changes in the glomeruli. However, the glycated haemoglobin level achieved in the CSII-treated group (8.7%) was not sufficient to stop the progression of morphological changes.

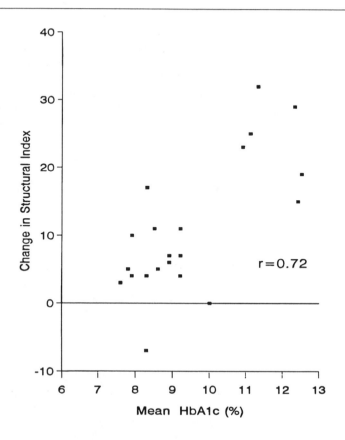

Figure 18-1. Results of a prospective study showing change in structural index (BMT/10 + Vv(matrix/glom) %) vs. mean HbA$_{1c}$ during 26-34 months in 21 IDDM-patients with microalbuminuria. Reference no. [5].

GLOMERULOPATHY AND ANTIHYPERTENSIVE TREATMENT

Antihypertensive treatment has been shown to have a beneficial effect on the course of nephropathy. Further, several recent data present evidence that administration of this treatment regimen in the stage of microalbuminuria to normotensive patients has protective effect [28].

To investigate the influence of angiotensin converting enzyme inhibitors (ACEI) or beta-blockers on renal structural changes in Type I diabetes, we studied 13 young normotensive patients with microalbuminuria [29]. Patients were randomized to either an ACEI (n=7) or a beta-blocker (n=6), and renal biopsies were taken before and after 36-48 months' treatment. As a reference group we used 9 patients on conventional insulin treatment and without antihypertensive treatment (AHT) who had renal biopsies previously taken with 26-34 months' intervals [26]. These patients had similar age, duration of diabetes and degree of microalbuminuria as those on AHT. We found that BMT, matrix star volume, diabetic glomerulopathy index (DGP, figure 18-2) [i.e. BMT/10+Vv(mat/glom)%] and interstitial fractional volume increased during follow-up in the reference group only. Microalbuminuria was normalised in both the ACEI-treated and the beta-blocker-treated groups, but not in the reference group. Mean HbA_{1c} during the study period did not differ between groups, whereas mean diastolic blood pressure was significantly lower in the antihypertensive groups than in the reference group. It was also found that mean diastolic blood pressure correlated significantly to the changes in BMT, DGP index and the interstitial expansion. Thus our data suggest that progression of *early* renal structural changes may be prevented or delayed during a 3 year period, by the use of either ACEI *or* beta-blocker. It is likely that this effect is due to maintenance of a normal or low blood pressure.

These results are somewhat in contrast to preliminary data from the ESPRIT study where ACEI were shown to reduce albuminuria but not affect the glomerulopathy changes [30]. It should be kept in mind though, that patients in the ESPRIT study had a longer diabetes duration and were older, but more important were in a more advanced stage of diabetic nephropathy than those included in our study.

We also studied the association between I/D polymorphism of the ACE-gene and progression of diabetic glomerulopathy in the same groups of patients referred to above, i.e those treated with either ACE-I or betablocker, and those without AHT. To extend the number of subjects another group of 9 patients on insulin pump treatment but without AHT, who likewise had renal biopsies previously performed, were included [27]. We found that eight patients had II-, 19 had ID-, and 3 had DD-genotypes, but only those with ID-or DD-genotypes showed any progression in BMT or DGP-index. Among patients with ID-or DD-genotypes progression of BM thickening and DGP-index was more marked in those without AHT than in those with any AHT. However, presence of the D-allele and not having AHT were both variables with an independent influence on the progression of BM thickening. These data indicate that microalbuminuric type 1 diabetic patients who are carriers of the D-allele do benefit of ACEI as well as of beta-blockers [31].

GLOMERULAR STRUCTURAL CHANGES VERSUS ALBUMIN EXCRETION

AER is an important parameter of kidney function in the early stages of nephropathy. In groups of diabetic patients representing a wide range of renal functional impairment significant correlations between glomerulopathy parameters and AER are found [1], and especially the correlation between mesangial expansion and AER has been underlined. This seems to reflect the fact that in the very advanced stages with marked proteinuria mesangial expansion is the dominant feature of the glomerulopathy. Within the range of microalbuminuria the correlation is less tight; however, positive associations have been described [5].

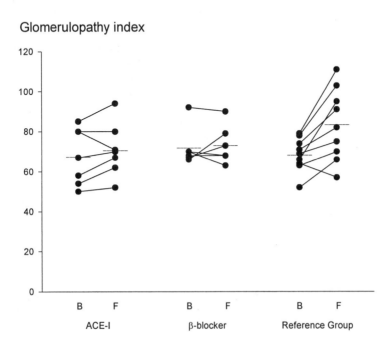

Fig 18-2. Glomerulopathy index (as in fig. 18-1) in baseline (B) and follow-up biopsies (F) in three groups treated with ACEI, beta-blocker or conventional insulin treatment. The increase in the reference group is statistically significant (p=0.007) and this group is significantly different from the two other groups (p=0.02 and 0.03 respectively).

In a study dealing with young normo-albuminuric patients it was found that a subset exhibiting microalbuminuria at the time of kidney biopsy had more advanced changes than those patients in the lower normoalbuminuric range [12]. One of our series has been followed for six years after the baseline biopsy. It was revealed that primarily BMT, but also systolic blood pressure and mean 6-year HbA_{1c} contributed to the variation in AER

[32]. In conflict with these observations are the reports mentioned above of rather advanced glomerulopathy in cases with low grade microalbuminuria [8,33,34], and even in normoalbuminuria [8,13]. It seems that these somewhat atypical cases with concurrently rather low GFR and AER are predominantly female Type 1 diabetes patients with long duration. In one of the series [34] a high frequency of totally occluded glomeruli was found, and enlargement of the vascular pole area in the open glomeruli was marked [35]. This change may represent a compensation to falling GFR and might influence the level of AER. Diabetic patients with a slow development of nephropathy may exhibit a deviating structural pattern where changes of arterioles and arteries (diabetic macroangiopathy) play an important role.

It is still unclear whether the elevation of blood pressure observed in diabetic nephropathy precedes, develops in parallel with or follows the initial increment of AER [28]. In our prospective study none of the patients had arterial hypertension (>150/90 mmHg), but 24 hours ambulatory blood pressure was not measured [8]. No associations between blood pressure (BP) and glomerular parameters were found, neither at baseline nor at follow-up, but all patients had BP within a fairly narrow range. This might indicate that BP has little impact on the initiation of structural lesions. But as mentioned above, systolic blood pressure at baseline of the prospective study correlated with the level of AER 6 years later. Also, Chavers et al. reported on a group of MA-patients with AER in the medium range (65 µg/min) with elevated BP (and/or reduced GFR) and found that they had more advanced structural changes than MA-patients with normal BP and GFR [36].

MECHANISMS OF ALBUMINURIA

Even if correlation between albumin excretion and structural lesions have been observed we still lack the deeper insight into the mechanisms behind the increment in albumin leakage. The increase in BM thickness in itself is unlikely to be responsible for the increased albumin excretion rate, but qualitative changes, e.g. reduced negative charge and/or presence of large pores, which develop concomitantly with the increase in thickness, may be decisive.

The urinary excretion of negatively charged proteins, e.g. albumin, is restricted by the negatively charged basement membrane. In the aforementioned prospective study [27] the charge selectivity index (clearances of IgG/IgG_4) was not associated with BM thickness at the beginning of the study. However, a striking correlation was found between the increase of BM thickness and the loss of charge selectivity during the study [37]. This may imply that the increase in BM thickness takes place concomitant with qualitative changes (e.g. loss of negative charge).

It is not known which substances that are responsible for the early thickening of BM and matrix expansion in diabetes. In the BM collagen IV predominates quantitatively, while laminin and heparan-sulphate proteoglycan probably play an important role as well. The mesangial matrix contains in addition collagen V, fibronectin, and chondroitin/dermatan sulfate proteoglycans [38]. Short-term experimental studies show that hyperglycaemia induces increased production of most of the aforementioned proteins [39-41], increased levels of the proteins' respective mRNA [42,43], increased matrix synthesis [44], and reduced amount of heparan-sulphate proteoglycan [45,46]. Furthermore, hyperglycaemia leads to accumulation of advanced glycated end products of proteins (AGE). These glycated proteins do contribute to the formation of pathological tissue deposits [47]. In our study [27] the level of serum-AGEs at the start of the study was related to the changes in structural parameters during the study period [48].

An interesting observation in advanced glomerulopathy [49] and occasionally also in the early stage in microalbuminuric patients is capillary loops with extremely thin and fluffy BM, contrasting markedly the other capillaries in the biopsies. They may be an expression of a compensatory glomerular growth, setting in at this early stage, and could represent the large pores.

The BM-thickening develops in parallel with matrix expansion. Matrix changes, quantitative and qualitative, may interfere with the function of the mesangial cells [50]. Mesangial cell function plays a role in many aspects of glomerular physiology [51] and one immediate consequence of the matrix expansion is that the distance between mesangial cells increases. This may impair the cell to cell interaction.

Altogether, the present data indicate that the increased loss of albumin across the glomerular filtration barrier is a sign associated with early structural lesions of diabetic glomerulopathy and that the further development can be arrested or at least slowed by intensive insulin and/or antihypertensive treatment.

REFERENCES

1.   Mauer SM, Steffes MW, Ellis EN, Sutherland DE, Brown DM, Goetz FC. Structural-functional relationships in diabetic nephropathy. J Clin Invest 1984; 74:1143-1155.

2.   Østerby R. Research methodologies related to renal complications: structural changes. In Research Methodologies in Human Diabetes, Part 2, Mogensen CE, Standl E, eds. Berlin, New York: Walter de Gruyter, 1995; pp 289-09

3.   Østerby R, Gundersen HJ. Glomerular size and structure in diabetes mellitus. 1. Early abnormalities. 1975; 11:229-229.

4.   Gundersen HJ, Østerby R. Glomerular size and structure in diabetes mellitus. 2. Late abnormalities. Diabetologia 1977;13:43-48.

5.   Bangstad H-J, Østerby R, Dahl-Jørgensen K, et al. Early glomerulopathy is present in young Type 1 (insulin-dependent) diabetic patients with microalbuminuria. Diabetologia 1993; 36: 523-529.

6.   Rudberg S, Østerby R, Dahlquist G, Nyberg G, Persson B. Predictors of renal morphological changes in the early stage of microalbuminuria in adolescents with IDDM. Diabetes Care 1997;20:265-271.

7.   Østerby R, Bangstad H-J, Rudberg S. Structural changes in microalbuminuria. Effect of intervention. Nephrology Dialysis Transplantation [Abstract] 1998; 13: 1067-68..

8.   Fioretto P, Steffes MW, Mauer SM. Glomerular structure in nonproteinuric IDDM patients with various levels of albuminuria. Diabetes 1994; 43: 1358-1364.

9.	Østerby R. Early phases in the development of diabetic nephropathy. Acta Med Scand 1975; Suppl.574 : 1-80.

10.	Steffes MW, Sutherland DER, Goetz FC, Rich SS, Mauer SM. Studies of kidney and muscle biopsies in identical twins discordant for type 1 diabetes mellitus. N Engl J Med 1985; 312: 1281-1287.

11.	Walker JD, Close CF, Jones SL, et al. Glomerular structure in type I (insulin-dependent) diabetic patients with normo- and microalbuminuria. Kidney Int 1992; 41: 741-748.

12.	Berg UB, Torbjørnsdotter TB, Jaremko G, Thalme B. Kidney morphological changes in relation to long-term renal function and metabolic control in adolescents with IDDM. Diabetologia 1998; 41. 1047-1056.

13.	Ellis EN, Warady BA, Wood EG, Hassanein R, Richardson WP, Lane PH et al. Renal structural-functional relationship in early diabetes mellitus. Pediatr Nephrol 1997;11:584-591.

14.	Ziyadeh FN, Goldfarb S. The diabetic renal tubulointerstitium. In Dodd S, ed: Current topics in pathology. Springer-Verlag, Berlin; 1995: 175-201.

15.	Lane PH, Steffes MW, Fioretto P, Mauer SM. Renal interstitial expansion in insulin-dependent diabetes mellitus. Kidney Int 1993; 43: 661-667.

16.	Østerby R, Bangstad H-J, Nyberg G, Walker JD, Viberti GC. A quantitative ultrastructural study of juxtaglomerular arterioles in IDDM patients with micro- and normoalbuminuria. Diabetologia 1995; 38: 1320-1327.

17.	Gulmann C, Rudberg S, Østerby R. Renal arterioles in patients with type I diabetes and microalbuminuria before and after treatment with antihypertensive drugs. Virchows Arch 1999; 434: 523-528.

18.	Gulmann C, Rudberg S, Nyberg G, Østerby R. Enlargement of the juxtaglomerular apparatus in insulin-dependent diabetes mellitus patients with microalbuminuria. Virchows Arch 1998; 433: 63-67.

19.	Rasch R. Prevention of diabetic glomerulopathy in streptozotocin diabetic rats by insulin treatment. Glomerular basement membrane thickness. Diabetologia 1979; 16: 319-324.

20.	Rasch R. Prevention of diabetic glomerulopathy in streptozotocin diabetic rats by insulin treatment. The mesangial region. Diabetologia 1979; 17: 243-248.

21.	Kern TS, Engerman RL. Kidney morphology in experimental hyperglycemia. Diabetes 1987; 36: 244-249.

22.	Petersen J, Ross J, Rabkin R. Effect of insulin therapy on established diabetic nephropathy in rats. Diabetes 1988; 37: 1346-1350.

23.	Bilous RW, Mauer SM, Sutherland DER, Najarian JS, Goetz FC, Steffes MW. The effect of pancreas transplantation on the glomerular structure of renal allografts in patients with insulin-dependent diabetes. N Engl J Med 1989; 321: 80-85.

24.	Barbosa J, Steffes MW, Connett J, Mauer M. Hyperglycemia is causally related to diabetic renal lesions. Diabetes 1992; 41: 9A.

25.	Wilczek H, Jaremko G, Tyden G, Groth CG. Evolution of diabetic nephropathy in kidney grafts. Transplantation 1995; 59: 51-57.

26.	Fioretto P, Steffes MW, Sutherland DER, Goetz FC, Mauer M. Reversal of lesions of diabetic nephropathy after pancreas transplantation. N Eng J Med 1998; 339: 69-75.

27.	Bangstad H-J, Østerby R, Dahl-Jørgensen K, Berg KJ, Hartmann A, Hanssen KF. Improvement of blood glucose control retards the progression of morphological changes in early diabetic nephropathy. Diabetologia 1994; 37: 483-490

28.   Mogensen CE. Microalbuminuria, blood pressure and diabetic renal disease. Origin and development of ideas. Diabetologia 1999; 42: 263-285.

29.   Rudberg S, Østerby R, Bangstad HJ, Dahlquist G, Persson B. Effect of angiotensin converting enzyme inhibitor or beta-blocker on glomerular structural changes in young microalbuminuric patients with Type I (insulin-dependent) diabetes mellitus. Diabetologia 1999; 42: 589-595.

30.   Baines LA, White KE, MacLeod JM, Bilous RW. Angiotensin converting enzyme inhibitors reduce albuminuria but do not affect glomerular structure in Type 1 diabetic nephropathy. Diabetes 1999; Suppl. 48: A36

31.   Rudberg S, Rasmussen LM, Bangstad H-J, Østerby R. Influence of insertion/deletion polymorphism in the angiotensin converting enzyme gene on the progression of diabetic glomerulopathy in IDDM patients with microalbuminuria. Diabetologia 1999;42: Suppl 1: A 269.

32.   Bangstad H-J, Østerby R, Hartmann A, Berg TJ, Hanssen KF. Severity of glomerulopathy predicts long-term urinary albumin excretion rate in patients with Type 1 diabetes and microalbuminuria. Diabetes Care 1999; 22: 314-319.

33.   Lane PH, Steffes MW, Mauer SM. Glomerular structure in IDDM women with low glomerular filtration rate and normal urinary albumin excretion. Diabetes 1992; 41: 581-586.

34.   Østerby R, Schmitz A, Nyberg G, Asplund J. Renal structural changes in insulin dependent diabetic patients with albuminuria. Comparison of cases with onset of albuminuria after short and long duration. APMIS 1998; 106: 361-370.

35.   Østerby R, Asplund J, Bangstad H-J et al. Glomerular volume and the glomerular vascular pole area in patients with insulin-dependent diabetes mellitus. Virchow Arch 1997; 431:351-357.

36.   Chavers BM, Bilous RW, Ellis EN, Steffes MW, Mauer SM. Glomerular lesions and urinary albumin excretion in Type 1 diabetes without overt proteinuria. N Engl J Med 1989; 320: 966-970.

37.   Bangstad H-J, Kofoed-Enevoldsen A, Dahl-Jørgensen K, Hanssen KF. Glomerular charge selectivity and the influence of improved blood glucose control in Type 1 diabetic patients with microalbuminuria. Diabetologia 1992; 35: 1165-1170.

38.   Silbiger S, Crowley S, Shan Z, Brownlee M, Satriano J, Schlondorff D. Nonenzymatic glycation of mesangial matrix and prolonged exposure of mesangial matrix to elevated glucose reduces collagen synthesis and proteoglycan charge. Kidney Int 1993; 43: 853-864.

39.   Brownlee M, Spiro RG. Glomerular basement membrane metabolism in the diabetic rat: in vivo studies. Diabetes 1979; 28: 121-125.

40.   Cagliero E, Roth T, Roy S, Lorenzi M. Characteristics and mechanisms of high-glucose-induced overexpression of basement membrane components in cultured human endothelial cells. Diabetes 1991; 40: 102-110.

41.   Roy S, Sala R, Cagliero E, Lorenzi M. Overexpression of fibronectin induced by diabetes or high glucose: phenomenon with a memory. Proc Natl Acad Sci USA 1990; 87: 404-408.

42.   Ledbetter S, Copeland EJ, Noonan D, Vogeli G, Hassel JR. Altered steady-state mRNA levels of basement membrane proteins in diabetic mouse kidneys and thromboxane synthase inhibition. Diabetes 1990; 39: 196-203.

43.   Poulsom R, Kurkinen M, Prockop DJ, Boot-Handford RP. Increased steady-state levels of laminin B1 mRNA in kidneys of long term streptozotocin-diabetic rats. J Biol Chem 1988; 263: 10072-10076.

44. Ayo SH, Radnik RA, Garoni JA, Glass II WF, Kreisberg JI. High glucose causes an increase in extracellular matrix proteins in cultured mesangial cells. Am J Pathol 1990; 136: 1339-1348.

45. Shimomura H, Spiro RG. Studies on the macromolecular components of human glomerular basement membrane and alterations in diabetes: decreased levels of heparan sulfate proteoglycan and laminin. Diabetes 1987; 36: 374-381.

46. Olgemöller B, Schwabbe S, Gerbitz KD, Schleicher ED. Elevated glucose decreases the content of a basement associated heparan sulphate proteoglycan in proliferating cultured porcine mesangial cells. Diabetologia 1992; 35: 183-186.

47. Brownlee M, Vlassara H, Cerami A. Nonenzymatic glycosylation and the pathogenesis of diabetic complications. Ann Intern Med 1984; 101: 527-537.

48. Berg TJ, Torjesen PA, Bangstad H-J, Bucala R, Østerby R, Hanssen KF. Advanced glycosylation end products predict changes in the kidney morphology in patients with insulin dependent diabetes mellitus. Metabolism 1997; 46: 661-665.

49. Østerby R, Nyberg G. New vessel formation in the renal corpuscles in advanced diabetic glomerulopathy. J Diabetic Compl 1987; 1: 122-127.

50. Kashgarian M, Sterzel RB. The pathobiology of the mesangium. Kidney Int 1992; 41: 524-529.

51. Hawkins NJ, Wakefield D, Charlesworth JA. The role of mesangial cells in glomerular pathology. Pathology 1990; 22: 24-32.

19.   RENAL STRUCTURE IN TYPE 2 DIABETIC PATIENTS   WITH MICROALBUMINURIA

Paola Fioretto, Michele Dalla Vestra, Alois Saller and Michael Mauer.
Department of Medical and Surgical Sciences and Center of the National Research Council for the Study of Aging, University of Padova, Italy;
Department of Pediatrics, University of Minnesota, Minneapolis, MN, USA.

RENAL STRUCTURAL CHANGES IN DIABETIC NEPHROPATHY

Although 80% or more of diabetic patients receiving renal replacement therapy have type 2 diabetes [1-5], the renal pathology and natural history of diabetic nephropathy (DN) in type 2 diabetes has been studied much less intensely than in type 1 diabetes and thus many important questions remain unclear. The clinical manifestations of DN, proteinuria, declining glomerular filtration rate (GFR) and increasing blood pressure, are similar in type 1 and type 2 diabetes [6-7], as they are in many other renal diseases; nevertheless whether these clinical features are the consequences of similar underlying renal lesions is not entirely known. In type 1 diabetes it is generally accepted that the most important structural changes, leading to progressive renal function loss occur in the glomerulus [8-13]; concomitantly and roughly in proportion to the degree of glomerulopathy, the glomerular arterioles, tubules and interstitium also undergo structural changes, including hyalinosis of the arteriolar wall, thickening and reduplication of tubular basement membranes, tubular atrophy and interstitial expansion and fibrosis [8-14]. These extraglomerular lesions become progressive and severe only when glomerulopathy is far advanced. Quantitative morphometric studies have demonstrated that the lesion most closely related to the decline in renal function in type 1 diabetes is mesangial expansion, caused predominantly by mesangial matrix accumulation [12, 15]. We have also observed, in sequential renal biopsies of type 1 diabetic patients performed 5 years apart, that the only structural change associated with increasing albuminuria was mesangial expansion [13]; glomerular basement membrane (GBM) width, interstitial expansion and the number of globally sclerosed glomeruli did not change over 5 years in this group of patients in transition from normo to microalbuminuria or from microalbuminuria to overt nephropathy. Thus in type 1 diabetes severe arteriolar, tubular and interstitial lesions are rare unless advanced diabetic glomerulopathy is present.

Mogensen C.E. (ed.), THE KIDNEY AND HYPERTENSION IN DIABETES MELLITUS.
Copyright© 2000 by Kluwer Academic Publishers, Boston ● Dordrecht ● London. All rights reserved.

When overt nephropathy develops in patients with type 1 diabetes for at least 10 years, advanced diabetic glomerulopathy is almost always present, while non-diabetic renal diseases are very uncommon in such patients [Fioretto and Mauer, unpublished data]. In proteinuric type 2 diabetic patients, in contrast, the prevalence of non diabetic renal lesions has been reported to be high (approximately 30%). Parving et al reported that 23% of type 2 diabetic patients with proteinuria had non-diabetic glomerulopathies, which these authors classified as minimal lesion nephropathy, mesangio-proliferative glomerulonephritis (GN) and sequelae of GN [16]. Heterogeneity in renal lesions has also been reported by Gambara et al, who found that only 37% of proteinuric type 2 diabetic patients had typical changes of DN [17]. In a more recent study from the same authors, 46% of the patients had typical diabetic nephropathy, whereas 18% had superimposed non-diabetic renal diseases [18]. Khan et al observed the presence of non diabetic renal disease in 42% of 153 type 2 patients with overt nephropathy [19]; the occurrence of non diabetic renal disease was much lower (12%) in the series of 33 proteinuric patients studied by Olsen and Mogensen [20]. However in all these studies, with the exception of the study of Parving, patients were referred to the nephrologist and kidney biopsies were performed for clinical indications; thus many of these renal biopsies were presumably performed because the patient's clinical course was considered to be atypical for diabetic nephropathy. These studies, therefore, may not describe the usual type 2 patients with diabetic nephropathy, but those with an unusual clinical course. The different results may reflect also differences in the indications for kidney biopsy. A large autopsy study on type 2 diabetic patients did not confirm a high incidence of non-diabetic renal diseases [21]. Thus the available data on renal structure in type 2 diabetic patients with proteinuria have heretofore been contradictory.

Quantitative morphometric studies in type 2 diabetes are scarce; in Japanese type 2 diabetic patients with a wide range of renal function, morphometric measures of diabetic glomerulopathy showed correlations to renal functional parameters similar to those observed in type 1 diabetes [22]. However, more recent studies suggest a significant incidence of normal glomerular structure among microalbuminuric and proteinuric Japanese type 2 diabetic patients [23]. Diabetic glomerulopathy was estimated by Østerby et al. in caucasian type 2 proteinuric diabetic patients [24]. All the morphometric glomerular parameters were, on average, abnormal. However some patients had glomerular structure within the normal range. In type 1 diabetic patients with overt nephropathy, on the other hand, glomerular structure was always severely altered [12, 24 and Fioretto and Mauer, unpublished data]. We have recently studied a group of caucasian type 2 diabetic patients, and found that, although diabetic glomerular structural parameters were more altered on average in patients with microalbuminuria and macroalbuminuria than in those with normoalbuminuria, several patients had normal glomerular structure despite abnormal albumin excretion rate [25]; also compared to patients with type 1 diabetes and similar renal function, diabetic glomerulopathy was less advanced in patients with type 2 diabetes. Albumin excretion rate was directly related to both GBM width (r=0.47, p<0.001) and Vv(mes/glom) (r=0.44, p<0.001); GFR was inversely related to Vv(mes/glom) (r=0.47, p<0.001) but not to GBM width. Although these structural/functional relationships were significant in type 2 diabetes, they were imprecise and less strong than in type 1 diabetes [12]. Thus these findings suggest that also in type 2 diabetes mesangial expansion is a crucial structural change, leading to loss of renal function. However glomerular lesions are less advanced in type 2 than type 1 diabetic patients and a substantial number of type 2 diabetic patients have normal glomerular structure despite abnormal albumin excretion rate. These data are in agreement with those in Pima Indians where, in a much smaller group, the authors did not find significant differences in glomerular ultrastructure between patients with long-term type 2 diabetes with normoalbuminuria and those with microalbuminuria [26]. Diabetic glomerulopathy parameters were more severely altered only in patients with proteinuria. These results were true for mesangial fractional volume, GBM width and also for foot process width and the number of podocytes per glomerulus. Thus the authors concluded that in Pima indians podocyte loss and increase in foot process width are important in the progression to overt nephropathy. Nevertheless, as for type 1 diabetes [27], the changes in podocytes occur late in the course of diabetic renal disease, and are probably involved more in the mechanisms of progression than in those of genesis and early development [26, 27].

MICROLABUMINURIA IN TYPE 2 DIABETES
Microalbuminuria (MA) antedates clinical proteinuria in both type 1 [28-30] and type 2 diabetes [31, 32]. The predictive value of MA was thought to be quite different in type 1 and type 2 diabetes in that only approximately 20% of type 2 patients with MA progressed to overt nephropathy over a decade of follow-up in contrast to over 80% of type 1 diabetic patients [32]. In fact MA in type 2 diabetes is considered a better predictor of cardiovascular mortality than of end stage renal disease [31, 33, 34]. However, in more recent studies, approximately 40% of type 2 diabetic patients with MA progressed to overt nephropathy over a decade and a similar progression rate was observed in patients with type 1 diabetes [35, 36]. The different predictive value of MA to overt nephropathy in the studies performed 2 decades ago and in the more recent ones may reflect a change in the natural history of renal disease in diabetes. The low predictive value of MA for overt nephropathy in type 2 diabetes may in part be accounted for by the high mortality from cardiovascular disease, which can interrupt the progression to clinical nephropathy. However, other explanations are tenable, including the possibility that MA in type 2 diabetes, at least in a subset of patients, may not be associated with the same underlying abnormalities which are so common in patients with type 1 diabetes and MA. Nonetheless, to date there is no full explanation to the clinical observation that only a subgroup of type 2 diabetic patients with MA progresses to overt nephropathy, while in the majority renal function remains stable. It can be hypothesized that MA in type 2 diabetic patients may be either consequent to diabetic glomerulopathy, as in type 1 diabetes, and progress to overt nephropathy, or be due to other renal lesions or reflect altered vascular permeability due to regional or generalized endothelial dysfunction [7, 37]. The structural basis for MA in type 1 diabetes has been studied by us and others and it is now established that when albuminuria exceeds 30 µg/min diabetic glomerulopathy, with thickening of the GBM and mesangial expansion is

usually well established [38]. Only one study had evaluated renal structure in MA type 2 diabetics [39]; surprisingly these authors, who had earlier described diagnostic heterogeneity in proteinuric type 2 diabetic patients [17], reported that all 16 MA type 2 diabetic patients had classic diabetic glomerulopathy.

For these reasons we undertook the study of renal function and structure in MA type 2 diabetic patients in order to describe the renal structural concomitants of this functional disturbance. The light microscopy results of this study [40, 41] are summarized here.

RENAL STRUCTURE IN MICROALBUMINURIC TYPE 2 DIABETIC PATIENTS

Study design and patient population
We invited patients with type 2 diabetes to participate in a longitudinal study of renal structural-functional relationships. Patients were admitted to the University of Padova for research evaluation of renal structure and function; kidney biopsy in this study was never performed for clinically indicated diagnostic purposes. Patients were defined as MA when albumin excretion rate (AER) was ≥ 20 µg/min but <200 µg/min in at least two of three consecutive sterile 24 hour urine collections. To date light microscopic slides from 53 MA patients have been evaluated [40, 41]. Thirty-five of the 53 patients (all caucasians) were males. Age was 58 ± 8 years (Mean$\pm$1SD), known diabetes duration was 11 ± 7 years and HbA1c was $8.3\pm1.8\%$. GFR, determined by the plasma clearance of [51] Cr-EDTA [42], was 99 ± 28 ml/min/1.73 m^2 and AER was 61 (20-199) µg/min (median, range). Patients were defined hypertensive when blood pressure values exceed 140/85 mm Hg [43], or when on antihypertensive therapy regardless of BP levels. Using these criteria all but 9 patients were receiving antihypertensive therapy, and the majority of them were on ACE-inhibors. Overall, according to the criteria described above, 78% of these patients were hypertensive.

Renal structure
Percutaneous kidney biopsies were performed in all patients, and renal tissue immediately fixed and embedded for light, electron and immunofluorescence microscopy studies [44]. For comparison, kidney biopsies were obtained from 36 (17 M/19F) kidney donors at the time of renal transplantation, at the University of Minnesota; these controls were matched for age with the diabetic patients (age: 55.7 ± 7 years).

Light microscopy
The initial reading of the biopsy material made apparent the inadequacy of existing descriptive systems, which had largely been based on observations of research biopsies in type 1 diabetes. In fact 50 consecutive type 1 diabetic patients with at least 10 years of diabetes duration and overt nephropathy that we have reviewed had obvious diabetic glomerulopathy [Fioretto and Mauer, unpublished data] and diabetic glomerulopathy is

also usually quite advanced in MA type 1 diabetic patients. In this series, however, many type 2 patients with MA either did not have glomerulopathy, or had only mild mesangial expansion by light microscopy; in fact the majority of the MA type 2 diabetic patients had normal or near normal glomerular structure, with or without tubulo-interstitial and arteriolar changes.

Thus we proposed a new classification system which included 3 major groups:

Category I: Normal or near normal renal structure.
These patients (15 M/7F, 41%) had biopsies which were normal or showed mild mesangial expansion, tubulo-interstitial changes or arteriolar hyalinosis (Figure 19-1A).

Category II: Typical diabetic nephropathology.
These patients (9M/5F, 26%) had established diabetic lesions with approximately balanced severity of glomerular, tubulo-interstitial and arteriolar changes. This picture is typical of that seen in type 1 diabetic patients with obvious light microscopic DN changes (Figure 19-1B).

Category III: Atypical patterns of renal injury.
These patients (11M/6F, 33%) had relatively mild diabetic glomerular changes with disproportionately severe renal structural changes including:
(a) Tubular atrophy, tubular basement membrane thickening and reduplication and interstitial fibrosis (tubulo-interstitial lesions) (Figure 19-1C).
(b) Advanced glomerular arteriolar hyalinosis commonly associated with atherosclerosis of larger vessels (Figure 19-1D).
(c) Global glomerular sclerosis.

In Category III group these patterns were present in all possible combinations (Figures 19-1C and 19-1D); however important tubulo-interstitial changes were observed in all but 1 patient who had very severe arteriolar hyalinosis lesions. These tubulo-interstitial lesions were often associated with arteriolar changes and in some patients with global glomerulosclerosis.

In the age matched control group, 3/36 subjects had important tubulo-interstitial changes. Several normal controls had mild arteriolar hyalinosis lesions; 6 controls had more advanced arteriolar lesions, sometimes comparable to those observed in patients in categories II and III.

We found no cases of definable non diabetic renal disease in this series of 53 patients. The difference between our results and those of previous reports in proteinuric type 2 diabetic patients (see above) may be best explained by the study design, in that patients in the present study had kidney biopsies performed on the basis of a research protocol as opposed to biopsies performed for clinical indications often based upon atypical course.

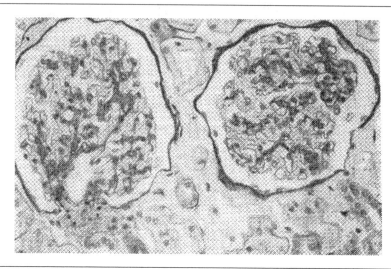

Figure 19-1A. Glomeruli from a patient in category C I. Glomerular structure is near normal with mild mesangial expansion (PAS).

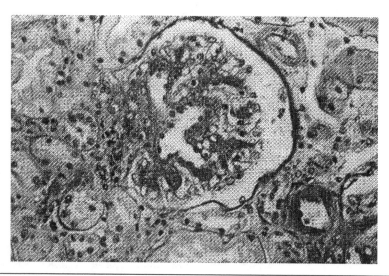

Figure 19-1B. Glomerulus from a patient in category C II, with well established diabetic glomerulopathy. Diffuse mesangial expansion, moderate ateriolar hyalinosis, and mild interstitial fibrosis are present (PAS).

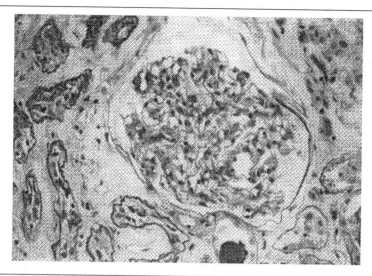

Figure 19-1C. Glomerulus from a patient in category C III (a) with near normal glomerular structure and TBM thickening, tubular atrophy and severe interstitial fibrosis (PAS).

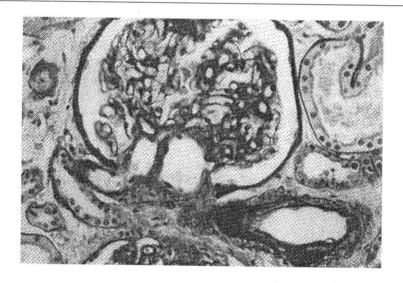

Figure 19-1D. Glomerulus from a patient in category C III (b) with mild mesangial expansion and severe arteriolar hyalinosis, affecting both afferent and efferent glomerular arterioles (PAS).

Clinical features in relation to patterns of lesions

Age was similar in the three groups; known duration of type 2 diabetes was different among groups, with CII and CIII patients having longer duration than CI [14±6 and 13±8 yrs vs 7±3, p<0.05 for both]. HbA1c levels were significantly different among groups with CII patients having the highest HbA1c values. Body mass index (BMI) was also different (ANOVA, p<0.02); BMI was only mildly increased in CII patients (26±4) and was significantly greater in CI (30±4) and CIII (29±3) than in CII patients(t-tests, p<0.05 for both). AER levels were similar in the three groups (median: 56, 58 and 69 μg/min respectively); GFR was lower in CII (86±37 ml/min/1.73 m^2) than in CI (109±19) and CIII patients (96±20, p<0.05 for both). Systolic and diastolic blood pressure values were similar in the three groups as was the prevalence of hypertension (84%, 73% and 79%, respectively).

Diabetic retinopathy was present in all CII patients (background in 6 and proliferative in 8). None of the patients in CI and CIII had proliferative retinopathy, while background diabetic retinopathy was observed in 9 of 22 CI and 6 of 17 CIII patients. Thus, all CII patients had diabetic retinopathy and all patients with proliferative retinopathy had "typical" diabetic nephropathy lesions.

From the clinical features, the three groups we hypothesize that the "atypical" patterns of renal injury observed in many of our patients are probably related to hyperglycemia. This suggests that hyperglycemia may cause different patterns of renal injury in older type 2 compared to younger type 1 diabetic patients. The tubulo-interstitial and vascular changes could also be related to ageing, atherosclerosis and systemic hypertension. However, hypertension was present in almost all patients in all 3 structural categories, and "per se" cannot account for the different lesions observed in category III. Further, mean age was similar in category II and III patients (60 years), despite the different patterns of renal injury in the two groups, and our observations in a large number of age-matched normal controls argue that normal aging is not sufficient to explain most of the renal structural changes observed in C III patients. One possibility is that the heterogeneity in renal structure might reflect the heterogeneous nature of type 2 diabetes "per se". Thus patients with "typical" DN lesions had longer known diabetes duration, worse metabolic control and they all had diabetic retinopathy. Interestingly, their BMI only slightly exceeded normal values, as opposed to the clearly increased BMI values in CI and CIII patients. This suggests that the different underlying pathophysiologic mechanisms responsible for type 2 diabetes in these groups of patients may also underlie different renal pathophysiologic mechanisms or responses. Another possibility is that some of the heterogeneity in renal structure seen in these studies may represent interactions of diabetes and ageing, particularly among CIII patients.

A remarkably high number of MA type 2 diabetic patients (41%) had normal or near normal renal structure (C I). They tended to be younger and to have shorter diabetes duration than patients with renal lesions (categories II and III). Although we do not have an explanation for the abnormal AER in these patients, it is possible that MA in this subset is a manifestation of generalized endothelial dysfunction rather than of established renal structural damage. The predictive significance of MA on the subsequent development of renal, retinal and macrovascular complications in these patients would be of great clinical and theoretical interest to elucidate in longitudinal studies.

ENDOTHELIAL FUNCTION IN RELATION TO RENAL STRUCTURE

Since MA is not associated with renal structural changes in a substantial subset of type 2 diabetic patients, we considered the possibility that MA in these patients could be consequent to endothelial dysfunction. To test this hypothesis we measured von Willebrand factor (vWF) plasma levels, an endothelial-derived protein indicative of endothelial function, in a group of MA patients who also had a research kidney biopsy performed [45]. Thirty-two patients were studied and, contrary to our hypothesis, vWF plasma levels were significantly increased only in patients with renal structural abnormalities [both CII (typical) and CIII (atypical) patterns] and was normal in patients with normal renal structure (CI) [45]. The results of this study do not provide an explanation for MA in patients without renal injury, and the nature of MA in these patients remains unknown. vWF plasma levels, however, represent only one measure of endothelial function, and further physiologic studies are necessary. Nevertheless, from these studies on vWF and renal structure we propose that there are two types of MA in type 2 diabetes: one associated with increased vWF plasma levels, established renal structural lesions and, frequently, diabetic retinopathy, and the other characterized by normal vWF plasma levels, normal renal structure and absent or mild diabetic retinopathy [45, 46]. Whether these two types of MA have different prognostic implications for end stage renal disease and cardiovascular events deserves longitudinal studies.

CONCLUSIONS

These studies, far from clarifying the mechanisms responsible for MA in type 2 diabetic patients, clearly demonstrate the complexity and the problematic nature of this renal functional abnormality in these patients. These results should also encourage and stimulate further investigations and new directions of research. Thus, to better understand the pathophysiologic mechanisms responsible for MA in type 2 diabetes we are currently studying the relationships between renal lesions and macrovascular disease [47]. Studies on the interaction of aging and type 2 diabetes on renal structure and function would also be of interest particularly in the subset of MA patients with disproportionally severe tubulo-interstitial lesions. Also a better understanding of tubular function needs to be developed in these patients [41].

Finally, longitudinal detailed renal structural and functional studies of these patients are crucial to the understanding of the clinical implications of these complex processes.

REFERENCES

1. Cordonnier DJ, Zmirou D, Benhamou PY, Halimi S, Ledoux F, Guiserix J. Epidemiology, development and treatment of end-stage renal failure in type 2 diabetes. The case of mainland France and of overseas French territories. Diabetologia 1993; 36: 1109-1112.
2. Stephen SGW, Gillaspry JA, Clyne D, Mejia A, Pollok VE. Racial differences in the incidence of end stage renal disease in type 1 and type 2 diabetes mellitus. Am J Kidney Dis 1990; 15: 562-567.
3. Ritz E, Nowack R, Fliser D, et al. Type II diabetes mellitus: is the renal risk adequately appreciated? Nephrol Dial Transplant 1991; 6: 679-682.
4. Catalano C, Postorino M, Kelly PJ. Diabetes mellitus and renal replacement therapy in Italy: prevalence, main characteristic and complications. Nephrol Dial Transplant 1990; 5: 788-796.
5. Mauer M, Mogensen CE, Friedman E. Diabetic Nephropathy. In: Schrier RW, Gottschalk CW (eds). Diseases of the kidne, 6th edn. Little Brown& Co. 1996, Vol 3, 2019-2062.
6. Mogensen CE, Shmitz A, Christiensen CK. Comparative renal pathophysyology relevant to IDDM and NIDDM patients. Diabetes Metab Rev 1988; 4: 453.
7. Schmitz A. Nephropathy in non-insulin dependent diabetes mellitus and perspectives for intervention. Diab Nutr Metab 1995; 7: 135-148.
8. Mauer SM, Steffes MW, Brown DM. The kidney in diabetes. Am J Med 1981; 70: 603-612.
9. Fioretto P, Mogensen CE, Mauer SM. Diabetic nephropathy. In: Pediatric nephroplogy, ed by Holliday MA, Barratt TM, Avner ED, New York, Williams and Wilkins, 1994; 576-585.
10. Lane PH, Steffes MW, Fioretto P, Mauer SM. Renal interstitial expansion in insulin-dependent diabetes mellitus. Kidney Int 1993; 43: 661-67.
11. Gellman DD, Pirani CL, Soothill JF, Muehrcke RC, Maduros W, Kark RM. Structure and funtion in diabetic nephropathy: the importance of diffuse glomerulosclerosis. Diabetes 1959; 8: 251-256.
12. Mauer SM, Steffes MW, Ellis EN, Sutherland DER, Brown DM, Goetz FC. Structural functional relationships in diabetic nephropathy. J Clin Invest 1984; 74: 1143-55.
13. Fioretto P, Steffes MW, Sutherland DER, Mauer M. Sequential renal biopsies in IDDM patients: structural factors associated with clinical progression. Kidney Int 1995; 48:1929-1935.
14. Brito P, Fioretto P, Drummund K, Kim Y, Steffes MW, Basgen JM, Sisson-Ross S, Mauer M. Proximal tubular basement membrane width in insulin-dependent diabetes mellitus. Kidney Int 1998; 53:754-761.
15. Steffes MW, Bilous RW, Sutherland DER, Mauer SM. Cell and matrix components in the glomerular mesangium in type I diabetes. Diabetes 1992; 41: 679-84.
16. Parving H-H, Gall M-A, Skøtt P, Jørgensen HE, Løkkegaard H, Jørgensen F, Nielsen B, Larsen S. Prevalence and causes of albuminuria in non-insulin-dependent diabetic patients. Kidney Int 1992; 41: 758-762.
17. Gambara V, Mecca G, Remuzzi G, Bertani T. Heterogeneous nature of renal lesions in type II diabetes. JASN 1993; 3: 1458-1466.
18. Ruggenenti P, Gambara V, Perna A, Bertani T, Remuzzi G. The nephropathy of NIDDM: predictors of outcome relative to diverse patterns of renal injury. JASN 1998; 9: 2336-2343.
19. Kahn S, Seghal V, Appel GB, D'Agati V. Correlates of diabetic and non-diabetic renal disease in NIDDM. JASN 1995; 6: 451 (abs).

20. Olsen S, Mogensen CE. Non-diabetic renal disease in NIDDM proteinuric patients may be rare in biopsies from clinical practice. Diabetologia 1996; 39: 1638-1645.

21. Waldherr R, Ilkenhans C, Ritz E. How frequent is glomerulonephritis in diabetes mellitus type II? Clinical Nephrology 1992; 37: 271-273.

22. Hayashi H, Karasawa R, Inn H et al. An electron microscopic study of glomeruli in Japanese patients with non-insulin dependent diabetes mellitus. Kidney Int 1992; 41: 749-757.

23. Moiya T, Moriya R, Yajima Y, Steffes MW, Mauer M. Urinary albumin excretion is a weaker predictor of diabetic nephropathy lesions in Japanese NIDDM patients than in Caucasian IDDM patients. JASN, 1997, 8: 116A (abs).

24. Østerby R, Gall MA, Schmitz A, Nielsen FS, Nyberg G, Parving HH. Glomerular structure and function in proteinuric type 2 (non insulin dependent) diabetic patients. Diabetologia 1993; 36: 1064-1070.

25. Fioretto P, Mauer M, Bortoloso E, Barzon I, Saller A, Dalla Vestra M, Abaterusso C, Baggio B, Nosadini R. Glomerular ultrastructure in type 2 diabetes. JASN 1998, 9: 114A (abs).

26. Patgalunan ME, Miller PL, Jumping-Eagle S, Nelson RG, Myers BD, Rennke HC, Coplon NS, Meyer TW. Podocyte loss and progressive glomerular injury in type 2 diabetes. J Clin Invest 1997; 99: 342-348.

27. Ellis EN, Steffes MW, Chavers BM, Mauer SM. Observations of glomerular epithelial cell structure in patients with type 1 diabetes mellitus. Kidney Int 1987; 32: 736-741.

28. Viberti GC, Hill RD, Jarrett RJ, Argyropoulos A, Mahmud U, Keen H. Microalbuminuria as a predictor of clinical nephropathy in insulin-dependent diabetes mellitus. Lancet 1982 i: 1430-32.

29. Parving H-H, Oxenbøll B, Svensen PAA, Christiansen JS, Andersen AR. Early detection of patients at risk of developing diabetic nephropathy: a longitudinal study of urinary albumin excretion. Acta Endocrinol Copenh 1982; 7, 100: 550-52.

30. Mogensen CE, Christensen CK. Predicting diabetic nephropathy in insulin-dependent diabetic patients. N Engl J Med 1986; 331: 89-93.

31. Mogensen CE. Microalbuminuria predicts clinical proteinuria and early mortality in maturity-onset diabetes. N Engl J Med 1984; 310: 356-360.

32. Mogensen CE. Microalbuminuria as a predictor of clinical diabetic nephropathy. Kidney Int 1987; 31: 673-689.

33. Schmitz A, Vaeth M. Microalbuminuria: a major risk factor in type 2 diabetes. A 10 year follow-up study of 503 patients. Diab Med 1988; 5: 126-134.

34. Jarrett RJ, Viberi GC, Argyropoulos A, Hill RD, Mahmud U, Murrells TJ. Microalbuminuria predicts mortality in non-insulin-dependent diabetes. Diab Med 1984; 1: 17-19.

35. Forsblom CM, Groop P-H, Ekstrand A, Groop LC. Predictive value of microalbuminuria in patients with insulin dependent diabetes of long duration. Br Med J 1992; 305: 1051-1053.

36. Rossing P, Hougaard P, Borch-Johnsen K, Parving H-H. Progression from microalbuminuria to diabetic nephropathy in IDDM. JASN 1997; 8: 117A, (abs).

37. Stehouwer CDA, Nauta JJP, Zeldenrust GC, Hackeng WHL, Donker AJM, den Ottolander GJH (1992). Urinary albumin excretion, cardiovascular disease, and endothelial dysfunction in non-insulin dependent diabetes mellitus. Lancet 1992; 340: 319-323.

38. Fioretto P, Steffes MW, Mauer M. Glomerular structure in non proteinuric IDDM patients with various levels of albuminuria. Diabetes 1994; 43: 1358-1364.

39.   Ruggenenti P, Mosconi L, Bianchi L, Cortesi L, Camparna M, Pagani G, Mecca G, Remuzzi G. Long-term treatment with either Enalapril or Nitrendipine stabilizes albuminuria and increases glomerular filtration rate in non-insulin-dependent diabetic patients. Am J Kidney Dis 1994; 24: 753-761.

40.   Fioretto P, Mauer M, Brocco E, Velussi M, Frigato F, Muollo B, Sambataro M, Abaterusso C, Baggio B, Crepaldi G, Nosadini R. Patterns of renal injury in type 2 (non insulin dependent) diabetic patients with microalbuminuria. Diabetologia 1996; 39: 1569-1576.

41.   Brocco E, Fioretto P, Mauer M, Saller A, Carraro A, Frigato F, Chiesura-Corona M, et al. Renal structure and function in non-insulin dependent diabetic patients with microalbuminuria. Kidney Int 1997; 63: S155-158.

42.   Sambataro M, Thomaseth K, Pacini G, et al. Plasma clearance of 51 Cr-EDTA provides a precise and convenient technique for measurement of glomerular filtration rate in diabetic humans. JASN 1996; 7: 118-127.

43.   The Fifth Report of the Joint National Committee on Detection, Evaluation, and Treatment of High Blood Pressure. Arch Int Med 1993; 153: 154-183.

44.   Ellis EN, Basgen JM, Mauer SM, Steffes MW. Kidney biopsy technique an evaluation. In Methods in Diabetes Research, Volume II Clinical Methods. Clarke WL, Larner J, Pohl SL, Eds. New York, John Wiley & Sons, 1986; 633-47.

45.   Fioretto P, Stehouwer CDA, Mauer M, Chiesura-Corona M, Brocco E, Carraro A, Bortoloso E, van Hinsberg V, Crepaldi G, Nosadini R. Heterogeneous nature of microalbuminuria in NIDDM: studies of endothelial function and renal structure. Diabetologia 1998; 41: 233-236.

46.   Stehower CDA, Yudkin JS, Fioretto P, Nosadini R. How heterogeneous is microalbuminuria in diabetes mellitus? The case for 'benign' and 'malignant' microalbuminuria. Nephrol Dial Transplant 1998; 13: 2751-2754.

47.   Saller A, Dalla Vestra M, Bombonato G, Sacerdoti D, Chiesura-Corona M, Marangon A, Fioretto P, Crepaldi G, Nosadini R. The role of macrovascular disease in the pathogenesis of renal damage in type 2 diabetic patients. Diabetologia 1999; 42, S1: A268 (abs).

20.   NEPHROPATHY IN NIDDM PATIENTS, PREDICTORS OF OUTCOME

Piero Ruggenenti, M.D.* and Giuseppe Remuzzi, M.D.*°
* Mario Negri Institute for Pharmacological Research, and Unit of Nephrology and
Dialysis, Azienda Ospedaliera, Ospedali Riuniti di Bergamo and
° Mario Negri Institute for Pharmacological Research, Bergamo, Italy

THE RELEVANCE OF THE PROBLEM

Nephropathy is a major cause of illness and death of patients with non insulin dependent diabetes mellitus (NIDDM), the excess being confined to proteinuric patients due to complications of end-stage renal disease (ESRD), but even more to cardiovascular events [1]. On the other hand diabetic nephropathy is the single most common cause of ESRD in the United States and more than one third of all patients enrolled in the Medicare ESRD program are actually diabetics [2]. It derives that costs of renal replacement therapy for diabetics alone is a major public health issue, approaching already epidemic proportions for NIDDM patients in Western countries [3,4].

The continuous increase in the number of diabetics needing renal replacement therapy (twice the annual rate of ESRD from other conditions [2,3]) depends on one hand from growing number of patients suffering diabetes (in particular NIDDM), as well as from the constant improvement in health care facilities that allows more and more patients to live long enough to progress to ESRD. Once on renal replacement therapy, however, mortality among diabetics is 1.5 to 2.5 times higher than in nondiabetics [4] so that less than 20% of diabetics survive for 5 years on dialysis [3,4]. These disturbing epidemiology again highlights the absolute need to identify potentially treatable risk factors in order to delay or even completely prevent the progression of diabetic nephropathy toward ESRD and need of replacement therapy. This is a major issue in NIDDM since, so far, the natural history of nephropathy in NIDDM patients has been more difficult to characterize than in IDDM. This is particularly true of Caucasians in whom the onset of NIDDM is difficult to detect and occurs at an advanced age. The confounding factors include an effect of aging per se to lower the GFR [5], a high frequency of co-existent renal disease unrelated to diabetes beyond the age of 50 years [6-8], and a high mortality rate from cardiovascular disease [9]. The latter phenomenon limits the full expression of the natural history of diabetic nephropathy, since only a minority of such patients progress to ESRD before premature cardiovascular death [9].

Mogensen C.E. (ed.), THE KIDNEY AND HYPERTENSION IN DIABETES MELLITUS.
Copyright© 2000 by Kluwer Academic Publishers, Boston ● Dordrecht ● London. All rights reserved.

INCIPIENT NEPHROPATHY

Microalbuminuria and progression to overt nephropathy

Microalbuminuria predicts progression to macroalbuminuria and renal failure (overt nephropathy) in either IDDM and NIDDM [10]. In 1984 Mogensen found that over 9 years the risk of progression to macroalbuminuria was only 22% in NIDDM [9] as compared with 80% in IDDM patients with microalbuminuria. However, more recent studies in non-European series found that the predictive value of microalbuminuria is comparable in IDDM and NIDDM. Indeed, Nelson and coworkers found that over four year the cumulative incidence of macroalbuminuria was 37% in microalbuminuric Pima Indians [11]. This is in agreement with the five-year incidence of 42% reported by Ravid et al [12] in young Jewish patients with NIDDM and microalbuminuria at baseline. Probably, the younger age of patients in both these series as compared to that in the Mogensen study (approximately 20 years difference) allowed a larger proportion of diabetics to live enough to progress to overt nephropathy [13].

Whether the onset of microalbuminuria predicts a progressive decline in GFR is unclear. Although the Nelson's study found that in microalbuminuric Pima Indians the GFR was stable over time [11], a progressive reduction in renal function, reflected by an increase in serum creatinine concentration, was reported in the Ravid's series [12]. Of note, in a recent series of hypertensive NIDDM patients with microalbuminuria, slight GFR depression at baseline and effective blood pressure control either with an ACE inhibitor or with a calcium channel blocker, the GFR was remarkably stable or even improving over more than two years follow-up [14].

Microalbuminuria and cardiovascular disease

Apart from predicting overt nephropathy, microalbuminuria also predicts mortality, specifically cardiovascular mortality, at least in white patients [9]. The competing risk of cardiac death and progression to renal failure may explain, at least in part, the Mogensen's findings of a lower predictive value of microalbuminuria for the development of overt nephropathy in NIDDM as compared with IDDM patients [9]. Indeed, in one series, over 10 years only 3% of microalbuminuric NIDDM diabetics died from uremia, while 58% did from cardiac causes [15]. Higher urinary albumin excretion rates were found in NIDDM patients with coronary heart disease both at the time the diagnosis of diabetes was made and later on. The association between microalbuminuria and heart disease and mortality is also seen in non diabetic population [10,16]. The "Steno hypothesis" postulates that albuminuria points to a more widespread disturbance of the endothelial cell function in diabetic and perhaps in non-diabetic patients with albuminuria [17]. Thus, endothelial cell barrier dysfunction in the macrocirculation (i.e.: in the coronaries) allows the transudation of plasma proteins (including lipoproteins) into the vessel wall where might promote the atherogenetic process. The idea of an endothelial cell dysfunction finds some preliminary support in studies showing that albuminuric NIDDM patients have a higher von Willebrand factor concentration than patients without albuminuria [18].

OVERT NEPHROPATHY

Genetic predictors of progression
Congenital and acquired factors can contribute to the progression of overt nephropathy in NIDDM [19]. Among the several genes that might account for different individual and racial susceptibility to nephropathy in IDDM as well as in NIDDM, those of the Renin Angiotensin System have been extensively investigated since an increased synthesis of Angiotensin II might in theory contribute to progressive renal injury either by affecting glomerular hemodynamics and size-selectivity, and by promoting growth of glomerular cells [20]. Plasma and tissue angiotensin II levels depend from the ACE activity which, in turn, is related to the insertion (I)/deletion (D) polymorphism of the ACE gene. The highest ACE plasma levels are found in diabetics with the DD genotype, the lowest in those with the II genotype, being the ID genotype associated with intermediate levels [21]. However, the predictive value of the I/D genotype is poorly established so far. Most studies suffered the limits of a cross-sectional design, others provided contrasting results because of the limited sample size and the etherogeneity of the outcome parameters considered, including micro-or macroalbuminuria in some instances, serum creatinine or progression to dialysis in others. Recently, however, the longitudinal study by Yoshida and coworkers [22] provided convincing evidence that NIDDM patients with the DD genotype had a higher incidence of progressive disease and a faster progression to ESRD, as compared to those with the ID and II genotype. These findings were further corroborated by data of a metanalysis in more than 4,700 diabetics that showed a significant association between the D allele and the risk of nephropathy, either in Asian and Caucasian series [23]. These data, however, should be considered with caution, since, as a general rule, the metanalysis findings may suffer the limits of publication bias. Thus, only properly designed prospective studies with an adequate sample size and including even genes of other determinants of Angiotensin II production or activity - such as angiotensinogen and angiotensin II type I receptor - will probably definitely address this important issue.

Acquired predictors of progression
Poor metabolic control is a recognized risk factor for nephropathy and other chronic complications of IDDM and NIDDM. However, the contribution of chronic hyperglycemia to progression of NIDDM nephropathy is not so clear, at least after persistent albuminuria has developed [19]. The role of dyslipidemia is also controversial, since higher serum cholesterol levels are associated with a faster disease progression either in IDDM and in NIDDM. However, finding that lipid lowering agents had no impact on GFR decline either in IDDM and NIDDM proteinuric patients, seems to challenge the possibility of a direct and independent contribution of hypercholesterolemia on the outcome of overt nephropathy [24]. A possible explanation of this apparent inconsistency is that hypercholesterolemia is commonly associated with overt proteinuria that, in turn, is the actual promoter of progression because of the chronic nephrotoxic effect of enhanced protein traffic [25]. On the other hand, recent evidence is available that some lipid lowering agents (namely HmGCoA inhibitors or

statins) may exert a specific renoprotective effect - independent of that potentially associated to blood cholesterol reduction - in experimental models of diabetic [26] and non diabetic [27] chronic nephropathies. For sure, an important role is recognized for systemic hypertension, and all the epidemiologic data show that effective blood pressure control is associated with a slower disease progression, possibly because of a concomitant amelioration of intracapillary hypertension. Some studies suggest that even smoking may act as a progression promoter in both IDDM and NIDDM patients with proteinuria [28,29], possibly by increasing systemic blood pressure and/or contributing to glomerular hyperfiltration, as documented in IDDM [30].

The role of proteinuria and glomerular involvement
At variance with IDDM - where overt proteinuria is almost invariably the clinical counterpart of typical diabetic glomerulopathy - in NIDDM the appearance of macroalbuminuria may reflect different patterns of renal injury, including typical diabetic-like lesions (in one to two thirds of cases), nephroangiosclerosis, or forms of glomerular disease of non-diabetic type [7,8]. A recent study [31] showed that in proteinuric NIDDM patients, the rate of renal disease progression was rather independent of the type of underlying glomerular lesions (Figure 20-1, Left Panel), but instead consistently predicted by the level of urinary protein excretion rate (Figure 20-1, Right Panel). In particular, higher were the urinary protein excretion values at baseline, higher was the risk of doubling base-line serum creatinine or ESRD in the follow-up. Even more important, a cut-off value of base-line urinary protein excretion rate was identified that segregated progressors from non-progressors. Thus, patients with urinary proteins ≤2g/24 hours had a stable serum creatinine and a 100% kidney survival at 5 years, while those with urinary proteins >2g/24 hours had a 92 % risk to progress to terminal renal failure over the same period. Among progressors, quantification of a global score of tissue injury (i.e.: the sum of the scores of glomerular diffuse or nodular sclerosis, glomerular ischemia, arteriolosclerosis, arteriolar hyalinosis, interstitial fibrosis, and tubular atrophy) was of further help to reliably predict disease outcome. Thus, higher was the injury score - independently of the pattern of the histologic lesions - higher the risk of progression. In particular, patients with a global score of tissue injury <7 never doubled their serum creatinine nor progressed to ESRD over the follow-up, whereas those with a score > 13 progressed to ESRD with a median kidney survival time of only 1.6 years. Of interest, in the above series, urinary protein excretion rate was the only independent clinical predictor, in addition to serum creatinine, of disease progression (Table 20-1). Noteworthy, failure for arterial blood pressure, HbA1C and blood glucose values to predict kidney survival was most likely related to the good control of hypertension and diabetes in the overall study population and within each of the considered subgroups. Thus, either base-line and follow-up systolic/diastolic blood pressure, HbA1C and blood glucose levels, as well as antidiabetic (in particular insulin) and antihypertensive (in particular ACE inhibitor) therapy were comparable in the different subgroups. Thus, neither biases in hypertension and diabetes control accounted for the remarkable differences in renal disease progression demonstrated in three subgroups (tertiles) with different levels of base-line urinary protein excretion rate. In

addition, the histologic classes were similarly represented in the 3 tertiles of base-line proteinuria, which renders extremely unlikely that different renal outcomes were actually dependent on different patterns of glomerular involvement, rather than on degree of proteinuria.

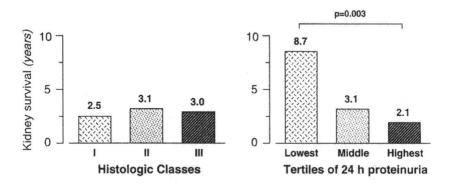

Figure 20-1: Risk of doubling of base-line serum creatinine or progression to end stage renal disease (ESRD) in macroalbuminuric NIDDM patients for different classes of glomerular changes (Left Panel) and for different tertiles of base-line 24 hour urinary protein excretion rate (Right Panel). Classes I, II, and III identify patients with typical diabetic glomerulopathy, nephroangiosclerosis and other glomerulopathies of non-diabetic type, respectively

Consistent with the above considerations were data that at multivariate analysis, base-line urinary protein excretion, but not the pattern of glomerular lesions, predicted the risk of progression during the subsequent follow-up (Table 20-1).

Noteworthy, in the above series of NIDDM patients and in a previous series of patients with non-diabetic renal disease [32], the median kidney survival time (30 months vs. 28 months, respectively) was virtually identical for comparable levels of baseline urinary proteins (4.2±3.2 vs. 5.3±2.4 g/24 h, respectively), again independently of the underlying glomerular disease. Altogether, these findings are consistent with the possibility that protein traffic is a major determinant of disease progression [25] and are remarkably consistent with data in Asian NIDDM patients that among a series of risk factors (including family history of hypertension, higher diastolic blood pressure, low serum albumin concentration and current smoking) proteinuria was by far the strongest predictor of progression to ESRD [33]. Of note, independently of all the above parameters, a proteinuria above 2.5 per day was associated with a five-fold higher risk of ESRD as compared to a proteinuria of 2.5 g per day or less [33]. Thus, several evidences

Parameter	Univariate	Multivariate
Demographic		
Age	0.09	0.13
Gender	0.52	0.15
Clinical		
Systolic Blood Pressure	0.20	0.74
Diastolic Blood Pressure	0.94	0.55
Blood Glucose	0.44	0.49
Serum creatinine	0.003	0.0003
24-h urinary protein excretion	0.04	0.04
Insulin therapy	0.28	0.37
ACE inhibitor therapy	0.46	0.72
Histologic		
Class	0.31	0.50
Global score	0.0001	0.02
Glomerular sclerosis	0.0001	0.12
Percent sclerotic glomeruli	0.004	0.26
Interstitial fibrosis	0.0002	0.33
Arteriolar hyalinosis	0.006	0.06

Table 20-1. Univariate and multivariate analysis of the correlation between baseline demographic, clinical or histologic parameters and risk of doubling baseline creatinine or ESRD.

converge to indicate that in NIDDM quantification of urinary protein excretion is enough to identify patients at risk of progression. Among progressors, a renal biopsy combined to precise quantification of urinary protein excretion, can help predicting the risk of terminal renal failure and the median time to dialysis. In particular, patients with no risk and patients inexorably destined to ESRD can be reliably identified. Of note, this important information can be safely obtained, as documented by the fact that in our previous series only one out of 70 biopsied patients required a blood transfusion because of symptomatic bleeding [30].

THE SEVERITY OF ALBUMINURIA AS A PREDICTOR OF RESPONSE TO RENOPROTECTIVE THERAPY

Early detection of increased urinary albumin excretion rate may have major clinical implications since epidemiologic data and results of several prospective, randomized trials clearly document that at the stage of microalbuminuria (incipient nephropathy) ACE inhibitors may exert a specific renoprotective effect and delay or prevent progression to overt nephropathy either in normotensive and in hypertensive NIDDM patients [34-38]. This conclusion is consistent with the results of a meta-regression analysis of 77 published studies showing that ACE inhibitors were more effective than ß-blockers or calcium channel blockers on microalbuminuria [39].

Response to therapy is quite different in macroalbuminuric NIDDM patients. Thus, unlike in IDDM, in NIDDM tight metabolic control has no significant impact on disease progression, as consistently documented by all the available prospective studies (reviewed in ref. 19], with the exception of a single one [40]. Similarly, all major observational studies failed to show an effect of protein intake on the rate of decline in GFR [19]. Even more impressive, are data on the remarkably different response to ACE inhibitor therapy. Unlike in overt nephropathy of IDDM [41,42] - and in most proteinuric nephropathies of non-diabetic type [43] - in overt nephropathy of NIDDM, evidence that ACE inhibitors reduce protein traffic, and effectively limit progression to ESRD has never been consistently obtained, so far. Actually, the opposite was true. A recent study [44] found that in NIDDM patients with overt nephropathy - despite a pattern of renal changes and levels of renal insufficiency and glomerular barrier dysfunction comparable to those reported in a previous series of IDDM patients with typical glomerulopathy [42] - ACE inhibitors failed to ameliorate glomerular size-selectivity and to reduce proteinuria. Failure to limit protein traffic may explain why, altogether, controlled studies so far available with adequate follow-up and repeated measurements of GFR consistently failed to show any favorable effect of ACE inhibitor therapy in NIDDM patients with overt nephropathy [34,45]. On the same line is the evidence that in this type of patients ACE inhibitors also failed to limit progression to ESRD [30].

A possible explanation for the poor response to ACE inhibition therapy is that at the stage of overt nephropathy of NIDDM, renal structural changes may already be very advanced and diffuse, involving thickening of the basement membrane, broadening of the foot processes, and diffuse sclerotic changes. It is tempting to speculate that these types of glomerular lesions that develop with time in NIDDM patients can reach an extent that prevents pharmacological treatments from achieving the desired effect on membrane sieving functional properties [44]. Thus, despite biopsy evidence of typical diabetic glomerulopathy, the same level of renal insufficiency and the same pattern of glomerular barrier size-selective dysfunction, the response to ACE inhibition in NIDDM versus IDDM patients with overt nephropathy appears to be different. Clearly, these data do not justify a generalized use of ACE inhibitors in proteinuric NIDDM patients, just because they are beneficial in IDDM. In particular, if one considers the high prevalence of renovascular disease, and the potential risk of ACE inhibitor-associated acute renal failure and life-threatening hyperkalemia in this setting, drawbacks of such an approach appear obvious. On the other hand, the above findings serve to emphasize the importance of early detection of albuminuria, ideally at the stage of microalbuminuria, when NIDDM patients may gain a benefit from ACE inhibition therapy comparable to that clearly documented in IDDM.

CONCLUSIONS

Efforts aimed at early detection of renal involvement in IDDM seem worthwhile. Today, microalbuminuria can be measured with tests that are reproducible, acceptable, and harmless to the patient. In addition, there seems to be an advantageous cost-benefit ratio in screening and early treatment. The World Health Organization and the International Diabetes Federation have recommended (St. Vincent Declaration) that all diabetics aged 12 to 70 years should be screened for microalbuminuria at least once a year. Regular monitoring of patients who result positive ensures that renal and extra-renal complications are identified early and preventive intervention therapy instituted, including good metabolic control, raised blood pressure correction, and Renin Angiotensin System inhibition [45]. Once overt nephropathy develops, in NIDDM patients a renal biopsy may help to establish a precise diagnosis of the underlying glomerular disease, but is not necessary to predict outcome or guide the treatment, provided that an acute or rapidly progressive glomerulonephritis can be reasonably excluded on clinical ground. Large scale multicenter trials are now in progress and will say within few years whether inhibition of the Renin Angiotensin system may slow the progression of overt nephropathy in NIDDM as effectively as in IDDM.

REFERENCES

1. Striker GE, Agodoa LL, Held P, Doi T, Conti F, Striker L: Kidney disease of diabetes mellitus (diabetic nephropathy): perspectives in the United States. J Diabetes Complications 5:51-52,1991
2. The United States Renal Data System: USRDS 1994 Annual Data Report, The National Institutes of Health, National Institute of Diabetes and Digestive and Kidney Diseases. Bethesda, MD 1994
3. Renal Data System: USRDS 1997 annual data report. National Institute of Diabetes and Digestive and Kidney Diseases. Bethesda, MD 1997
4. Pastan S, Bailey J: Dialysis therapy. N Engl J Med 338:1428-1437,1998
5. Palmer BF, Levi M: Effect of aging on renal function and disease. In: Brenner's & Rector's *The Kidney*. Vol. 2, edited by Brenner BM, 5th ed. Philadelphia, W.B. Saunders Company, 1996, pp 2274-2296
6. Ruggenenti P, Remuzzi G: The diagnosis of renal involvement in non-insulin-dependent diabetes mellitus. Curr Opin Nephrol Hypertens 6:141-145,1997
7. Gambara V, Mecca G, Remuzzi G, Bertani T: Heterogeneous nature of renal lesions in type II diabetes. J Am Soc Nephrol 3:1458-1466,1993
8. Parving H-H, Gall M-A, Skott P, Jorghensen HE, Lokkegaard H, Jorgens F, Nielsen B, Larsen S: Prevalence and causes of albuminuria in non-insulin-dependent diabetic patients. Kidney Int 41:758-762,1992
9. Mogensen CE: Microalbuminuria predicts clinical proteinuria and early mortality in maturity-onset diabetes. N Engl J Med 310:356-360,1984
10. Mogensen CE, Keane WF, Bennett PH, Jerums G, Parving H-H, Passa P, Steffes MW, Striker GE, Viberti GC: Prevention of diabetic renal disease with special reference to microalbuminuria. Lancet 346:1080-1084,1995

11. Nelson RG, Bennett PH, Beck GJ, et al. for the Diabetic Renal Disease Study Group: Development and progression of renal disease in Pima Indians with non-insulin-dependent diabetes mellitus. N Engl J Med 335:1636-1642,1996

12. Ravid M, Savin H, Jutrin I, Bental T, Katz B, Lishner M: Long term stabilizing effect of angiotensin-converting enzyme inhibition on plasma creatinine and on proteinuria in normotensive type II diabetic patients. Ann Intern Med 118:577-581,1993

13. Parving H-H: Initiation and progression of diabetic nephropathy. N Engl J Med 335:1682-1683,1996

14. Mosconi L, Ruggenenti P, Perna A, Mecca G, Remuzzi G: Nitrendipine and enalapril improve albuminuria and glomerular filtration rate in non-insulin dependent diabetes. Kidney Int 49 (Suppl.55): S-91-S-93, 1996

15. Schmitz A, Vaeth M: Microalbuminuria a major risk factor in non-insulin-dependent diabetes. A 10-year follow-up study of 503 patients. Diabetic Med 5:126-134,1988

16. Striker GE: Report on a workshop to develop management recommendations for the prevention of progression in chronic renal disease (Bethesda, April, 1994). Nephrol Dial Transplant 10:290-292,1995

17. Deckert T: Nephropathy and coronary death. The fatal twins in diabetes mellitus. Nephrol Dial Transplant 9:1069-1071,1994

18. Nielsen FS, Rossing P, Bang L, Smidt UM, Svendsen TL, Gall MA, Parving H-H: Endothelial dysfunction in NIDDM patients with and without nephropathy. J Am Soc Nephrol 5:380,1994 (abstract)

19. Parving H-H: Renoprotection in diabetes: genetic and non-genetic risk factors and treatment. Diabetologia 41:745-759,1998

20. Parving H-H, Osterby R, Anderson PW, Hsueh WA: Diabetic nephropathy. In: Brenner's & Rector's *The Kidney*. Vol. 2, edited by Brenner BM, 5th ed. Philadelphia, W.B. Saunders Company, 1996, pp 1864-1892.

21. Rigat B, Hubert C, Corvol P, Soubrier F: PCR detection of the insertion/deletion polymorphism of the human angiotensin converting enzyme gene (DCP1) (dipeptidyl-carboxy peptidose 1). Nucleic Acids Res 20 1992

22. Yoshida H, Kuriyama S, Atsumi Y, et al.: Angiotensin I converting enzyme gene polymorphism in non-insulin-dependent diabetes mellitus. Kidney Int 50:657-664,1996

23. Fujisawa T, Ikegami H, Kawaguchi Y, Hamada Y, Ueda H, Shintani M, Fukuda M, Ogihara T: Meta-analysis of association of insertion/deletion polymorphism of angiotensin I-converting enzyme gene with diabetic nephropathy and retinopathy. Diabetologia 41:47-53,1998

24. Nielsen S, Schmitz O, Moller N, et al.: Renal function and insulin sensitivity during simvastatin treatment in type 2 (non-insulin-dependent) diabetic patients with microalbuminuria. Diabetologia 36:1079-1086,1993

25. Remuzzi G, Bertani T: Pathophysiology of progressive nephropathies. N Engl J Med 339:1448-1456,1998.

26. Han DC, Lee SK, Hwang SD, Lee HB: Lovastatins prevents glomerulosclerosis in streptozotocin-induced diabetic uninephrectomized rats (abstract); Kidney Int 44: 1181, 1993

27. Lee SK, Jin SY, Han DC, Hwang SD, Lee HB: Effects of delayed treatment with enalapril and/or lovastatin on the progression of glomerulosclerosis in 5/6 nephrectomized rats; Nephrol Dial Transplant 8: 1338-1343, 1993

28. Orth SR, Ritz E, Schrier RW: The renal risk of smoking. Kidney Int 51:1669-1677,1997

29. Sawicki PT, Didjurgeit U, Muhllauser I, Bender R, Heinemann L, Berger M: Smoking is associated with progression of diabetic nephropathy. Diabetes Care 17:126-131,1994

30.   Hansen HP, Rossing P, Jacobsen P, Jensen BR, Parving H-H: The acute effect of smoking on systemic haemodynamics, kidney and endothelial function in insulin-dependent diabetic patients with microalbuminuria. Scand J Clin Lab Invest 56:393-399,1996

31.   Ruggenenti P, Gambara V, Perna A, Bertani T, Remuzzi G: The nephropathy of non-insulin dependent diabetes: predictors of outcome relative to diverse patterns of renal injury. J Am Soc Nephrol 9:2336-2343,1998

32.   The GISEN Group: Randomised placebo-controlled trial of effect of ramipril on decline in glomerular filtration rate and risk of terminal renal failure in proteinuric, non-diabetic nephropathy. Lancet 349:1857-1863,1997

33.   Yokoyama H, Tomonaga O, Hirayama M, Ishii A, Takeda M, Babazono T, Ujihara U, Takahashi C, Omori Y: Predictors of the progression of diabetic nephropathy and the beneficial effect of angiotensin-converting enzyme inhibitors in NIDDM patients. Diabetologia 40:405-411,1997

34.   Ruggenenti P, Remuzzi G: Anti-hypertensive agents and incipient diabetic nephropathy. In: The Diabetes Annual/9, edited by Marshall SM, Home PD, Rizza RA, Amsterdam, Elsevier Science B.V., 1995, pp 295-317.

35.   Ruggenenti P, Remuzzi G: The renoprotective action of angiotensin-converting enzyme inhibitors in diabetes. Exp Nephrol 4:53-60,1996

36.   Mengel MC, Segal R: Renal protective effects of enalapril in hypertensive NIDDM: role of baseline albuminuria. Kidney Int 45:S150,1994

37.   Trevisan R, Tiengo A: Effect of low-dose ramipril on microalbuminuria in normotensive or mild hypertensive non-insulin dependent diabetic patients. Am J Hypertens 8:876-883,1995

38.   Sano T, Kawamura T, Matsumae H, et al.: Effects of long-term enalapril treatment on persistent micro-albuminuria in well-controlled hypertensive and normotensive NIDDM patients. Diabetes Care 17:420-424,1994

39.   Kasiske BL, Kalil RSN, Ma JZ, Liao M, Keane WF: Effects of antihypertensive therapy on the kidney in patients with diabetes: a meta-regression analysis. Ann Intern Med 118:129,1993

40.   Wu M, Yu C, Yang C-W, et al.: Poor pre-dialysis glycaemic control is a predictor of mortality in type II diabetic patients on maintenance haemodialysis. Nephrol Dial Transplant 12:2105-2110,1997

41.   Morelli E, Loon N, Meyer TW, Peters W, Myers BD: Effects of converting-enzyme inhibition on barrier function in diabetic glomerulopathy. Diabetes 39:76-82,1990

42.   Remuzzi A, Ruggenenti P, Mosconi L, Pata V, Viberti G, Remuzzi G: Effect of low-dose enalapril on glomerular size-selectivity in human diabetic nephropathy. J Nephrol 6:36-43,1993

43.   Ruggenenti P, Remuzzi G: Angiotensin-converting enzyme inhibitor therapy for non-diabetic progressive renal disease. Curr Opin Nephrol Hypertens 6:489-495,1997

44.   Ruggenenti P, Mosconi L, Sangalli F, Casiraghi F, Gambara V, Remuzzi G, Remuzzi A: Glomerular size-selective dysfunction in NIDDM is not ameliorated by ACE inhibition or calcium channel blockade. J Am Soc Nephrol 55:984-994,1999

45.   Nielsen FS, Rossing P, Gall MA, Skott P, Smidt UM, Parving H-H: Long-term effect of lisinopril and atenolol on kidney function in hypertensive NIDDM subjects with diabetic nephropathy. Diabetes 46:1182-1188,1997

46.   American Diabetes Association: Clinical Practice Recommendations 1999. Diabetic nephropathy. Diabetes Care 22 (Suppl.1):S66-S69,1999

21. ADVANCED GLYCATION END-PRODUCTS AND DIABETIC RENAL DISEASE

Mark E. Cooper and George Jerums
University of Melbourne, Austin & Repatriation Medical Centre, West Heidelberg, Australia

Since there is chronic hyperglycaemia in diabetes, there is an acceleration of the Maillard or browning reaction [1]. This is a spontaneous reaction between glucose and proteins, lipids or nucleic acids, particularly on long-lived proteins such as the collagens [1]. There is a sequence of biochemical reactions, many of which are still poorly defined, leading to the formation of a range of advanced glycation end-products (AGEs), some of which are fluorescent. These modified long-lived tissue proteins are formed as a result not only of glycation but also oxidative processes and many of these AGEs are now considered glycoxidation products [2]. Over the last decade, an increasing number of AGEs have been identified [3]. However, the identity of the AGEs linked to diabetic complications and in particular to renal disease has not been clearly determined. Of particular interest is the hypothesis that diet derived AGEs may also be involved in tissue AGE accumulation [4].

Initial studies involved assessment of AGEs by measuring their specific fluorescence in tissue homogenates. It was clearly shown that these fluorescent AGEs were increased in the aorta from diabetic rats [5]. Further studies were performed in diabetic animals and confirmed increased AGEs in the diabetic kidney [6, 7] and retina [8], sites of diabetic microvascular disease. In clinical studies, Monnier et al were able to demonstrate increased AGE levels with age, diabetic patients having an even further increase in AGE levels, as assessed by specific fluorescence [9]. In addition, levels of collagen-linked fluorescence from human skin increased with the severity of retinopathy, suggesting that there is a link between the severity of complications and cumulative exposure to hyperglycaemia [9]. However, in that study, the trend for collagen-linked fluorescence to be linked with levels of proteinuria did not reach statistical significance.

More recently, other techniques have been developed to assay AGEs. Non-fluorescent AGEs such as carboxymethylysine (CML) have been assayed and a relationship between this AGE and diabetic complications has been shown [10]. Using a radioreceptor assay, Makita et al have reported increased AGE levels in diabetic patients, particularly in the setting of renal impairment [11]. Various antibodies to AGEs have now been developed and using a variety of immunohistochemical techniques, increased AGE levels have been reported in both human and experimental diabetes [12, 13]. Our own group using a radioimmunoassay has detected increased AGE levels in the diabetic kidney [13] and using immunohistochemistry we have localised this increase in AGE levels to the glomerulus [14]. Beisswenger et al have used an ELISA technique to detect AGEs in serum and noted increased AGE levels in diabetic patients with complications including retinopathy and nephropathy [15].

AGE RECEPTORS

Over the last few years, a number of AGE binding sites have been identified. The first binding site to be cloned has been termed RAGE and was initially identified in endothelial cells [16]. Our own group has detected RAGE in various other sites including the kidney, retina, nerve and blood vessels, sites of diabetes associated vascular injury [14]. Further studies have suggested that RAGE has a central role in the development of vascular disease in diabetes by influencing various pathological processes including expression of adhesion molecules involved in mononuclear cell recruitment and hyperpermeability [17, 18]. Vlassara's group has cloned at least 3 different proteins which bind to AGEs [19]. The role of these proteins remains an area of intensive investigation and it has been postulated that they may mediate a range of functions including clearance of AGEs and activation of intracellular messengers such as protein kinase C [19]. These AGE-binding sites have been identified in cultured mesangial cells [19]. Other proteins such as lysozyme can also bind AGEs [20] but the significance of these ligand-receptor interactions has still not been fully delineated. Our own group has identified AGE binding sites in proximal tubules which appear to be upregulated in diabetes [21]. However, the molecular identity of these AGE binding sites has not yet been determined. It is still uncertain whether these AGE-binding proteins act primarily to clear AGEs which would be viewed as a beneficial effect or whether they are mainly involved in activating a range of pathological processes which lead to diabetic complications.

AGEs AND CYTOKINES

In vitro AGEs have been shown to activate a range of cytokines which may be relevant to diabetic complications. In the non-diabetic mouse, *in vivo* injection of *in vitro* prepared AGEs has been shown to not only lead to increased gene expression of TGFß and type IV collagen in the kidney [22] but also to lead to histological changes with some resemblance to diabetic nephropathy [23]. These changes included mesangial expansion and glomerulosclerosis. Our group has shown that activation of gene expression of the prosclerotic cytokine, TGFß1 is closely linked to AGE accumulation in blood vessels [24]. Furthermore, the inhibitor of advanced glycation, aminoguanidine, prevented diabetes associated overexpression of TGFß1 and type IV collagen in these blood vessels [24]. AGEs have been also shown to activate vascular endothelial growth factor (VEGF) [25, 26], a cytokine implicated in diabetes associated retinal neovascularisation and increased vascular permeability [27]. It is not yet known if these effects also occur in the kidney, a major site of VEGF production [28].

AGEs,- RECEPTORS AND CYTOKINES

It is likely that AGEs lead to diabetic complications via both receptor and receptor-independent pathways. It is postulated that AGEs activate a range of cytokines which mediate important pathological processes involved in tissue remodelling including cell adhesion, extracellular matrix accumulation, vascular permeability and cell proliferation (Fig. 21-1). This involves cytokines such as the anti-adhesin, SPARC [29], adhesins such as VCAM-1 [17], the prosclerotic cytokine, TGFß1 [24], vascular endothelial growth factor [25] and PDGF, a cytokine which promotes cell proliferation [30].

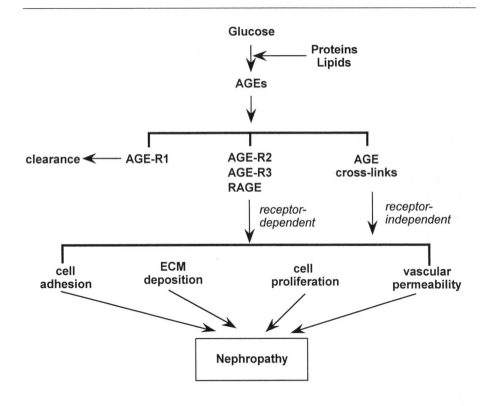

Fig. 21.1.

INHIBITION OF ADVANCED GLYCATION

Pharmacological inhibitors of AGE-dependent pathways have been developed. Aminoguanidine is a hydrazine derivative which prevents AGE formation [5]. This effect has been attributed to its ability to bind to reactive dicarbonyl and aldehyde products of early glycation and glycoxidation such as 3-deoxyglucosone [2]. Aminoguanidine has been shown in experimental models of diabetes to not only reduce tissue AGE levels but also to retard the development of neuropathy, retinopathy and nephropathy [7, 8, 31]. Our own studies in the streptozotocin diabetic rat have shown that aminoguanidine, administered for 32 weeks from the induction of diabetes, retarded the development of albuminuria and mesangial expansion [7]. Aminoguanidine therapy also prevented diabetes-related increases in fluorescent AGEs.

Subsequent studies in our laboratory have explored whether aminoguanidine is more effective when administered early or late in the evolution of experimental diabetic nephropathy. Four groups of diabetic rats were studied over 32 weeks, one receiving no therapy, the second receiving aminoguanidine throughout, the third receiving aminoguanidine for the first 16 weeks only and the fourth receiving aminoguanidine for the last 16 weeks [13]. Untreated diabetic rats showed an exponential increase in albuminuria over the 8 month study period whereas rats treated with aminoguanidine showed decreased levels of albuminuria, in proportion to the duration of treatment. This study confirmed that *in vivo* generation of AGEs in the kidney is time dependent and closely linked to the development of experimental diabetic nephropathy. New, more selective, potent inhibitors of advanced glycation have been developed recently which, unlike aminoguanidine, do not appear to inhibit NO synthase [32, 33]. These agents have been shown to inhibit renal AGE accumulation [33].

Of particular interest are the thiazolium compounds such as phenacylthiazolium bromide (PTB) which react with and cleave covalent, AGE-derived protein cross-links [34]. More recently, another chemically related cross-link breaker, ALT-711, has been reported to reverse diabetes induced increases in large artery stiffness [35]. If PTB or related compounds can be shown to have similar effects in the kidney, this would provide a conceptual basis for the reversal of AGE-mediated tissue damage, which till now has been regarded as irreversible.

CLINICAL STUDIES

Makita et al. have shown that the highest levels of AGEs are observed in patients with end-stage renal disease, in the absence or presence of diabetes [11]. Furthermore, aminoguanidine, as outlined previously, has been shown in experimental studies to attenuate the development of diabetic nephropathy. Therefore, a range of clinical studies are in progress focussing on the role of aminoguanidine in end-stage renal disease and in diabetic patients with nephropathy [36]. Two separate phase III studies known as ACTION 1 and ACTION 2 have now been completed and involve evaluation of the effects of aminoguanidine in type I and type II diabetic patients with overt proteinuria and impaired renal function [37].

Preliminary findings from the ACTION 1 study suggest that aminoguanidine treatment was associated with a trend towards attenuating an increase in serum creatinine and a statistically significant decrease in proteinuria, diastolic blood pressure and lipid levels [URL: www.alteonpharma.com/pimag1.htm]. The final results of these clinical trials as well as planned studies with newer inhibitors of advanced glycation are awaited with interest. It is anticipated that the findings of these and other studies using inhibitors of advanced glycation will have direct relevance to the management of diabetic patients with renal disease. Furthermore, these agents have the potential to influence other diabetic vascular complications.

REFERNCES

1. Brownlee M. Lilly Lecture 1993. Glycation and diabetic complications. Diabetes 1994; 43: 836-41.
2. Fu MX, Wells-Knecht KJ, Blackledge JA, Lyons TJ, Thorpe SR, Baynes JW. Glycation, glycoxidation, and cross-linking of collagen by glucose. Kinetics, mechanisms, and inhibition of late stages of the Maillard reaction. Diabetes 1994; 43: 676-683.
3. Wells-Knecht KJ, Brinkmann E, Wells-Knecht MC, Litchfield JE, Ahmed MU, Reddy S, Zyzak DV, Thorpe SR, Baynes JW. New biomarkers of maillard reaction damage to proteins. Nephrol Dial Transplantation 1996; 11 (Suppl 5): 41-47.
4. Koschinsky T, He CJ, Mitsuhashi T, Bucala R, Liu C, Buenting C, Heitmann K, Vlassara H. Orally absorbed reactive glycation products (glycotoxins) - an environmental risk factor in diabetic nephropathy. Proc Natl Acad USA 1997; 94: 6474-6479.
5. Brownlee M, Vlassara H, Kooney A, Ulrich P, Cerami A. Aminoguanidine prevents diabetes-induced arterial wall protein cross-linking. Science 1986; 232: 1629-1632.
6. Nicholls K, Mandel T. Advanced glycosylation end products in experimental murine diabetic nephropathy: effect of islet grafting and of aminoguanidine. Lab Invest 1989; 60: 486-489.
7. Soulis-Liparota T, Cooper M, Papazoglou D, Clarke B, Jerums G. Retardation by aminoguanidine of development of albuminuria, mesangial expansion, and tissue fluorescence in streptozocin-induced diabetic rat. Diabetes 1991; 40: 1328-34.
8. Hammes H, Martin S, Federlin K, Geisen K, Brownlee M. Aminoguanidine treatment inhibits the development of experimental diabetic retinopathy. Proc Natl Acad Sci USA 1991; 88: 11555-11558.
9. Monnier V, Vishwanath V, Frank K, Elmets G, Dauchot P, Kohn R. Relation between complications of type I diabetes mellitus and collagen-linked fluorescence. N Engl J Med 1986; 314: 403-408.
10. Dyer DG, Dunn JA, Thorpe SR, Bailie KE, Lyons TJ, McCance DR, Baynes JW. Accumulation of Maillard reaction products in skin collagen in diabetes and aging. J Clin Invest 1993; 91: 2463-9.
11. Makita Z, Radoff S, Rayfield EJ, Yang Z, Skolnik E, Delaney V, Friedman EA, Cerami A, Vlassara H. Advanced glycosylation end products in patients with diabetic nephropathy. N Engl J Med 1991; 325: 836-842.
12. Makita Z, Bucala R, Rayfield EJ, Friedman EA, Kaufman AM, Korbet SM, Barth RH, Winston JA, Fuh H, Manogue KR, et al. Reactive glycosylation endproducts in diabetic uraemia and treatment of renal failure. Lancet 1994; 343: 1519-22.

13.   Soulis T, Cooper ME, Vranes D, Bucala R, Jerums G. The effects of aminoguanidine in preventing experimental diabetic nephropathy are related to duration of treatment. Kidney Int 1996; 50: 627-634.

14.   Soulis T, Thallas V, Youssef S, Gilbert RE, McWilliam B, Murray-McIntosh RP, Cooper ME. Advanced glycation end products and the receptor for advanced glycated end products co-localise in organs susceptible to diabetic microvascular injury: immunohistochemical studies. Diabetologia 1997; 40: 619-628.

15.   Beisswenger PJ, Makita Z, Curphey TJ, Moore LL, Jean S, Brinck Johnsen T, Bucala R, Vlassara H. Formation of immunochemical advanced glycosylation end products precedes and correlates with early manifestations of renal and retinal disease in diabetes. Diabetes 1995; 44: 824-9.

16.   Schmidt A, Vianna M, Gerlach M, Brett J, Ryan J, Kao C, Esposito H, Hegarty W, Hurley W, Clauss M, Wang F, Pan Y, Tsang T, Stern D. Isolation and characterisation of two binding proteins for advanced glycation end products from bovine lung which are present on the endothelial cell surface. J Biol Chem 1992; 267: 14987-14997.

17.   Schmidt AM, Hori O, Chen JX, Li JF, Crandall J, Zhang J, Cao R, Yan SD, Brett J, Stern D. Advanced glycation endproducts interacting with their endothelial receptor induce expression of vascular cell adhesion molecule-1 (VCAM-1) in cultured human endothelial cells and in mice. A potential mechanism for the accelerated vasculopathy of diabetes. J Clin Invest 1995; 96: 1395-1403.

18.   Wautier JL, Zoukourian C, Chappey O, Wautier MP, Guillausseau PJ, Cao R, Hori O, Stern D, Schmidt AM. Receptor-mediated endothelial cell dysfunction in diabetic vasculopathy. Soluble receptor for advanced glycation end products blocks hyperpermeability in diabetic rats. J Clin Invest 1996; 97: 238-243.

19.   Li Y, Mitsuhashi T, Wojciechowicz D, Shimizu N, Li J, Stitt A, He C, Banerjee D, Vlassara H. Molecular identity and distribution of advanced glycation endproducts receptors: Relationship of p60 to OST-48 and p90 to 80K-H membrane proteins. Proc Natl Acad Sci USA 1996; 93: 11047-11052.

20.   Li YM, Tan AX, Vlassara H. Antibacterial activity of lysozyme and lactoferrin is inhibited by binding of advanced glycation-modified proteins to a conserved motif. Nature Medicine 1995; 1: 1057-1061.

21.   Youssef S, Nguyen DT, Soulis T, Panagiotopoulos S, Jerums G, Cooper ME. Effect of diabetes and aminoguanidine therapy on renal advanced glycation end-product binding. Kidney International 1999; 55: 907-916.

22.   Yang CW, Vlassara H, Peten EP, He CJ, Striker GE, Striker LJ. Advanced glycation end products up-regulate gene expression found in diabetic glomerular disease. Proc Natl Acad Sci USA 1994; 91: 9436-9440.

23.   Vlassara H, Striker LJ, Teichberg S, Fuh H, Li YM, Steffes M. Advanced glycation end products induce glomerular sclerosis and albuminuria in normal rats. Proc Natl Acad Sci USA 1994; 91: 11704-11708.

24.   Rumble JR, Cooper ME, Soulis T, Cox A, Wu L, Youssef S, Jasik M, Jerums G, Gilbert R. Vascular hypertrophy in experimental diabetes: role of advanced glycation end products. J Clin Invest 1997; 99: 1016-1027.

25.   Yamagishi S, Yonekura H, Yamamoto Y, Katsuno K, Sato F, Mita I, Ooka H, Satozawa N, Kawakami T, Nomura M, Yamamoto H. Advanced glycation end products-driven angiogenesis in vitro. J Biol Chem 1997; 272: 8723-8730.

26.   Lu M, Kuroki M, Amano S, Tolentino M, Keough K, Kim I, Bucala R, Adamis AP. Advanced glycation end products increase retinal vascular endothelial growth factor expression. J Clin Invest 1998; 101: 1219-1224.

27. Gilbert RE, Vranes D, Berka JL, Kelly DJ, Cox A, Wu LL, Stacker SA, Cooper ME. Vascular endothelial growth factor and its receptors in control and diabetic rat eyes. Lab Invest 1998; 78: 1017-1027.

28. Cooper ME, Vranes D, Youssef S, Stacker SA, Cox AJ, Rizkalla B, Casley DJ, Kelly DJ, Bach LA, Gilbert RE. Increased renal expression of VEGF and its receptor VEGFR-2 in experimental diabetes. Diabetes 1999; 48: 2229-39.

29. Gilbert RE, McNally PG, Cox A, Dziadek M, Rumble J, Cooper ME, Jerums G. SPARC Gene Expression is Reduced in Early Diabetes Related Kidney Growth. Kidney Int 1995; 48: 1216-1225.

30. Isaka Y, Fujiwara Y, Ueda N, Kaneda Y, Kamada T, Imai E. Glomerulosclerosis induced by in vivo transfection of transforming growth factor-beta or platelet-derived growth factor gene into the rat kidney. J Clin Invest 1993; 92: 2597-601.

31. Kihara M, Schmelzer JD, Poduslo JF, Curran GL, Nickander KK, Low PA. Aminoguanidine effects on nerve blood flow, vascular permeability, electrophysiology, and oxygen free radicals. Proc Natl Acad Sci USA 1991; 88: 6107-11.

32. Kochakian M, Manjula BN, Egan JJ. Chronic dosing with aminoguanidine and novel advanced glycosylation end product formation inhibitors ameliorates cross-linking of tail tendon collagen in streptozotocin-induced diabetic rats. Diabetes 1996; 45: 1694-1700.

33. Soulis T, Sastra S, Thallas V, Mortensen SB, Wilken M, Clausen JT, Bjerrum OJ, Petersen H, Lau J, Jerums G, Boel E, Cooper ME. A novel inhibitor of advanced glycation end-product formation inhibits mesenteric vascular hypertrophy in experimental diabetes. Diabetologia 1999; 42: 472-479.

34. Vasan S, Zhang X, Zhang X, Kapurniotu A, Bernhagen J, Teichberg S, Basgen J, Wagle D, Shih D, Terlecky I, Bucala R, Cerami A, Egan J, Ulrich P. An agent cleaving glucose-derived protein crosslinks in vitro and in vivo. Nature 1996; 382: 275-8.

35. Wolffenbuttel BHR, Boulanger CM, Crijns FRL, Huijberts MSP, Poitevin P, Swennen GNM, Vasan S, Egan JJ, Ulrich P, Cerami A, Levy BI. Breakers of advanced glycation end products restore large artery properties in experimental diabetes. Proc Natl Aced Sci USA 1998; 95: 4630-4634.

36. Bucala R, Vlassara H. Advanced glycosylation end products in diabetic renal and vascular disease. Am J Kidney Dis 1995; 26: 875-88.

37. Wuerth J-P, Bain R, Mecca T, Park G, Cartwright K, Pimagedine Investigator Group. Baseline data from the Pimagedine Action trials. Diabetologia 1997; 40 (Suppl 1): A548.

22. PROTEIN KINASE C IN DIABETIC RENAL INVOLVEMENT, THE PERSPECTIVE OF ITS INHIBITION

Annarita Gabriele, Daisuke Koya[1] and George L. King[2]
Endocrinology Division, Department of Clinical Science, La Sapienza University, Rome 00161 Italy,
[1]Third Department of Medicine, Shiga University of Medical Science, Seta, Otsu Shiga 520-21, Japan
[2]Research Division, Joslin Diabetes Center, Department of Medicine, Harvard Medical School, Boston, MA 02215, USA

The Diabetes Control and Complications Trial (DCCT) and, more recently, the United Kingdom Prospective Diabetes Study (UKPDS) reported that the strict maintenance of euglycemia by intensive insulin treatment can delay the onset and slow the progression of diabetic nephropathy, respectively, in patients with type 1 and type 2 diabetes mellitus [1,2], suggesting that the adverse effects of hyperglycemia on metabolic pathways are main cause of long-term complications in diabetes such as kidney disease. The importance of hyperglycemia in the development of diabetic nephropathy is supported by the results of Heilig et al. who have found that the overexpression of glucose transporter 1 (GLUT1) into glomerular mesangial cells enhanced the production of extracellular matrix components which can contribute mesangial expansion and finally glomerulosclerosis, even in normal glucose levels [3]. Multiple biochemical mechanisms have been proposed to explain the adverse effects of hyperglycemia. Activation of diacylglycerol (DAG)-protein kinase C (PKC) pathway [4,5], enhanced polyol pathway related with myo-inositol depletion [6], altered redox state [7], overproduction of advanced glycation end products [8], and enhanced growth factor and cytokine production [9,10] have all been proposed as potential cellular mechanisms by which hyperglycemia induces the chronic diabetic complications.

In this article, evidence regarding the activation of DAG-PKC pathway will be briefly reviewed (Fig. 22 -1). The possibility that changes in PKC activities could be causing diabetic vascular complications has been discussed frequently due to the finding that PKC activation can increase vascular permeability, extracellular matrix synthesis, contractility, leukocyte attachment, cell growth, and angiogenesis [11-13]. All of these vascular functions have been reported to be abnormal in the diabetic state. When the

DAG levels and PKC activities were first quantitated, we and Craven et al. showed that elevating glucose concentration from 5 to 20 mM increased both DAG and PKC levels in vascular cells or tissue including renal glomeruli, retina, and aorta [14-17]. Possible activation of DAG-PKC has also been reported in the liver and skeletal muscle of insulin resistant diabetic animals, suggesting that the activation of DAG-PKC signal transduction pathway by hyperglycemia may also induce insulin resistance in those tissues. Activation of PKC and membrane β2-isoform have been recently shown to be increased in monocytes from type 2 diabetic patients and in healthy people in which an acute rise of plasma glucose was induced [18]. Furthermore, the normalization of circulating plasma glucose by insulin infusion, in diabetic patients, resulted in a slight reduction of PKC activity. These data therefore indicate that PKC activation in type 2 diabetes is largely accounted for by hyperglycemia and monocyte PKC activation may be responsible for the accelerated atherosclerosis in type 2 diabetic patients [18].

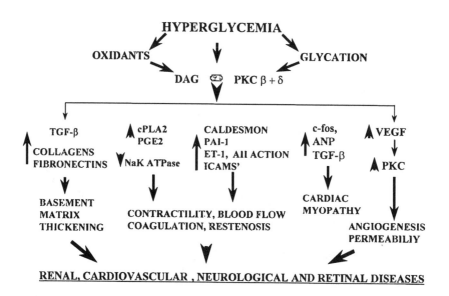

Figure 22'-1: Diagram of the effects of DAG-PKC activation in diabetes vascular complications.

It is not surprising that the activation of PKC could affect such a wide range of tissues since PKC is a family of serine and threonine kinases which act as intracellular signal transduction system for many cytokines and hormones [11,12]. Different PKC isoforms are also one of the major downstream targets for lipid signaling molecules and can be classified according to their structure differences. Conventional PKC isoforms (α, $\beta 1$, $\beta 2$, γ) are sensitive to both Ca++ and DAG whereas new PKC isoforms (δ, ϵ, η, θ, μ) are sensitive to DAG but insensitive to Ca++ due to the loss of Cl region. Atypical PKC isoforms (ς, λ) may also be sensitive to other phospholipids such as the products of phosphatidylinositol-3-kinase.

The sources of cellular DAG are multiple with the majority derived from the hydrolysis of polyphosphoinositides or phosphatidylcholine by phospholipase C or D, respectively [11,12,13]. The mechanism by which PKC is activated by diabetes and by hyperglycemia appears to be related to increase in de novo synthesis of DAG through glycolytic pathway [14,15]. It is also possible that the increases in free fatty acids in diabetic state may enhance DAG levels.

We and others have found the activation of DAG-PKC pathway in glomeruli of diabetic rats and cultured mesangial cells exposed to high glucose concentrations [14,16,19]. Vitamin E treatment in animal models of diabetes induced regression of renal hyperfiltration associated with normalization of DAG/PKC pathway through activation of DAG kinase [20].

Multiple PKC isoforms are activated in each vascular tissue of diabetic animal models. Among them PKC-β isoforms appear to be most consistently increased. Using immunoblotting study we have reported that PKC-α and $\beta 1$ isoforms exhibited a greater increase, in vivo, in membranous fractions isolated from diabetic rat glomeruli and, in vitro, in mesangial cells exposed to elevated glucose levels [19], whereas PKC-$\beta 2$ was reported to be preferentially activated in aorta and heart of diabetic rats [17]. Interestingly, Kikkawa et al. have reported that PKC-ς as well as PKC-α was activated in rat glomerular mesangial cells exposed to high glucose concentrations [9], although the mechanism for PKC-ς activation, which is independent on DAG, is unclear.

Functionally, the activation of DAG-PKC pathway has been correlated with many vascular changes in enzymatic activities, gene expressions, contractility, extracellular matrix synthesis, and cell growth and differentiation. To determine those vascular or renal dysfunctions which are due to specifically the activation of PKC-β isoform, we have designed a specific inhibitor to PKC-β isoform (LY333531) and studied its effect on glomerular cells or tissues from diabetic animals. The specificity of PKC-β inhibitor LY333531 was evaluated by in vitro study to examine the PKC isoform-induced phosphorylation of myelin basic protein. LY333531 inhibited PKC-$\beta 1$ and $\beta 2$ with a half-maximal inhibitory constant (IC50) of 4.5 and 5.9 nM, respectively, whereas the IC50 was 250 nM or greater for other PKC isoforms [16]. Furthermore, its specifity was confirmed in vivo study to examine the phosphorylation of PKC α and $\beta 1$, which has been shown to correspond to PKC isoform specific activation, in isolated glomeruli from control and slreptozotocin-induced diabetic rats with or without LY333531 (10 mg/kg body wt/day) [19]. Diabetes enhanced phosphorylation of both PKC α and $\beta 1$ by 60 and 75%, respectively. PKC-β specific inhibitor LY333531 prevented the increase in phosphorylation of PKC-$\beta 1$ but not PKC-α, suggesting the specific PKC-β isoform inhibition of LY333531 even in vivo [19].

The effect of PKC-β isoform inhibitor, LY333531, on renal hemodynamics were examined first. These functional parameters included glomerular filtration rates (GFR) and urinary albumin excretion rates (UAE). Treatment with LY333531 orally at the onset of diabetes normalized GFR and glomerular PKC activity in a dose-dependent manner [16]. Treatment with LY333531 also ameliorated the increase in urinary albumin excretion rate in diabetic rats 12 weeks after the onset of diabetes [16], suggesting that PKC-β activation may cause the early hemodynamic and histological abnormalities which have been implicated to be responsible for glomerular injury leading to the progression of diabetic nephropathy. Vitamin E treatment in diabetic rats reduced renal DAG levels, normalized PCK-β activation and glomerular filtration rates [20]. High-dose vitamin E treatment in type 1 diabetic patients, with <10 years duration of disease and no microalbuminuria, significantly normalized renal hyperfiltration. Diabetic patients with the highest creatinine clearances and poorest glycemic control showed the most marked normalization in response to vitamin E treatment [21].

One possible mechanism to explain renal hyperfiltration is the increase in vasodilatory prostanoids such as prostaglandin (PG) E2 and PGI2 which have been noted in the kidney of diabetic patients and animals with glomerular hyperfiltration [23,24]. We have reported that the possible overproduction of glomerular PGE2 in the glomeruli of diabetic rats could be due to an enhanced synthesis of arachidonic acid via the activation of cytosolic phospholipase A2 (cPLA2) by PKC since specific inhibitor of PKC-β isoform was able to decrease PGE and arachidonic acid release by hyperglycemia [19]. Haneda et al. have found that the increase in mitogen-activated protein kinase (MAPK) activity, which was dependent on diabetes-induced activation of PKC pathway, was able to enhance cPLA2 activity, resulting in increase in arachidonic acid release in glomerular mesangial cells exposed to elevated glucose levels [25]. Williams et al. have also reported similar findings showing that PKC activation by glucose increased PGE2 production through cPLA2 and it was normalized in the presence of PKC inhibitors such as H-7 or staurosporine in glomerular mesangial cells [6]. Those results strongly support that diabetes-induced hyperfiltration could be due to an overproduction of vasodilatory prostanoids through the activation of cPLA2 which was due to the activation of PKC-MAPK pathway. In addition, Igarashi et al. identified p38 MAP kinase as a possible target, in vascular cells, which can be activated by high glucose levels and diabetes [27]. Its activation is mediated by either PKC-dependent or -independent pathways, with the latter induced significantly by levels of hyperglycemia not usually observed clinically. At moderate and commonly encountered levels of hyperglycemia, p38 MAP kinase was activated by PKC-β isoform-dependent processes [27].

Another important biochemical change induced by DAG-PKC activation is the inhibition of Na+-K+ ATPase, an integral component of the sodium pump, which is involved in the maintenance of cellular integrity and functions such as contractility, growth, and differentiation [28]. Its inhibition has been well established in the vascular and neural tissues of diabetic patients and diabetic experimental animals [6]. However, the mechanisms by which hyperglycemia can inhibit Na+-K+ ATPase is still unclear especially regarding the role of PKC. We have found that PKC activation induced by diabetes or hyperglycemia can lead to the inhibition of Na+-K+ ATPase and PKC-β inhibitor prevented the decrease of Na+-K+ATPase induced by hyperglycemia, suggesting the importance of PKC-β activation in the development of mesangial or glomerular dysfunctions which are due to the inhibition of Na+-K+ ATPase activity in diabetes [19].

One of the most important glomerular pathological changes in diabetic nephropathy is structural alterations including glomerular hypertrophy, basement membrane thickening, and mesangial expansion due to accumulation of extracellular matrix components such as collagen and fibronectin [29]. A close relation is also found between mesangial expansion and the declining surface area available for glomerular filtration. Thus, the mechanisms responsible for mesangial expansion are closely related to the formation of nodular glomerulosclerosis, resulting in end stage diabetic nephropathy.

Although multiple mechanisms are probably involved in causing mesangial expansion, many studies have recently focused on the role of transforming growth factor β (TGF-β), a multifunctional cytokine, in the regulation of extracellular matrix production in diabetic nephropathy [9,10]. TGF-β can stimulate the production of extracellular matrix such as type IV collagen, fibronectin and laminin in cultured mesangial cells and epithelial cells [30,31]. Increase in gene and protein expressions of TGF-β were found in glomeruli from diabetic animal models as well as diabetic patients [32,33,34], suggesting that overexpression of TGF-β might be responsible for the development of mesangial expansion in diabetic nephropathy. This hypothesis was strengthen by the fact that inhibition of TGF-β activity with neutralizing antibody attenuates the increase in mRNA expressions of type IV collagen and fibronectin in renal cortex and glomeruli of diabetic animal models [35,36]. Since PKC is well known stimulator for synthesis of type IV collagen and fibronectin [37], it has been postulated that PKC activation might be involved in the enhancement of TGF-β expression in diabetes. To substantiate this hypothesis, we have examined the effect of PKC-β inhibitor LY333531 on the gene expressions of TGF-β1, type IV collagen, and fibronectin in glomeruli of control and diabetic rats [19]. In the glomeruli of diabetic rats, the expression of TGF-β1 mRNA was significantly increased compared to control rats [19]. Treatment with LY333531 abrogated the enhanced glomerular expression of TGF-β mRNA in diabetic rats [19]. LY333531 also prevented mRNA overexpression of extracellular matrix components such as type IV collagen and fibronectin in the glomeruli of diabetic rats, again supporting the importance of PKC-β activation and TGF-β expression in causing extracellular matrix protein overproduction. TGF-β driven matrix synthesis has been recently showed to be mediated by connective tissue growth factor (CTGF), a pro-fibrotic factor, which Murphy et al showed to be expressed in renal cortex and glomeruli of rat kidneys with diabetic nephropathy and to be induced in primary human mesangial cells exposed to high glucose levels, through TGF-β1-dependent and PKC dependent pathways [38].

In summary, a great deal of evidence have accumulated to indicate a pivotal role of PKC-β isoform activation in causing many of the pathophysiological abnormalities associated with the development and progression of diabetic nephropathy and the vascular diseases. The ability of PKC-β specific inhibitor LY333531 to prevent diabetes induced glomerular hyperfiltration, increase in albuminuria inhibition of Na+-K+ ATPase, and glomerular overexpression of TGF-β and extracellular matrix components suggested that PKC-β activation induced by diabetes lies in intracellular signaling pathway leading to these abnormalities. The availability of PKC-β inhibitor LY333531 provided an important insight into the molecular pathogenesis of diabetic nephropathy. Clinical studies using PKC-β inhibitor LY333531 which are ongoing will determine the therapeutic usefulness of PKC-β inhibition in diabetic complications.

Since vitamin E treatment has been shown to be beneficial in normalizing renal hemodynamics without changing glycemic control, vitamin E treatment may potentially provide additional risk reductions for the development of nephropathy in addition to those achievable through intensive insulin therapy alone.

ACKNOWLEDGEMENTS
Studies were supported by National Institutes of Health grants, NIH ROI-EY0510 and EY9178

REFERENCES
1.   The Diabetes Control and Complications Trial Research Group: The effect of intensive treatment of diabetes on the development and progression of long-term complications in insulin-dependent diabetes mellitus. N Engl J Med 329:977-986, 1993
2.   UK Prospective Diabetes Study Group: Intensive blood-glucose control with sulphonylureas or insulin compared with conventional treatment and risk of complications in patients with type 2 diabetes (UKPDS 33). Lancet 352, 9131: 837-853, 1998
3.   Heilig CW, Concepeion LA, Riser BL, Freytag 80, Zhu M, Cortes P: Overexpression of glucose transporters in rat mesangial cells cultured in a normal glucose milieu mimics the diabetic phenotype J Clin Invest 96:1802-1814, 1995
4.   King GL, Ishii H, Koya D: Diabetic vascular dysfunctions: A model of excessive activation of protein kinase C. Kidney Int 52:S77-S85, 1997
5.   DeRubertis FR, Craven PA: Activation of protein kinase C in glomerular cells in diabetes. Mechanisms and potential link to the pathogenesis of diabetic glomerulopathy. Diabetes 43: 1-8, 1994
6.   Greene D, Lattimer SA, Sima AAF: Sorbitol, phosphoinositides and sodium-potassium-ATPase in the pathogenesis of diabetic complications. N Engl J Med 316: 599-606, 1987
7.   Williamaon JR, Chang K, Frangos M, Hasan KS, Ido Y, Kawamura T, Nyengaard JR, Van den Enden M, Kilo C, Tilton RG: Hyperglycemic pseudohypoxia and diabetic complications. Diabetes 42: 801-813, 1993
8.   Brownlee M, Cerami A, Vlassara H: Advanced glycosylation end products in tissue and the biochemical basis of diabetic complications N Engl J Med 318: 1315-I321, 1988
9.   Sharama K, Ziyadeh FN: Hyperglycemia and diabetic kidney disease Mechanisms and potential link to the pathogenesis of diabetic glomerulopathy. Diabetes 43: 1-8, 1994

10. Mogyorosi A, Ziyadeh FN: Update on pathogenesis, markers and management of diabetic nephropathy. Curt Opin Nephrol Hyperten 5:243-253, 1996

11. Nishizuka Y: Intracellular signaling by hydrolysis of phospholipids and activation of protein kinase C. Science: 258: 607-614, 1992

12. Nishizuka Y: Protein kinase C and lipid signaling for sustained cellular responses. FASEB J 9:484-496, 1995

13. Liacovitch M, Cantley LC: Lipid second messengers. Cell 77:329-334, 1994

14. Craven PA, Davidson CM, DeRubertis FR: Increase in diacylglycerol mass in isolated glomeruli by glucose from de novo synthesis of glycerolipids. Diabetes 39:667-674, 1990

15. Inoguchi T, PuX, Kunisaki M, Higashi S, Feener EP, King GL: Insulin's effect on protein kinase C and diacylglycerol induced by diabetes and glucose in vascular tissue. Am J Physiol 267: E369-E379, 1994

16. Ishii H., Jirousek MR, Koya D, Takagi C, Xia P, Clermont A, Bursell S-E, Kem TS, Ballas LM, Heath WF, Stramm LE, Feener EP, King GL: Amelioration of vascular dysfunctions in diabetic rats by an oral PKC-β inhibitor. Science, 272: 728-731, 1996

17. Inoguchi T, Battan R, Handler E, Sportsman JR, Heath WF, King GL: Preferential elevation of protein kinase C $\beta2$ and diacylglycerol levels in the aorta and heart of diabetic rats: differential reversibility to glycemic control by islet cell transplantation. Proc Natl Acad Sci USA 89: 11059-11063, 1992

18. Ceolotto G, Gallo A, Miola M, Sartori M, Trevisan R, Del Prato S, Semplicini A, and Avogaro A. Protein Kinase C activity is acutely regulated by plasma glucose concentration in human monocytes in vivo. Diabetes, 48: 1316-1322, 1999

19. Koya D, Jirousek MR, Lin Y-W, Ishii H, Kuboki K, King GL: Characterization of PKC-β isoform activation on the gene expression of transforming growth factor β, extracellular matrix components, and prostanoids in the glomeruli of diabetic rats. J Clin Invest, 100:115-126, 1997

20. Koya D, Lee 1-K, Ishii H, Kanoh H, King GL. Prevention of glomerular dysfunction in diabetic rats by treatment with d-α-tocopherol. J Am Soc Nephrol 8:426-435, 1997

21. Bursell S-E, Clermont AC, Aiello LP, Aiello LM, Schlossman DK, Feener EP, Lafel L, King GL. High-dose vitamin E Supplementation normalizes retinal blood flow and creatinine clearance in patients with type 1 diabetes. Diabetes Care, 22, 8:1245-1251

22. Kikkawa R, Haneda M, Uzu T, Koya D, Sugimoto T, Shigeta Y: Translocation of protein kinase C and in rat glomerular mesangial cells cultured under high glucose conditions. Diabetologia 37:838-841, 1994

23. Craven PA, Caines MA, DeRubertis FR: Sequential alterations in glomerular prostaglandin and thromboxane synthesis in diabetic rats: relationship to the hyperfiltration of early diabetes. Metabolism 36:95-103, 1987

24. Perico N, Benigni A, Gabanelli M, Piccinelli A, Rog M, Riva CD, Remuzzi G: Atrial natriuretic peptide and prostacyclin synergistically mediate hyperfiltration and hyperfusion of diabetic rats. Diabetes 41:533-538

25. Haneda M, Araki S-1, Togawa M, Sugimoto T, Isono M, Kikkawa R: Mitogen-activated protein kinase cascade is activated in glomeruli of diabetic rats and glomerular mesangial cells cultured under high glucose conditions. Diabetes 46: 84-853, 1997

26. Williams B, Schreier RW: Glucose-induced protein kinase C activity regulates arachidonic acid release and eicosanoid production by cultured glomerular mesangial cells. J Clin Invest 92: 2889-2896, 1993

27. lgarashi M, Wakasaki H, Takahara N, Ishii H, Jiang Z-Y, Yamauchi T, Kuboki K, Meier M, Rhodes CJ and King GL. Glucose or diabetes activates p38 mitogen-activated protein kinase via different pathways. J Clin Invest 103:185-195, 1999

28. Vasilets LA, Schwarz W: Structure function relationships of cation binding in Na+/K+-ATPase. Biochim Biophys Acta 1154:201-222,1993

29. Ziyadeh FN: The extracellular matrix in diabetic nephropathy. Am J Kidney Dis 22:736-744, 1993

30. MacKay K, Striker LJ, Stauffer JW, Agodoa LY, Striker GE: Transforming growth factor murine glomerular receptors and responses of isolated glomerular cells. J Clin Invest 83:1160-1167, 1989

31. Nakamura T, Miller D, Ruoslahti E, Border WA: Production of extracellular matrix by glomerular epithelial cells is regulated by transforming growth factor-β. Kidney Int 41:1213-1221, 1992

32. Yamamoto T, Nakamura T, Noble NA, Ruoslahti E, Border WA: Expression of transforming growth factor β is elevated in human and experimental diabetic nephropathy, Proc Natl Acad Sci USA 90:1814-1818, 1993

33. Nakamura T, Fukui M, Ebihara 1, Osada S, Nagaoka I, Tomino Y, Koide H: mRNA expression of growth factors in glomeruli from diabetic rats. Diabetes 42:450-456, 1993

34. Sharina K, Ziyadeh FN: Renal hypertrophy is associated with upregulation of TGF-β1 gene expression in diabetic BB rat and NOD mouse. Am J Physiol 267:F1094-F 1 10 1, 1994

35. Ziyadeh FN, Sharma K Ericksen M, Wolf G: Stimulation of collagen gene and protein synthesis in murine mesangial cells by high glucose is mediated by autocrine activation of transforming growth factor P. J Clin Invest 93:536-542, 1994

36. Sharma K, Jin Y, Gua J, Ziyadeh FN: Neutralization of TGF-β by anti-TGF-β antibody attenuates kidney hypertrophy and the enhanced extracellular matrix gene expression in STZ-induced diabetic mice. Diabetes 45:522-530, 1996

37. Fumo P, Kuncio GS, Ziyadeh FN: PKC and high glucose stimulates collagen (IV) transcriptional activity in a reporter mesangial cell line. Am J Physiol 267: F632-F638, 1994

38. Murphy M, Godson C, Cannon S, Kato S, Mackenzie HS, Martin F, and Brady HR. Suppression subtractive hybridization identifies high glucose levels as a stimulus for expression of connective tissue growth factor and other genes in human mesangial cells. J Biol Chem 274, 9:5830-5834

23.   BIOCHEMICAL ASPECTS OF DIABETIC NEPHROPATHY

Cora Weigert and Erwin D. Schleicher
Department of Medicine, Division of Endocrinology, Metabolism and Pathobiochemistry, University of Tübingen, Germany

The dominant histological feature of diabetic nephropathy is the thickening of the glomerular basement membrane (GBM) and expansion of the mesangial matrix [1-3]. The changes correlate strongly with the clinical onset of proteinuria, hypertension and kidney failure. Although more than 50 years have elapsed since Kimmelstiel and Wilson [4] described in diabetic glomeruli the distinctive periodic acid-schiff (PAS)-reactive nodular deposits, progress in elucidating the pathobiochemistry has been slow. Recent investigations with electron microscopic, immunochemical and biochemical methods have led to an improved understanding of the structure-function relationship of the glomerular filtration unit in normal and pathological conditions [5].

MOLECULAR STRUCTURE AND FUNCTION OF GLOMERULAR EXTRACELLULAR MATRIX

The extracellular matrix of the glomerulus consists of the basement membrane interposed between endothelial and epithelial cells and the closely adjoining extracellular matrix surrounding the mesangial cells. The structural and functional properties of the matrix components are summarized in table 23-1. The basement membrane representing the size and charge selective area of the filtration unit is composed of a filamentous network of collagen type IV fibrils. Immunohistochemical studies revealed that the collagen IV chains are inhomogenously distributed within the glomerulus. The α1,α2-chains are primarily detected in the mesangial matrix whereas the α3,α4-chains are exclusively found in the glomerular basement membrane [6]. The basement membranes also contain a proteoglycan which consists of three heparan sulfate side chains covalently attached to the protein core [10,11]. It has been convincingly shown that the negatively charged heparan sulfate chains form the anionic barrier of the glomerular filtration unit [5,12,13]. A detailed review of this heparan sulfate proteoglycan (HSPG) and its changes in diabetes is given in the following chapter. The traces of fibronectin found in normal glomerular matrices are probably derived from plasma since the tissue specific fibronectin A+ which contains the extra domain A is not detected in normal glomeruli [14]. The mesangial matrix, although developmentally and morphologically distinct from the glomerular basement membrane, contains essentially the same components but in different distributions.

Several functions of the matrix components can now be explained by features of these components on the molecular level. Specific cell-matrix adhesion molecules which are intercalated in the cellular plasma membrane recognize well-defined amino acid sequences found in collagen, laminin and fibronectin [9,15]. Furthermore, these adhesion molecules (integrins) which are in contact with the cytoskeleton influence cell migration and cell proliferation. Changes in matrix composition may therefore alter cellular adhesion, migration and proliferation and thus influencing repair processes [15]. The finding that HSPG by virtue of its side chains specifically binds polypeptide growth factors like basic fibroblast growth factor (bFGF) or transforming growth factor ß (TGF-ß) is important in this context. It has been suggested that the matrix-bound growth factors may act as a reservoir for vascular repair mechanisms [16]. The anti-proliferative role of heparan sulfate on mesangial cells underlines the possible importance of this proteoglycan in glomerular matrix [17].

Table 23-1.
Structure and function of the major components of the glomerular basement membrane and mesangial matrix

Component	Structure	Function
Collagen type IV	Triplehelix with non-helical segments; 5 different chains with approximately 1700 amino acids are known [6,9]	Mechanical scaffold; Size selective filter; Binding to cell adhesion molecules
	Chains are unequally distributed in the glomerular matrix [6]	
Collagen type VI	3 different chains [8]	Formation of microfibrils
Laminin	3 different poly-peptide chains MW 800 KD [9]	Cell adhesion Integrin binding
Heparan sulfate Proteoglycan (HSPG)	Coreprotein MW 470 KD [7,10] 3 heparan sulfate side chains	Integrin binding Charge selective filter Antiproliferative Binding of humoral factors

STRUCTURAL AND FUNCTIONAL GLOMERULAR ALTERATIONS IN DIABETES

The first major change after the onset of diabetes is the increased volume of the whole kidney [18] and the glomeruli [19]. These hypertrophical glomeruli have normal structural composition. After a few years the amount of glomerular matrix material is increased [1,3]. Biochemical determinations indicate an increased amount of collagen in the glomerular extracellular matrices [20]. More recently, an increase in collagen type VI in the glomerular matrix of diabetic patients has been documented [21]. On the basis of immunochemical measurement, it has become evident that the HSPG content of glomerular matrix is lower in diabetic patients [22] consistent with previous chemical analyses of the heparan sulfate chains [23,24]. These immunochemical measurements, although yielding reliable quantitative values, were performed with preparations of glomerular matrices which contain firstly, both the basement membrane and the mesangial matrix and secondly a mixture of glomeruli which may be affected to a variable degree. Therefore, immunohistochemical studies have been performed to distinguish the changes within the different compartments of the glomerulus and between the individual glomeruli.

These immunohistochemical studies, summarized in table 23-2, indicate that in diabetic kidneys with slight lesions only a minor increase in all basement membrane components was found except for HSPG. More pronounced diffuse glomerulosclerosis showed a further increase in basement membrane components, especially collagen IV $\alpha1,\alpha2$-chains in the expanded mesangial matrix. However, HSPG which was entirely absent from the enlarged matrix could only be observed in the periphery of the glomeruli. The staining of collagen IV $\alpha3,\alpha4$-chain showed a similar distribution as found for HSPG however, with intense staining of the thickened glomerular basement membrane [6]. To this stage of nephropathy the accumulation of excess matrix material can be attributed to quantitative changes of the components present in normal glomeruli. In contrast, pronounced nodular lesions exhibited a strong decrease of collagen IV $\alpha1,\alpha2$-chains, laminin, and HSPG which were only detectable in the periphery of the noduli. Staining sequential sections with collagen VI antiserum or PAS revealed coincidence of both stainings indicating that the noduli consist mostly of collagen type VI [8]. Peripheral areas of these noduli were also positive for collagen III which was not detected in earlier lesions. It appears that in diffuse glomerulosclerosis an increase in normal matrix components occurs while the nodular glomerulosclerosis is characterized by qualitative changes (table 23-2). Morphological and structural changes occurring in the interstitium, tubuli or glomerular arterioles are a concomitant of diabetic nephropathy [1].

The likelihood that increased matrix content occurring in diffuse glomerulosclerosis is the consequence of increased synthesis coupled with decreased degradation is supported by *in vivo* and *in vitro* studies of collagen metabolism in glomeruli obtained from diabetic animals [20,25,26]. An increased synthesis was unequivocally demonstrated by extracellular matrix gene expression. Fukui et al. [27] showed increased steady state mRNA levels of the collagen IV $\alpha 1$-chain, laminin B1 and B2 and fibronectin while the collagen I $\alpha 1$-chain was unchanged in the kidneys of diabetic rats after one month of diabetes. The message for HSPG was decreased after induction of diabetes and increased steadily afterwards. The changes in mRNA levels which preceded the glomerular matrix expansion could be prevented by normalisation of blood glucose by insulin treatment. Recent *in situ* hybridization studies revealed that mRNA transcript levels of $\alpha_1(IV)$ collagen are increased more than twofold in glomerular and proximal tubular cells in long-term (12 months) diabetic rats [28]. In the glomerulum, mainly mesangial cells showed enhanced $\alpha_1(IV)$ collagen expression. The $\alpha_1(IV)$ collagen deposition in the mesangial matrix was similarly increased. Chronic treatment with a modified heparin preparation completely prevented the increased $\alpha_1(IV)$ collagen deposition and expression and the overt albuminuria in diabetic rats. Taken together, these results indicate that the increased synthesis of collagen IV, laminin and fibronectin is the biochemical correlate of the expansion of the mesangial matrix and the thickening of glomerular basement membrane observed histologically. The occurrence of decreased degradation of matrix components has also been documented [26].

Table 23-2.
Changes of glomerular matrix composition in different stages of diabetic glomerulosclerosis (GS)*

	diffuse GS		nodular GS	
	GBM	mesangium	GBM	Mesangium
Laminin	↑	↑	↑	↓
collagen IV				
α1,α2-chain	↑	↑	↑	↓
α3,α4-chain	↑	-	↑	↑
HSPG	↓→	↓	↓	
Fibronectin A+	-	n.d.	-	↑
collagen III	-	-[1]	-	↑[2]
collagen VI	↓	↑[3]	↓	↑↑

↑ = increased; ↓ = decreased; → = unchanged; - = not detectable; *see also [6-8]; n.d. = not determined; [1]traces in late diffuse GS; [2]only peripheral; [3]focally

Extensive studies have shown that the changes in glomerular ultrastructure are closely associated with renal function [2,3]. Comparing the immunohistochemical findings with clinical data Nerlich et al. [7] found that the increase in the glomerular matrix components was consistently associated with impaired renal filter function. Late stage nodular glomerulosclerosis associated with decrease of all basement membrane components, and increase in collagen III and VI coincided with severe renal insufficiency. In all cases, even in early diffuse glomerulosclerosis, HSPG was decreased.

INVOLVEMENT OF GROWTH FACTORS IN THE DEVELOPMENT OF DIABETIC NEPHROPATHY

The morphological changes occurring in diabetic micro- and macroangiopathy have led to the idea that growth hormone or other growth factors may play an active role in mediating these alterations [29]. In a recent study with experimental animals Nakamura et al. [30] demonstrated the gene expression of different growth factors including TGF-ß, bFGF and platelet derived growth factor in glomeruli of diabetic rats within 4 weeks after induction of diabetes. The gene expression was relatively specific since other growth factors like IGF-I were unchanged. Insulin treatment partially ameliorated the induction of growth factors. In a related study Yamamoto et al. [14] reported that in glomeruli of diabetic rats there is a slow, progressive increase in the expression of TGF-ß mRNA and TGF-ß protein. A more recent report showed that the induction of glomerular TGF-β1synthesis is significant after 14 days of diabetes indicating that the increased TGF-β1 production is an early event in diabetes [31]. A key action of TGF-ß is the induction of extracellular matrix production and specific matrix proteins, and these matrix proteins were increased in diabetic rat glomeruli. Corresponding changes were found in patients with diabetic nephropathy, whereas glomeruli from normal subjects or individuals with other glomerular diseases were essentially negative. These findings suggest that TGF-ß plays a pivotal role in the glomerular matrix expansion that occurs in diabetic nephropathy. A causal relationship between TGF-ß expression and matrix accumulation in the acute model of glomerular nephritis was proven by preventing matrix accumulation with TGF-ß antiserum [32,33]. Furthermore, addition of oligonucleotides antisense to TGF-β1 attenuated the high glucose-induced matrix production indicating that hyperglycemia induces TGF-β1 synthesis in mesangial cells [34]. Recently, the involvement of TGF-ß1 was confirmed by tissue specific expression of the TGF-ß1 gene in the kidney of transgenic mice. Overproduction of TGF-ß1 in the juxta-glomerular apparatus resulted in local accumulation of extracellular matrix proteins including collagen type IV and laminin and thickening of the basement membrane [35].

HYPERGLYCAEMIA AND THE PATHOGENESIS OF DIABETIC GLOMERULOPATHY

The biochemical events leading to the quantitative and finally qualitative alterations of the glomerular matrix and to the induction of growth factors are currently under intensive investigation. Epidemiological studies indicate that the development of diabetic nephropathy is linked to hyperglycaemia [36,37]. Recent reports support this hypothesis demonstrating that hyperglycaemia increases the expression of several genes, which play causative roles in the pathogenesis of diabetic glomerulopathy. Three pathobiochemical pathways activated by elevated glucose levels are favoured in the current discussion.

The first possibility involves the direct action of high glucose on the cells. Ayo and coworkers reported that prolonged exposure to high glucose concentrations leads to an increase in collagen IV, laminin and fibronectin synthesis on the protein and mRNA level in mesangial cells [38]. Furthermore, mesangial cells exposed to elevated glucose synthesize less HSPG [39]. Studies with epithelial, endothelial and mesangial cells revealed that all three cell types of the glomerulus produce more collagen type IV when exposed to elevated glucose levels [40]. Periodic changes in glucose concentration, simulating more closely disordered glucose homeostasis, lead to enhanced synthesis of collagen type III and IV compared to continuous low or high glucose environment. The data indicate the deleterious effects of fluctuating glucose levels on the development of diabetic glomerulosclerosis [41]. Studies with mesangial cells overexpressing glucose transporters provide a more direct evidence for the involvement of glucose in matrix production [42]. Mesangial cells stable transfected with the human glucose transporter 1 gene, the main isoform expressed by these cells, had an increased glucose uptake (5-fold) and net utilization (43-fold) and exerted enhanced synthesis of matrix components when cultured in <u>normal</u> glucose concentration. Thus increased cellular glucose flux enhances matrix production in mesangial cells. Furthermore, in mesangial cells expressing normal levels of glucose transporters exposure to 20 mM glucose for 3 days stimulates the expression of glucose transporter 1 thereby increasing basal glucose uptake [43]. These *in vitro* experiments suggest that hyperglycaemia rather than hyperinsulinaemia or hyperosmolarity is the cause of enhanced matrix synthesis [38,40]. Moreover, an elevated expression of TGF-ß1 as a key molecule in the pathogenesis of diabetic nephropathy has also been linked to hyperglycaemia [33, 34].

Recent data show that hyperglycaemia stimulates gene expression of matrix proteins and TGF-ß1 by increasing the activity of the corresponding promoters (table 23-3). These studies using promoter fragments fused to reporter genes such as luciferase indicate an activation of the murine and human TGF-ß1 promoter by high glucose [44,45]. The fibronectin promoter is stimulated additively by high glucose and TGF-ß1 [46]. TGF-ß1 itself is known to activate promoters of several genes, including the promoters for α2 collagen type I [47], type IV [48], laminin [49] and in an autocrine loop transcription of its own gene [50]. Similarly TGF-ß1 increases the activity of the HSPG promoter [51], while hyperglycaemia caused a decrease in HSPG expression [52]. The most frequently found transcription factors which may mediate the high glucose- and TGF-ß1-induced promoter activation are members of the AP-1 family. Consensus sequences for AP-1 have been found in the promoters of the different collagen types, fibronectin and TGF-ß1 and confirmed to be responsible for the high glucose- or TGF-ß1-mediated transcriptional activation [45-47,49,50].

Several reports demonstrate the activation of AP-1 by hyperglycaemia. AP-1 proteins are regulated by enhanced expression and phosphorylation, both of which can alter the composition of the transcription factor complex which binds to promoter sequences. The transcripts and protein levels of the AP-1 family members c-Jun and c-Fos are elevated in mesangial cells cultured in high glucose [53].

Table 23-3.
Regulation of gene expression of matrix proteins and TGF-ß1 by hyperglycaemia and TGF-ß1. Involved transcription factors are shown in brackets.

Gene	Promoter activity induced by			
	TGF-ß1		Hyperglycaemia	
TGF-ß1	+	(AP1)	+	(AP-1)
Fibronectin	+	(AP-1)	+	(AP-1)
collagen I α2	+	(AP-1)	?	
collagen IV α2	+	(Sp1)	?	
laminin	+	(AP-1)	?	
HSPG	+	(NF-1)	-	?

+= increased promoter activity, -= decreased promoter activity, ?= effect not known , transcription factor not known. AP-1 activating protein-1; Sp1 stimulatory protein1; NF-1 nuclear factor-1.

Posttranslational activation is shown by increased DNA binding activity of AP-1 proteins derived from mesangial cells exposed to elevated glucose concentrations, which is not due to differences in the protein level [54] and by phosphorylation of the AP-1 related transcription factor CREB after treatment of mesangial cells with high glucose and TGF-ß1 [55]. These findings give rise to the question, which protein kinase cascades are activated by hyperglycaemia and involved in the upregulation of genes by AP-1. Among the several distinct mitogen-activated protein kinases (MAPK) the extracellular signal regulated kinases (ERK1/2), the Jun N-terminal kinases and the p38 MAP kinases were shown to mediate enhanced gene expression and posttranslational phosphorylation of AP-1 proteins. The activity of ERK 1/2 is enhanced in mesangial cells cultured in high glucose [56], whereas a recent report demonstrated an elevated activity of p38 MAP kinase in mesangial-like aortic smooth muscle cells after exposure to 16.5 mM glucose [57]. In both studies the activation of protein kinase C (PKC) is necessary for the stimulation of the MAP kinases by high glucose. The involvement of PKC is in accordance with several reports which provide evidence for a role of glucose-induced activation of PKC in the elevated synthesis of matrix components [58,59]. Application of a PKC inhibitor (preferentially inhibiting the ß-isoform) ameliorated the glomerular filtration rate, albumin excretion rate and retinal circulation in diabetic rats in a dose-responsive manner, in parallel with its inhibition of PKC activities [60]. Two metabolic pathways responsible for high glucose-induced PKC activation are discussed. One involves the metabolism of glucose to diacylglycerol, a known PKC activator [61], while the other involves the biosynthetic hexosamine pathway [62], which may also activate PKC [63]. In addition, stimulation of MAPK activity by TGF-ß1 is linked to PKC activation [64]. The proposed molecular mechanism of hyperglycaemia-induced matrix synthesis in mesangial cells is shown in figure 23-1. Another group of transcription factors which is responsible for TGF-ß1-mediated gene expression is the Smad family. These signal molecules are activated by direct interaction with the TGF-ß1 receptors at intracellular sites of the receptor leading to their nuclear translocation and enhanced transcription of genes containing TGF-ß1 response elements. The Smads cooperate with Jun proteins and c-Fos by direct binding or by cross talk between different DNA binding sites resulting in transcriptional activation of TGF-ß1 target genes [65,66]. The role of this synergism in hyperglycaemia-induced gene expression is unknown.

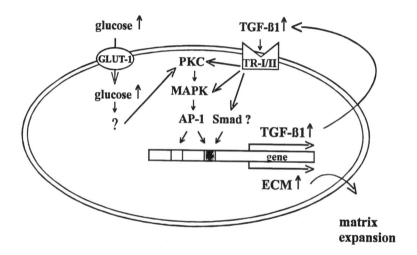

Fig. 23-1 Proposed molecular mechanism of the hyperglycaemia-induced matrix synthesis in mesangial cells. Elevated glucose entering the cell via the glucose transporter 1 (GLUT 1) activates the protein kinase C (PKC) and mitogen-activated protein kinases (MAPK) leading to enhanced expression and/or phosphorylation of proteins of the activating protein 1 complex (AP-1). Since the promoters of extracellular matrix (ECM) proteins and TGF-ß1 contain AP-1 binding sites the expression of these genes is induced. TGF-ß1 acting auto-/paracrine further enhances ECM synthesis via binding to the TGF-ß1 receptor (TR-I/II) and activation of AP-1 through the PKC-MAPK pathway. The Smad familiy of signal transducers may be involved. By this vicious cycle overproduction of matrix is maintained also after hyperglycaemic periods.

The second pathomechanism linking elevated glucose levels with diabetic glomerulopathy may be the non-enzymatic glycosylation (glycation) of matrix proteins which are freely accessible to glucose. The extend of glycation is dependent on proteins' half lives and the mean glucose level of the patient during the life time of the respective protein [67,68]. The amount of glycation in these tissues seemed to be related to the extend and severity of the patients' late complications [68]. More recent approaches suggest that the development of diabetic late complications may be linked to the formation of advanced glycosylation end-products (AGE-products) [69]. These AGE-products, such as carboxymethyl-lysine, pentosidine and malondialdehyde-lysine, accumulate in expanded mesangial matrix and nodular lesions as shown in renal tissue from patients with diabetic nephropathy [70]. The cellular effects of AGE-products are mediated by specific binding to cell surface molecules of which the receptor for advanced glycation end-products (RAGE) is well characterized [71]. Expression of RAGE is increased in kidneys from patients with diabetic nephropathy [72]. Furthermore, AGE-products and their receptors co-localize in the renal glomerulus of rats with experimental diabetes [73]. Although upregulation of mesangial TGF-ß1 synthesis with concomitant increase of extracellular matrix production by AGEs has been shown [74], the main action of the AGE-RAGE system not only in terms of diabetic nephropathy is to cause chronic cellular activation and oxidative stress. The RAGE expression is enhanced by a positive feedback loop via activation of the transcription factor NF-kB [71], perpetuating the stimulatory event and leading to cellular perturbation. In this stage the cells are highly susceptible for further stress stimuli resulting in chronic inflammation and accelerated sclerosis .

The third pathochemical mechanism involves intracellular formation of sorbitol from glucose catalysed by aldose reductase [75]. Chronic hyperglycaemia leads to sorbitol accumulation in a variety of tissues like peripheral neurons, lense and renal tubuli [76]. The initial hypothesis that sorbitol accumulation causes tissue damage is unlikely to operate in kidney [37]. The inositol depletion theory suggested by Greene and coworkers explains tissue damages as impairment of myo-inositol uptake leading to a decrease of phosphatidyl-inositides in the cell membrane [75]. Although the cellular inositol uptake is competitively inhibited by D-glucose [77] and non-competitively inhibited by hyperosmolar intracellular sorbitol [78], recent studies showed that cells may counterregulate inositol depletion [79,80]. Thus, it is not generally agreed that the increase in intracellular sorbitol is the cause of the impaired function of the affected tissues in diabetes. Furthermore, after treatment of diabetic rats for six months with the aldose reductase inhibitor tolrestat only a slight reduction in the urinary albumin excretion rate was observed indicating that other mechanism are operating in diabetic nephropathy [81].

ANGIOTENSIN II AND DEVELOPMENT OF DIABETIC GLOMERULOPATHY

Angiotensin II is the dominant effector of the renin-angiotensin system (RAS). Angiotensin II regulates salt and water balance, blood pressure, and the vascular tone. Several recent studies have provided clear evidence that angiotensin-converting enzyme (ACE)-inhibitors slow the progression of diabetic nephropathy by mechanisms mainly independent from reduction of systemic blood pressure [82,83]. Thus, angiotensin II exerts non-hemodynamic effects on the kidney which may contribute to the enhanced extracellular matrix production in diabetic glomerulopathy [84]. The profibrogenetic actions of angiotensin II have been shown by several laboratories.

In vitro studies with cultured mesangial and proximal tubular cells revealed striking similarities between the effects of high glucose exposure and angiotensin II treatment [84,85]. Angiotensin II stimulates TGF-ß1 synthesis and matrix component production at both the mRNA and protein level through engagement of the angiotensin type 1 (AT1)-receptor in mesangial cells. The increased extracellular matrix protein expression depends on bioactivity and *de-novo* synthesis of TGF-ß, since administration of neutralizing antibodies to TGF-ß or TGF-ß antisense oligonucleotides blocked this cellular response to angiotensin II [84,85]. Recent studies with mesangial-like smooth muscle cells showed the involvement of MAPK and AP-1 in angiotensin II-induced TGF-ß1 expression [86]. Furthermore, angiotensin II activated PKC in mesangial and proximal tubular cells through AT1-receptors [82]. Taken together, these non-hemodynamic effects of angiotensin II on TGF-ß1 synthesis and matrix production in renal cells are quite similiar to those of hyperglycaemia and could explain the protective effects of ACE-inhibitor therapy on development of diabetic glomerulopathy independent of the blood pressure lowering activity. However, little is known about the interaction of hyperglycaemia and angiotensin II. The dysregulation of the renin-angiotensin system in diabetes is not well characterized and multiple investigations gave no clear hint that the intrarenal angiotensin II-system is activated in patients susceptible to diabetic nephropathy [82]. Moreover, the AT1-receptors are downregulated in diabetic renal disease [82]. It remains to be shown whether high glucose and angiotensin II act independent through different pathways or whether they potentiate the response of renal cells to the other signal. *In vitro* studies in mesangial-like smooth muscle cells suggest a simultaneous action of high glucose and angiotensin II. The MAP kinases ERK1/2 and p38 are additively activated by both stimuli resulting in an enhanced effect on transcription factor AP-1 activity compared to high glucose or angiotensin II treatment alone [87]. A recent report linking hyperglycaemia to increased angiotensin II generation demonstrated that high glucose stimulates angiotensin II production in mesangial cells and that the high glucose-induced TGF-ß1 synthesis, mesangial matrix accumulation, and decrease in collagenase activity is reversed by losartan, a AT1-receptor antagonist [88]. These data give rise to the hypothesis, that antagonizing the effects of angiotensin II, e.g. in ACE-inhibitor therapy, interfere not only with the renin-angiotensin-system but may ameliorate hyperglycaemia-induced pathomechanisms which are mediated in part by angiotensin II and resulting in development of diabetic nephropathy. The proposed signal transduction pathways stimulated by hyperglycaemia and angiotensin II and possible interactions are summarized in figure 23-2.

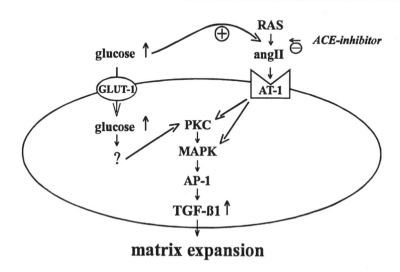

matrix expansion

Fig. 23-2 Proposed molecular mechanism of the hyperglycaemia- and angiotensin II-induced TGF-ß1 expression. Elevated glucose entering the cell via the glucose transporter 1 (GLUT 1) activates the protein kinase C (PKC) and activating protein 1 (AP-1) which in turn initiates the gene expression shown in Fig. 23-1. After binding to the angiotensin receptor 1 (AT-1) angiotensin II (Ang II) may stimulate the matrix synthesis by activation of the same signal transduction pathway. Elevated glucose may also increase Ang II production. Inhibition of the renin-angiotensin-system (RAS) by application of angiotensin converting enzyme (ACE) inhibitors is indicated.

ACKNOWLEDGEMENTS
The work from the author's laboratory was supported by the Deutsche Forschungsge-meinschaft (Schl 239/6-2). The critical comments of Drs. R. Lehmann and R. Lammers are gratefully acknowledged.

REFERENCES

1. Mauer SM, Ellis E, Bilous RW, Steffes MW. »The pathology of diabetic nephropathy.« In *Complications of Diabetes Mellitus*, Draznin B, Melmed S, LeRoith D, eds. New York: Alan R Liss Inc., 1989; pp 95-101.

2. Mauer SM, Steffes MW, Ellis EN, Sutherland DER, Brown DM, Goetz FC. Structural-functional relationships in diabetic nephropathy. J Clin Invest 1984; 74: 1143-1155.

3. Østerby R, Gall MA, Schmitz A, Nielsen FS, Nyberg G, Parving H-H. Glomerular structure and function in proteinuric type 2 (non-insulin-dependent) diabetic patients. Diabetologia 1993; 36: 1064-1070.

4. Kimmelstiel P, Wilson C. Intercapillary lesions in the glomeruli of the kidney. Am J Pathol 1936; 12: 83-89.

5. Farquhar MG. »The glomerular basement membrane: A selective macromolecular filter.« In *Cell Biology of Extracellular Matrix*, Hay E, ed. New York, London: Plenum Press, 1981; pp 335-378.

6. Kim Y, Kleppel M, Butkowski R, Mauer M, Wieslander J, Michael A. Differential expression of basement membrane collagen chains in diabetic nephropathy. Am J Pathol 1991; 138: 413-420.

7. Nerlich A, Schleicher E. Immunohistochemical localization of extracellular matrix components in human diabetic glomerular lesions. Am J Pathol 1991; 139: 889-899.

8. Nerlich A, Schleicher ED, Wiest I, Specks U, Timpl R. Immunohistochemical localization of collagen VI in diabetic glomeruli. Kidney Int 1994, 45: 1648-1656.

9. Timpl R. Structure and biological activity of basement membrane proteins. Eur J Biochem 1989; 180: 487-503.

10. Kallunki P, Tryggvason K. human basement membrane heparan sulfate proteoglycan core protein: A 467-kD protein containing multiple domains resembling elements of the low density lipoprotein receptor, laminin, neural cell adhesion molecules, and epidermal growth factor. J Cell Biol 1992; 116: 559-571.

11. Schleicher ED, Wagner EM, Olgemöller B, Nerlich AG, Gerbitz KD. Characterization and localization of basement membrane-associated heparan sulphate proteoglycan in human tissues. Lab Invest 1989; 61: 323-332.

12. Stow JL, Sawada H, Farquhar MG. Basement membrane heparan sulfate proteoglycans are concentrated in the laminae rarae and in podocytes of the rat renal glomerulus. Proc Natl Acad Sci USA 1985; 82: 3296-3300.

13. van den Born J, van den Heuvel PWJ, Bakker MAH, Veerkamp JH, Assmann KJM, Berden JHM. A monoclonal antibody against GBM heparan sulfate induces an acute selective proteinuria in rats. Kidney Int 1992; 41: 115-123.

14. Yamamoto T, Nakamura T, Noble NA, Ruoslahti E, Border WA. Expression of transforming growth factor ß is elevated in human and experimental diabetic nephropathy. Proc Natl Acad Sci USA 1993; 90: 1814-1818.

15. Ruoslahti E. »Extracellular matrix in the regulation of cellular functions.« In *Cell to Cell Interaction*, Burger MM, Sordat B, Zinkernagel RM, eds. Basel: Karger, 1990; pp 88-98.

16. d'Amore PA. Modes of FGF release in vivo and in vitro Cancer and Metastasis Reviews 1990; 9: 227-238.

17. Wright TC, Casellot JJ, Diamond JR, Karnovsky MJ. »Regulation of cellular proliferation by heparin and heparan sulfate.« In *Heparin*, Lane DA, Lindahl U, eds. London: Edward Arnold, 1989; pp 295-316.

18. Steffes MW, Østerby R, Chavers B, Mauer, MS. Mesangial expansion as a central mechanism for loss of kidney function in diabetic patients. Diabetes 1989; 38: 1077-1081.

19. Østerby R, Gundersen HJG. Glomerular size and structure in diabetes mellitus: early abnormalities. Diabetologia 1975; 11: 225-259.

20. Spiro RG. »Pathogenesis of diabetic glomerulopathy: a biochemical view.« In *The Kidney and Hypertension in Diabetes Mellitus*, Mogensen CE, ed. Boston: Martinus Nijhoff Publishing, 1988; pp 117-130.

21. Mohan PS, Carter WG, Spiro RG. Occurrence of type VI collagen in extracellular matrix of renal glomeruli and its increase in diabetes. Diabetes 1990; 39: 31-37.

22. Shimomura H, Spiro RG. Studies on macromolecular components of human glomerular basement membrane and alterations in diabetes: decreased levels of heparan sulfate proteoglycan. Diabetes 1987; 36: 374-381.

23. Parthasarathy N, Spiro RG. Effect of diabetes on the glycosaminoglycan component of the human glomerular basement membrane. Diabetes 1982; 31: 738-741.

24. Schleicher E, Wieland OH. Changes of human glomerular basement membrane in diabetes mellitus. Eur J Clin Chem Clin Biochem 1984; 22: 223-227.

25. Haneda M, Kikkawa R, Horide N, Togawa M, Koya D, Kajiwara N, Ooshima A, Shigeta Y. Glucose enhances type IV collagen production in cultured rat glomerular mesangial cells. Diabetologia 1991; 34: 198-200.

26. Schaefer RM, Paczek L, Huang S, Teschner M, Schaefer L, Heidland A. Role of glomerular proteinases in the evolution of glomerulosclerosis. Eur J Clin Chem Clin Biochem 1992; 30: 641-646.

27. Fukui M, Nakamura T, Ebihara I, Shirato I, Tomino Y, Koide H. ECM gene expression and its modulation by insulin in diabetic rats. Diabetes 1992; 41: 1520-1527.

28. Ceol M, Nerlich A, Baggio B, Anglani A, Sauer U, Schleicher E, Gambaro G. Increased glomerular α_1 (IV) collagen expression and deposition in long-term diabetic rats is prevented by chronic glycosminoglycan treatment. Lab Invest 1996; 74; 484-495.

29. Flyvbjerg A. Growth factors and diabetic complications. Diabetic Med 1990; 7: 387-390.

30. Nakamura T, Fukui M, Ebihara I, Osada S, Nakaoka I, Tomino Y, Koide H. mRNA Expression of growth factors in glomeruli from diabetic rats. Diabetes 1993; 42: 450-456.

31. Park IS, Kiyomoto H, Abboud SL, Abboud HE. Expression of transforming growth factor-beta and type IV collagen in early streptozotocin-induced diabetes. Diabetes 1997; 46: 473-480.

32. Border WA, Okuda S, Languino LR, Sporn MB, Ruoslahti E. Suppression of experimental glomerulonephritis by antiserum against transforming growth factor beta 1. Nature 1990; 346: 371-374.

33. Sharma K, Ziyadeh FN. Perspectives in diabetes.Hyperglycemia and diabetic kidney disease. The case for transforming growth factor-β as a key mediator. Diabetes 1995; 44: 1139-1146.

34. Kolm V, Sauer U, Olgemöller B, Schleicher ED. High glucose-induced TGF-beta 1 regulates mesangial production of heparan sulfate proteoglycan.Am J Physiol 1996; 270 : F812-21.

35.   Wogensen L, Nielsen CB, Hjorth, P, Rasmussen LM, Nielsen AH, Gross K, Sarvetnick N, Ledet T: Under control of the Ren-1^c promoter, locally produced transforming growth factor-ß1 induces accumulation of glomerular extracellular matrix in transgenic mice. Diabetes 1999; 48: 182-192.

36.   Kern TS, Engerman TL. Arrest of glomerulopathy in diabetic dogs by improved diabetic control. Diabetologia 1990; 21: 178-183.

37.   Larkins RG, Dunlop ME. The link between hyperglycaemia and diabetic nephropathy. Diabetologia 1992; 35: 499-504.

38.   Ayo SH, Radnik RA, Glass IIWF, Garoni JA, Rampt ER, Appling DR, Kreisberg JI. Increased extracellular matrix synthesis and mRNA in mesangial cells grown in high-glucose medium. Am J Physiol 1990; 260: F185-F191.

39.   Olgemöller B, Schwaabe S, Gerbitz KD, Schleicher ED. Elevated glucose decreases the content of a basement membrane associated proteoglycan in proliferating mesangial cells. Diabetologia 1992; 35: 183-186.

40.   Danne T, Spiro MJ, Spiro RG. Effect of high glucose on type IV collagen production by cultured glomerular epithelial, endothelial, and mesangial cells. Diabetes 1993; 42: 170-177.

41.   Takeuchi A, Throckmorton DC, Brogden AP, Yoshizawa N, Rasmussen H, Kashgarian M. Periodic high extracellular glucose enhances production of collagens III and IV by mesangial cells. Am Physiol Soc 1995; 268: F13-F19.

42.   Heilig CW, Concepcion LA, Riser BL, Freytag SO, Zhu M, Cortes P. Overexpression of glucose transporters in rat mesangial cells cultured in a normal glucose milieu mimics the diabetic phenotype. J Clin Invest 1995; 96: 1802-1814.

43.   Heilig CW, Liu, Y, England RL, Freytag, SV, Gilbert, JD, Heilig KO, Zhu M, Concepcion, LA, Brosius III FC: D-Glucose stimulates mesangial cell GLUT1 expression and basal and IGF-1-sensitive glucose uptake in rat mesangial cells. Diabetes 1997, 46: 1030-1039.

44.   Hofman BB, Sharma K, Zhu Y, Ziyadeh FN: Transcriptional activation of transforming growth factor-ß1 in mesangial cell culture by high glucose concentration. Kidney Int 54:1107-1116, 1998

45.   Weigert C, Pfeiffer A, Haering H, Schleicher E: Glucose-induced activation of the TGF-ß1 promoter in mesangial cells (Abstract). Diabetologia 1998; 41: Suppl. 1: A297.

46.   Kreisberg JI, Garoni JA, Radnik R, Ayo SH: High glucose and TGF-ß1 stimulate fibronectin gene expression through a cAMP response element. Kidney Int 1994, 46: 1019-1024.

47.   Chung KY, Agarwal A, Uitto J, Mauviel A: An AP-1 binding sequence is essential for regulation of the human alpha2(I) collagen (COL1A2) promoter activity by transforming growth factor-beta. J Biol Chem 1996, 271: 3272-3278.

48.   Kuncio GS, Alvarez R, Li S, Killen PD, Neilson EG: Transforming growth factor-beta modulation of the alpha 1(IV) collagen gene in murine proximal tubular cells. Am J Physiol 1996, 271: F120-125.

49.   Virolle T, Monthouel MN, Djabari Z, Ortonne JP, Meneguzzi G, Aberdam D: Three activator protein-1-binding sites bound by the Fra2.JunD complex cooperate for the regulation of murine laminin alpha3A (lama3A) promoter activity by transforming growth factor-beta. J Biol Chem 1998, 273: 17318-17325.

50. Kim S-J, Angel P, Lafyatis R, Hattori K, Kim KY, Sporn MB, Karin M, Roberts AB: Autoinduction of transforming growth factor ß1 is mediated by the AP-1 complex. Mol Cell Biol 1990,10: 1492-1497.

51. Iozzo RV, Pillarisetti J, Sharma B, Murdoch AD, Danielson KG, Uitto J, Mauviel A: Structural and functional characterization of the human perlecan gene promoter. Transcriptional activation by transforming growth factor-beta via a nuclear factor 1-binding element. J Biol Chem 1997, 272: 5219-28.

52. Kanwar YS, Liu ZZ, Kumar A, Usman MI, Wada J, Wallner EI: D-glucose-induced dysmorphogenesis of embryonic kidney. J Clin Invest 1996, 98: 2478-88.

53. Kreisberg JI, Radnik RA, Ayo SH, Garoni J, Saikumar P: High glucose elevates c-fos and c-jun transcripts and proteins in mesangial cell cultures. Kidney Int 1994, 46: 105-112.

54. Wilmer WA, Cosio FG: DNA binding of activator protein-1 is increased in human mesangial cells cultured in high glucose concentrations. Kidney Int 1998, 53:1172-1181.

55. Kreisberg JI, Radnik RA, Kreisberg SH: Phosphorylation of cAMP responsive element binding protein after treatment of mesangial cells with high glucose plus TGFß or PMA. Kidney Int 1996, 50: 805-810.

56. Haneda M, Araki S-I, Togawa M, Sugimoto T, Isono M, Kikkawa R: Activation of mitogen-activated protein kinase cascade in diabetic glomeruli and mesangial cells cultured under high glucose conditions. Kidney Int 1997; Suppl 60: 66-69

57. Igarashi M, Wakasaki H, Takahara N, Ishii H, Zhen YJ, Yamauchi T, Kuboki K, Meier M, Rhodes CJ, King GL: Glucose or diabetes activate p38 mitogen-activated protein kinase via different pathways. J Clin Invest 103: 185-195, 1999

58. Ayo SH, Radnik R, Garoni JA, Troyer DA, Kreisberg JA. High glucose increases diacylglycerol mass and activates protein kinase C in mesangial cells. Am J Physiol 1991; 261: F571-F577.

59. Craven PA, DeRubertis FR. Protein kinase C is activated in glomeruli from streptozotocin diabetic rats. Possible mediation by glucose. J Clin Invest 1989; 83: 1667-1675.

60. Ishii H, Jirousek MR, Koya D, Takagi C, Xia P, Clermont A, Bursell SE, Kern TS, Ballas LM, Heath WF, Stramm LE, Feener EP, King GL. Amelioration of vascular dysfuntions in diabetic rats by an oral PKC beta inhibitor. Science 1996; 272: 728-731.

61. Inoguchi T, Battan R, Handler E, Sportsman JR, Heath WF, King GL: Preferential elevation of protein kinase C bII and diacylglycerol levels in the aorta and heart of diabetic rats: differential reversibility to glycemic control by islet cell transplantation. Proc Natl Acad Sci USA 1992, 89: 11059-11063.

62. Kolm-Litty V, Sauer U, Nerlich A, Lehmann R, Schleicher ED: High glucose-induced transforming growth factor ß1 production is mediated by the hexosamine pathway in porcine glomerular mesangial cells. J Clin Invest 1998, 101:160-169.

63. Kolm-Litty V, Tippmer S, Haering H-U, Schleicher E: Glucosamine induces translocation of protein kinase C isoenzymes in mesangial cells. Exp Clin Endocrinol Diabetes 1998, 106: 377-383.

64. Palcy S, Goltzman D: Protein kinase signalling pathways involved in the up-regulation of the rat alpha 1(I) collagen gene by transforming growth factor beta1 and bone morphogenetic protein 2 in osteoblastic cells. Biochem J 1999, 343: 21-27.

65. Liberati NT, Datto MB, Frederick JP, Shen X, Wong C, Rougier-Chapman EM, Wang XF: Smads bind directly to the Jun family of AP-1 transcription factors. Proc Natl Acad Sci USA 1999, 96: 4844-4849

66.   Wong C, Rougier-Chapman EM, Frederick JP, Datto MB, Liberati NT, Li JM, Wang XF: Smad3-Smad4 and Ap-1 complexes synergize in transcriptional activation of the c-Jun promoter by transforming growth factor beta. Mol Cell Biol 1999, 19: 1821-1830

67.   Brownlee M, Cerami A, Vlassara H. Advanced glucosylation end products in tissue and the biochemical basis of diabetic complications. N Engl J Med 1988; 318: 1315-1321.

68.   Vogt BW, Schleicher ED, Wieland OH. ε-Aminolysine bound glucose in human tissues obtained at autopsy: increase in diabetes mellitus. Diabetes 1982; 31: 1123-1127.

69.   Ledl F, Schleicher E. New aspects of the Maillard reaction in foods and in the human body. Angew Chem Intern Ed Engl 1990; 29: 565-594.

70.   Suzuki D, Miyata T, Saotome N, Horie K, Inagi R, Yasuda Y, Uchida K, Izuhara Y, Yagame M, Sakai H, Kurokawa K: Immunohistochemical evidence for an increased oxidative stress and carbonyl modifications of proteins in diabetic glomerular lesions. J Am Soc Nephrol 1999, 10: 822-832

71.   Schmidt AM, Yan SD, Wautier J-L, Stern D: Activation of receptor for advanced glycation end products. Circ Res 1999, 84: 489-497.

72.   Bierhaus A, Ritz E, Nawroth PP: Expression of receptors for advanced glycation end-products in occlusive vascular and renal disease. Nephrol Dial Transplant 1996, 11 Suppl 5:87-90.

73.   Soulis T, Thallas V, Youssef S, Gilbert RE, McWilliam BG, Murray-McIntosh RP, Cooper ME: Advanced glycation end products and their receptors co-localise in rat organs susceptible to diabetic microvascular injury. Diabetologia 1997, 40: 619-628

74.   Pugliese G, Pricci F, Romeo G, Pugliese F, Mene P, Giannini S, Cresci B, Galli G, Rotella CM, Vlassara H, Di Mario U: Upregulation of mesangial growth factor and extracellular matrix synthesis by advanced glycation end products via a receptor-mediated mechanism. Diabetes 1997, 46: 1881-1887

75.   Greene D. The pathogenesis and its prevention of diabetic neuropathy and nephropathy. Metabolism 1988; 37: suppl. 1: 25-29.

76.   Schmolke M, Schleicher E, Guder WG. Renal sorbitol, myo-inositol and glycerophosphorylcholine in streptozotocin-diabetic rats. Eur J Clin Chem Clin Biochem 1992; 30: 607-614.

77.   Olgemöller B, Schwaabe S, Schleicher ED, Gerbitz KD. Competitive inhibition by glucose of myo-inositol incorporation into cultured porcine mesangial cells. Biophys Biochem Acta 1990; 1052: 47-52.

78.   Li W, Chan LS, Khatami M, Rockey JH: Non-competitive inhibition of myo-inositol transport in cultured bovine retinal capillary pericytes by glucose and reversal by sorbinil. Biochim Biophys Acta 1986; 857: 198-208.

79.   Guzman NJ, Crews FT. Regulation of inositol transport by glucose and protein kinase C in mesangial cells. Kidney Int 1992; 42: 33-40.

80.   Olgemöller B, Schleicher E, Schwaabe S, Gerbitz KD. Upregulation of myo-inositol transport compensates for competitive inhibition by glucose. Diabetes 1993; 42: 1119-1125.

81.   Mc Caleb ML, Mc Kean ML, Hohman TC, Laver N, Robinson WG. Intervention with aldose reductase inhibitor, tolrestat, in renal and retinal lesions of streptozotocin diabetic rats. Diabetologia 1991; 34: 659-701.

82.   Wolf G, Ziyadeh FN: The role of angiotensin II in diabetic nephropathy: emphasis on nonhemodynamic mechanisms. Am J Kid Disease 1997, 29: 153-163

83. Mogensen CE: Microalbuminuria, blood pressure and diabetic renal disease: origin and development of ideas. Diabetologia 1999, 42: 263-285.

84. Wolf G: Angiotensin II is involved in the progression of renal disease: importance of non-hemodynamic mechanisms. Nephrologie 1998, 19: 451-456

85. Kagami S, Border WA, Miller DE, Noble NA: Angiotensin II stimulates extracellular matrix protein synthesis through induction of transforming growth factor-beta expression in rat glomerular mesangial cells. J Clin Invest 1994, 93: 2431-2437

86. Hamaguchi A, Shokei K, Izumi Y, Zhan Y, Yamanaka S, Iwao H: Contribution of extracellular signal-regulated kinase to angiotensin II-induced transforming growth factor-ß1 expression in vascular smooth muscle cells. Hypertension 1999, 34: 126-131.

87. Natarajan R, Scott S, Bai W, Yerneni KKV, Nadler J: Angiotensin II signaling in vascular smooth muscle cells under high glucose conditions. Hypertension 1999, 33: 378-384

88. Singh R, Alavi N, Singh AK, Leehey DJ: Role of angiotensin II in glucose-induced inhibition of mesangial matrix degradation. Diabetes 1999, 48: 2066-2073

24. PATHOGENESIS OF DIABETIC GLOMERULOPATHY: THE ROLE OF GLOMERULAR HEMODYNAMIC FACTORS

Sharon Anderson, M.D. and Radko Komers, M.D., Ph.D.
Division of Nephrology and Hypertension, Oregon Health Sciences University, Portland, OR, U.S.A.

INTRODUCTION

Glomerular hyperfiltration in insulin-dependent (Type 1) diabetes mellitus of short duration has been recognized for many years [1-3], with increments in renal plasma flow (RPF) and nephromegaly [3]. With the finding of early hyperfiltration, Stalder and Schmid proposed that these early functional changes may predispose to the subsequent development of diabetic glomerulopathy [1]. Further support for the hypothesis that renal hyperperfusion and hyperfiltration contribute to diabetic glomerulopathy came from the finding of diabetic glomerulopathy only in the non-stenosed kidney in the setting of unilateral renal artery stenosis [4].

Although glomerular hyperperfusion and hyperfiltration have long been recognized in early Type 1 diabetes [1-3], similar studies have only recently been performed in the much larger patient population with non-insulin-dependent (Type 2) diabetes. Studies reveal a wide range of renal hemodynamics in this group, but provide clear evidence for elevations of GFR and RPF in significant proportions of patients of Caucasian, Native- and African-American origin [5-11]. Furthermore, compelling evidence for the presence of renal hemodynamic abnormalities in Type 2 diabetes has been recently reported by Nelson, et al [12]. In that study, conducted in Pima Indians, transition from impaired glucose tolerance to Type 2 diabetes was accompanied by a 30% increase in glomerular filtration rate (GFR). An increase in GFR has been also reported in obesity, a condition which often accompanies Type 2 diabetes [13].

Alterations in renal hemodynamics in diabetes are also associated with loss of renal functional reserve, i.e., the ability to increase GFR in response to amino acid infusion or to an ingestion of a meal rich in protein [14]. These maneuvers may identify altered renal hemodynamics in a subset of patients whose basal GFR values are within the normal range.

It has been proposed that the glomerular hyperfunction of early Type 1 diabetes predicts the later development of overt nephropathy and diabetic glomerulopathy [15,16], while others have failed to document such a relationship [17-19]. The reasons

Mogensen C.E. (ed.), THE KIDNEY AND HYPERTENSION IN DIABETES MELLITUS.

for these disparate findings are as yet unclear. Likewise, the role of the glomerular hyperfiltration observed in Type 2 diabetic patients in the subsequent development of nephropathy remains to be established in longitudinal studies. However, preliminary results indicate a reduction in GFR over the first 2 years after diagnosis, with the greatest changes in the younger patients with initial GFR values greater than 120 ml/min [20]. Despite the controversy in human diabetes concerning the significance of hyperfiltration in the subsequent development of overt nephropathy, extensive experimental data provides considerable insight into the importance of hemodynamic factors in the initiation and progression of diabetic glomerulopathy [21,22].

RENAL HEMODYNAMICS IN EXPERIMENTAL DIABETES MELLITUS

Several animal models with spontaneous or induced diabetes have been used to study the role of altered hemodynamics in the development of diabetic glomerulopathy [21-24]. As in Type 1 diabetic patients, diabetic rats tend to exhibit reduced values for whole kidney GFR during periods of severe uncontrolled hyperglycemia; single nephron (SN) GFR and plasma flow rates are also normal or reduced in animals in such catabolic states [24]. In the more clinically applicable model of moderate hyperglycemia, whole kidney GFR and SNGFR increase by about 40% as compared to normal rats [24-26]. Reductions in intrarenal vascular resistances result in elevation of the glomerular capillary plasma flow rate, Q_A. Despite normal blood pressure levels, transmission of systemic pressures to the glomerular capillaries is facilitated by proportionally greater reduction in afferent compared to efferent arteriolar resistances. Consequently, the glomerular capillary hydraulic pressure (P_{GC}) rises. Thus, the observed single nephron hyperfiltration results from both glomerular capillary hyperperfusion and hypertension [24-26]. In longterm studies, diabetic rats develop morphologic changes reminiscent of those in the diabetic human, including glomerular basement membrane thickening, renal and glomerular hypertrophy, mesangial matrix thickening and hyaline deposition, and ultimately glomerular sclerosis [25-30].

Evidence that these glomerular hemodynamic maladaptations contribute to the development and progression of diabetic glomerulopathy has been shown by studies involving maneuvers which aggravate or ameliorate glomerular hyperperfusion and hyperfiltration, without affecting metabolic control. Uninephrectomy, which increases SNGFR, Q_A and P_{GC} in normal rats, accelerates the development of albuminuria and glomerular sclerosis in diabetic rats [31]. Intensification of glomerular lesions is observed in the unclipped kidney of diabetic rats with two-kidney Goldblatt hypertension, while the clipped kidney is substantially protected from glomerular injury [32]. Diabetic renal injury is similarly amplified by augmentation of dietary protein content, which increases glomerular perfusion and filtration [25].

In contrast, dietary protein restriction, which reduces SNGFR, Q_A and P_{GC} in other models, has clarified the role of hemodynamic factors in diabetic glomerulopathy. In long-term diabetes, low protein diets limits SNGFR by reducing the elevated P_{GC} and Q_A, and virtually prevents albuminuria and glomerular injury. In contrast, diabetic rats fed a high protein diet exhibit glomerular capillary hyperfiltration, hyperperfusion and hypertension, and marked increases in albuminuria and glomerular morphologic injury [25]. As there were no differences in metabolic control between the various groups, this study provided clear evidence that amelioration of the maladaptive glomerular hemodynamic pattern could prevent diabetic renal disease could dramatically lower the risk of diabetic glomerulopathy.

MECHANISMS OF HYPERFILTRATION IN DIABETES

The pathogenesis of diabetic hyperfiltration is multifactorial. Numerous mediators for this effect have been proposed (Table 24-1), and are briefly reviewed here. The metabolic milieu may contribute: hyperglycemia and/or insulinopenia *per se* [23,33], together with augmented growth hormone and glucagon levels [34,35]. Reduction of plasma glucose with initial institution of therapy reduces GFR in both Type 1 and 2 diabetes [33,36]. In moderately hyperglycemic diabetic rats, normalization of blood glucose levels reverses hyperfiltration [37], and insulin infusion reduces P_{GC} [38]. A recent report suggested that the lack of C-peptide in diabetic rats also contributes to hyperfiltration [39]. In contrast, insulin infusion sufficient to produce hyperinsulinemia, with euglycemia, increases P_{GC} and hyperfiltration in normal rats [40]. Further, infusion of blood containing early glycosylation products reproduces glomerular hyperfiltration in normal rats [41].

Table 24-1

POTENTIAL MEDIATORS OF DIABETIC HYPERFILTRATION
Factors affecting predominantly afferent arteriolar tone
      Hyperglycemia/insulinopenia
      Advanced glycosylation end products
      Atrial natriuretic peptide and extracellular fluid volume expansion
      Nitric oxide and blunted tubulo-glomerular feedback
      Vasodilator prostaglandins
      Increased plasma ketone bodies, organic acids
      Increased plasma glucagon levels
      Increased plasma levels of growth hormone and insulin-like growth factor-1
      Impaired afferent arteriolar voltage-gated calcium channels
      Altered responsiveness or receptor density to catecholamines/angiotensin II/TxA$_2$
Factors affecting predominantly efferent arteriolar tone
      Increased activity of the RAS, endothelin, and vasoconstrictor prostanoids
Miscellaneous factors
      Protein kinase C
      Increased sodium reabsorption upstream from macula densa
      Increased kallikrein-kinin activity
      Abnormalities in calcium metabolism
      Vascular endothelial growth factor
      Abnormal myo-inositol metabolism
      Tissue hypoxia/abnormalities in local vasoregulatory factors

---

Apart from the above mentioned mechanisms which are closely related to the diabetic metabolic milieu, there is substantial evidence suggesting that renal hemodynamic alterations are a consequence of imbalance between the vasoactive humoral systems controlling the glomerular microcirculation. It is assumed that the balance between the factors influencing afferent arteriolar tone is shifted towards vasodilators, whereas the opposite would be expected on the efferent arteriole. Atrial natriuretic peptide (ANP), with its glomerular actions characterized by afferent dilation and efferent constriction, represents one of the promising candidates for mediating diabetic hyperfiltration. Plasma ANP levels are elevated in diabetes [42], and blockade of ANP action with an antibody [42] or a specific receptor antagonist [43] blunts hyperfiltration in diabetic rats. It is likely that altered levels of ANP in diabetes are a consequence of an increase in total exchangeable body sodium and a hypervolemic state [44,45], although resistance to ANP, as described by Fioretto, et al [46], may be also involved. In any case, these observations suggest that sodium homeostasis is an important factor in the pathogenesis of hyperfiltration. This is further underscored by studies showing that amelioration of hyperfiltration in diabetic rats can be achieved by sodium restriction [47,48].

Nitric oxide (NO) is a potent dilator acting on both afferent and efferent arterioles, presumably with predominant afferent actions *in vivo* [49].   In mammalian tissues, including the kidney, NO is synthesized by a family of isoenzymes known as nitric oxide synthases (NOS).   Inhibition of NO synthesis with non-specific NOS inhibitors (which affect all NOS isoforms) decreases GFR in hyperfiltering diabetic rats [50-53]. More recent studies have attempted to identify the contributions of individual NOS isoforms in this process. We have recently focused on renal hemodynamic roles of the neuronal NOS (nNOS, NOS1). This isoform is of particular interest in the diabetic kidney.   Under physiological conditions, NOS1-derived NO counteracts afferent vasoconstrictor signals mediated by the tubuloglomerular feedback mechanism (TGF), thus contributing to the control of P_{GC} [54]. We have recently demonstrated increased sensitivity of the renal vascular tree to the systemic NOS1 inhibition in diabetic rats [55]. Furthermore, we found complete amelioration of hyperfiltration in response to intrarenal NOS1 inhibition, as well as increased immunohistochemical expression of NOS1 in macula densa regions of diabetic kidneys [56]. These observations identified NOS1-derived NO as an important player in the pathogenesis of hyperfiltration in diabetes, and are in accordance with previous reports showing blunting of the TGF mechanism in diabetic rats [57,58]. However, as recently suggested by Vallon, et al [59], reduced TGF activity resulting in hyperfiltration may be simply a result of increased Na^{+} tubular reabsorption via Na^{+}/glucose cotransport, leading to reduced electrolyte delivery to the distal nephron. There is also recent evidence suggesting that activity of the endothelial NOS isoform (NOS3) may be increased, and contribute to renal NO hyperproduction in diabetes [60,61]. Unlike the other two isoforms, inducible NOS (NOS2) seems to play a minimal role in renal hemodynamics in diabetes. Selective inhibition of NOS2 with L-iminoethyl-lysine did not influence renal function in hyperfiltering diabetic rats [61] Furthermore, the enzyme is not expressed in renal cortex during the hyperfiltering state, both in rats with or without insulin treatment [61, 62, Komers and Anderson, unpublished observations]. In addition to "primary" dysregulation of NO synthesis, the

NO-mediated alterations in renal hemodynamics may be related to increased activity of factors which act as NO-dependent vasodilators. Very recently, De Vriese, et al [63] reported that neutralization of vascular endothelial growth factor (VEGF) with an antibody ameliorates diabetic hyperfiltration. This factor, which has been implicated in non-hemodynamic pathways in the pathogenesis of diabetic complications, possesses vasomotor effects mediated by NO [64].

Enhanced activity of vasodilator prostaglandins is another mechanism proposed as a mediator of diabetic hyperfiltration, as prostaglandin synthetase inhibition results in significant reductions in SNGFR, Q_A and P_{GC} [65]. Diabetes-related abnormalities of other vasodilator mechanisms have also been suggested, with findings of activation of the kallikrein-kinin system [66-68]. However, studies with kinin receptor antagonists have thus far proven inconsistent [69-71].

With respect to the delicate balance between dilators and constrictors in the control of glomerular hemodynamics, reduced afferent or mesangial actions of vasoconstrictor systems may also contribute. These mechanisms include reduced glomerular receptor sites for the vasoconstrictive Ang II and thromboxane [72,73], and altered vascular responsiveness to catecholamines and Ang II [74-76].

The role of vasoconstrictor systems is, however, more complex. In apparent contrast to the reduced preglomerular and glomerular actions of some of these systems, inhibition of vasoconstrictor systems, such as the RAS [77], endothelin (ET) [78], or thromboxane A_2 (TxA$_2$) [79,80], has beneficial effects on the development of nephropathy, including amelioration of diabetic hyperfiltration. The most plausible explanation for this phenomenon is that the reduction of hyperfiltration by inhibition of these substances is achieved, at least in part, by inhibition of their efferent arteriolar actions. This also suggests that, unlike the preglomerular vasculature, diabetes is associated with normal or increased efferent actions of vasoconstrictors. Supporting this view are our whole kidney data showing an increase in the renal hemodynamic response to Ang II in diabetic rats [75]. Moreover, we also found that diabetic animals demonstrated a renal vasodilatory response and a decrease in filtration fraction in response to Ang II receptor blockade [55]. It should be noted that similar to the glomerular microcirculatory pattern in general, renal hemodynamic responses to various effectors or inhibitors in experimental diabetes are largely dependent on the degree of metabolic control and insulin treatment. These differences may explain some disparate findings of studies exploring the activities of vasoactive systems in diabetes.

There is convincing evidence suggesting a role for activation of the protein kinase C (PKC) enzyme family in the pathogenesis of diabetic complications. Importantly, some of these iso-enzymes are not only activated by hyperglycemia via de novo synthesis of diacylglycerol, but also operate in signaling cascades of some vasoactive peptides, such as Ang II. Amelioration of hyperfiltration, associated with an overall renoprotective effect in the diabetic kidney, was observed in studies with newly available inhibitors of PKC [81].

Non-humoral mechanisms may be also involved. Functional impairment of renal afferent arteriolar voltage-gated calcium channels may result in decreased vascular tone [82]. Increased activity of the polyol pathway and related disturbances in cellular myo-inositol metabolism have been implicated in the pathogenesis of several diabetic microangiopathic complications. Dietary myo-inositol supplementation and pharmacologic inhibition of aldose reductase sometimes [83], though not always [84], prevents renal hypertrophy, hyperfiltration and proteinuria in diabetic rats.

ROLE OF GLOMERULAR HYPERTENSION

Of the glomerular hemodynamic determinants of hyperfiltration, the available evidence suggests that glomerular capillary hypertension plays the key role in progression of renal injury. Long-term protection against albuminuria and glomerular sclerosis was obtained in normotensive diabetic rats by angiotensin converting enzyme inhibitor (ACEI) therapy in doses which modestly lowered systemic blood pressure, but selectively normalized P_{GC}, without affecting the supranormal SNGFR and Q_A [26]. Studies in a variety of experimental models, including diabetes, have consistently shown that interventions which control glomerular capillary hypertension are associated with marked slowing of the development of structural injury [85].

Little is yet known of the exact mechanism(s) by which glomerular capillary hypertension eventuates in structural injury. Recently, innovative new techniques using a variety of *in vitro* systems have been developed to address this question. These studies postulate that glomerular hemodynamic factors modify the growth and activity of glomerular component cells, inducing the elaboration or expression of cytokines and other mediators which then stimulate mesangial matrix production and promote structural injury. For instance, increased shear stress on endothelial cells enhances activity of such mediators as endothelin [86], nitric oxide [87,88], transforming growth factor-ß [89], and several cellular adhesion molecules [90,91], and modulates release of platelet derived growth factor [90,91]. Altered hemodynamics also influence mesangial cells: it has been postulated that expansion of the glomerular capillaries, and stretching of the mesangium in response to hypertension, might translate high P_{GC} into increased mesangial matrix formation [94]. Evidence for this mechanism comes from observations in microperfused rat glomeruli, in which increased hydraulic pressure was associated with increased glomerular volume; and in cultured mesangial cells, where cyclic stretching resulted in enhanced synthesis of protein, total collagen, collagen IV, collagen I, laminin, fibronectin, and transforming growth factor-ß (TGF-ß) [94-97]. Of particular relevance to diabetes, the accumulation of extracellular matrix caused by any degree of mechanical strain is aggravated in a milieu of high glucose concentration [98]. Additionally, growing mesangial cells under pulsatile conditions has been reported to stimulate protein kinase C, calcium influx, and proto-oncogene expression [99], and Ang II receptor and angiotensinogen mRNA levels [95], as well as altered extracellular matrix protein processing enzymes [100,101]. Recently, it has been noted that mediators of oxidant stress are induced by shear stress in vascular smooth muscle cells [102], as well as mechanical stretch in proximal tubular cells [103]. More evidence comes from the recent finding that application of pressure (comparable to elevated glomerular pressures in vivo) enhances mesangial cell matrix synthesis in cultured cells [104].

Given these new techniques, the cellular mechanisms by which glomerular hypertension leads to structural injury are in process of being elucidated.

ANTIHYPERTENSIVE THERAPY IN EXPERIMENTAL DIABETES

Further support for the notion that glomerular capillary hypertension constitutes a central mechanism of glomerular injury in experimental diabetes comes from studies comparing differing antihypertensive agents [21]. Of the agents studied, ACEI have consistently limited injury parameters (albuminuria and glomerular sclerosis) in normotensive diabetic rats, uninephrectomized diabetic rats, and diabetes superimposed on genetic hypertension [26,105-110], as well as in diabetic dogs [111]. In studies where glomerular hemodynamics were measured, the protection afforded by ACEI was associated with reduction of P_{GC}, due to preferential reduction of efferent arteriolar tone.

In contrast, conflicting results have been reported for antihypertensive regimens which fail to control glomerular hypertension. Agents such as dihydropyridine calcium channel blockers, -blockers and combinations of vasodilators and diuretics ("triple therapy") have not resulted in structural and functional protection in experimental diabetes with any consistency [106-111]. Failure to exert longterm control of glomerular hypertension has frequently been found to contribute to lack of protection with these alternate agents.

That the beneficial effects of ACEI are due in large part to limitation of Ang II formation has been confirmed in studies showing that the beneficial hemodynamic [112] and structural [113] effects can be reproduced with specific Ang II receptor antagonists. Ang II possesses a number of physiological actions. Limitation of several of these have been postulated to contribute to the protective effect of ACEI, including control of systemic and glomerular hypertension; decreased mesangial and tubular macromolecular and solute transfer; decreased proteinuria with improved glomerular permselectivity; and limitation of glomerular hypertrophy and microvascular growth. Although experimental diabetes is characterized by glomerular enlargement, longterm protection with ACEI has been observed without consistent limitation of glomerular size [105,106,108]. The proposed beneficial mechanisms of ACEI are, however, not mutually exclusive. Indeed, though less emphasized, the renin-angiotensin system is now thought to participate in pathogenesis of tubulointerstitial injury, as well as glomerular injury, in the setting of diabetes. As has been recently reviewed, hyperglycemia and the renin-angiotensin system may act synergistically to promote fibrosis in the diabetic kidney, by mechanisms beyond hemodynamic factors [114].

Although the role of aggressive control of hypertension in the preservation of renal function in diabetic nephropathy is clear, clinical studies directly comparing different antihypertensive agents have remained somewhat controversial. Earlier meta-analyses [115,116] and clinical trials [117] suggested a superior ability of ACEI to slow the pace of diabetic nephropathy, as compared to other antihypertensive agents. However, more recent reports indicate that this issue is still debatable [118,119].

Elucidation of the complex mechanisms that contribute to diabetic hyperfiltration remains a challenge. Many genetic, metabolic and hemodynamic factors act in concert with the end result of glomerular obsolescence. The enormity of the clinical problem of nephropathy in this highly susceptible patient population mandates continued intense research into pathogenetic mechanisms, and approaches to specific therapy of patients at risk for renal disease.

REFERENCES

1. Stalder G, Schmid R. 1959. Severe functional disorders of glomerular capillaries and renal hemodynamics in treated diabetes mellitus during childhood. Ann Paediatr, 193:129-138.

2. Ditzel J, Junker K. 1972. Abnormal glomerular filtration rate, renal plasma flow and renal protein excretion in recent and short-term diabetes. Br Med J, 2:13-19.

3. Mogensen CE, Andersen MJF. 1973. Increased kidney size and glomerular filtration rate in early juvenile diabetes. Diabetes, 22:706-712.

4. Berkman J, Rifkin H. 1973. Unilateral nodular diabetic glomerulosclerosis (Kimmelstiel-Wilson). Metabolism, 22:715-722.

5. Vora J, Dolben J, Dean J, Williams JD, Owens DR, Peters JR. 1992. Renal hemodynamics in newly presenting non-insulin-dependent diabetics. Kidney Int, 41:829-835.

6. Myers BD, Nelson RG, Williams GW, et al. 1991. Glomerular function in Pima Indians with non-insulin-dependent diabetes mellitus of recent origin. J Clin Invest, 88:524-530.

7. Palmisano JJ, Lebovitz HE. 1989. Renal function in Black Americans with type II diabetes. J Diab Compl, 3:40-44.

8. Nelson RG, Bennett PH, Beck GJ, Tan M, Knowler WC, Mitch WE, Hirschman GH, Myers BD. 1996. Development and progression of renal disease in Pima Indians with non-insulin-dependent diabetes mellitus. New Engl J Med, 335:1636-1642.

9. Nowack R, Raum E, Blum W, Ritz E. 1992. Renal hemodynamics in recent-onset Type II diabetes. Am J Kidney Dis, 20:342-347

10. Ritz E, Stefanski A. 1996. Diabetic nephropathy in Type II diabetes. Am J Kidney Dis, 27:167-194.

11. Wirta O, Pasternack A, Laippala P, Turjanmaa V. 1996. Glomerular filtration rate and kidney size after six years disease duration in non-insulin-dependent diabetic subjects. Clin Nephrol, 45:10-71.

12. Nelson RG, Tan M, Beck GJ, Bennett PH, Knowler WC, Mitch WE, Blouch K, Myers BD. 1999. Changing glomerular filtration with progression from impaired glucose tolerance to Type II diabetes mellitus. Diabetologia, 42:90-93.

13. Hall JE, Brands MW, Henegar JR, Sheck EW. 1998. Abnormal kidney function as a cause and a consequence of obesity hypertension. Clin Exp Pharmacol Physiol, 25:58-64.

14. Sackmann H, Tran-Van T, Tack T, Hanaire-Broutin H, Tauber JP, Ader JL. 1998. Renal functional reserve in IDDM patients. Diabetologia, 41:86-93.

15. Mogensen CE. 1986. Early glomerular hyperfiltration in insulin-dependent diabetics and late nephropathy. Scand J Clin Lab Invest, 46:201-206.

16. Rudberg S, Persson B, Dahlquist G. 1992. Increased glomerular filtration rate as a predictor of diabetic nephropathy - an 8 year prospective study. Kidney Int, 41:822-828.

17. Lervang H-H, Jensen S, Borchner-Mortensen J, Ditzel J. 1988. Early glomerular hyperfiltration and the development of late nephropathy in type 1 (insulin-dependent) diabetes mellitus. Diabetologia, 31:723-729.

18.   Yip JW, Jones SL, Wiseman M, Hill C, Viberti GC. 1996. Glomerular hyperfiltration in the prediction of nephropathy in IDDM. A 10-year followup study. Diabetes, 45:1729-1733.

19.   Mogensen CE. 1994. Glomerular hyperfiltration in human diabetes. Diabetes Care, 17:770-775.

20.   Vora JP, Dolben J, Williams JD, Peters JR, Owens DR. 1993. Impact of initial treatment on renal function in newly-diagnosed type 2 (non-insulin-dependent) diabetes mellitus. Diabetologia, 36:734-740

21.   Anderson S. 1992. Antihypertensive therapy in experimental diabetes. J Am Soc Nephrol, 3 (Suppl 1):S86-S90.

22.   O'Donnell MP, Kasiske BL, Keane WF. 1986. Glomerular hemodynamics and structural alterations in experimental diabetes. FASEB J, 2:2339-2347.

23.   Park SK, Meyer TW. 1995. The effect of hyperglycemia on glomerular function in obese Zucker rats. J Lab Clin Med, 125:501-507.

24.   Hostetter TH, Troy JL, Brenner BM. 1981. Glomerular hemodynamics in experimental diabetes mellitus. Kidney Int, 19:410-415.

25.   Zatz R, Meyer TW, Rennke HG, Brenner BM. 1985. Predominance of hemodynamic rather than metabolic factors in the pathogenesis of diabetic glomerulopathy. Proc Natl Acad Sci (USA), 82:5963-5967.

26.   Zatz R, Dunn BR, Meyer TW, Anderson S, Rennke HG, Brenner BM. 1986. Prevention of diabetic glomerulopathy by pharmacological amelioration of glomerular capillary hypertension. J Clin Invest, 77:1925-1930.

27.   Seyer-Hansen K. 1983. Renal hypertrophy in experimental diabetes mellitus. Kidney Int, 23:643-646.

28.   Seyer-Hansen K, Hansen J, Gundersen HJG. 1980. Renal hypertrophy in experimental diabetes. A morphometric study. Diabetologia, 18:501-505.

29.   Steffes MW, Brown DM, Basgen JM, Mauer SM. 1980. Amelioration of mesangial volume and surface alterations following islet transplantation in diabetic rats. Diabetes, 29:509-515.

30.   Mauer SM, Michael AF, Fish AJ, Brown DM. 1972. Spontaneous immunoglobulin and complement deposition in glomeruli of diabetic rats. Lab Invest, 27:488-494.

31.   O'Donnell MP, Kasiske BL, Daniels FX, Keane WF. 1986. Effect of nephron loss on glomerular hemodynamics and morphology in diabetic rats. Diabetes, 35:1011-1015.

32.   Mauer SM, Steffes MW, Azar S, Sandberg SK, Brown DM. 1978. The effect of Goldblatt hypertension on development of the glomerular lesions of diabetes mellitus in the rat. Diabetes, 27:738-744.

33.   Christiansen JS, Gammelgaard J, Tronier B, Svendsen PA, Parving H-H. 1982. Kidney function and size in diabetics before and during initial insulin treatment. Kidney Int, 21:683-688.

34.   Parving H-H, Christiansen JS, Noer I, Tronier B, Mogensen CE. 1980. The effect of glucagon infusion on kidney function in short-term insulin-dependent juvenile diabetics. Diabetologia, 19:350-354.

35.   Christiansen JS, Gammelgaard J, Orskov H, Andersen AR, Telmer S, Parving H-H. 1980. Kidney function and size in normal subjects before and during growth hormone administration for one week. Eur J Clin Invest, 11:487-490.

36.   Vora J, Dolben J, Williams JD, Peters JR, Owens DR. 1993. Impact of initial treatment on renal function in newly-diagnosed Type 2 (non-insulin-dependent) diabetes mellitus. Diabetologia, 36:734-740.

37. Stackhouse S, Miller PL, Park SK, Meyer TW. 1990. Reversal of glomerular hyperfiltration and renal hypertrophy by blood glucose normalization in diabetic rats. Diabetes, 39:989-995.

38. Scholey JW, Meyer TW. 1989. Control of glomerular hypertension by insulin administration in diabetic rats. J Clin Invest, 83:1384-1389.

39. Sjoquist M, Huang W, Johansson BL. 1998. Effects of C-peptide on renal function at the early stage of experimental diabetes. Kidney Int, 54:758-764.

40. Tucker BJ, Anderson CM, Thies RS, Collins RC, Blantz RC. 1992. Glomerular hemodynamic alterations during acute hyperinsulinemia in normal and diabetic rats. Kidney Int, 42:1160-1168.

41. Sabbatini M, Sansone G, Uccello F, Giliberti A, Conte G, Andreucci VE. 1992. Early glycosylation products induce glomerular hyperfiltration in normal rats. Kidney Int, 42:875-881.

42. Ortola FV, Ballermann BJ, Anderson S, Mendez RE, Brenner BM. 1987. Elevated plasma atrial natriuretic peptide levels in diabetic rats. J Clin Invest, 80:670-674.

43. Zhang PL, Mackenzie HS, Troy JL, Brenner BM. 1994. Effects of an atrial natriuretic peptide receptor antagonist on glomerular hyperfiltration in diabetic rats. J Am Soc Nephrol, 4:1564-1570.

44. Feldt-Rasmussen B. 1987. Central role for sodium in the pathogenesis of blood pressure changes independent of angiotensin, aldosterone and catecholamines in Type 1 (insulin-dependent) diabetes mellitus. Diabetologia, 30:610-617.

45. O'Hare JA, Ferris BJ, Brady D, Twomey B, O'Sullivan DJ. 1985. Exchangable sodium and renin in hypertensive diabetic patients with and without nephropathy. Hypertension, 7 [Suppl II]: II-43-II-48.

46. Fioretto P, Sambataro M, Cipollina MR, Giorato C, Carraro A, Opocher G, Sacerdoti D, Brocco E, Morocutti A, Mantero F. 1992. Role of atrial natriuretic peptide in the pathogenesis of sodium retention in IDDM with and without glomerular hyperfiltration. Diabetes, 41:936-945.

47. Bank N, Lahorra MA, Aynedjian HS, Wilkes BM. 1988. Sodium restriction corrects hyperfiltration of diabetes. Am J Physiol, 254: F668-F676.

48. Allen TJ, Waldron MJ, Casley D, Jerums G, Cooper ME. 1997. Salt restriction reduces hyperfiltration, renal enlargement, and albuminuria in experimental diabetes. Diabetes, 46:119-124.

49. Deng A, Baylis C. 1993. Locally produced EDRF controls preglomerular resistance and ultrafiltration coefficient. Am J Physiol, 264: F212-F215.

50. Bank N, Aynedjian HS. 1993. Role of EDRF (nitric oxide) in diabetic renalhyperfiltration. Kidney Int, 43:1306-12.

51. Tolins JP, Shultz PJ, Raij L, Brown DM, Mauer SM. 1993. Abnormal renal hemodynamic response to reduced renal perfusion pressure in diabetic rats: role of NO. Am J Physiol, 265: F886-95.

52. Mattar AL, Fujihara CK, Ribeiro MO, de Nucci G, Zatz R. 1996. Renal effects of acute and chronic nitric oxide inhibition in experimental diabetes. Nephron, 74:136-43

53. Komers R, Allen TJ, Cooper ME. 1994. Role of endothelium-derived nitric oxide in the pathogenesis of the renal hemodynamic changes of experimental diabetes. Diabetes, 43:1190-1197.

54. Wilcox CS, Welch WJ, Murad F, Gross SS, Taylor G, Levi R, Schmidt HH. 1992. Nitric oxide synthase in macula densa regulates glomerular capillary pressure. Proc Natl Acad Sci, 89: 11993-11997.

55. Komers R, Oyama TT, Chapman JG, Allison KM, Anderson S. 2000. Effects of systemic inhibition of neuronal nitric oxide synthase (NOS1) in diabetic rats. Hypertension, 35: 655-661.

56. Komers R, Lindsley JN, Oyama TT, Allison KM, Anderson S. Role of neuronal nitric oxide synthase (NOS1) in the pathogenesis of renal hemodynamic changes in diabetes. Submitted.

57. Blantz RC, Peterson OW, Gushwa L, Tucker BJ. 1982. Effect of modest hyperglycemia on tubuloglomerular feedback activity. Kidney Int, 22 (Suppl 12):S206-S212.

58. Vallon V, Blantz RC, Thomson S. 1995. Homeostatic efficiency of tubuloglomerular feedback is reduced in established diabetes mellitus in rats. Am J Physiol, 269:F876-F883.

59. Vallon V, Richter K, Blantz RC, Thomson S, Osswald H. 1999. Glomerular hyperfiltration in experimental diabetes mellitus: potential role of tubular reabsorption. J Am Soc Nephrol,10:400A (Abstract).

60. Sugimoto H, Shikata K, Matsuda M, Kushiro M, Hayashi Y, Hiragushi K, Wada J, Makino H. 1998. Increased expression of endothelial cell nitric oxide synthase (ecNOS) in afferent and glomerular endothelial cells is involved in glomerular hyperfiltration of diabetic nephropathy. Diabetologia, 41: 1426-1434.

61. Veelken R, Hilgers KF, Hartner A, Haas A, Bohmer KP, Sterzel RB. 2000. Nitric oxide synthase isoforms and glomerular hyperfiltration in early diabetic nephropathy. J Amer Soc Nephrol, 11: 71-79.

62. Sugimoto H, Shikata K, Wada J, Horiuchi S, Makino H. 1999. Advanced glycation end products-cytokine-nitric oxide sequence pathway in the development of diabetic nephropathy: aminoguanidine ameliorates the overexpression of tumour necrosis factor-alpha and inducible nitric oxide synthase in diabetic rat glomeruli. Diabetologia, 42:878-886.

63. De Vriese, R. Tilton, R. Vanholder, N. Lameire. 1999. Hyperfiltration and albuminuria in diabetes: role of vascular endothelial growth factor (VEGF). J Am Soc Nephrol, 10: 677A (Abstract).

64. Kroll J, Waltenberger J. 1999. A novel function of VEGF receptor-2 (KDR): rapid release of nitric oxide in response to VEGF-A stimulation in endothelial cells. Biochem Biophys Res Commun, 265: 636-639.

65. Jensen PK, Steven K, Blaehr H, Christiansen JS, Parving H-H. 1986. Effects of indomethacin on glomerular hemodynamics in experimental diabetes. Kidney Int, 29:490-495.

66. Mayfield RK, Margolius HS, Levine JH, Wohltmann HJ, Loadholt CB, Colwell JA. 1984. Urinary kallikrein excretion in insulin-dependent diabetes mellitus and its relationship to glycemic control. J Clin Endocrinol Metab 59:278-286.

67. Jaffa AA, Miller DH, Bailey GS, Chao J, Margolius HS, Mayfield RK. 1987. Abnormal regulation of renal kallikrein in experimental diabetes. Effects of insulin in prokallikrein synthesis and activation. J Clin Invest, 80: 1651-1659.

68. Campbell DJ, Kelly DJ, Wilkinson-Berka JL, Cooper ME, Skinner SL. 1999. Increased bradykinin and "normal" angiotensin peptide levels in diabetic Sprague-Dawley and transgenic (mRen-2)27 rats. Kidney Int, 56:211-21

69. Jaffa AA, Rust PF, Mayfield RK. 1995. Kinin, a mediator of diabetes-induced glomerular hyperfiltration. Diabetes, 44:156-160.

70. Vora JP, Oyama TT, Thompson MM, Anderson S. 1997. Interactions of the kallikrein-kinin and renin-angiotensin systems in experimental diabetes. Diabetes, 46:107-112.

71. Komers R, Cooper ME. 1995. Acute renal hemodynamic effects of ACE inhibition in diabetic hyperfiltration: role of kinins. Am J Physiol, 268:F588-F594.

72. Ballermann BJ, Skorecki KL, Brenner BM. 1984. Reduced glomerular angiotensin II receptor density in early untreated diabetes mellitus in the rat. Am J Physiol, 247:F110-F116.

73. Wilkes BM, Kaplan R, Mento PF, Aynedjian H Macica CM, Schlondorff D, Bank N. 1992. Reduced glomerular thromboxane receptor sites and vasoconstrictor responses in diabetic rats. Kidney Int, 41:992-999.

74. Christlieb AR. 1974. Renin, angiotensin and norepinephrine in alloxan diabetes. Diabetes, 23:962-970.

75. Kennefick TM, Oyama TT, Thompson MM, Vora JP, Anderson S. 1996. Enhanced renal sensitivity to angiotensin actions in diabetes mellitus in the rat. Am J Physiol, 271:F595-F602.

76. Ohishi K, Okwueze MI, Vari RC, Carmines PK. 1994. Juxtamedullary microvascular dysfunction during the hyperfiltration stage of diabetes mellitus. Am J Physiol, 267:F99-F105.

77. Anderson S, Rennke H, Brenner BM. 1992. Nifedipine versus fosinopril in uninephrectomized diabetic rats. Kidney Int, 41: 891-897.

78. Benigni A, Colosio V, Brena C, Bruzzi I, Bertani T, Remuzzi G. 1998. Unselective inhibition of endothelin receptors reduces renal dysfunction in experimental diabetes. Diabetes, 47:450-456.

79. Craven PA, Melhem MF, De Rubertis FR. 1992. Thromboxane in the pathogenesis of glomerular injury in diabetes. Kidney Int, 42:937-946.

80. Kontessis PS, Jones SL, Barrow SE, Stratton PD, Alessandrini P, De Cosmo S, Ritter JM, Viberti JC. 1993. Effect of thromboxane sythase inhibitor on renal function in diabetic nephropathy. J Lab Clin Med, 121:415-423.

81. Ishii H, Jirousek MR, Koya D, Takagi C, Xia P, Clermont A, Bursell SE, Kern TS, Ballas LM, Heath WF, Stramm LE, Feener EP, King GL. 1996. Amelioration of vascular dysfunctions in diabetic rats by an oral PKC beta inhibitor. Science, 272:728-731

82. Carmines PK, Ohishi K, Ikenaga H. 1996. Functional impairment of renal afferent arteriolar voltage-gated calcium channels in rats with diabetes mellitus. J Clin Invest, 98:2564-2571.

83. Goldfarb S, Ziyadeh FN, Kern EFO, Simmons DA. 1991. Effects of polyol-pathway inhibition and dietary myo-inositol on glomerular hemodynamic function in experimental diabetes mellitus in rats. Diabetes, 40:465-471.

84. Daniels BS, Hostetter TH. 1989. Aldose reductase inhibition and glomerular abnormalities in diabetic rats. Diabetes, 38:981-986.

85. Anderson S. 1993. Pharmacologic interventions in experimental animals. In Prevention of Progressive Chronic Renal Failure. El Nahas AM, Mallick NP, Anderson S, eds. Oxford: Oxford Univ. Press, 1993.

86. Kuchan MJ, Frangos JA. 1993. Shear stress regulates endothelin-1 release via protein kinase C and cGMP in cultured endothelial cells. Am J Physiol, 264:H150-H156.

87. Buga GM, Gold ME, Fukuto JM, Ignarro LJ. 1991. Shear stress-induced release of nitric oxide from endothelial cells grown on beads. Hypertension, 17:187-193.

88. Awolesi MA, Sessa WC, Sumpio BE. 1995. Cyclic strain upregulates nitric oxide synthesis in cultured bovine aortic endothelial cells. J Clin Invest, 96:1449-1454.

89. Ohno M, Cooke JC, Dzau VJ, Gibbons GH. 1995. Fluid shear stress induces endothelial transforming growth factor beta-1 transcription and production. Modulation by potassium-channel blockade. J Clin Invest, 95:1363-1369.

90. Nagel T, Resnick N, Atkinson WJ, Dewey CF, Jr, Gimbrone, MA, Jr. 1994. Shear stress selectively upregulates intercellular adhesion molecule-1 expression in cultured human vascular endothelial cells. J Clin Invest, 94:885-891.

91. Sugimoto H, Shikata K, Hirata K, Akiyama K, Matsuda M, Kushiro M, Hayashi Y, Miyatake N, Miyasaka M, Makino H. 1997. Increased expression of intercellular adhesion molecule-1 (ICAM-1) in dibetic rat glomeruli: glomerular hyperfiltration is a potential mechanism of ICAM-1 upregulation. Diabetes, 46:2075-2081.

92. Ott MJ, Olson JL, Ballermann BJ. 1995. Chronic *in vitro* flow promotes ultrastructural differentiation of endothelial cells. Endothelium, 3:21-30.

93. Malek AM, Gibbons GH, Dzau VJ, Izumo S. 1993. Fluid shear stress differentially modulates expression of genes encoding basic fibroblast growth factor and platelet-derived growth factor B chain in vascular endothelium. J Clin Invest 92:2013-2021.

94. Riser BL, Cortes P, Zhao X, Bernstein J, Dumler F, Narins RG. 1992. Intraglomerular pressure and mesangial stretching stimulate extracellular matrix formation in the rat. J Clin Invest, 90:1932-1943.

95. Becker BN, Yasuda T, Kondo S, Vaikunth S, Homma T, Harris RC. 1994. Mechanical stretch/relaxation stimulates a cellular renin-angiotensin system in cultured rat mesangial cells. Exp Nephrol, 6:57-66

96. Harris RC, Haralson MA, Badr KF. 1992. Continuous stretch-relaxation in culture alters rat mesangial cell morphology, growth characteristics, and metabolic activity. Lab Invest, 66:548-554.

97. Riser BL, Cortes P, Heilig C, Grondin J, Ladson-Wofford S, Patterson D, Narins RG. 1996. Cyclic stretching force selectively up-regulates transforming growth factor-ß isoforms in cultured rat mesangial cells. Am J Pathol, 148:1915-1923.

98. Cortes P, Zhao X, Riser BL, Narins RG. 1997. Role of glomerular mechanical strain in the pathogenesis of diabetic nephropathy. Kidney Int, 51:57-68.

99. Homma T, Akai Y, Burns KD, Harris RC. 1992. Activation of S6 kinase by repeated cycles of stretching and relaxation in rat glomerular mesangial cells. J Biol Chem, 267:23129-23135.

100. Yasuda T, Kondo S, Homma T, Harris RC. 1996. Regulation of extracellular matrix by mechanical stress in rat glomerular mesangial cells. J Clin Invest 98:1991-2000

101. Harris RC, Akai Y, Yasuda T, Homma T. 1995. The role of physical forces in alterations of mesangial cell function. Kidney Int 45 (Suppl 45):S17, 1995

102. Wagner CT, Durante W, Christodoulide N, Hellums JD, Schafer AI. 1997. Hemodynamic forces induce the expression of heme oxygenase in cultured vascular smooth muscle cells. J Clin Invest, 100:589-596.

103. Ricardo SD, Ding G, Eufemio M, Diamond JR. 1997. Antioxidant expression in experimental hydronephrosis: role of mechanical stretch and growth factors. Am J Physiol, 272:F789-F798.

104. Mattana J, Singhal PC. 1995. Applied pressure modulates mesangial cell proliferation and matrix synthesis. Am J Hypertension, 8:1112-1120.

105. Anderson S, Rennke HG, Garcia DL, Brenner BM. 1989. Short and long term effects of antihypertensive therapy in the diabetic rat. Kidney Int, 36:526-532.

106. Anderson S, Rennke HG, Brenner BM. 1992. Nifedipine versus fosinopril in uninephrectomized diabetic rats. Kidney Int, 41:891-897.

107. Cooper ME, Rumble JR, Allen TJ, et al. 1992. Antihypertensive therapy and experimental diabetic nephropathy. Kidney Int, 41:898-903.

108. Fujihara C, Padilha RM, Zatz R. 1992. Glomerular abnormalities in long-term experimental diabetes. Diabetes, 41:286-293.

109.   Geiger H, Bahner U, Vaaben W, et al. 1992. Effects of angiotensin-converting enzyme inhibition in diabetic rats with reduced renal function. J Lab Clin Med, 120:861-867.

110.   O'Brien R, Cooper ME, Jerums G, Doyle AE. 1993. The effects of perindopril and triple therapy in a normotensive model of diabetic nephropathy. Diabetes, 42:604-609.

111.   Brown SA, Walton CL, Crawford P, Bakris GL. 1993. Long-term effects of antihypertensive regimens on renal hemodynamics and proteinuria. Kidney Int, 43:1210-1218.

112.   Anderson S, Jung FF, Ingelfinger JR. 1993. Renal renin-angiotensin system in diabetes: functional, immunohistochemical, and molecular biologic correlations. Am J Physiol, 265:F477-F486.

113.   Remuzzi A, Perico N, Amuchastegui CS, Malanchini B, Mazerska M, Battaglia C, Bertani C, Remuzzi G. 1993. Short- and long-term effect of angiotensin II receptor blockade in rats with experimental diabetes. J Am Soc Nephrol, 4:40-49.

114.   Wolf G, Ziyadeh N. 1997. The role of angiotensin II in diabetic nephropathy: emphasis on nonhemodynamic mechanisms. Am J Kidney Dis, 29:153-163.

115.   Kasiske BL, Kalil RSN, Ma JZ, Liao M, Keane WF. 1993. Effect of antihypertensive therapy on the kidney in patients with diabetes: a meta-regression analysis. Ann Intern Med, 118:129-138.

116.   Böhlen L, de Courten M, Weidmann P. 1994. Comparative study of the effect of ACE-inhibitors and other antihypertensive agents on proteinuria in diabetic patients. Am J Hypertension, 7:84S-92S.

117.   Lewis EJ, Hunsicker LG, Bain RP, Rohde RD. 1993. The effect of angiotensin-converting-enzyme inhibition on diabetic nephropathy. New Engl J Med, 329:1456-1462.

118.   Nielsen FS, Rossing P, Gall MA, Skott P, Smidt UM, Parving H-H. 1997. Long-term effects of lisinopril and atenolol on kidney function in hypertensive NIDDM subjects with diabetic nephropathy. Diabetes, 46: 1182:-88.

119.   Tarnow L, Rossing P, Jensen C, Parving H-H. 1999. Long-term renoprotective effect of nisoldipine and lisinopril in type 1 diabetic patients with diabetic nephropathy [abstract]. J Am Soc Nephrol, 10:134A.

25. AN UPDATE ON THE ROLE OF GROWTH FACTORS IN THE DEVELOPMENT OF DIABETIC KIDNEY DISEASE

Allan Flyvbjerg, MD, DSc
Medical Research Lab. M (Diabetes and Endocrinology) and Medical Department M (Diabetes and Endocrinology), Institute of Experimental Clinical Research, University of Aarhus, Aarhus Kommunehospital, DK-8000 Aarhus C, Denmark

INTRODUCTION

Various growth factors have been proposed to be players in different areas of diabetes mellitus including a possible relationship to the characteristic changes in metabolism and development of complications. In particular, growth hormone (*GH*) and insulin-like growth factors (*IGFs*) system have a long and distinguished history with relation both to the diabetic metabolic aberration and the pathogenesis of diabetic angiopathy. The published evidence covering this area has recently been reviewed [1-3]. Further, substantial evidence has suggested that some growth factors (i.e. *GH* and *IGFs*, epidermal growth factor (*EGF*), transforming growth factor β (*TGF-β*), platelet derived growth factor (*PDGF*), tumor necrosis factor α (*TNF-α*) and fibroblastic growth factors (*FGFs*)) have conceivable effects on the development of renal complications in diabetes as reviewed in *The Kidney and Hypertension in Diabetes Mellitus, 2th Edition, 1994* [4]. The present review is an update of the topic with emphasis on *three* of the above mentioned growth factor systems and a new promising candidate, i.e. vascular endothelial growth factor (VEGF). The first part of the review presents an update for a definite role of the GH/IGF system in the pathogenesis of the renal changes in experimental diabetes with focus on the renoprotective effects of long-acting somatostatin analogues and GH-receptor antagonists. In the second and third part, an update of the literature suggesting a causal role for EGF and TGF-β in the patogenesis of diabetic renal changes is presented and in the fourth part the new evidence of VEGF being involved in the development of diabetic kidney disease is given.

GROWTH HORMONE (GH) AND INSULIN-LIKE GROWTH FACTORS (IGFs)

The GH/IGF system constitutes a complex system of peptides in the circulation, extracellular space and in most tissues. Essentially all members of the axis are present in the kidney and IGF-I mRNA and peptide have been demonstrated in collecting tubules and the thin limb of Henle's loop [5-7], specific IGF-I receptors have been demonstrated in glomeruli and tubules of the kidney [8,9] and, in addition, all six IGF binding proteins (IGFBPs) are present in the kidney [7,10-12]. Several of the components of the renal GH/IGF axis are increased in experimental diabetes and may be involved in early diabetic renal changes and possibly also in the development of long-term diabetic renal changes (for review see 13-15]. Thus, the *early* diabetic renal hypertrophy is preceded by a transient increase in kidney IGF-I content with a peak 24-48 hours after diabetes induction [16-18]. Further, IGF-I accumulation and renal hypertrophy are directly pro-portional to the blood glucose levels in rats [19]. The demonstrated increase in kidney IGF-I is not likely caused by local production, as IGF-I mRNA levels are unaltered during the phase of early kidney growth [18,20] or even decreased [21,22]. Changes in GH binding protein (GHBP), GH- and IGF-I receptor number and affinity have been investigated in early experimental diabetes and reported to be unchanged (14,23], however, in *long-term* diabetes a sustained increase in renal GHBP mRNA and IGF-I receptor mRNA is seen [14,20,22]. The possible role of IGFBPs in renal IGF-I accumulation and *early* renal growth has been examined in diabetic rats using Western ligand blotting [24]. Diabetes induction was followed by a transient local increase in a 30 kDa IGFBP species (containing IGFBP-1) in the kidney [24]. The transient increase in the IGFBPs occured in parallel with the transient increase in kidney IGF-I content and thus preceded the diabetic renal growth. In addition, an early and sustained increase in renal IGFBP-1 and IGFBP-5 mRNAs is seen in *long-term* diabetic rats with a diabetes duration for six months [7,14]. In conclusion, these experimental data indicate that GH, IGF-I, and IGFBPs are involved in the development of both early and late diabetic renal changes. Further, this knowledge has stimulated testing of existing drugs with specific action on the GH/IGF system and innovation in drug development with potential use in the treatment of diabetic nephropathy.

MANIPULATION OF THE ALTERED GH/IGF AXIS IN DIABETIC KIDNEY DISEASE

Long-acting somatostatin analogues
The hypothesis that somatostatin and its long-acting analogues could be used in the treatment of subjects with diabetes mellitus was initially based on the expected benefit of suppressing elevated circulating GH levels in order to minimize their deleterious effects on diabetic metabolic abberration and to prevent development of long-term diabetic complications. The biological half-life of native somatostatin is too short to allow its use in clinical therapy and accordingly, long-acting somatostatin analogues (e.g. octreotide and lanreotide) have been developed and opened the possiblity of performing experi-mental and clinical trials. In *short-term experimental diabetes* octreotide administration for seven days from diabetes onset completely inhibits the initial renal hypertrophy and the kidney IGF-I accumulation in rats [17]. Further, lanreotide in a dose similar to the octreotide dose given above has been demonstrated to inhibit renal glomerular growth as

well [25]. When a lower octreotide dose is used a partial inhibition of the diabetes associated renal growth is seen, which may suggest a dose dependent effect of octreotide on renal IGF-I accumulation and diabetic renal growth [26]. Series of recent experiments has shown that early intervention with somatostatin analogues after diabetes onset seems crucial for achievement of full inhibitory effects on morphological changes. If initiation of octreotide treatment is postponed as short as 3 to 9 days after diabetes induction the early diabetic renal hypertrophy is only partly inhibited, indicating that early intervention with somatostatin analogues is important [27]. Similar results were observed in a study in which octreotide treatment was initiated for 3 weeks after a period of untreated diabetes for 3 or 6 months, as a tendency only towards a reduction in renal volume was observed [28]. The effects of somatostatin analogues on circulating and local IGFBPs in diabetes have only been examined sparsely. Lanreotide has been shown to inhibit the diabetes associated increase in serum 30 kDa IGFBP species (containing IGFBP-1) in rats and further to reduce serum IGFBP-3 [25]. In addition, octreotide inhibits the increased renal levels of IGFBP-1 mRNA levels in early experimental diabetes, with no effect on hepatic IGFBP-1 mRNA levels [29]. This is in contrast to the effect of octreotide on IGFBP-1 mRNA levels in non-diabetic rats, in which a dose dependent stimulatory effect of octreotide on hepatic IGFBP-1 mRNA is seen along with unchanged renal IGFBP-1 mRNA levels [30]. Accordingly, it may be hypothesized that somatostatin analogues may prevent some of the classic early diabetic renal changes by inhibiting the renal IGF-I accumulation through mechanisms involving effects on renal IGFBPs. The effects of somatostatin analogue treatment on diabetic renal morphological and functional changes have also been examined in *long-term experimental diabetes*. Six months octreotide treatment from the day of diabetes induction is followed by significant reductions of increase in kidney weight, kidney IGF-I levels, and urinary albumin excretion (UAE) when compared to untreated diabetic rats [31]. In addition, diabetic rats treated for 5 weeks with octreotide from diabetes onset showed a reduction in renal glomerular growth [33]. However, when octreotide treatment for 14 weeks was initiated in unilaterally nephrectomized diabetic rats on the day of diabetes induction 3 days after the nephrectomy, no effect of octreotide treatment on renal hypertrophy, UAE or glomerular hyperfiltration was observed [33]. The lack of effect of octreotide treatment on renal hypertrophy in this situation may be due to the late intervention as IGF-I accumulation had already peaked in the remaining kidney following uninephrectomy [16]; or to the low octreotide dose used [16]. In studies by Igarashi et al. [34,35] octreotide treatment for 2-3 weeks was followed by diminished kidney hypertrophy and albuminuria in uninephrectomized-diabetic rats following an untreated diabetes period of 15 weeks. A recent study from our group aimed at examining the effect of 3 weeks treatment with octreotide and an angiotensin-converting enzyme inhibitor (ACEi)(captopril) either alone or in combination following 3 months of untreated diabetes [36]. Octreotide treatment alone and in combination with captopril induced a significant reduction in kidney weight compared to placebo treated diabetic animals [36]. Further, the combined treatment of octreotide and captopril was followed by a significant reduction in UAE compared to placebo treated diabetic rats giving evidence for a definite effect of the combined treatment with octreotide and captopril on manifest experimental diabetic renal changes [36].

Clinical studies of native somatostatin and its analogues and their possible effects on kidney function and hypertrophy have progressed since Vora et al. [37], using intravenous native somatostatin, observed an immediate reduction in urinary flow, renal plasma flow (RPF) and glomerular filtration rate (GFR) in control subjects and patients with insulin dependent diabetes mellitus (IDDM). Acute infusion (2 to 3 hours) of the somatostatin analogue, octreotide, to IDDM diabetic patients induced a reduction in RPF and GFR, and in addition plasma GH and glucagon decreased significantly [38]. However, in another study only a trend towards lowering GFR and no effect on serum GH was observed following octreotide infusion [39]. In more long-term studies octreotide administration for 12 weeks in eleven IDDM patients induced a significant decrease in the elevated GFR along with a reduction in total kidney volume. Three of the patients were reexamined 12 weeks after cessation of octreotide treatment, and their GFR had risen to the level at the start of the study [40]. In a recent study, the effect of lanreotide was examined in hyperfiltrating IDDM patients for a treatment period of nine months [41]. In lanreotide-treated patients, a decrease in GFR and RPF was observed after three months, with no significant difference after nine months [41]. It has to be noted, however, that only four patients were included in each of the lanreotide- and placebo-treated groups [41]. So far no published clinical studies have yet appeared on the possible long-term effects of somatostatin analogues on UAE in IDDM patients.

GH-receptor antagonists
Recently, a series of highly specific antagonists of the GH action has been developed for the potential therapeutic use in various conditions, including diabetes mellitus. Initially it was shown that alteration of single amino acids in the third α-helix of bovine (b)GH (residues 109-126) results in a GH antagonist [42-44]. *In vitro* experiments showed that this new group of GH antagonists binds to the GH receptor with the same affinity as native GH, but *in vivo* a phenotypic dwarf animal characterized by low circulating IGF-I levels and a proportional body composition develops when the GH antagonist is expressed in transgenic mice [42-44]. Recent studies have reported renoprotective effects of two of these GH antagonists in long-term diabetic transgenic mice that express the GH antagonist (bGH-G119R or hGH-G120R) [45-47]. Compared with transgenic diabetic mice expressing wild-type bGH or bGH, the diabetic mice expressing GH antagonists showed lesser glomerular damage [45,46], no increase in total urine protein [45], no glomerular hypertrophy [47] and no increase in glomerular $\alpha1$ type IV collagen mRNA levels [47]. The inhibitory effects of GH antagonists in transgenic mice were seen without alteration in glycemic control as similar levels in blood glucose, insulin and Hb_{A1c} were seen in the different diabetic animals expressing wild-type bGH, GH antagonists or bGH [45,46]. Theoretically, however, GH antagonist transgenic mice may be less susceptible to diabetic renal changes because of effects of GH receptor blockade and low circulating IGF-I levels before the induction of diabetes. Furthermore, the renal effects might be mediated indirectly through the low serum IGF-I levels *per se* at the time of diabetes induction. In order to elucidate the potential usefulness of GH

antagonists as a therapeutic agent in diabetic kidney disease in terms of tolerance and specificity, we recently performed a series of studies with exogenous administration of a long-acting GH antagonist (G120K-PEG) to diabetic mice [48-50]. In the initial experiment non-diabetic and STZ-diabetic mice were treated with the GH antagonist for one month after diabetes induction [48]. In GH antagonist-treated diabetic mice, renal IGF-I accumulation, renal enlargement, and glomerular hypertrophy were abolished, and further the diabetes-associated increase in UAE was reduced [48]. These effects were achieved through a specific mechanism at the renal GH receptor level, as no effect of treatment was seen on changes in body weight, food consumption, metabolic control, serum GH or IGF-I [48]. The same results were recently confirmed in non-obese diabetic (NOD) mice [49]. In a recently conducted experiment the effect of GH antagonism alone or in combination with ACEi treatment was examined on manifest renal changes in NOD mice [50]. Preliminary results showed that GH antagonist treatment was equally potent to ACEi treatment in reducing UAE [50]. No *clinical studies* have yet appeared on the effects of this new group of GH-receptor antagonists on metabolism and diabetic complications in diabetic patients.

EPIDERMAL GROWTH FACTOR (EGF)

The kidney is one of the main sites of EGF synthesis and recent studies have suggested that the kidney is also a target organ of EGF [51]. The presence of EGF receptors has been demonstrated in several segments of the nephron [52], and EGF administered *in vivo* systemically or directly into the renal artery increases urine flow and urinary sodium and potassium excretion [53]. The demonstration of acute effects of EGF on renal function [54,55] opens some intriguing possibilities for a physiological role of EGF in the kidney. Although one study [51] reported reduced urinary EGF excretion after reduction of renal mass, others reported increased urinary EGF excretion [56], increased renal EGF synthesis and a transiently increased amount of immunoreactive EGF in distal kidney tubules after unilateral nephrectomy [57].

In *experimental diabetes* a possible role for EGF in the *early* renal enlargement has been proposed. In a study by Guh et al. [58] a pronounced elevation in diurnal urine EGF excretion was seen, while no significant change was observed in renal EGF within the first 7 days after induction of diabetes. These findings were confirmed in a recent study by Gilbert et al. [59] where unchanged levels of kidney and plasma EGF were reported, within the first week after induction of diabetes, along with a three fold increase in urinary EGF excretion. In addition, renal EGF mRNA as measured both by Northern blotting and in situ hybridization, was increased by 4-8 times [59]. These studies implicate that EGF may play a role as a renotropic factor in early experimental diabetes.

So far no studies have been published on changes in the renal EGF content or EGF excretion in *long-term experimental diabetes*. However, several cross-sectional *clinical studies* have studied the possible role of EGF in diabetic nephropathy by measuring the urinary excretion of EGF in IDDM patients with and without incipient/overt nephropathy [60-63] and in NIDDM patients with incipient nephropathy

[64]. In general, reduced urinary excretion of EGF is found in patients with elevated UAE in comparison with non-diabetic controls [60,61]. A significant inverse correlation between urinary excretion of EGF and UAE was reported in two studies [60,61], while absent in one study [62]. A consistent finding is, however, that urinary excretion of EGF correlates positively with GFR [60,62] and creatinine clearance [63]. In a study in NIDDM patients with incipient diabetic nephropathy, the effect of an ACE-inhibitor (enalapril) and an calcium antagonist (nitrendipine) on UAE and urinary EGF excretion was examined [64]. Interestingly, enalapril significantly reduced UAE and increased urinary EGF excretion, while nitrendipine had no significant effect on any of these parameters [64]. These studies demonstrate that the urinary excretion of EGF diminished with increasing nephron impairment, and that renal tubular function, as judged by urinary EGF excretion, is reduced early in the development of diabetic kidney disease. The decrease in urinary EGF excretion with decreasing renal function is not specific for the renal changes seen in diabetic patients as it is also seen in patients with various *non-diabetic glomerulopathies* [65].

TRANSFORMING GROWTH FACTOR-β (TGF-β)

TGF-β is a prominent member of a family of cell regulatory proteins and is unique among growth factors in its broad effects on extracellular matrix. TGF-β is a 25 kDa polypeptide, synthesized as an inactive precursor protein which may bind to a 125 kDa TGF-β binding protein, and is proteolytically changed into its active form. The kidney is both producing TGF-β and a target of TGF-β action, as both mRNA TGF-β, the active protein, and TGF-β receptors have been demonstrated in all cell types of the glomerulus [66-68] and by proximal tubule renal cells [69,70]. *In vitro*, TGF-β has been shown to modulate extracellular matrix production and interestingly both glomerular mesangial and epithelial cells increase synthesis of extracellular matrix proteins including protoglycans, fibronectin, type IV collagen and laminin in response to TGF-β [71-73]. In addition, TGF-β inhibits the synthesis of collagenases and stimulates tissue production of metalloproteinase inhibitors [74-76]. Both these mechanisms could lead to a reduced degradation of ECM and possibly contribute to matrix accumulation. Evidence has been published recently for TGF-β playing a role in different forms of kidney diseases characterized by changes in structure and ECM. In cultured glomerular cells obtained from immunologically induced glomerulonephritis, increased amounts of active TGF-β can be detected [77]. Furthermore, both the administration of an antibody raised against

TGF-β [78] or decorin [79], a natural inhibitor of TGF-β, to glomerulonephritic rats suppresses glomerular matrix production and prevents matrix accumulation in injured glomeruli. In addition, there is evidence for TGF-β playing a role in the development of *diabetic nephropathy*. High glucose concentrations increase TGF-β1 mRNA levels in both cultured mesangial cells and proximal tubular cells in vitro [66-70]. Further, the elevated glucose levels in vitro stimulate TGF-β gene expression and bioactivity, cellular hypertrophy and collagen transcription in proximal tubules [69] in addition to increased mesangial production of heparan sulfate proteoglycan [80].

In addition to the in vitro experiments mentioned above interesting experiments have been published recently on changes in renal TGF-β in *early experimental diabetes* in vivo. In a study performed in STZ-diabetic rats, an increase in glomerular TGF-β mRNA was reported as early as 24 hours after the onset of hyperglycaemia [81]. The animals were followed for up to two weeks with a sustained rise for the whole period and a three-fold increase in glomerular TGF-β levels could be demonstrated by use of immunohistochemistry [81]. Intensive insulin treatment to normalize blood glucose levels attenuated the rise in glomerular TGF-β expression [81]. Increased renal levels of TGF-β mRNA in the early course of diabetes associated renal hypertrophy have also been described both in the NOD mouse [82,83] and the diabetic BB rat [82]. In addition, a sustained increase in glomerular TGF-β mRNA levels in *long-term STZ-diabetic rats* with a diabetes duration for up to 24 weeks has been described [66]. Finally, in a non-diabetic transgenic mouse model overexpressing glomerular TGF-β1, accumulation of extracellular matrix components (i.e. laminin and collagen IV) is observed [84].

Two *clinical studies* have been published dealing with changes in the renal expression of the TGF-β system [85,86]. Initially increased TGF-β immunostaining was described in glomeruli obtained from diabetic subjects [85]. This observation was confirmed and further extended in a recent study, in which increased glomerular and tubulointerstitial levels of all three TGF-β isoforms were reported in diabetic nephropathy, but also in several other conditions characterized by accumulation of extracellular matrix (i.e. IgA nephropathy, focal and segmental glomerulosclerosis, crescentic glomerulonephritis and lupus nephritis)[86]. Further, a positive correlation between TGF-β, fibronectin and plasminogen activator inhibitor-1 levels in glomeruli and tubulointerstitium was reported [86]. These studies support the hypothesis that glucose induced rise in renal TGF-β expression and peptide in the kidney may be responsible for some of the renal changes that precede the development of diabetic nephropathy.

MANIPULATION OF THE ALTERED TGF-β AXIS IN DIABETIC KIDNEY DISEASE

Neutralizing antibodies
Data supporting the hypothesis that the glucose induced rise in renal TGF-β expression and peptide may be responsible for some of the renal changes that follow the development of diabetic nephropathy, have been published recently in studies using neutralizing antibodies. *In vitro* the glucose mediated increase in type IV collagen synthesis in mesangial cells is dependent on the autocrine action of TGF-β1, as neutralizing antibodies to TGF-β attenuate the rise [87]. Further, in a recent study *in vivo*, administration of a neutralizing TGF-β1,2,3 antibody to STZ-diabetic mice for nine days attenuated the elevated renal TGF-β1 and TGF-β Type II receptor mRNA levels and reduced both the diabetes associated renal/glomerular growth and enhanced renal expression of collagen IV and fibronectin [88].

Angiotensin converting enzyme (ACE) inhibition

It has been suggested that activation of the renal TGF-β system in diabetes may be mediated, besides a direct stimulatory effect of hyperglycaemia *per se*, through activation of the renin-angiotensin system, because exposure of mesangial cells *in vitro* to angiotensin II stimulates the expression of TGF-β and extracellular matrix proteins [89]. Further a recent study examined the effect of an ACEi (captopril) on high-glucose induced changes in the TGF-β system and growth in LLC-PK$_1$ cells, a porcine kidney cell line analogous to the proximal tubule cell [90]. In this cell system high glucose increased TGF-β1 mRNA, TGF-β Type receptor I and II protein expressions and cellular hypertrophy, while cellular mitogenesis was inhibited. Captopril dose-dependently decreased TGF-β Type I and II receptor protein expressions and cellular hypertrophy, increased cellular hyperplasia while TGF-β mRNA was unchanged [90]. In a recent *in vivo* study the effect of ACE inhibition (ramipril) on the interstitial expression of TGF-β1 and matrix accumulation was examined in STZ-diabetic rats [91]. Using different techniques it was shown that the diabetes associated tubularinterstitial increase in TGF-β1 and collagen IV (both mRNA and protein) was prevented by ACE inhibition. Further, a recent study from our group has aimed at examining the possible effect of ACE-inhibition on the intrarenal (i.e. in particular the glomerular) changes in all TGF-β isoforms (TGF-β 1,2,3) and TGF-β receptors (Type I, Type II, Type III) in experimental diabetes [92]. STZ-diabetic and non-diabetic rats were treated for two and four weeks with enalapril or placebo. Enalapril partially prevented the diabetes associated renal hypertrophy and fully the increase in 24h UAE. Further, enalapril treatment decreased the glomerular levels of TGF-β Type I and TGF-β Type III receptor isoforms to values below non-diabetic control level while treatment decreased the glomerular TGF-β Type II receptor level to almost undetectable levels. The glomerular expression of the TGF-β isoforms were not dramatically influenced by treatment. These findings suggest that the TGF-β axis operating through a complex intrarenal system, may be a significant mediator of the renal changes observed in experimental diabetes. Moreover, ACE inhibition has pronounced inhibitory effects on the elevated levels of the TGF-β receptors required for intracellular signaling through this growth factor system. These findings suggest a possible new mechanism of action for ACEi's.

Protein kinase C β (PKC β) inhibition.

Based on *in vitro* experiments, it has been proposed that high glucose-induced PKC activation in glomerular cells is followed by increased TGF-β activity. In a recent study, antioxidant administration by alfa-tocopherol to mesangial cells exposed to high glucose blocked the increase in PKC, TGF-β and matrix accumulation, but without altering the effect of TGF-β induced matrix production [93]. *In vivo* experiments with administration of a specific PKC β isoform inhibitor (LY 333531) to STZ-diabetic rats for three months abolished the diabetes associated increase in glomerular TGF-β1 mRNA, matrix accumulation and UAE, suggesting that hyperglycaemia-induced PKC β activation might be involved in the mediation of abnormal glomerular and mesangial functions, such as overproduction of TGF-β and matrix components [94]. However, in a recent study from our group, administration of the same specific PKC β isoform inhibitor (LY

333531) for one month to STZ-diabetic rats showed renoprotective effects, without effect on any components of the intrarenal TGF-β system [95]. In contrast to the study referenced above [94], our study included a full characterization of changes in all TGF-β isoforms and receptors, thus indicating that the renoprotective effects of PKC β inhibition *in vivo* may not strictly be mediated through the TGF-β system.

Advanced glycation endproduct (AGE) inhibition
In a recent study in an *experimental diabetic* NIDDM model renal TGF-β1 mRNA and glomerular TGF-β1 immunoreactivity was reported to be elevated over a diabetes duration of 9 to 68 weeks [96]. Oral administration of a new AGE-inhibitor (OPB-9195) for up to 68 weeks reduced the increased renal levels of TGF-β1 mRNA and protein to normal, along with normalization of diabetes-associated renal collagen IV accumulation and a diminuation of increased UAE [96].

VASCULAR ENDOTHELIAL GROWTH FACTOR (VEGF)
The group of VEGFs consists of at least five different isoforms of homodimeric glycoproteins [97]. Further, at least two high-affinity receptors (VEGFR-1 and -2) have been described [98]. Essentially all VEGF isoforms and both receptors are expressed in the kidney. *In vitro* mesangial cells, glomerular endothelial cells, vascular smooth muscle cells, proximal and distal tubular cells are capable of producing VEGF [99-102]. The today most potent stimulator of VEGF is hypoxia [103], but in mesangial cells angiotensin II has been shown to stimulate VEGF, a process that is blocked by coincubation of losartan, an angiotensin 1 receptor antagonist [102].

In the recent study in the *experimental diabetic* NIDDM model described above [96], renal VEGF mRNA and glomerular VEGF immunoreactivity was reported to be elevated over a diabetes duration of 9 to 68 weeks [96]. In another study, changes in renal VEGF levels were described in STZ-diabetic rats with a diabetes duration of 3 and 32 weeks [104]. VEGF mRNA and protein were localized mainly to the glomerular epithelial cells and VEGFR-2 mRNA mainly to glomerular endothelial cells [104]. VEGF mRNA and peptide were increased in diabetic animals at both timepoints examined, while the expression of VEGFR-2 and VEGF receptor binding were increased only at 3 weeks [104].

In one *clinical study* serum VEGF levels in children and adolescents with IDDM were not different from the levels in non-diabetic controls [105]. Further, another clinical study describing VEGF expression in renal biopsy specimens from patients with different kidney diseases, included a small number of 5 patients with diabetic nephropathy [106]. The results from these preliminary data indicated that glomerular VEGF expression was highly expressed in the patients with mildest sclerotic changes, while decreased with increasing sclerosis [106].

MANIPULATION OF THE ALTERED VEGF AXIS IN DIABETIC KIDNEY DISEASE

Neutralizing antibodies

Data supportive for the hypothesis that an enhanced renal VEGF system may be responsible for the diabetes-associated renal changes, have recently been published in an elegant study using an anti-VEGF monoclonal neutralizing antibody in STZ-diabetic rats [107]. Six weeks treatment with the neutralizing VEGF antibody fully abolished the diabetes-associated   hyperfiltration and partially the increase in UAE [107]. VEGF antibody treatment had no effect on metabolic control in diabetic animals and no renal effects of treatment were seen in non-diabetic controls [107].

Advanced glycation endproduct (AGE) inhibition

In the study by Tsuchida et al. described above in an animal model of NIDDM [96], it was shown that long-term AGE-inhibitor (OPB-9195) treatment of diabetic animals abolished the enhance renal VEGF mRNA and glomerular VEGF immunoreactivity along with renoprotection [96].

SUMMARY AND CONCLUSIONS

This review has collected recent facets of evidence for the significance of growth factors in the development of diabetic kidney disease. The knowledge we have today indicates that growth factors, through a complex system may be responsible for both *early* and *long-term* renal changes in experimental diabetes. Further insight into these processes may be useful in the future development of new antagonists for trial in the treatment of diabetic kidney disease.

Acknowledgements

The work was supported by the Danish Medical Research Council (#9700592), The Danish Kidney Foundation, the Ruth König Petersen Foundation, the Danish Diabetes Association, the Novo Foundation, the Nordic Insulin Foundation, the Johanne and Aage Louis Petersen Foundation, the Institute of Experimental Clinical Research, University of Aarhus, Denmark and the Aarhus University-Novo Nordisk Center for Research in Growth and Regeneration (Danish Medical Research Council Grant #9600822).

REFERENCES

1.   Flyvbjerg A, Frystyk J, Sillesen IB, Ørskov H. Growth hormone and insulin-like growth factor I in experimental and human diabetes. In: Alberti KGMM, Krall LP (Eds), Diabetes Annual/6, Elsevier Science Publishers B.V., Amsterdam 1991; pp. 562-590.
2.   Growth hormone and insulin-like growth factor I in human and experimental diabetes. Flyvbjerg A, Ørskov H, Alberti KGMM (Eds), John Wiley & Sons, Chichester 1993; pp. 1-322.

3. International symposium on glucose metabolism and growth factors. Flyvbjerg A, Alberti KGMM, Froesch ER, De Meyts P, von zür Mühlen A, Ørskov H (Eds), Metabolism 1995; 44 [Suppl 4]: pp. 1-123.

4. Flyvbjerg A, Nielsen B, Skjærbæk C, Frystyk J, Grønbæk H, Ørskov H. Roles of growth factors in diabetic kidney disease. In: Mogensen CE (Ed), The Kidney and Hypertension in Diabetes Mellitus, 2nd Edition, Kluwer Academic Publishers, Boston, Dordrecht, London, 1994, pp. 233-243.

5. Bortz JD, Rotwein P, DeVol D, Bechtel PJ, Hansen VA, Hammerman MR. Focal expression of insulin-like growth factor I in rat kidney collecting duct. J Cell Biol 1988; 107: 811-819.

6. Flyvbjerg A, Marshall SM, Frystyk J, Rasch R, Bornfeldt KE, Arnqvist H, Jensen PK, Pallesen G, Ørskov H. Insulin-like growth factor I in initial renal hypertrophy in potassium-depleted rats. Am J Physiol 1992; 262: F1023-F1031.

7. Landau D, Chin E, Bondy C, Domene H, Roberts CT, Grønbæk H, Flyvbjerg A, LeRoith D. Expression of insulin-like growth factor binding proteins in the rat kidney: Effects of long-term diabetes. Endocrinology 1995; 136: 1835-1842.

8. Arnqvist HJ, Ballermann BJ, King GL. Receptors for and effects of insulin and IGF-I in rat glomerular mesangial cells. Am J Physiol 1988; 254: C411-C416.

9. Pillion DJ, Haskell JF, Meezan E . Distinct receptors for insulin-like growth factor I in rat renal glomeruli and tubules. Am J Physiol 1988; 255: E504-E512.

10. Chin E, Bondy C. Insulin-like growth factor system gene expression in the human kidney. J Clin Endocrinol Metab 1992; 75: 962-968.

11. Shimasaki S, Shimonaka M, Zhang HP, Ling N. Identification of five different insulin-like growth factor binding proteins (IGFBPs) from adult rat serum and molecular cloning of a novel IGFBP-5 in rat and human. J Biol Chem 1991; 266: 10646-10653.

12. Shimasaki S, Gao L, Shimonaka M, Ling N. Isolation and molecular cloning of insulin-like growth factor-binding protein-6. Mol Endocrinol 1991; 5: 938-948.

13. Flyvbjerg A. The growth hormone/insulin-like growth factor axis in the kidney: Aspects in relation to chronic renal failure. J Pediatr Endocrinol 1994; 7: 85-92.

14. Flyvbjerg A, Landau D, Domene H, Hernandez L, Grønbæk H, LeRoith D. The role of growth hormone, insulin-like growth factors (IGFs), and IGF-Binding proteins in experimental diabetic kidney disease. Metabolism 1995; 44: 67-71.

15. Flyvbjerg A. Role of growth hormone, insulin-like growth factors (IGFs) and IGF-binding proteins in the renal complications of diabetes. Kidney Int 1997; 52 [Suppl 60]: S12-S19.

16. Flyvbjerg A, Thorlacius-Ussing O, Næraa R, Ingerslev J, Ørskov H. Kidney tissue somatomedin C and initial renal growth in diabetic and uninephrectomized rats. Diabetologia 1988; 31: 310-314.

17. Flyvbjerg A, Frystyk J, Thorlacius-Ussing O, Ørskov H. Somatostatin analogue administration prevents increase in kidney somatomedin C and initial renal growth in diabetic and uninephrectomized rats. Diabetologia 1989; 32: 261-265.

18. Flyvbjerg A, Bornfeldt KE, Marshall SM, Arnqvist HJ, Ørskov H. Kidney IGF-I mRNA in initial renal hypertrophy in experimental diabetes in rats. Diabetologia 1990; 33: 334-338.

19. Flyvbjerg A, Ørskov H. Kidney tissue insulin-like growth factor I and initial renal growth in diabetic rats: relation to severity of diabetes. Acta Endocrinol (Copenh) 1990; 122: 374-378.

20. Werner H, Shen Orr Z, Stannard B, Burguera B, Roberts CT Jr, LeRoith D. Experimental diabetes increases insulin-like growth factor I and II receptor concentration and gene expression in kidney. Diabetes 1990; 39: 1490-1497.

21. Bornfeldt KE, Arnqvist HJ, Enberg B, Mathews LS, Norstedt G. Regulation of insulin-like growth factor-I and growth hormone receptor gene expression by diabetes and nutritional state in rat tissues. J Endocrinol 1989; 122: 651-656.

22. Weiss O, Anner H, Nephesh I, Alayoff A, Bursztyn M, Raz I. Insulin-like growth factor I (IGF-I) and IGF-I receptor gene expression in the kidney of chronically hypoinsulinemic rat and hyperinsulinemic rat. Metabolism 1995; 44: 982-986.

23. Marshall SM, Flyvbjerg A, Frystyk J, Korsgaard L, Ørskov H. Renal insulin-like growth factor I and growth hormone receptor binding in experimental diabetes and after unilateral nephrectomy in the rat. Diabetologia 1991; 34: 632-639.

24. Flyvbjerg A, Kessler U, Dorka B, Funk B, Ørskov H, Kiess W. Transient increase in renal insulin-like growth factor binding proteins during initial kidney hypertrophy in experimental diabetes in rats. Diabetologia 1992; 35: 589-593.

25. Grønbæk H, Nielsen B, Frystyk J, Flyvbjerg A, Ørskov H. Effect of lanreotide, a somatostatin analogue, on diabetic renal hypertrophy, kidney and serum IGF-I and IGF binding proteins. Exp Nephrol 1996; 4: 295-303.

26. Steer KA, Sochor M, Kunjara S, Doepfner W, McLean P. The effect of a somatostatin analogue (SMS 201-995) on the concentration of phosphoribosyl pyrophosphate and the activity of the pentose phosphate pathway in the early renal hypertrophy of experimental diabetes in the rat. Biochem Med Metab Biol 1988; 39: 226-233.

27. Grønbæk H, Nielsen B, Frystyk J, Ørskov H, Flyvbjerg A. Effect of octreotide on experimental diabetic renal and glomerular growth: Importance of early intervention. J Endocrinol 1995; 147: 95-102.

28. Grønbæk H, Nielsen B, Østerby R, Harris AG, Ørskov H, Flyvbjerg A. Effect of octreotide and insulin on manifest renal and glomerular hypertrophy and urinary albumin excretion in long-term experimental diabetes in rats. Diabetologia 1995; 38: 135-144.

29. Weiss O, Rubinger D, Nephesh I, Moshe R, Raz I. The influence of octreotide on the IGF system gene expression in the kidney of diabetic rats [Abstract]. Diabetologia 1995; 38: A206.

30. Flyvbjerg A, Schuller AGP, van Neck JW, Groffen C, Ørskov H, Drop SLS. Stimulation of hepatic insulin-like growth factor binding protein-1 and -3 gene expression by octreotide in rats. J Endocrinol 1995; 147: 545-551.

31. Flyvbjerg A, Marshall SM, Frystyk J, Hansen KW, Harris AG, Ørskov H. Octreotide administration in diabetic rats: effects on renal hypertrophy and urinary albumin excretion. Kidney Int 1992; 41: 805-812.

32. Iwasaki S. Octreotide suppresses the kidney weight and glomerular hypertrophy in diabetic rats. Nippon Jinzo Gakkai Shi 1993; 35: 247-255.

33. Muntzel M, Hannedouche T, Niesor R, Noel LH, Souberbielle JC, Lacour B, Drueke T. Long-term effects of a somatostatin analogue on renal haemodynamics and hypertrophy in diabetic rats. Clin Sci 1992; 83: 575-581.

34. Igarashi K, Ito S, Shibata A. Effect of a somatostatin analogue (SMS 201-995) on urinary albumin excretion in streptozotocin-induced diabetic rats. J Japan Diab Soc 1990; 33: 531-538.

35. Igarashi K, Nakazawa A, Tani N, Yamazaki M, Ito S, Shibata A. Effect of a somatostatin analogue (SMS 201-995) on renal function and excretion in diabetic rats. J Diab Compl 1991; 5: 181-183.

36. Grønbæk H, Vogel I, Lancranjan I, Flyvbjerg A, Ørskov H. Effect of octreotide, captopril, or insulin on manifest long-term experimental diabetic renal changes. Kidney Int 1998; 53: 173-180.

37.   Vora J, Owens DR, Luzio SD, Atiea J, Ryder R, Hayes TM. Renal response to intravenous somatostatin in insulin-dependent diabetic patients and normal subjects. J Clin Endocrinol Metab 1987; 64: 975-979.

38.   Pedersen MM, Christensen SE, Christiansen JS, Pedersen EB, Mogensen CE, Ørskov H. Acute effects of a somatostatin analogue on kidney function in type 1 diabetic patients. Diab Med 1990; 7: 304-309.

39.   Krempf M, Ranganathan S, Remy JP, Charbonnel B, Guillon J. Effect of a long acting somatostatin analogue (SMS 201-995) on high glomerular filtration rate in insulin dependent diabetic patients. Int J Clin Pharmacol Ther Toxicol 1990; 28: 309-311.

40.   Serri O, Beauregard H, Brazeau P, Abribat T, Lambert J, Harris A, Vachon L. Somatostatin analogue, octreotide, reduces increased glomerular filtration rate and kidney size in insulin-dependent diabetes. JAMA 1991; 265: 888-892.

41.   Jacobs ML, Derkx FH, Stijnen T, Lamberts SW, Weber RF. Effect of long-acting somatostatin analog (somatulin) on renal hyperfiltration in patients with IDDM. Diabetes Care 1997; 20: 632-636.

42.   Chen WY, Wight DC, Wagner TE, Kopchick JJ. Expression of a mutated bovine growth hormone gene suppresses growth of transgenic mice. Proc Natl Acad Sci USA 1990; 87: 5061-5065.

43.   Chen WY, Wight DC, Chen N-Y, Coleman TA, Wagner TE, Kopchick JJ. Mutations in the third α-helix of bovine growth hormone dramatically affect its intracellular distribution in vitro and growth enhancement in transgenic mice. J Biol Chem 1991; 266: 2252-2258.

44.   Chen WY, White ME, Wagner TE, Kopchick JJ. Functional antagonism between endogenous mouse growth hormone (GH) and a GH analog results in dwarf transgenic mice. Endocrinology 1991; 129: 1402-1408.

45.   Chen N-Y, Chen WY, Bellush L, Yang C-W, Striker LJ, Striker GE, Kopchick JJ. Effects of streptozotocin treatment in growth hormone (GH) and GH antagonist transgenic mice. Endocrinology 1995; 136: 660-667.

46.   Chen N-Y, Chen WY, Kopchick JJ. A growth hormone antagonist protects mice against streptozotocin induced glomerulosclerosis even in the presence of elevated levels of glucose and glycated hemoglobin. Endocrinology 1996; 137: 5163-5165.

47.   Liu Z-H, Striker LJ, Phillips C, Chen N-Y, Chen Y, Kopchick JJ, Striker GE. Growth hormone expression is required for the development of diabetic glomerulosclerosis in mice. Kidney Int 1995; 48 [Suppl 51]: S37-S38.

48.   Flyvbjerg A, Bennett WF, Rasch R, Kopchick JJ, Scarlett JA. Inhibitory effect of a growth hormone receptor antagonist (G120K-PEG) on renal enlargement, glomerular hypertrophy and urinary albumin excretion in experimental diabetes in mice. Diabetes 1999; 48: 377-382.

49.   Segev Y, Landau D, Rasch R, Flyvbjerg A, Phillip M. Growth hormone receptor antagonism prevents early renal changes in nonobese diabetic mice. J Am Soc Nephrol 1999; 10: 2374-2381.

50.   Flyvbjerg A, Rasch R. Effect of growth hormone (GH) receptor antagonist (G120K-PEG) treatment on manifest renal changes in non obese diabetic (NOD) mice (Abstract). J Am Soc Nephrol 1999; 10: A3444.

51.   Olsen PS, Nexø E, Poulsen SS, Hansen HF, Kirkegaard P. Renal origin of rat urinary epidermal growth factor. Reg Pept 1984; 10: 37-45.

52.   Gustavson B, Cowley G, Smith JA, Ozanne B. Cellular localization of human epidermal growth factor receptor. Cell Biol Int Rep 1984; 8: 649-658.

53.   Scoggins BA, Butkus A, Coghlan JP, et al. In vivo cardiovascular, renal and endocrine effects of epidermal growth factor in sheep. In: Labrie F, Prouix L (Eds), Endocrinology, Elsevier Science Publishers B.V., Amsterdam 1984; pp. 573-576.

54.   Stanton RC, Seifter JL. Epidermal growth factor rapidly activates the hexose monophosphate shunt in kidney cells. Am J Physiol 1988; 253: C267-C271.

55.   Vehaskari VM, Hering-Smith KS, Moskowitz DW, Weirer ID, Hamm LL. Effect of epidermal growth factor on sodium transport in the cortical collecting tubules. Am J Physiol 1989; 256: F803-F809.

56.   Jørgensen PE, Kamper A-L, Munck O, Strandgaard S, Nexø E. Urinary excretion of epidermal growth factor in living human kidney doners and their recipients. Eur J Clin Invest 1995; 25: 442-446.

57.   Jennische E, Andersson G, Hansson HA. Epidermal growth factor is expressed by cells in the distal tubulus during postnephrectomy renal growth. Acta Physiol Scand 1987; 129: 449-450.

58.   Guh JY, Lai YH, Shin SJ, Chuang LY, Tsai JH. Epidermal growth factor in renal hypertrophy in streptozotocin-diabetic rats. Nephron 1991; 59: 641-647.

59.   Gilbert RE, Cox A, McNally PG, Wu LL, Dziadek M, Cooper ME, Jerums G. Increased epidermal growth factor in experimental diabetes related renal growth. Diabetologia 1997; 40: 778-785.

60.   Mathiesen ER, Nexø E, Hommel E, Parving H-H. Reduced urinary excretion of epidermal growth factor in incipient and overt diabetic nephropathy. Diab Med 1989; 6: 121-126.

61.   Dagogo-Jack S, Marshall SM, Kendall-Taylor P, Alberti KGMM. Urinary excretion of human epidermal growth factor in the various stages of diabetic nephropathy. Clin Endocrinol (Oxf) 1989; 31: 167-173.

62.   Meulen CG, Bilo HJ, van Kamp GJ, Gans RO, Donker AJ. Urinary epidermal growth factor excretion is correlated to renal function loss per se and not to the degree of diabetic renal failure. Netherlands J Med 1994; 44: 12-17.

63.   Lev-Ran A, Hwang DL, Miller JD, Josefsberg Z. Excretion of epidermal growth factor (EGF) in diabetes. Clin Chim Acta 1990; 192: 201-206.

64.   Josefsberg Z, Ross SA, Lev-Ran A, Hwang DL. Effects of enalapril and nitrendipine on the excretion of epidermal growth factor and albumin in hypertensive NIDDM patients. Diab Care 1995; 15: 690-693.

65.   Mattila AL, Pasternack A, Viinikka L, Perheentupa B. Subnormal concentrations of urinary epidermal growth factor in patients with kidney disease. J Clin Endocrinol Metab 1986; 62: 1180-1183.

66.   Nakamura T, Fukui M, Ebihara E, Osada S, Nagaoka I, Tomino Y, Koide H. mRNA expression of growth factors in glomeruli from diabetic rats. Diabetes 1993; 42: 450-456.

67.   Ziyadeh FN, Chen Y, Davila A, Goldfarb S. Self limited stimulation of mesangial cell growth in high glucose: autocrine activation of TGF-β reduces proliferation but increases mesangial matrix. Kidney Int 1992; 42: 647-656.

68.   Choi ME, Eung-Gook K, Ballerman BJ. Rat mesangial cell hypertrophy in response to transforming growth factor β1. Kidney Int 1993; 44: 948-958.

69.   Ziyadeh FN, Snipes ER, Watanabe M, Alvarey RJ, Goldfarb S, Haverty TP. High glucose induces cell hypertrophy and stimulates collagen gene transcription in proximal tubule. Am J Physiol 1990; 259: F704-F714.

70.   Rocco MV, Chen Y, Goldfarb S, Ziyadeh FN. Elevated glucose stimulates TGF-β gene expression and bioactivity in proximal tubules. Kidney Int 1992; 41: 107-114.

71.   Nakamura T, Miller D, Rouslahti E, Border WA. Production of extracellular matrix by glomerular epithelial cells is regulated by transforming growth factor β1. Kidney Int 1992; 41: 1213-1221.

72.   Humes HD, Nakamura T, Cieslinski DA, Miller D, Emmons RV, Border WA. Role of protoglycans and cytoskeleton in the effects of TGF-β1 on renal proximal tubule cells. Kidney Int 1993; 43: 575-584.

73.   Roberts AB, McCune BK, Sporn MB. TGF-β1: Regulation of extracellular matrix. Kidney Int 1992; 41: 557-559.

74.   Davies M, Thomas GJ, Martin J, Lovett DH. The purification and characterisation of a glomerular basement membrane degrading neutral proteinase from the rat mesangial cells. Biochem J 1988; 251: 419-425.

75.   Edwards DR, Murphy G, Reynolds JJ, Whitman SE, Docherty AJP, Angel P, Heath JK. Transforming growth factor beta modulates the expression of collagenase and metalloproteinase inhibitor [Abstract]. EMBO J 1987; 6: 1899.

76.   Lovett DH, Marti HP, Martin J, Grond J, Kashfarian DH. Transforming growth factor β1 stimulates mesangial cell synthesis of the 72 kD type IV collagenase independent of TIMP-1 [Abstract]. J Am Soc Nephrol 1991; 1: 578.

77.   Okuda S, Languino LR, Ruoslahti E, Border WA. Elevated expression of transforming growth factor-β and proteoglycan production in experimental glomerulonephritis. Possible role in expansion of the mesangial matrix. J Clin Invest 1990; 86: 453-462.

78.   Border WA, Okuda S, Languino LR, Sporn MB, Ruoslahti E. Suppression of experimental glomerulonephritis by antiserum against transforming growth factor β1. Nature 1990; 346: 371-374.

79.   Border WA, Noble NA, Yamamoto T, Harper JR, Yamaguchi Y, Pierschbacher MD, Ruoslahti E. Natural inhibitor of transforming growth factor-β protects against scarring in experimental kidney disease. Nature 1992; 360: 361-364.

80.   Kolm V, Sauer U, Olgemoller B, Schleicher ED. High glucose-induced TGF-β1 regulates mesangial production of heparan sulphate proteoglycan. Am J Physiol 1996; 70: F812-F821.

81.   Shankland SJ, Scholey JW. Expression of transforming grwoth factor β1 during diabetic renal hypertrophy. Kidney Int 1994; 46: 430-442.

82.   Sharma K, Ziyadeh FN. Renal hypertrophy is associated with upregulation of TGF-β1 gene expression in diabetic BB rat and NOD mouse. Am J Physiol 1994; 67: F1094-F1101.

83.   Pankewycz OG, Guan J-X, Kline Bolton W, Gomez A, Benedict JF. Renal TGF-β regulation in spontaneously diabetic NOD mice with correlations in mesangial cells. Kidney Int 1994; 46: 748-758.

84.   Wogensen L, Nielsen CB, Hjort P, Rasmussen LM, Nielsen AH, Gross K, Sarvetnick N, Ledet T. Under control of the Ren-1c promoter, locally produced transforming growth factor-β1 induces accumulation of glomerular extracellular matrix in transgenic mice. Diabetes 1999; 48: 182-192.

85.   Yamamoto T, Nakamura T, Noble NA, Ruoslahti E, Border WA. Expression of transforming growth factor is elevated in human and experimental diabetic glomerulopathy. Proc Natl Acad Sci USA 1993; 90: 1814-1818.

86.   Yamamoto T, Noble NA, Cohen AH, Nast CC, Hishida A, Gold LI, Border WA. Expression of transforming growth factor-β isoforms in human glomerular diseases. Kidney Int 1996; 49: 461-469.

87.   Ziyadeh FN, Sharma K, Ricksen N, Wolf G. Stimulation of collagen gene expression and protein synthesis in murine mesangial cells by high glucose is mediated by autocrine activation of transforming growth factor β. J Clin Invest 1994; 93: 536-542.
88.   Sharma K, Jin Y, Guo J, Ziyadeh FN. Neutralization of TGF-β by anti-TGF-β antibody attenuates kidney hypertrophy and the enhanced extracellular matrix gene expression in STZ-induced diabetic mice. Diabetes 1996; 45: 522-530.
89.   Kagami S, Border WA, Miller DE, Noble NA. Angiotensin II stimulates extracellular matrix protein synthesis through induction of transforming growth factor-β expression in rat glomerular mesangial cells. J Clin Invest 1994; 93: 2431-2437.
90.   Guh JY, Yang ML, Yang YL, Chang CC, Chuang LY. Captopril reverses high-glucose-induced growth effects on LLC-PK$_1$ cells partly by decreasing transforming growth factor-β receptor protein expression. J Am Soc Nephrol 1996; 7: 1207-1215.
91.   Gilbert RE, Cox A, Wu LL, Allen TJ, Hulthen L, Jerums G, Cooper ME. Expression of transforming growth factor β1 and type IV collagen in the renal tubulointerstitium in experimental diabetes: effects of angiotensin converting enzyme inhibition. Diabetes 1998; 47: 414-422.
92.   Flyvbjerg A, Hill C, Grønbæk H, Logan A. Effect of ACE-inhibition on renal TGF-β type II receptor expression in experimental diabetes in rats [Abstract]. J Am Soc Nephrol 1999; 10: A3444.
93.   Studer RK, Craven PA, DeRubertis FR. Antioxidant inhibition of protein kinase C-signaled increases in transforming growth factor-β in mesangial cells. Metabolism 1997; 46: 918-925.
94.   Koya D, Jirousek MR, Lin Y-W, Ishii H, Kuboki K, King G. Characterization of protein kinase C β isoform activation on the gene expression of transforming growth factor-β, extracellular matrix components and prostanoids in the glomeruli of diabetic rats. J Clin Invest 1997; 100: 115-126.
95.   Flyvbjerg A, Hill C, Nielsen B, Logan A. Effect of protein kinase C β inhibition on renal morphology, urinary albumin excretion and renal transforming growth factor β in experimental diabetes in rats [Abstract]. J Am Soc Nephrol 1999; 10: A3445.
96.   Tsuchida K, Makita Z, Yamagishi S, Atsumi T, Miyoshi H, Obara S, Ishida M, Ishikawa S, Yasumura K, Koike T. Suppression of transforming growth factor beta and vascular endothelial growth factor in diabetic nephropathy in rats by a novel advanced glycation end product inhibitor, OPB-9195. Diabetologia 1999; 42: 579-588.
97.   Tisher E, Mitchell R, Hartman T, Silva M, Gospodarowicz D, Fiddes JC, Abraham JA. The human gene for vascular endothelial growth factor. Multiple protein forms are encoded through alternative exon splicing. J Biol Chem 1991; 266: 11947-11954.
98.   Neufeld G, Cohen T, Gengrinovitch S, Poltorak Z. Vascular endothelial growth factor (VEGF) and its receptors. FASEB J 1999; 13: 9-22.
99.   Brown LF, Berse B, Tognazzi K, Manseau EJ, van de Water L, Senger DR, Dvorak HF, Rosen S. Vascular permeability factor mRNA and protein expression in human kidney. Kidney Int 1992; 42: 1457-1461.
100.   Simon M, Grone HJ, Johren O, Kullmer J, Plate KH, Risau W, Fuchs E.Expression of vascular endothelial growth factor and its receptors in human renal ontogenesis and in adult kidney. Am J Physiol 1995; 268: F240-F250.
101.   Grone HJ, Simon M, Grone EF. Expression of vascular endothelial growth factor in renal vascular disease and renal allografts. J Pathol 1995; 177: 259-267.

102. Pupilli C, Lasagni L, Romagnani P, Bellini F, Mannelli M, Misciglia N, Mavilia C, Vellei U, Villari D, Serio M. Angiotensin II stimulates the synthesis and secretion of vascular permeability factor/vascular endothelial growth factor in human mesangial cells. J Am Soc Nephrol 1999; 10: 245-255.

103. Shweiki D, Itin A, Soffer D, Keshet E. Vascular endothelial growth factor induced by hypoxia may mediate hypoxia-initiated angiogenesis. Nature 1992; 359: 843-845.

104. Cooper ME, Vranes D, Youssef S, Stacker SA, Cox AJ, Rizkalla B, Casley DJ, Bach LA, Kelly DJ, Gilbert RE. Increased renal expression of vascular endothelial growth factor (VEGF) and its receptor VEGFR-2 in experimental diabetes. Diabetes 1999; 48: 2229-2239.

105. Malamitsi-Puchner A, Sarandakou A, Tziotis J, Dafogianni C, Bartsocas CS. Serum levels of basic fibroblast growth factor and vascular endothelial growth factor in children and adolescents with Type 1 diabetes mellitus. Pediatr Res 1998; 44: 873-875.

106. Shulman K, Rosen S, Tognazzi K, Manseau EJ, Brown LF. Expression of vascular permeability factor (VPF/VEGF) is altered in many glomerular diseases. J Am Soc Nephrol 1996; 7: 661-666.

107. De Vriese A, Tilton R, Vanholder R. Hyperfiltration and albuminuria in diabetes: Role of vascular endothelial growth factor (VEGF)[Abstract]. J Am Soc Nephrol 1999;10: A3434.

26.   TRANSFORMING GROWTH FACTOR-β AND OTHER CYTOKINES IN EXPERIMENTAL AND HUMAN NEPHROPATHY

Sheldon Chen, M. Carmen Iglesias de la Cruz, Motohide Isono, and Fuad N. Ziyadeh
Penn Center for Molecular Studies of Kidney Diseases, Renal-Electrolyte and Hypertension Division, Department of Medicine, University of Pennsylvania, Philadelphia, PA 19104-6144, USA

Genetic, hemodynamic, and metabolic factors are important in the pathogenesis of diabetic nephropathy. This chapter, complementing the coverage of related chapters in this book, will focus on some of the metabolic mediators, especially the various cytokines and growth factors, with particular focus on the transforming growth factor-β (TGF-β). Various mediator factors and signal transduction pathways interact in an intricate circuitry of autocrine, paracrine, and even endocrine mechanisms when the kidney is chronically exposed to high ambient glucose concentrations. The effects of high glucose on renal cells may arise because of increased metabolism of glucose through the polyol pathway [1], increased *de novo* synthesis of diacylglycerol (DAG) with activation of protein kinase C (PKC) [2, 3], activation of the hexosamine pathway [4], or increased nonenzymatic glycation of proteins [5, 6]. Recent studies have demonstrated the importance of many soluble mediators in diabetic renal disease (reviewed in [7, 8]) including platelet-derived growth factor (PDGF), endothelin, angiotensin II (AII), prostanoids, insulin-like growth factor-I (IGF-I), leptin, and vascular endothelial growth factor (VEGF). Some features of these mediators will be highlighted here, after providing a detailed account of the crucial role that TGF-β plays in the pathogenesis of diabetic nephropathy. Additionally, the discussion will summarize the evidence linking the diverse mediators to the overactivity of the TGF-β system in diabetic renal disease.

OVERVIEW OF THE TGF-β SYSTEM
The TGF-β superfamily is comprised of over 40 related proteins, including the three mammalian isoforms of TGF-β (-β1, -β2, and -β3), the activins, and the bone morphogenetic proteins [9]. The past decade has witnessed an expansive literature supporting important roles for the TGF-β family in several types of kidney diseases. In

pathophysiological states, the renal TGF-β system plays a central role in cell growth and differentiation, chemotaxis (of fibroblasts, monocytes, and neutrophils), and stimulation of various extracellular matrix molecules [10]. In particular, TGF-β promotes renal cell hypertrophy and stimulates glomerular and tubular production of a host of extracellular matrix molecules [11, 12].

The matrix-stimulating effects of TGF-β involve several key systems: 1) stimulation of gene expression of matrix molecules such as fibronectin, proteoglycans, and several collagen isotypes; 2) inhibition of matrix degradation via a dual-pronged pathway of suppressing the expression and activity of serine, thiol, and metalloproteinases (e.g., plasminogen activator, collagenase, elastase, stromelysin) as well as stimulating tissue inhibitors of metalloproteinases (TIMPs) and plasminogen activator inhibitor-1 (PAI-1) [13]; and 3) upregulation of integrins (the cell receptors of extracellular matrix), thereby enhancing the ability of cells to interact with specific matrix proteins. Additionally, excess TGF-β activity is important in mediating fibroproliferative disorders because of its potent chemotactic properties for macrophages and fibroblasts and its ability to stimulate proliferation of fibroblasts (including renal interstitial cells) under certain conditions.

The three mammalian isoforms of TGF-β share similar actions *in vitro* but not *in vivo* [9, 14]. This is partly due to differences in developmental regulation and tissue-specific expression. In the adult kidney, TGF-β1 has been described in tubular epithelial cells (both proximal and distal), in interstitial cells, and to a lesser extent in glomerular mesangial, endothelial, and epithelial cells. TGF-β3 follows a similar pattern of expression but in quantitatively lower amounts. The TGF-β2 protein is largely restricted to the juxtaglomerular apparatus where it may play an important role in renin metabolism (reviewed in [7, 15]). It should be kept in mind that non-renal cells like platelets, macrophages, and vascular smooth muscle cells can also contribute to the overall TGF-β activity in the kidney. Unless otherwise specified, the discussion in this chapter will focus on the ubiquitous TGF-β1 isoform.

The active form of TGF-β1 is a homodimer of two cysteine-rich 12.5 kDa polypeptide subunits derived from the C-terminal end of the gene product and linked by a single disulfide bond. This mature, active form is capable of binding to its receptor and propagating a signal [16]. TGF-β is secreted as latent complexes, and these in turn exist in soluble forms or insoluble forms bound to extracellular matrix constituents [17, 18]. The latent complex is composed of the mature TGF-β dimer linked non-covalently to a latency-associated peptide (LAP), which is also encoded by the TGF-β gene [19]. LAP imparts latency by blocking TGF-β binding to the signaling receptor. In certain tissues including the glomerulus, the latent complex exists in covalent association with the product of another gene, the latent TGF-β binding protein (LTBP). In the kidney, tubular epithelial cells secrete the small latent complex (mature TGF-β1 + LAP), while glomerular parenchymal and arteriolar cells secrete the large latent complex (mature TGF-β1 + LAP + LTBP) [20]. This pattern of tissue expression implies potentially important differences in activation and functional regulation of the TGF-β system between the glomerular/vascular compartment and the tubular compartment.

Activation of latent TGF-β *in vivo* is largely controlled by proteases (e.g., plasmin) that cleave the LAP from the bioactive TGF-β dimer [21]. Plasmin-mediated activation of TGF-β involves the binding of the latent form to a mannose-6-phosphate receptor on the cell surface and then the concerted action of transglutaminase and plasmin to remove LAP. A protease-independent conformational change of the latent complex can also occur when thrombospondin (TSP), derived from the alpha-granules of platelets, allows the active TGF-β moiety to bind to its cell surface receptor. As will be discussed later, the TSP system may partly explain how TGF-β1 can be activated in mesangial cells by high ambient glucose. Activation of TGF-β *in vitro* can be achieved by treatment with acid (pH4) and heat (80°C) or detergents.

The three TGF-β isoforms share a common receptor system and an intracellular signalling cascade [22]. Virtually all cell types produce one or more isoforms of TGF-β and express TGF-β receptors. Three major types of TGF-β receptors have been identified: type I (also called Alk5), type II, and type III (also called betaglycan). Type III lacks an identifiable cytoplasmic signalling domain and may act to enhance the delivery of TGF-β on the cell surface to the signalling receptor. A molecule similar to betaglycan that is found on endothelial cells is called endoglin. Signalling begins when TGF-β engages the type II receptor, also called the primary receptor since it directly binds ligand. The ligand-bound type II receptor then binds to the type I receptor to form a heterotetramer. Within this complex, the type II receptor phosphorylates the type I receptor at a serine/glycine rich domain. This enables the type I receptor to phosphorylate further downstream signalling molecules and is thus considered the *sine qua non* event in TGF-β signalling [23]. The serine-threonine kinase activity of the TGF-β receptor complex is believed to be necessary for the profibrotic and antiproliferative actions of TGF-β [22, 24].

The TGF-β receptors transduce their signals through novel intracellular proteins called Smad proteins [25, 26]. Receptor-activated Smad2 and Smad3 are specific for the TGF-β isoforms [27] (while Smad1 and Smad5 are specific for other ligands such as the bone morphogenetic proteins). Phosphorylation of Smad2 or Smad3 by the type I receptor allows them to interact with Smad4 (also called DPC4), a different member of the Smad family that does not get phosphorylated by the type I receptor. The Smad2-Smad4 or Smad3-Smad4 complex translocates into the nucleus and interacts with other transcription factors, including FAST-1, CBP (cyclic AMP-response element-binding protein), and AP-1, to effect a coordinated transcriptional response from many different genes. Such target genes contain Smad-specific binding sequences in their promoter. A third type of Smad proteins is inhibitory in action; Smad6 and Smad7 can inhibit the binding of Smad2 or Smad3 to the type I receptor [28]. Recent evidence also suggests that the transcription factors Ski and Sno are involved in antagonizing TGF-β signalling by interfering with the nuclear actions of Smad2-Smad4 or Smad3-Smad4 complexes. Experimental evidence indicates that the Smad pathway is directly involved in cell cycle regulation by TGF-β, but other intracellular signalling pathways such as the mitogen-activated protein (MAP) kinase cascades may also participate. Likewise, Smad proteins and possibly other unrelated signalling molecules may mediate some of the other functions of TGF-β such as stimulation of extracellular matrix production.

As will be discussed later in relation to diabetic kidney disease, TGF-β production is stimulated by high ambient glucose, glycated proteins, as well as a host of cytokines and growth factors such as the mitogen PDGF and the vasoactive agents AII, thromboxane, and endothelin. Dysregulation of the TGF-β system in profibrotic states often represents an unregulated degree of tissue repair that swings the balance toward excess scar deposition. This is exacerbated by the fact that TGF-β1 has the peculiar ability to induce its own production, thereby amplifying the fibroproliferative response in a positive feedback fashion.

EFFECTS OF HIGH AMBIENT GLUCOSE IN RENAL CELL CULTURE SYSTEMS

Increased renal extracellular matrix production in diabetes is the result of increased synthesis and/or decreased degradation rates [11, 29, 30]. To model the effects of diabetes on the kidney, researchers have grown various renal cell types in tissue culture under high ambient glucose conditions. High glucose stimulates proximal tubular and mesangial cell hypertrophy [31, 32]. It also stimulates the production of connective tissue molecules such as fibronectin and collagens in proximal tubular cells and glomerular mesangial, epithelial, and endothelial cells [31, 33-39]. Recent cell culture studies have also demonstrated that renal cortical fibroblasts produce excess collagen type I under high glucose conditions [40]. In rat mesangial cell culture, periodically elevated glucose levels increase collagen production to a greater extent than persistently elevated glucose concentrations [41]. This more closely mimics the fluctuation of blood glucose levels *in vivo* and may highlight the detrimental effects of labile hyperglycemia on the pathogenesis of diabetic glomerulosclerosis. The critical factor for renal cell damage is the intracellular accumulation and metabolism of glucose rather than simply the increased extracellular concentration of glucose. This is supported by experiments involving mesangial cells transfected with the human glucose transporter GLUT1 gene [42]. Such cells demonstrate markedly stimulated glucose uptake and metabolism and enhanced matrix synthesis even when the extracellular glucose concentration is normal.

Other effects of high glucose on extracellular matrix metabolism in human glomerular mesangial and epithelial cells involve a significant decrease in heparan sulfate proteoglycan (HSPG) synthesis and alterations in the sulfation pattern [43, 44]. These may cause profound changes in charge- and size-permselectivity of the glomerular basement membrane (GBM) that are believed to contribute to diabetic proteinuria *in vivo*.

ACTIVATION OF THE TGF-β SYSTEM IN RENAL CELLS CULTURED IN HIGH GLUCOSE

We were the first to postulate that increased renal TGF-β bioactivity is important in the pathogenesis of diabetic nephropathy [45]. Several studies have concluded that high glucose induces biochemical alterations that stimulate the production of TGF-β and other intermediary growth factors [7, 8, 15, 40, 46]. Studies employing neutralizing anti-TGF-β antibodies have provided convincing evidence that the prosclerotic and hypertrophic effects of high ambient glucose in cultured renal cells are largely mediated by autocrine production and activation of TGF-β. In particular, such studies have involved glomerular mesangial cells [32, 36], glomerular epithelial cells [39], proximal tubular cells [31, 47, 48], and renal cortical fibroblasts [40]. Neutralizing anti-TGF-β antibodies also reverse the downregulation of collagenase activity in rat mesangial cells grown in high glucose [49]. TGF-β1 antisense oligonucleotides [38] have been used to attenuate the increased synthesis of extracellular matrix and to reverse the inhibition of cell proliferation caused by high ambient glucose. Additionally, high ambient glucose upregulates TGF-β receptor mRNAs and proteins in cultured murine mesangial cells and porcine LLC-PK1 tubular epithelial cells [50-52].

Multiple explanations may be provided for how high glucose stimulates TGF-β. Transcriptional activation of the TGF-β1 gene by high ambient glucose has been demonstrated in mouse mesangial cells [53]. The promoter of the mouse or human TGF-β1 gene has a consensus nucleotide sequence termed 'glucose response element' that seems to be the target for transcriptional activation by high glucose [53]. The TGF-β1 promoter also has multiple AP-1-like consensus sites which respond to phorbol-ester/PKC stimulation [54]. High ambient glucose increases DAG content and activates PKC in glomeruli isolated from diabetic rats and in cultured mesangial cells [2, 55-58]. DAG, like phorbol esters, activates several isoforms of PKC [59]. Increased PKC activity in the diabetic state may lead to activation of the MAP kinase cascades such as extracellular signal-regulated kinase (ERK) [60, 61] and p38 MAP kinase [62]. Activation of PKC may also result in increased production of the AP-1 transcription complex (Jun and Fos) [63]. The AP-1 binding sequence is essential for regulation of the promoter activity of many relevant genes including the α2 chain of collagen type I [64] and TGF-β1 itself [54]. The mRNA level of *c-fos* is increased in glomeruli isolated from diabetic rats [65] and also in mesangial cells cultured in high glucose [66]. Furthermore, increased DNA binding of AP-1 is reported in human mesangial cells cultured in high glucose [67]. Importantly, Kim et al. have demonstrated that TGF-β1 protein positively autoregulates the expression of TGF-β1 mRNA in an AP-1-dependent fashion [68]. This positive, autoinductive feedback loop greatly exaggerates the profibrogenic potential of TGF-β1 in progressive kidney diseases including diabetic nephropathy.

Another type of positive feedback loop may exist involving TGF-β1 and the transmembrane glucose transporter, GLUT1. Evidence now suggests that TGF-β1 can upregulate GLUT1 at both the message and protein levels in mesangial cells [69]. High glucose raises TGF-β1 levels, which increase GLUT1 and thus cellular glucose uptake, which in turn can lead to metabolic changes that increase TGF-β1 production further. In this way, a high ambient glucose level accentuates its effects by increasing intracellular glucose uptake and metabolism.

A recent study [4] using porcine mesangial cells has suggested that high glucose-induced TGF-β1 production is mediated by the hexosamine pathway. D-glucosamine, a structural analog of D-glucose, enhances the production of TGF-β and fibronectin proteins and promotes the conversion of latent TGF-β to the active form. Inhibition by antisense oligonucleotides or substrate analogs of enzymes in the hexosamine pathway prevents the high glucose-induced increase in TGF-β1 expression and bioactivity in mesangial cells.

High glucose may indirectly stimulate the TGF-β system through other intermediate molecules such as TSP, an extracellular matrix glycoprotein that activates latent TGF-β. In the presence of high glucose, cultured human mesangial cells increase production of TSP [70]. Elevated concentrations of TSP in turn stimulate the formation of both active TGF-β and fibronectin. A neutralizing anti-TGF-β antibody blocks fibronectin production indicating that TGF-β mediates TSP-induced fibronectin [70]. Thus the TSP pathway participates in the post-translational modification of TGF-β in the diabetic state.

TGF-β appears to exert some of its profibrotic effects through connective tissue growth factor (CTGF). This cysteine-rich peptide stimulates fibroblasts to divide and to synthesize collagen. Not surprisingly, its expression is markedly increased in several disorders of renal fibrosis including diabetic nephropathy [71]. The technique of suppression subtractive hybridization has recently identified CTGF as a component of the stimulatory effects of high glucose on human mesangial cells [72]. The addition of TGF-β1 to mesangial cells also triggers CTGF expression, and high glucose appears to induce CTGF partly through a TGF-β-dependent pathway [72]. Other experiments involving the normal rat kidney (NRK) fibroblast cell line have shown that blockade of CTGF with antisense oligonucleotides or with anti-CTGF antibodies effectively abolishes TGF-β stimulated collagen synthesis [73]. CTGF thus acts downstream of TGF-β to promote fibrosis by certain cell types [74]. However, whether CTGF will prove to be an etiologic agent of renal fibrosis in diabetic kidney disease will have to await interventional studies designed to block its actions in experimental models.

TGF-β IN EXPERIMENTAL DIABETIC KIDNEY DISEASE

Elevated renal TGF-β mRNA and protein levels have been found in various experimental animal models of insulin-dependent diabetes mellitus [75]. In streptozotocin (STZ)-diabetic rats, increased mRNA and protein levels of TGF-β1 and type IV collagen have been demonstrated by *in situ* hybridization and immunohistochemistry within 7 days of diabetes onset [76]. Similarly, renal cortical TGF-β expression is upregulated within a few days of development of diabetes in other models of spontaneous type 1 diabetes such as the BB rat and the NOD mouse [77]. This event coincides with the development of kidney hypertrophy [77], which is likely linked to the increased expression of TGF-β1 and type II TGF-β receptor in the mouse kidney [78]. TGF-β is upregulated not only in early but also in later stages of disease in spontaneous and STZ-induced diabetic animals [79-82]. Moreover, STZ-induced diabetes in rats results in decreased glomerular cathepsin and metalloprotease activities, factors which contribute to the accumulation of extracellular matrix molecules [83]. In agreement with this finding, glomeruli from STZ-diabetic rats demonstrate persistently upregulated TGF-β1 mRNA and protein levels in association with a relentless increase in extracellular matrix components for up to 40 weeks of diabetes [84-87].

Hyperglycemia is required for upregulation of TGF-β and extracellular matrix production since restoration of normoglycemia by high-dose insulin attenuates the renal cortical [78] and glomerular [76] expression of these molecules.

The importance of the renal TGF-β system in diabetic kidney disease is shown by the significant attenuation of glomerular and renal hypertrophy achieved by short-term treatment (9 days) of STZ-diabetic mice with neutralizing monoclonal antibodies against all three isoforms of TGF-β [78]. It is interesting to note that in this model the mRNA expression of TGF-β1 and the type II TGF-β receptor in the renal cortex is increased after just 3 days of diabetes, and this is associated with increased urinary levels of total (active plus latent) TGF-β [78]. The increased mRNA levels of the α1 chain of type IV collagen and fibronectin in the kidney were significantly attenuated by intraperitoneal treatment of the diabetic mice with anti-TGF-β antibodies [78]. In fact, long-term anti-TGF-β antibody therapy *in vivo* (for 8 weeks) effectively prevents renal insufficiency and mesangial matrix expansion in the *db/db* mouse, a model of type 2 diabetes [88]. Recent studies in diabetic rats have demonstrated marked attenuation of glomerular overexpression of mRNAs encoding TGF-β1, collagen type IV, and fibronectin following chronic treatment with a novel PKC-β selective inhibitor [82]. Together, these studies highlight the importance of the renal TGF-β system in the chronic manifestations of diabetic kidney disease such as glomerulosclerosis and renal insufficiency.

HUMAN DIABETIC KIDNEY DISEASE AND TGF-β

Studies have shown that the TGF-β system is upregulated in kidney tissue derived from patients with diabetic nephropathy. Immunostaining for the three isoforms of TGF-β is increased in both the glomeruli and tubulointerstitium of patients with established diabetic kidney disease [84, 89, 90]. TGF-β immunostaining is also enhanced in other glomerular diseases characterized by secondary tubulointerstitial fibrosis, and this is associated with increased staining of the extracellular matrix proteins tenascin and fibronectin whose production is also TGF-β-dependent [89]. The technique of reverse transcriptase-polymerase chain reaction has detected markedly increased glomerular expression of TGF-β1 mRNA in renal biopsy specimens from diabetic patients with nephropathy [91]. The level of glomerular TGF-β1 mRNA expression correlated closely with the degree of hyperglycemia, as measured by glycosylated hemoglobin and by severity of the sclerosis index.

Corroborative studies using cell culture systems derived from the human kidney have found, as in rodent renal cells, that high ambient glucose media upregulate gene expression of TGF-β in mesangial [92] and proximal tubular cells [93].

A recent study [94] was designed to determine if diabetic patients have enhanced renal production of TGF-β. Aortic, renal vein, and urinary levels of TGF-β were measured in 14 type 2 diabetic and 11 non-diabetic control patients undergoing elective coronary artery catheterization. Both groups were roughly matched with regard to the range of renal function and to the presence of hypertension and proteinuria. Renal blood flow was measured to calculate net mass balance across the kidney. The gradient of TGF-β1 concentration across the renal vascular bed was positive in the diabetic patients indicating net renal production of TGF-β1, whereas the gradient was negative in the non-diabetic patients indicating net renal TGF-β1 extraction. (Renal production of immunoreactive endothelin tended to be higher, but not significantly, in diabetic patients.) When the renal TGF-β1 mass balance was calculated, a similar pattern was observed with approximately 1000 ng/min of TGF-β1 added to the circulation by the kidney in the diabetic group and approximately 3500 ng/min removed from the circulation in the non-diabetic group. In addition, urinary levels of bioassayable TGF-β were increased four-fold in the diabetic versus non-diabetic patients. The increased urinary TGF-β was not simply a consequence of enhanced urinary permeability to albumin as diabetic patients both with and without microalbuminuria had enhanced TGF-β urinary excretion. These results support the conclusion that the kidneys of diabetic patients overproduce TGF-β1 protein. The details of this phenomenon and the exact contribution of the different renal cell types to TGF-β1 production will need to be investigated in future studies.

In a *post-hoc* study, Sharma and co-workers [95] assessed whether treatment with captopril lowers serum levels of TGF-β1 in a small subset of patients with diabetic nephropathy previously enrolled in the Collaborative Study Group [96]. There was a significant decrease of 21% in serum TGF-β1 levels in the captopril-treated group after 6 months while there was a slight increase of 11% in the placebo group after the same period. Interestingly, the decrease in serum TGF-β1 levels in the captopril group correlated with stabilization of the glomerular filtration rate over the ensuing 2 year period, and this association was even more pronounced in the subset of patients with an initial glomerular filtration rate of less than 75 ml/min. These results suggest that TGF-β1 plays an important role in the progression of diabetic nephropathy and that converting enzyme inhibitor therapy may protect the kidney by lowering TGF-β1 production.

A recent genetic study found that the Thr263Ile mutation in the TGF-β1 gene is associated with the presence of diabetic nephropathy in type 1 diabetic patients [97]. The functional significance of this mutation is unknown.

Other Mediators in Diabetic Renal Disease

AII: An important concept that has emerged in diabetes research is the idea that AII not only mediates intraglomerular hypertension but also behaves as a growth factor that causes some of the hypertrophy and fibrosis seen in diabetic renal disease (reviewed in [46]). Much of the latter effect of AII appears to be mediated by TGF-β. Tissue culture studies have demonstrated that AII stimulates TGF-β1 production in proximal tubular cells [98] and mesangial cells [99]. Clinical conditions which are associated with upregulation of the renin-AII system often upregulate TGF-β expression. For example, a high intraglomerular hydrostatic pressure secondary to efferent arteriolar constriction by AII stretches the mesangial cell and stimulates it to produce TGF-β isoforms [100]. The renoprotective effect of angiotensin converting enzyme inhibitors [96, 101] may be partly related to the blockade of AII-induced TGF-β production in renal cells [98, 99]. Furthermore, captopril reverses the high glucose-induced growth effects on LLC-PK1 cells in culture partly by decreasing TGF-β receptor protein expression [51]. The renoprotective efficacy of captopril in patients with diabetic nephropathy seems to correlate with the reduction of serum TGF-β1 levels [95].

Endothelins: Glomerular expression of endothelin-1 (ET-1) mRNA is increased in STZ-diabetic rats [102] and the urinary level of ET-1 is elevated in the diabetic BB rat [102].   An endothelin receptor A antagonist, FR139317, when administered to STZ-diabetic rats, attenuated glomerular hyperfiltration and urinary protein excretion and decreased glomerular mRNA levels of collagens, laminins, tumor necrosis factor (TNF-α), PDGF-B, TGF-β1, and basic fibroblast growth factor (bFGF) [103].   Endothelin levels are higher in type 2 diabetic patients than in the general population [104], and levels are higher in type 2 diabetic patients with retinopathy than without retinopathy. Treatment with captopril reduces ET-1 levels in such patients [105] suggesting a role for AII in the upregulation of ET-1 in diabetes.

Thromboxane: Studies in experimental animal models have demonstrated increased renal thromboxane expression [106] and urinary excretion of thromboxane B2 shortly after the onset of diabetes [55, 107, 108].   The source of increased thromboxane production may be the diabetic glomerulus [109] and/or infiltrating platelets [110]. Addition of thromboxane analogs to mesangial cells in culture results in stimulation of fibronectin production [111], which appears to be mediated by PKC activation [56]. Inhibitors of thromboxane synthesis and its receptor have been found to ameliorate diabetes-induced albuminuria [109, 112] and mesangial matrix expansion [109], but they may not prevent thickening of the GBM [109, 113].

   It should be noted that exogenous prostaglandin E_2 (PGE$_2$) or drugs capable of increasing endogenous PGE$_2$ dose-dependently decrease the level of extracellur matrix protein and mRNA and also dampen TGF-β gene expression in cultured rat mesangial cells [114]. The net balance between the actions of vasoconstrictive and vasodilatory eicosanoids may determine whether TGF-β bioactivity is enhanced or diminished.

PDGF: PDGF-B expression is upregulated in glomeruli from diabetic rats [115] and is implicated in the link between high glucose levels and the TGF-β pathway. Studies in human mesangial cells have found that antibodies to PDGF inhibited high glucose-stimulated TGF-β1 mRNA [92]. A study in human proximal tubular cells found that high ambient glucose was sufficient to increase TGF-β1 mRNA levels but that PDGF was required to cause secretion and activation of the TGF-β protein [93]. Of interest is that the expression of the PDGF-B receptor is increased in mesangial and other vascular cells (such as vascular smooth muscle and capillary endothelial cells) exposed to high ambient glucose [116]. It appears that PDGF may be more important in advanced stages of human diabetic nephropathy. Urinary levels of PDGF-BB were markedly increased in diabetic patients with microalbuminuria or macroalbuminuria but not in diabetic patients without albuminuria [117].

   PDGF may also play a role in mediating glycation-stimulated matrix production in mesangial cells [118]. Neutralizing anti-PDGF antibody reduces the mRNA of the α1 chain of type IV collagen which is induced by advanced glycation end-products (AGEs) in cultured mouse mesangial cells [119].

IGF-I: A role for this factor in diabetic kidney disease has been suggested [120, 121] and is reviewed elsewhere in this book. Continuous, 12-week subcutaneous infusion of the somatostatin analog octreotide, which antagonizes the effects of growth hormone and IGF-I, has been reported to reduce renal volume and glomerular hyperfiltration in 11 normoalbuminuric, normotensive patients with type 1 diabetes [122]. Growth hormone may also play a role in mediating diabetic renal pathology. Transgenic mice overexpressing growth hormone have renal and glomerular hypertrophy with associated glomerulosclerosis similar to the histology of diabetic nephropathy [123]. A growth hormone receptor antagonist prevented renal hypertrophy and urinary albumin excretion in STZ-mice [124]. There is likely an important interaction or "cross-talk" among various growth factors, such as TGF-β, IGF-I, and PDGF, that may promote diabetic renal pathology (reviewed in [15]).

VEGF: This growth factor is implicated in the microvascular complications of diabetes, especially retinopathy, but its role in nephropathy remains speculative. VEGF is a homodimeric glycoprotein that exists in at least five different isoforms that are produced by differential exon splicing [125]. Smaller isoforms are freely soluble and larger isoforms are locally bound to extracellular matrix [126]. Virtually all cell types produce VEGF and they increase their secretion mostly in response to hypoxia to stimulate endothelial cell proliferation and new blood vessel formation (angiogenesis) [127]. VEGF, also known as vascular permeability factor (VPF), is 50,000 times more potent than histamine and it markedly increases microvascular endothelial permeability to macromolecules [128-130].

VEGF and its receptors are widely expressed in the kidney. The glomerular visceral epithelial podocyte expresses VEGF constitutively [131] and the collecting duct epithelial cell expresses it at a lower level [132]. Under hypoxic conditions, proximal and distal tubular epithelial cells, interstitial cells, and vascular smooth muscle cells synthesize VEGF [133]. The mesangial cell can be stimulated to produce VEGF by AII, an effect that is blocked by the AT1 receptor antagonist losartan [134]. Even the glomerular endothelial cell produces VEGF [135] resulting in an autocrine system. The two high-affinity receptors for VEGF, fms-like tyrosine kinase-1 (flt-1) and Kinase Domain Receptor/fetal liver kinase-1 (KDR/flk-1), appear to be mostly restricted to the endothelial cell, being found on pre- and post-glomerular vessels and on glomerular capillaries [136]. Mesangial cells also possess at least one form of the VEGF receptor [137].

In the normal kidney, VEGF may function to maintain the integrity of the glomerular endothelium and its fenestrations [138, 139]. During an ischemic or hypoxic injury, VEGF may help to alleviate decreased blood flow and restore vascular integrity [133]. The possibility that diabetes can increase renal VEGF/VPF production has led to the theory that this factor is one of the causes of albuminuria. However, experimental and clinical evidence to support this reasoning is currently lacking. Infusion of VEGF into isolated perfused rat kidneys did not change the glomerular permeability to albumin [140]. Nevertheless, the diabetic state results in the upregulation of many mediators that can stimulate the production of VEGF. High glucose itself stimulates vascular smooth muscle cells to augment VEGF expression [141] perhaps via glucose-induced PKC activation [142]. Phorbol esters stimulate mesangial cell VEGF production, [143] and inhibition of PKC blocks the signalling of VEGF [144]. Reactive oxygen species can induce VEGF in both endothelial cells [145] and vascular smooth muscle cells [146]. Various cytokines such as TGF-β [147], AII [134], IGF-I [148], bFGF [149], PDGF [150], and platelet activating factor (PAF) [151] all raise VEGF production. Mechanical stretch, the *in vitro* correlate of intraglomerular hypertension, also increases mesangial VEGF production via an AII-independent mechanism [152].

However, no one has yet convincingly demonstrated that increased VEGF is associated with proteinuria in either diabetes or other proteinuric diseases. In one study, type 1 diabetic children and adolescents were found to have similar serum VEGF levels as compared to healthy controls [153]. Even the patients with longer duration of diabetes and worse metabolic control did not have significantly increased serum VEGF levels. Another study examined VEGF expression in renal biopsy specimens with various diseases including diabetic nephropathy [154]. Five of the 47 cases had diabetes, and those glomeruli free of sclerosis displayed strong expression of VEGF while those with extensive sclerosis showed markedly decreased expression of VEGF. It is thus possible that early diabetes is characterized by increased glomerular VEGF and advanced diabetes is characterized by decreased VEGF.

The role of VEGF in the etiology of non-diabetic proteinuria is equally inconclusive. VEGF levels are not elevated in either Finnish nephropathy [155] or steroid-sensitive nephrotic syndrome [156]. However, in a rat model of bovine serum albumin-induced nephritis [157], VEGF and VEGF receptor mRNA expression increased proportionally with the severity of proteinuria.

Leptin: Leptin, a circulating hormone abundant in obese patients with or without type 2 diabetes, has recently been implicated as a contributor to glomerulosclerosis [158]. Leptin is made primarily by adipose cells and acts on the hypothalamus to reduce food intake and to increase energy expenditure [159]. Thus, higher body fat results in increased leptin production which then participates in a negative feedback loop that regulates body weight. Indeed, a spontaneous mutation in the *ob* gene which encodes leptin results in massive obesity in the *ob/ob* mouse [160]. Exogenous leptin treatment in this mouse corrects the obesity.

The *db/db* mouse contains a mutation that confers leptin resistance [161]. Specifically, the long form of the leptin receptor, Ob-Rb, is defective in the hypothalamus [162]. Such mice exhibit hyperphagia and rapid weight gain. With development of obesity, the mice become insulin-resistant and hyperglycemic. After several months, the *db/db* mouse develops renal lesions that are indistinguishable from those of human diabetic glomerulopathy [163]. Because kidney cells contain shorter forms of the leptin receptor that may transduce a discrete signal, it has been postulated [158] that hyperleptinemia in addition to hyperglycemia [164] may mediate the renal fibrogenic process in this mouse model of type 2 diabetes. Toward this end, our group recently studied the effects of exogenous leptin on the production of TGF-β and type IV collagen by the kidney [158]. Recombinant leptin added to cultures of rat glomerular endothelial cells enhanced TGF-β mRNA and protein expression. The cells possess the short form of the leptin receptor (Ob-Ra) and display activation of downstream signalling cascades in response to leptin binding. When leptin is infused into normal rats for 72 hours or 3 weeks, there is increased renal glomerular expression of TGF-β followed by increased type IV collagen expression, proteinuria, and segmental glomerulosclerosis.

MECHANISMS OF RENAL UPREGULATION OF THE TGF-β SYSTEM IN THE DIABETIC STATE IN RELATIONSHIP TO OTHER MEDIATORS

Vasoactive humoral factors such as AII, endothelins, and altered prostaglandin metabolism have all been implicated in the pathogenesis of diabetic nephropathy, and all these factors may upregulate the TGF-β/TGF-β receptor system in the diabetic kidney (reviewed in [7, 15]). AII is capable of stimulating TGF-β production in proximal tubular and mesangial cell cultures [98, 99]. Hyperglycemia acts in synergy with locally increased AII to stimulate renal hypertrophy and synthesis of extracellular matrix proteins (reviewed in [12]). In return, AII can potentiate the effects of high glucose by inhibiting proteinases responsible for protein turnover and stimulating TGF-β synthesis [12]. Moreover, hyperglycemia can enhance the expression of AII-receptors and prolong the half-life of AII itself by inhibiting AII-degrading enzymes. The net effect therefore is increased bioactivity of AII.

As reviewed above, endothelins may stimulate TGF-β production because endothelin receptor antagonists decrease the overexpression of glomerular TGF-β1 mRNA in diabetic rats [103]. Thromboxane has also been demonstrated to stimulate TGF-β production in mesangial cells [56].

The stimulus for chronic upregulation of TGF-β may be partly related to the presence of glycated proteins in long-standing diabetes [165, 166]. The early Amadori-glucose adducts of proteins such as serum albumin have been shown to stimulate TGF-β expression in mesangial cells [166]. Administration of AGE-modified proteins to normal mice elevates the mRNA levels of TGF-β1, α1(IV) collagen, and laminin B1. These increases are reversed by concomitant aminoguanidine therapy [167]. Exposure to glycated LDL increases TGF-β1 and fibronectin mRNA levels in cultured murine mesangial cells [168]. The increased fibronectin message is prevented by anti-TGF-β antibody treatment [168]. Finally, mesangial cells have specific receptors for AGE which may result in enhanced matrix and cytokine production [119, 169].

In addition to the metabolic factors listed above, hemodynamic and mechanical forces are operative in the diabetic state. The cyclical stretch/relaxation of mesangial cells in culture, which closely mimics increased glomerular pressure *in vivo* [100, 170, 171], has been associated with increased synthesis of TGF-β and extracellular matrix molecules. Fluid shear stress increases message expression and synthesis of the active form of TGF-β in cultured bovine aortic endothelial cells [172].

Oxidative stress, which occurs in diabetes, has been proposed as a link between hyperglycemia and diabetic complications [173]. There is increased generation of reactive oxygen species and free radicals in the kidneys of diabetic patients [174]. In cell culture, the addition of hydrogen peroxide can directly induce the expression of TGF-β in mesangial cells [175]. Antioxidant treatment with taurine prevents the accumulation of extracellular matrix in the kidney of STZ-induced diabetic rats [176].

Upregulation of the renal type II TGF-β receptor in the diabetic state represents another major pathway for enhanced bioactivity of the TGF-β system. High ambient glucose increases the expression of this receptor in mesangial cells [50]. Amadori glucose adducts of albumin also increase TGF-β type II receptor mRNA and protein levels in mesangial cell cultures [166]. Interestingly, captopril inhibits high glucose-mediated hypertrophy in tubular LLC-PK1 cells and also reduces the increased protein expression of types I and II TGF-β receptors [51].

Table 26-1: Mediators of Diabetic Renal Disease

I.   Genetic predisposition
II. Glomerular hemodynamic stress*
III. Metabolic Perturbations
    A. Non-enzymatic glycation of circulating or structural proteins
          Amadori-glucose adducts (e.g., of serum albumin)*
          Advanced glycosylation end-products (AGE)*
    B. Activation of pathways of glucose metabolism
          Polyol pathway (increased sorbitol)*
          Pentose phosphate shunt (increased UDP glucose)
          De novo synthesis of diacylglycerol and stimulation of protein kinase C*
          Disordered *myo*-inositol metabolism
          Altered cellular redox state* (increased $NADP^+/NADPH$, $NADH/NAD^+$)
          Hexosamine pathway*
          Oxidant injury*
    C. Activation of cytokines and growth factor systems
          Transforming growth factor-β*
          Angiotensin II*
          Endothelins*
          Thromboxane*
          Platelet-derived growth factor*
          Insulin-like growth factor-I
          Vascular endothelial growth factor
          Leptin*
(*Factors known to stimulate the transforming growth factor-β system)

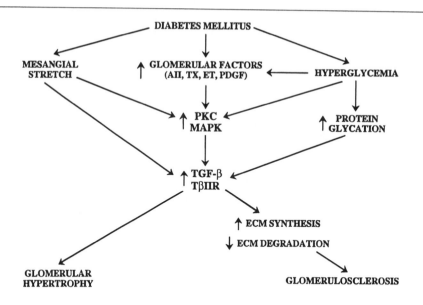

Figure 26-1. The central role of transforming growth factor-β (TGF-β.) in mediating glomerular hypertrophy and glomerulosclerosis in diabetic nephropathy. Several characteristics of the diabetic state (hyperglycemia; increased intraglomerular hydrostatic pressure and mesangial stretch; enhanced production of glomerular vasoactive agents and growth factors; and increased nonenzymatic glycation of proteins) activate the renal TGF-β/TGF-β receptor system. (PKC: protein kinase C; MAPK: mitogen-activated protein kinase; AII: angiotensin II; TX: thromboxane; ET: endothelin; PDGF: platelet-derived growth factor; TβIIR: TGF-β type II receptor; ECM: extracellular matrix).

CONCLUDING REMARKS:

The characteristic lesions of diabetic nephropathy such as renal hypertrophy, increased glomerular hypertension, and altered extracellular matrix metabolism may be intimately related to the effects of high ambient glucose on various growth factors and cytokines that are increased locally or in the circulation. Recent studies using cell culture techniques and experimental animal models have provided important insights into the pathogenetic mechanisms of diabetic nephropathy (Table 26-1).

Much attention has been devoted to clarifying the role of TGF-β as a mediator of kidney disease. The data we have reviewed strongly support the hypothesis that elevated renal production and/or activity of TGF-β predominantly mediate the renal hypertrophy and extracellular matrix expansion seen in experimental and human diabetic nephropathy (Figure 26-1). Ongoing genetic studies linking cytokines and growth factors, especially the TGF-β/TGF-β receptor system, may further shed light on the predictability of diabetic nephropathy in the population at risk.

In summary, TGF-β successfully fulfils all of Koch's postulates to qualify as a causative agent of diabetic nephropathy [177]: 1) High ambient glucose and recombinant TGF-β1 exert similar actions on renal cells (i.e., cell hypertrophy and increased extracellular matrix synthesis). 2) Increased amounts of TGF-β are produced in renal cells when grown in high glucose (e.g., mesangial, proximal tubular, and renal interstitial cells). 3) Increased renal production and urinary levels of TGF-β1 are observed in diabetic animals and humans. 4) Upregulation of TGF-β receptors is observed in the glomerular and tubular compartments of experimental diabetic animals. 5) Genetic manipulation to overexpress TGF-β1 leads to glomerulosclerosis and tubulointerstitial fibrosis. 7) Features of the diabetic state such as high levels of vasoactive agents (thromboxane, AII, and endothelin) in the glomerulus, increased levels of nonenzymatically-glycated proteins, and intraglomerular hypertension can all increase glomerular TGF-β1 production. 8) Patients with type 2 diabetes have increased renal production of TGF-β1 prior to established overt nephropathy, and the increased glomerular expression of TGF-β1 correlates with glycemic control. 9) Inhibition of TGF-β bioactivity using neutralizing anti-TGF-β antibodies or antisense TGF-β1 oligodeoxynucleotides reverses the glucose-stimulated matrix production in cultured renal cells. 10) Finally, systemic treatment with neutralizing panselective anti-TGF-β antibodies or antisense TGF-β1 oligodeoxynucleotides prevents the early manifestations of diabetic renal disease in STZ-diabetic mice and effectively prevents renal insufficiency and mesangial matrix expansion in type 2 diabetic *db/db* mice. It is hoped that future innovative therapies that rationally target the TGF-β system will vastly improve clinical outcomes in the twenty-first century beyond what is achievable with current practices [178].

ACKNOWLEDGMENTS

Supported in part by a grant from the Juvenile Diabetes Foundation International and by the National Institutes of Health (DK-44513, DK-45191, and DK-54608 to Dr. F. N. Ziyadeh and training grant DK-07006). Dr. S. Chen is a nephrology fellow at the University of Pennsylvania and is supported by the Juvenile Diabetes Foundation International. Dr. M. C. Iglesias de la Cruz is a visiting scholar at the University of Pennsylvania and is supported by the Ministerio de Educación y Cultura, Spain. Dr. M. Isono is a visiting scholar at the University of Pennsylvania and is supported by a fellowship grant from the Juvenile Diabetes Foundation International.

REFERENCES:

1.	Goldfarb S, Ziyadeh FN, Kern EFO, Simmons DA. Effects of polyol-pathway inhibition and dietary myo-inositol on glomerular hemodynamic function in experimental diabetes mellitus in rats. Diabetes 1991;40:465-471.

2.   DeRubertis FR, Craven PA. Activation of protein kinase C in glomerular cells in diabetes. Mechanisms and potential links to the pathogenesis of diabetic glomerulopathy. Diabetes 1994;43:1-8.

3.   Fumo P, Kuncio GS, Ziyadeh FN. PKC and high glucose stimulate collagen α1[IV] transcriptional activity in a reporter mesangial cell line. Am J Physiol 1994;267:F632-F638.

4.   Kolm-Litty V, Sauer U, Nerlich A, Lehmann R, Schleicher ED. High glucose-induced transforming growth factor beta-1 production is mediated by the hexosamine pathway in porcine glomerular mesangial cells. J Clin Invest 1998;101:160-169.

5.   Brownlee M, Vlassara H, Cerami A. Nonenzymatic glycosylation and the pathogenesis of diabetic complications. Ann Intern Med 1984;101:527-537.

6.   Cohen MP, Ziyadeh FN. Amadori glucose adducts modulate mesangial cell growth and collagen gene expression. Kidney Int 1994;45:475-484.

7.   Hoffman BB, Ziyadeh FN. The role of growth factors in the development of diabetic nephropathy. Curr Opin Endocrinol Diabetes 1996;3:322-329.

8.   Abboud HE. Growth factors and diabetic nephrology: An overview. Kidney Int Suppl 1997;60:S3-S6.

9.   Roberts AB, Kim S-J, Noma T, Glick AB, Lafyatis R, Lechleider R, Jaakowlew SB, Geiser A, O'Reilly MA, Danielpour D, Sporn MB. Multiple forms of TGF-beta: Distinct promoters and differential expression. In Clinical Applications of TGF-beta. Sporn MB and Roberts AB (ed.): Chichester, UK, Ciba Foundation Symposium, 1991, 7-28.

10.   Mozes MM, Bottinger EP, Jacot TA, Kopp JB. Renal expression of fibrotic matrix proteins and of transforming growth factor-beta (TGF-beta) isoforms in TGF-beta transgenic mice. J Am Soc Nephrol 1999;10:271-280.

11.   Ziyadeh FN. The extracellular matrix in diabetic nephropathy. Am J Kidney Dis 1993;22:736-744.

12.   Wolf G, Ziyadeh FN. Molecular mechanisms of diabetic renal hypertrophy. Kidney Int 1999;56:393-405.

13.   Laiho M, Saksela O, Andreasen PA, Keski-Oja J. Enhanced production and extracellular deposition of the endothelial-type plasminogen activator inhibitor in cultured human lung fibroblasts by transforming growth factor-beta. J Cell Biol 1986;103:2403-2410.

14.   MacKay K, Kondaiah P, Danielpour D, Austin HA 3d, Brown PD. Expression of transforming growth factor-beta-1 and beta-2 in rat glomeruli. Kidney Int 1990;38:1095-1100.

15.   Sharma K, Ziyadeh FN. Biochemical events and cytokine interactions linking glucose metabolism to the development of diabetic nephropathy. Semin Nephrol 1997;17:80-92.

16.   Hoffman M. Researchers get a first look at the versatile TGF-beta family. Science 1992;257:332.

17.   Miyazono K, Heldin CH. Latent forms of TGF-beta: Molecular structure and mechanisms of activation. In Clinical Applications of TGF-beta. Bock GR and Marsh J (ed.): Wiley, 1991, 81-92.

18.   Paralkar VM, Vukicevic S, Reddi AH. Transforming growth factor beta type 1 binds to collagen IV of basement membrane matrix: Implications for development. Dev Biol 1991;143:303-308.

19.   Wakefield LM, Winokur TS, Hollands RS, Christopherson K, Levinson AD, Sporn MB. Recombinant latent transforming growth factor beta-1 has a longer plasma half-life in rats than active transforming growth factor beta-1, and a different tissue distribution. J Clin Invest 1990;86:1976-1984.

20. Ando T, Okuda S, Tamaki K, Yoshitomi K, Fujishima M. Localization of transforming growth factor-beta and latent transforming growth factor-beta binding protein in rat kidney. Kidney Int 1995;47:733-739.

21. Flaumenhaft R, Abe M, Mignatti P, Rifkin DB. Basic fibroblast growth factor-induced activation of latent transforming growth factor-beta in endothelial cells: Regulation of plasminogen activator activity. J Cell Biol 1992;118:901-909.

22. Massague J, Attisano L, Wrana JL. The TGF-beta family and its composite receptors. Trends Cell Biol 1994;4:172-178.

23. Wrana JL, Attisano L, Wieser R, Ventura F, Massague J. Mechanism of activation of the TGF-beta receptor. Nature 1994;370:341-347.

24. Wieser R, Attisano L, Wrana JL, Massague J. Signaling activity of transforming growth factor-beta type II receptors lacking specific domains in the cytoplasmic region. Mol Cell Biol 1993;13:7239-7247.

25. Sekelsky JJ, Newfeld SJ, Raftery LA, Chartoff EH, Gelbart WM. Genetic characterization and cloning of mothers against dpp, a gene required for decapentaplegic function in Drosophila melanogaster. Genetics 1995;139:1347-1358.

26. Liu F, Hata A, Baker JC, Doody J, Carcamo J, Harland RM, Massague J. A human Mad protein acting as a BMP-regulated transcriptional activator. Nature 1996;381:620-623.

27. Zhang Y, Feng X, We R, Derynck R. Receptor-associated Mad homologues synergize as effectors of the TGF-beta response. Nature 1996;383:168-172.

28. Hayashi H, Abdollah S, Qiu Y, Cai J, Xu YY, Grinnell BW, Richardson MA, Topper JN, Gimbrone MA Jr, Wrana JL, Falb D. The MAD-related protein Smad7 associates with the TGF-beta receptor and functions as an antagonist of TGF-beta signaling. Cell 1997;89:1165-1173.

29. Ziyadeh FN. Renal tubular basement membrane and collagen type IV in diabetes mellitus. Kidney Int 1993;43:114-120.

30. Cohen MP, Ziyadeh FN. Role of Amadori-modified nonenzymatically glycated serum proteins in the pathogenesis of diabetic nephropathy. J Am Soc Nephrol 1996;7:183-190.

31. Ziyadeh FN, Snipes ER, Watanabe M, Alvarez RJ, Goldfarb S, Haverty TP. High glucose induces cell hypertrophy and stimulates collagen gene transcription in proximal tubule. Am J Physiol 1990;259:F704-F714.

32. Wolf G, Sharma K, Chen Y, Ericksen M, Ziyadeh FN. High glucose-induced proliferation in mesangial cells is reversed by autocrine TGF-beta. Kidney Int 1992;42:647-656.

33. Ayo SH, Radnik R, Garoni JA, Troyer DA, Kreisberg JI. High glucose increases diacylglycerol mass and activates protein kinase C in mesangial cell cultures. Am J Physiol 1991;261:F571-F577.

34. Ayo SH, Radnik RA, Glass WF 2d, Garoni JA, Rampt ER, Appling DR, Kreisberg JI. Increased extracellular matrix synthesis and mRNA in mesangial cells grown in high-glucose medium. Am J Physiol 1991;260:F185-F191.

35. Haneda M, Kikkawa R, Horide N, Togawa M, Koya D, Kajiwara N, Ooshima A, Shigeta Y. Glucose enhances type IV collagen production in cultured rat glomerular mesangial cells. Diabetologia 1991;34:198-200.

36. Ziyadeh FN, Sharma K, Ericksen M, Wolf G. Stimulation of collagen gene expression and protein synthesis in murine mesangial cells by high glucose is mediated by autocrine activation of transforming growth factor-beta. J Clin Invest 1994;93:536-542.

37. Wakisaka M, Spiro MJ, Spiro RG. Synthesis of type VI collagen by cultured glomerular cells and comparison of its regulation by glucose and other factors with that of type IV collagen. Diabetes 1994;43:95-103.

38. Kolm V, Sauer U, Olgemooller B, Schleicher ED. High glucose-induced TGF-beta-1 regulates mesangial production of heparan sulfate proteoglycan. Am J Physiol 1996;270:F812-F821.

39. van Det NF, Verhagen NA, Tamsma JT, Berden JH, Bruijn JA, Daha MR, van der Woude FJ. Regulation of glomerular epithelial cell production of fibronectin and transforming growth factor-beta by high glucose, not by angiotensin II. Diabetes 1997;46:834-840.

40. Han DC, Isono M, Hoffman BB, Ziyadeh FN. High glucose stimulates proliferation and collagen type I synthesis in renal cortical fibroblasts: Mediation by autocrine activation of TGF-beta. J Am Soc Nephrol 1999;10:1891-1899.

41. Takeuchi A, Throckmorton DC, Brogden AP, Yoshizawa N, Rasmussen H, Kashgarian M. Periodic high extracellular glucose enhances production of collagens III and IV by mesangial cells. Am J Physiol 1995;268:F13-F19.

42. Heilig C, Concepcion L, Riser BL, Freytag S. Overexpression of GLUT1 in rat mesangial cells: A new model to simulate diabetes. J Am Soc Nephrol 1994;5:965 [abstract].

43. van Det NF, van den Born J, Tamsma JT, Verhagen NA, Berden JH, Bruijn JA, Daha MR, van der Woude FJ. Effects of high glucose on the production of heparan sulfate proteoglycan by mesangial and epithelial cells. Kidney Int 1996;49:1079-1089.

44. Kasinath BS, Block JA, Singh AK, Terhune WC, Maldonado R, Davalath S, Kallgren MJ, Wanna L. Regulation of rat glomerular epithelial cell proteoglycans by high-glucose medium. Arch Biochem Biophys 1994;309:149-159.

45. Rocco MV, Ziyadeh FN. Transforming growth factor-beta: An update on systemic and renal actions. In Hormones, Autacoids, and the Kidney. Goldfarb S and Ziyadeh FN (ed.): New York, Churchill Livingstone, 1991, 391-410.

46. Wolf G, Ziyadeh FN. The role of angiotensin II in diabetic nephropathy: Emphasis on nonhemodynamic mechanisms. Am J Kidney Dis 1997;29:153-163.

47. Ziyadeh FN, Simmons DA, Snipes ER, Goldfarb S. Effect of myo-inositol on cell proliferation and collagen transcription and secretion in proximal tubule cells cultured in elevated glucose. J Am Soc Nephrol 1991;1:1220-1229.

48. Rocco MV, Chen Y, Goldfarb S, Ziyadeh FN. Elevated glucose stimulates TGF-beta gene expression and bioactivity in proximal tubule. Kidney Int 1992;41:107-114.

49. Song RH, Singh AK, Alavi N, Leehey DJ. Decreased collagenase activity of mesangial cells incubated in high glucose media is reversed by neutralizing antibody to transforming growth factor-beta. J Am Soc Nephrol 1994;5:972 [abstract].

50. Mogyorosi A, Hoffman BB, Guo J, Jin Y, Ericksen M, Sharma K, Ziyadeh FN. Elevated glucose concentration stimulates expression of the type II receptor in glomerular mesangial cells. J Am Soc Nephrol 1996;7:1875 [abstract].

51. Guh JY, Yang ML, Yang YL, Chang CC, Chuang LY. Captopril reverses high-glucose-induced growth effects on LLC-PK1 cells partly by decreasing transforming growth factor-beta receptor protein expressions. J Am Soc Nephrol 1996;7:1207-1215.

52. Riser BL, Ladson-Wofford S, Sharba A, Cortes P, Drake K, Guerin CJ, Yee J, Choi ME, Segarini PR, Narins RG. TGF-beta receptor expression and binding in rat mesangial cells: Modulation by glucose and cyclic mechanical strain. Kidney Int 1999;56:428-439.

53. Hoffman B, Sharma K, Zhu Y, Ziyadeh F. Transcriptional activation of transforming growth factor-beta-1 in mesangial cell culture by high glucose concentration. Kidney Int 1998;54:1107-1116.

54. Kim SJ, Glick A, Sporn MB, Roberts AB. Characterization of the promoter region of the human transforming growth factor-beta-1 gene. J Biol Chem 1989;264:402-408.

55. Craven PA, DeRubertis FR. Protein kinase C is activated in glomeruli from streptozotocin diabetic rats. J Clin Invest 1989;83:1667-1675.

56. Studer RK, Negrete H, Craven PA, DeRubertis FR. Protein kinase C signals thromboxane induced increases in fibronectin synthesis and TGF-beta bioactivity in mesangial cells. Kidney Int 1995;48:422-430.

57. Negrete H, Studer RK, Craven PA, DeRubertis FR. Role for transforming growth factor-beta in thromboxane-induced increases in mesangial cell fibronectin synthesis. Diabetes 1995;44:335-339.

58. Babazono T, Kapor-Drezgic J, Dlugosz J, Whiteside C. Altered expression and subcellular localization of diacylglycerol-sensitive protein kinase C isoforms in diabetic rat glomerular cells. Diabetes 1998;47:668-676.

59. Zhang G, Kazanietz MG, Blumberg PM, Hurley JH. Crystal structure of the cys2 activator-binding domain of protein kinase C delta in complex with phorbol ester. Cell 1995;81:917-924.

60. Haneda M, Araki S, Togawa M, Sugimoto T, Isono M, Kikkawa R. Mitogen-activated protein kinase cascade is activated in glomeruli of diabetic rats and glomerular mesangial cells under high glucose conditions. Diabetes 1997;46:847-853.

61. Awazu M, Ishikura K, Hida M, Hoshiya M. Mechanisms of mitogen-activated protein kinase activation in experimental diabetes. J Am Soc Nephrol 1999;10:738-745.

62. Igarashi M, Wakasaki H, Takahara N, Ishii H, Jiang ZY, Yamauchi T, Kuboki K, Meier M, Rhodes CJ, King GL. Glucose or diabetes activates p38 mitogen-activated protein kinase via different pathways. J Clin Invest 1999;103:185-195.

63. de Groot RP, Auwerx J, Karperien M, Staels B, Kruijer W. Activation of junB by PKC and PKA signal transduction through a novel cis-acting element. Nucleic Acids Res 1991;19:775-781.

64. Chung KY, Agarwal A, Uitto J, Mauviel A. An AP-1 binding sequence is essential for regulation of the human alpha 2(I) collagen (COL1A2) promoter activity by transforming growth factor-beta. J Biol Chem 1996;271:3272-3278.

65. Shankland SJ, Scholey JW. Expression of growth-related protooncogenes during diabetic renal hypertrophy. Kidney Int 1995;47:782-788.

66. Kreisberg JI, Radnik RA, Ayo SH, Garoni J, Saikumar P. High glucose elevates c-fos and c-jun transcripts and proteins in mesangial cell cultures. Kidney Int 1994;46:105-112.

67. Wilmer WA, Cosio FG. DNA binding of activator protein-1 is increased in human mesangial cells cultured in high glucose concentrations. Kidney Int 1998;53:1172-1181.

68. Kim SJ, Angel P, Lafyatis R, Hattori K, Kim KY, Sporn MB, Karin M, Roberts AB. Autoinduction of transforming growth factor-beta-1 is mediated by the AP-1 complex. Mol Cell Biol 1990;10:1492-1497.

69. Inoki K, Haneda M, Maeda S, Koya D, Kikkawa R. TGF-beta-1 stimulates glucose uptake by enhancing GLUT1 expression in mesangial cells. Kidney Int 1999;55:1704-1712.

70. Tada H, Isogai S. The fibronectin production is increased by thrombospondin via activation of TGF-beta in cultured human mesangial cells. Nephron 1998;79:38-43.

71. Ito Y, Aten J, Bende RJ, Oemar BS, Rabelink TJ, Weening JJ, Goldschmeding R. Expression of connective tissue growth factor in human renal fibrosis. Kidney Int 1998;53:853-861.

72. Murphy M, Godson C, Cannon S, Kato S, Mackenzie HS, Martin F, Brady HR. Suppression subtractive hybridization identifies high glucose levels as a stimulus for expression of connective tissue growth factor and other genes in human mesangial cells. J Biol Chem 1999;274:5830-5834.

73. Duncan MR, Frazier KS, Abramson S, Williams S, Klapper H, Huang X, Grotendorst GR. Connective tissue growth factor mediates transforming growth factor beta-induced collagen synthesis: Down-regulation by cAMP. FASEB J 1999;13:1774-1786.

74. Grotendorst GR. Connective tissue growth factor: A mediator of TGF-beta action on fibroblasts. Cytokine Growth Factor Rev 1997;8:171-179.
75. Sharma K, Ziyadeh FN. Hyperglycemia and diabetic kidney disease. The case for transforming growth factor-beta as a key mediator. Diabetes 1995;44:1139-1146.
76. Park I, Kiyomoto H, Abboud S, Abboud H. Expression of transforming growth factor-beta and type IV collagen in early streptozotocin-induced diabetes. Diabetes 1997;46:473-480.
77. Sharma K, Ziyadeh FN. Renal hypertrophy is associated with upregulation of TGF-beta-1 gene expression in diabetic BB rat and NOD mouse. Am J Physiol 1994;267:F1094-F1101.
78. Sharma K, Jin Y, Guo J, Ziyadeh FN. Neutralization of TGF-beta by anti-TGF-beta antibody attenuates kidney hypertrophy and the enhanced extracellular matrix gene expression in STZ-induced diabetic mice. Diabetes 1996;45:522-530.
79. Pankewycz OG, Guan JX, Bolton WK, Gomez A, Benedict JF. Renal TGF-beta regulation in spontaneously diabetic NOD mice with correlations in mesangial cells. Kidney Int 1994;46:748-758.
80. Shankland SJ, Scholey JW. Expression of transforming growth factor-beta-1 during diabetic renal hypertrophy. Kidney Int 1994;46:430-442.
81. Yang S, Fletcher WH, Johnson DA. Regulation of cAMP-dependent protein kinase: Enzyme activation without dissociation. Biochem 1995;34:6267-6271.
82. Koya D, Jirousek MR, Lin YW, Ishii H, Kuboki K, King GL. Characterization of protein kinase C beta isoform activation on the gene expression of transforming growth factor-beta, extracellular matrix components, and prostanoids in the glomeruli of diabetic rats. J Clin Invest 1997;100:115-126.
83. Reckelhoff JF, Tygart VL, Mitias MM, Walcott JL. STZ-inducted diabetes results in decreased activity of glomerular cathepsin and metalloprotease in rats. Diabetes 1993;42:1425-1432.
84. Yamamoto T, Nakamura T, Noble N, Ruoslahti E, Border W. Expression of transforming growth factor-beta is elevated in human and experimental diabetic nephropathy. Proc Natl Acad Sci USA 1993;90:1814-1818.
85. Nakamura T, Fukui M, Ebihara I, Osada S, Nagaoka I, Tomino Y, Koide H. mRNA expression of growth factors in glomeruli from diabetic rats. Diabetes 1993;42:450-456.
86. Bertoluci MC, Schmid H, Lachat JJ, Coimbra TM. Transforming growth factor-beta in the development of rat diabetic nephropathy. A 10-month study with insulin-treated rats. Nephron 1996;74:189-196.
87. Han DC, Kim YJ, Cha MK, Song KI, Kim JH, Lee EY, Ha H, Lee HB. Glucose control suppressed the glomerular expression of TGF-beta-1 and the progression of experimental diabetic nephropathy. J Am Soc Nephrol 1996;7:1870 [abstract].
88. Ziyadeh FN, Hoffman BB, Guo J, Eltayeb BO, Han DC, Sharma K. Amelioration of renal insufficiency and excess matrix gene expression by chronic treatment with anti-TGF-beta antibody in db/db diabetic mice. J Am Soc Nephrol 1998;9:646A [abstract].
89. Yamamoto T, Noble NA, Cohen AH, Nast CC, Hishida A, Gold LI, Border WA. Expression of transforming growth factor-beta isoforms in human glomerular diseases. Kidney Int 1996;49:461-469.
90. Yoshioka K, Takemura T, Murakami K, Okada M, Hino S, Miyamoto H, Maki S. Transforming growth factor-beta protein and mRNA in glomeruli in normal and diseased human kidneys. Lab Invest 1993;68:154-163.
91. Iwano M, Kubo A, Nishino T, Sato H, Nishioka H, Akai Y, Kurioka H, Fujii Y, Kanauchi M, Shiiki H, Dohi K. Quantification of glomerular TGF-beta-1 mRNA in patients with diabetes mellitus. Kidney Int 1996;49:1120-1126.

92.   Di Paolo S, Gesualdo L, Ranieri E, Grandaliano G, Schena FP. High glucose concentration induces the overexpression of transforming growth factor-beta through the activation of a platelet-derived growth factor loop in human mesangial cells. Am J Path 1996;149:2095-2106.

93.   Phillips AO, Steadman R, Topley N, Williams JD. Elevated D-glucose concentrations modulate TGF-beta-1 synthesis by human cultured renal proximal tubular cells. The permissive role of platelet-derived growth factor. Am J Path 1995;147:362-374.

94.   Sharma K, Ziyadeh FN, Alzahabi B, McGowan TA, Kapoor S, Kurnik BRC, Kurnik PB, Weisberg LS. Increased renal production of transforming growth factor-beta-1 in patients with type II diabetes. Diabetes 1997;46:854-859.

95.   Sharma K, Eltayeb BO, Alzahabi B, Ziyadeh FN, Rhode R, Lewis EJ. Captopril-induced reduction in serum levels of TGF-beta-1 predicts long-term renoprotection in insulin-dependent diabetic patients. Am J Kidney Dis 1999;34:818-823.

96.   Lewis EJ, Hunsicker LG, Bain RP, Rohde RD. The effect of angiotensin-converting-enzyme inhibition on diabetic nephropathy. The collaborative study group. N Engl J Med 1993;329:1456-1462.

97.   Pociot F, Hansen PM, Karlsen AE, Langdahl BL, Johannesen J, Nerup J. TGF-beta-1 gene mutations in insulin-dependent diabetes mellitus and diabetic nephropathy. J Am Soc Nephrol 1998;9:2302-2307.

98.   Wolf G, Mueller E, Stahl RAK, Ziyadeh FN. Angiotensin II-induced hypertrophy of cultured murine proximal tubular cells is mediated by endogenous transforming growth factor-beta J Clin Invest 1993;92:1366-1372.

99.   Kagami S, Border WA, Miller DE, Noble NA. Angiotensin II stimulates extracellular matrix protein synthesis through induction of transforming growth factor-beta expression in rat glomerular mesangial cells. J Clin Invest 1994;93:2431-2437.

100.   Riser BL, Cortes P, Heilig C, Grondin J, Ladson-Wofford S, Patterson D, Narins RG. Cyclic stretching force selectively up-regulates transforming growth factor-beta isoforms in cultured rat mesangial cells. Am J Pathol 1996;148:1915-1923.

101.   Mogensen CE. Renoprotective role of ACE inhibitors in diabetic nephropathy. Br Heart J 1994;72:S38-S45.

102.   Morabito E, Corsico N, Arrigoni Martelli E. Endothelins urinary excretion is increased in spontaneously diabetic rats: BB/BB. Life Sci 1995;56:PL13-PL18.

103.   Nakamura T, Ebihara I, Fukui M, Tomino Y, Koide H. Effect of a specific endothelin receptor A antagonist on mRNA levels for extracellular matrix components and growth factors in diabetic glomeruli. Diabetes 1995;44:895-899.

104.   Takahashi K, Ghatei MA, Lam HC, O'Halloran DJ, Bloom SR. Elevated plasma endothelin in patients with diabetes mellitus. Diabetologia 1990;33:306-310.

105.   Ferri C, Laurenti O, Bellini C, Faldetta MRC, Properzi G, Santucci A, De Mattia G. Circulating endothelin-1 levels in lean non-insulin-dependent diabetic patients. Influence of ACE inhibition. Am J Hypertens 1995;8:40-47.

106.   Ledbetter S, Copeland EJ, Noonan D, Vogeli G, Hassell JR. Altered steady-state mRNA levels of basement membrane proteins in diabetic mouse kidneys and thromboxane synthase inhibition. Diabetes 1990;39:196-203.

107.   Craven PA, Caines MA, DeRubertis FR. Sequential alterations in glomerular prostaglandin and thromboxane synthesis in diabetic rats: Relationship to the hyperfiltration of early diabetes. Metabolism 1987;36:95-103.

108. Gambardella S, Andreani D, Cancelli A, Di Mario U, Cardamone I, Stirati G, Cinotti GA, Pugliese F. Renal hemodynamics and urinary excretion of 6-keto-prostaglandin F1alpha and thromboxane B2 in newly diagnosed type I diabetic patients. Diabetes 1988;37:1044-1048.

109. Craven PA, Melhem MF, DeRubertis FR. Thromboxane in the pathogenesis of glomerular injury in diabetes. Kidney Int 1992;42:937-946.

110. DeRubertis FR, Craven PA. Contribution of platelet thromboxane production to enhanced urinary excretion and glomerular production of thromboxane and to the pathogenesis of albuminuria in the streptozotocin-diabetic rat. Metabolism 1992;41:90-96.

111. Bruggeman LA, Horigan EA, Horikoshi S, Ray PE, Klotman PE. Thromboxane stimulates synthesis of extracellular matrix proteins in vitro. Am J Physiol 1991;261:F488-F494.

112. Matsuo Y, Takagawa I, Koshida H, Kawabata T, Nakamura M, Ida T, Zhou L, Marumo F. Antiproteinuric effect of a thromboxane receptor antagonist, S-1452, on rat diabetic nephropathy and murine lupus nephritis. Pharmacology 1995;50:1-8.

113. Hora K, Oguchi H, Furukawa T, Hora K, Tokunaga S. Effects of a selective thromboxane synthetase inhibitor OKY-046 on experimental diabetic nephropathy. Nephron 1990;56:297-305.

114. Pricci F, Pugliese G, Mene P, Romeo G, Romano G, Galli G, Casini A, Rotella CM, DiMario U, Pugliese F. Regulatory role of eicosanoids in extracellular matrix overproduction induced by long-term exposure to high glucose in cultured rat mesangial cells. Diabetologia 1996;39:1055-1062.

115. Fukui M, Nakamura T, Ebihara I, Makita Y, Osada S, Tomino Y, Koide H. Effects of enalapril on endothelin-1 and growth factor gene expression in diabetic rat glomeruli. J Lab Clin Med 1994;123:763-768.

116. Inaba T, Ishibashi S, Gotoda T, Kawamura M, Morino N, Nojima Y, Kawakami M, Yazaki Y, Yamada N. Enhanced expression of platelet-derived growth factor-beta receptor by high glucose. Involvement of platelet-derived growth factor in diabetic angiopathy. Diabetes 1996;45:507-512.

117. Fagerudd JA, Groop PH, Honkanen E, Teppo AM, Gronhagen-Riska C. Urinary excretion of TGF-beta-1, PDGF-BB and fibronectin in insulin-dependent diabetes mellitus patients. Kidney Int Suppl 1997;63:S195-S197.

118. Throckmorton DC, Brogden AP, Min B, Rasmussen H, Kashgarian M. PDGF and TGF-beta mediate collagen production by mesangial cells exposed to advanced glycosylation end products. Kidney Int 1995;48:111-117.

119. Doi T, Vlassara H, Kirstein M, Yamada Y, Striker GE, Striker LJ. Receptor-specific increase in extracellular matrix production in mouse mesangial cells by advanced glycosylation end products is mediated via platelet-derived growth factor. Proc Natl Acad Sci USA 1992;89:2873-2877.

120. Flyvbjerg A, Bornfeldt KE, Marshall SM, Arnqvist HJ, Orskov H. Kidney IGF-I mRNA in initial renal hypertrophy in experimental diabetes in rats. Diabetologia 1990;33:334-338.

121. Flyvbjerg A, Marshall SM, Frystyk J, Hansen KW, Harris AG, Orskov H. Octreotide administration in diabetic rats: Effects on renal hypertrophy and urinary albumin excretion. Kidney Int 1992;41:805-812.

122. Serri O, Beauregard H, Brazeau P, Abribat T, Lambert J, Harris A, Vachon L. Somatostatin analogue, octreotide, reduces increased glomerular filtration rate and kidney size in insulin-dependent diabetes. JAMA 1991;265:888-892.

123. Quaife CJ, Mathews LS, Pinkert CA, Hammer RE, Brinster RL, Palmiter RD. Histopathology associated with elevated levels of growth hormone and insulin-like growth factor I in transgenic mice. Endocrinology 1989;124:40-48.

124. Flyvbjerg A, Bennett WF, Rasch R, Kopchick JJ, Scarlett JA. Inhibitory effect of a growth hormone receptor antagonist (G120K-PEG) on renal enlargement, glomerular hypertrophy, and urinary albumin excretion in experimental diabetes in mice. Diabetes 1999;48:377-382.

125. Tischer E, Mitchell R, Hartman T, Silva M, Gospodarowicz D, Fiddes JC, Abraham JA. The human gene for vascular endothelial growth factor. Multiple protein forms are encoded through alternative exon splicing. J Biol Chem 1991;266:11947-11954.

126. Neufeld G, Cohen T, Gengrinovitch S, Poltorak Z. Vascular endothelial growth factor (VEGF) and its receptors. FASEB J 1999;13:9-22.

127. Shweiki D, Itin A, Soffer D, Keshet E. Vascular endothelial growth factor induced by hypoxia may mediate hypoxia-initiated angiogenesis. Nature 1992;359:843-845.

128. Senger DR, Connolly DT, Van de Water L, Feder J, Dvorak HF. Purification and NH_2-terminal amino acid sequence of guinea pig tumor-secreted vascular permeability factor. Cancer Res 1990;50:1774-1778.

129. Keck PJ, Hauser SD, Krivi G, Sanzo K, Warren T, Feder J, Connolly DT. Vascular permeability factor, an endothelial cell mitogen related to PDGF. Science 1989;246:1309-1312.

130. Conn G, Bayne ML, Soderman DD, Kwok PW, Sullivan KA, Palisi TM, Hope DA, Thomas KA. Amino acid and cDNA sequences of a vascular endothelial cell mitogen that is homologous to platelet-derived growth factor. Proc Natl Acad Sci USA 1990;87:2628-2632.

131. Brown LF, Berse B, Tognazzi K, Manseau EJ, Van de Water L, Senger DR, Dvorak HF, Rosen S. Vascular permeability factor mRNA and protein expression in human kidney. Kidney Int 1992;42:1457-1461.

132. Simon M, Grone HJ, Johren O, Kullmer J, Plate KH, Risau W, Fuchs E. Expression of vascular endothelial growth factor and its receptors in human renal ontogenesis and in adult kidney. Am J Physiol 1995;268:F240-F250.

133. Grone HJ, Simon M, Grone EF. Expression of vascular endothelial growth factor in renal vascular disease and renal allografts. J Pathol 1995;177:259-267.

134. Pupilli C, Lasagni L, Romagnani P, Bellini F, Mannelli M, Misciglia N, Mavilia C, Vellei U, Villari D, Serio M. Angiotensin II stimulates the synthesis and secretion of vascular permeability factor/vascular endothelial growth factor in human mesangial cells. J Am Soc Nephrol 1999;10:245-255.

135. Uchida K, Uchida S, Nitta K, Yumura W, Marumo F, Nihei H. Glomerular endothelial cells in culture express and secrete vascular endothelial growth factor. Am J Physiol 1994;266:F81-F88.

136. Simon M, Rockl W, Hornig C, Grone EF, Theis H, Weich HA, Fuchs E, Yayon A, Grone HJ. Receptors of vascular endothelial growth factor/vascular permeability factor (VEGF/VPF) in fetal and adult human kidney: Localization and [125I]VEGF binding sites. J Am Soc Nephrol 1998;9:1032-1044.

137. Takahashi T, Shirasawa T, Miyake K, Yahagi Y, Maruyama N, Kasahara N, Kawamura T, Matsumura O, Mitarai T, Sakai O. Protein tyrosine kinases expressed in glomeruli and cultured glomerular cells: Flt-1 and VEGF expression in renal mesangial cells. Biochem Biophys Res Commun 1995;209:218-226.

138. Jakeman LB, Winer J, Bennett GL, Altar CA, Ferrara N. Binding sites for vascular endothelial growth factor are localized on endothelial cells in adult rat tissues. J Clin Invest 1992;89:244-253.

139. Risau W. Angiogenesis and endothelial cell function. Arzneimittelforschung 1994;44:416-417.

140.   Klanke B, Simon M, Rockl W, Weich HA, Stolte H, Grone HJ. Effects of vascular endothelial growth factor (VEGF)/vascular permeability factor (VPF) on haemodynamics and permselectivity of the isolated perfused rat kidney. Nephrol Dial Transplant 1998;13:875-885.

141.   Natarajan R, Bai W, Lanting L, Gonzales N, Nadler J. Effects of high glucose on vascular endothelial growth factor expression in vascular smooth muscle cells. Am J Physiol 1997;273:H2224-H2231.

142.   Williams B, Gallacher B, Patel H, Orme C. Glucose-induced protein kinase C activation regulates vascular permeability factor mRNA expression and peptide production by human vascular smooth muscle cells in vitro. Diabetes 1997;46:1497-1503.

143.   Iijima K, Yoshikawa N, Connolly DT, Nakamura H. Human mesangial cells and peripheral blood mononuclear cells produce vascular permeability factor. Kidney Int 1993;44:959-966.

144.   Pal S, Claffey KP, Dvorak HF, Mukhopadhyay D. The von Hippel-Lindau gene product inhibits vascular permeability factor/vascular endothelial growth factor expression in renal cell carcinoma by blocking protein kinase C pathways. J Biol Chem 1997;272:27509-27512.

145.   Chua CC, Hamdy RC, Chua BH. Upregulation of vascular endothelial growth factor by H_2O_2 in rat heart endothelial cells. Free Radic Biol Med 1998;25:891-897.

146.   Ruef J, Hu ZY, Yin LY, Wu Y, Hanson SR, Kelly AB, Harker LA, Rao GN, Runge MS, Patterson C. Induction of vascular endothelial growth factor in balloon-injured baboon arteries. A novel role for reactive oxygen species in atherosclerosis. Circ Res 1997;81:24-33.

147.   Pertovaara L, Kaipainen A, Mustonen T, Orpana A, Ferrara N, Saksela O, Alitalo K. Vascular endothelial growth factor is induced in response to transforming growth factor-beta in fibroblastic and epithelial cells. J Biol Chem 1994;269:6271-6274.

148.   Goad DL, Rubin J, Wang H, Tashjian AH Jr, Patterson C. Enhanced expression of vascular endothelial growth factor in human SaOS-2 osteoblast-like cells and murine osteoblasts induced by insulin-like growth factor I. Endocrinology 1996;137:2262-2268.

149.   Hata Y, Rook SL, Aiello LP. Basic fibroblast growth factor induces expression of VEGF receptor KDR through a protein kinase C and p44/p42 mitogen-activated protein kinase-dependent pathway. Diabetes 1999;48:1145-1155.

150.   Nauck M, Roth M, Tamm M, Eickelberg O, Wieland H, Stulz P, Perruchoud AP. Induction of vascular endothelial growth factor by platelet-activating factor and platelet-derived growth factor is downregulated by corticosteroids. Am J Respir Cell Mol Biol 1997;16:398-406.

151.   Ahmed A, Dearn S, Shams M, Li XF, Sangha RK, Rola-Pleszczynski M, Jiang J. Localization, quantification, and activation of platelet-activating factor receptor in human endometrium during the menstrual cycle: PAF stimulates NO, VEGF, and FAKpp125. FASEB J 1998;12:831-843.

152.   Gruden G, Thomas S, Burt D, Zhou W, Chusney G, Gnudi L, Viberti G. Interaction of angiotensin II and mechanical stretch on vascular endothelial growth factor production by human mesangial cells. J Am Soc Nephrol 1999;10:730-737.

153.   Malamitsi-Puchner A, Sarandakou A, Tziotis J, Dafogianni C, Bartsocas CS. Serum levels of basic fibroblast growth factor and vascular endothelial growth factor in children and adolescents with type 1 diabetes mellitus. Pediatr Res 1998;44:873-875.

154.   Shulman K, Rosen S, Tognazzi K, Manseau EJ, Brown LF. Expression of vascular permeability factor (VPF/VEGF) is altered in many glomerular diseases. J Am Soc Nephrol 1996;7:661-666.

155. Haltia A, Solin ML, Jalanko H, Holmberg C, Miettinen A, Holthofer H. Mechanisms of proteinuria: Vascular permeability factor in congenital nephrotic syndrome of the Finnish type. Pediatr Res 1996;40:652-657.

156. Webb NJ, Watson CJ, Roberts IS, Bottomley MJ, Jones CA, Lewis MA, Postlethwaite RJ, Brenchley PE. Circulating vascular endothelial growth factor is not increased during relapses of steroid-sensitive nephrotic syndrome. Kidney Int 1999;55:1063-1071.

157. Horita Y, Miyazaki M, Koji T, Kobayashi N, Shibuya M, Razzaque MS, Cheng M, Ozono Y, Kohno S, Taguchi T. Expression of vascular endothelial growth factor and its receptors in rats with protein-overload nephrosis. Nephrol Dial Transplant 1998;13:2519-2528.

158. Wolf G, Hamann A, Han DC, Helmchen U, Thaiss F, Ziyadeh FN, Stahl RAK. Leptin stimulates proliferation and TGF-beta expression in renal glomerular endothelial cells: Potential role in glomerulosclerosis. Kidney Int 1999;56:860-872.

159. Hamann A, Matthaei S. Regulation of energy balance by leptin. Exp Clin Endocrinol Diabetes 1996;104:293-300.

160. Halaas JL, Gajiwala KS, Maffei M, Cohen SL, Chait BT, Rabinowitz D, Lallone RL, Burley SK, Friedman JM. Weight-reducing effects of the plasma protein encoded by the obese gene. Science 1995;269:543-546.

161. Maffei M, Fei H, Lee GH, Dani C, Leroy P, Zhang Y, Proenca R, Negrel R, Ailhaud G, Friedman JM. Increased expression in adipocytes of ob RNA in mice with lesions of the hypothalamus and with mutations at the db locus. Proc Natl Acad Sci USA 1995;92:6957-6960.

162. Chua SC Jr, Chung WK, Wu-Peng XS, Zhang Y, Liu SM, Tartaglia L, Leibel RL. Phenotypes of mouse diabetes and rat fatty due to mutations in the OB (leptin) receptor. Science 1996;271:994-996.

163. Cohen MP, Clements RS, Hud E, Cohen JA, Ziyadeh FN. Evolution of renal function abnormalities in the db/db mouse that parallels the development of human diabetic nephropathy. Exp Nephrol 1996;4:166-171.

164. Wolf G, Schroeder R, Thaiss F, Ziyadeh FN, Helmchen U, Stahl RAK. Glomerular expression of p27Kip1 in diabetic *db/db* mouse: Role of hyperglycemia. Kidney Int 1998;53:869-879.

165. Ziyadeh FN, Mogyorosi A, Kalluri R. Early and advanced non-enzymatic glycation products in the pathogenesis of diabetic kidney disease [editorial]. Exp Nephrol 1997;5:2-9.

166. Ziyadeh FN, Han DC, Cohen JA, Guo J, Cohen MP. Glycated albumin stimulates fibronectin gene expression in glomerular mesangial cells: Involvement of the transforming growth factor-beta system. Kidney Int 1998;53:631-638.

167. Yang C-W, Vlassara H, Peten EP, He C-J, Striker GE, Striker LJ. Advanced glycation end products up-regulate gene expression found in diabetic glomerular disease. Proc Natl Acad Sci USA 1994;91:9436-9440.

168. Ha H, Kamanna VS, Kirschenbaum MA, Kim KH. Role of glycated low density lipoprotein in mesangial extracellular matrix synthesis. Kidney Int Suppl 1997;60:S54-S59.

169. Skolnik EY, Yang Z, Makita Z, Radoff S, Kirstein M, Vlassara H. Human and rat mesangial cell receptors for glucose-modified proteins: Potential role in kidney tissue remodelling and diabetic nephropathy. J Exp Med 1991;174:931-939.

170. Riser BL, Cortes P, Zhao X, Bernstein J, Dumler F, Narins RG. Intraglomerular pressure and mesangial stretching stimulate extracellular matrix formation in the rat. J Clin Invest 1992;90:1932-1943.

171. Yasuda T, Kondo S, Homma T, Harris RC. Regulation of extracellular matrix by mechanical stress in rat glomerular mesangial cells. J Clin Invest 1996;98:1991-2000.
172. Ohno M, Cooke JP, Dzau VJ, Gibbons GH. Fluid shear stress induces endothelial transforming growth factor-beta-1 transcription and production. Modulation by potassium channel blockade. J Clin Invest 1995;95:1363-1369.
173. Baynes JW. Role of oxidative stress in development of complications in diabetes. Diabetes 1991;40:405-412.
174. Yaqoob M, McClelland P, Patrick AW, Stevenson A, Mason H, White MC, Bell GM. Evidence of oxidant injury and tubular damage in early diabetic nephropathy. QJM 1994;87:601-607.
175. Nath KA, Grande J, Croatt A, Haugen J, Kim Y, Rosenberg ME. Redox regulation of renal DNA synthesis, transforming growth factor-beta-1 and collagen gene expression. Kidney Int 1998;53:367-381.
176. Ha H, Yu MR, Kim KH. Melatonin and taurine reduce early glomerulopathy in diabetic rats. Free Radic Biol Med 1999;26:944-950.
177. Ziyadeh FN. Evidence for the involvement of transforming growth factor-beta in the pathogenesis of diabetic kidney disease: Are Koch's postulates fulfilled? Curr Pract Med 1998;1:87-89.
178. Mogensen CE, Christensen CK. Predicting diabetic nephropathy in insulin-dependent patients. N Engl J Med 1984;311:89-93.

27. BLOOD PRESSURE ELEVATION IN DIABETES: THE RESULTS FROM 24-h AMBULATORY BLOOD PRESSURE RECORDINGS

Klavs Würgler Hansen, Per Løgstrup Poulsen and Eva Ebbehøj
Aarhus Kommunehospital, Medical Dept. M, DK-8000 Aarhus, Denmark

Ambulatory blood pressure (BP) measurement permits assessment of BP in the patients own surroundings, during normal daily activities on the job and in the night. Previously semiautomatic monitors were used, which required manually inflation of the cuff [1], or direct (intra-arterial) BP measurement [2]. The first true ambulatory 24-h report of indirectly measured BP obtained with a portable and fully automatic monitor was published in 1975 [3]

The application of the technique to diabetic patients was first reported by Rubler in 1982 using an equipment weighing 3.07 kg [4]. The number of studies using ambulatory BP monitoring in diabetic patient in the eighties were moderate and with a few exceptions [4-7] focusing on autonomic neuropathy [8-13].

The knowledge from ambulatory BP measurement in general has recently been reviewed [14-18] and practical guidelines published [18-20]. Including the present one five reviews of ambulatory BP measurement in diabetes have appeared [21-24].

METHODOLOGICAL ASPECTS: A GUIDE TO THE CRITICAL READER.
The two most popular ways of obtaining automatic indirect BP records are either by use of an microphone in the cuff or by oscillometric technique [19,25]. Some monitors offers both options. While the manufacturer of the monitor is always stated in papers dealing with ambulatory BP monitoring, the technique is not necessarily described.

No monitor is perfect and even in monitors which have fulfilled national standards, major discrepancies between the monitors and values obtained by sphygmomanometry are observed in some of the patients. Some papers state that individually "calibration" of the monitor to each of the studied patients has been performed (by 3 to 5 simultaneous or sequential measurements). However, it is not possibly to calibrate a fully automatic monitor in strict terms (without returning to the manufacturer) and the word calibration is a misnomer in this context. The difference between auscultatory BP and the monitor can be evaluated in each patient (rather inaccurate) and this difference can either be accepted or not.

If the result of clinic BP measurement is provided it should be observed whether this is obtained by sphygmomanometry or by use of the same monitor as used for ambulatory measurements [26]. Only in the latter case are clinic and ambulatory values directly comparable.

Although more sophisticated methods exist [27,28], the diurnal variation of BP is usually reported as the night/day ratio. Obviously this must be based on individual information of the night period, otherwise the ratio is overestimated [29].

The term "non-dipper" has become a popular short term for a person who do not describe a normal reduction of BP at night. A commonly used definition of a "non-dipper" requires a relative reduction of night blood pressure less than 10 % of the day value for both systolic and diastolic BP [30]. Unfortunately no consensus exist. In addition the proportion of non-dippers also depends on the definition of night and day time which should be based on individiual information of time for going to bed and rising rather than fixed periods. If individual information is not available the use of "short fixed intervals" have been proposed [31].

Patients who are hypertensive by clinic measurements but shows a normal ambulatory BP are designated "white coat hypertensive" [32]. This term is well understood in literature although "isolated clinic hypertension" may be more precise [33]. The effect of the "white coat" was originally described as a transient (5 min) elevation of BP [33]. At present the "white coat effect" is usually calculated as the difference (clinic BP - day time BP) [34]. The proportion of white coat hypertensive subjects in a hypertensive population depends on:

i: The definition of hypertension (usually clinic BP > 140/90 mmHg)

ii: How carefully the hypertensive subjects are identified (if patients are labelled as hypertensive based on only one clinic BP the frequency of white coat hypertension is high, if a several clinic BP measurements -as recommended- are obtained at different occasions before diagnosis, the frequency is lower).

iii: The definition of a normal ambulatory BP (if the cut off limit for a normal ambulatory BP is defined as a day time BP < 131/86 mmHg the freqency of white coat hypertension is lower than for a cut off limit of BP < 140/90 mmHg).

iiii: The presence of other selection criteria related to clinic BP level or possible end organ signs. (The frequency of white coat hypertension is higher in a population with mild hypertension than in a population with moderate or severe hypertension even if the white coat effect is higher in the latter group [34]). If a hypertensive population are selected on the basis of criteria which may be related to elevated BP (i.e. albuminuria or retinopathy in diabetes) the proportion of patients who fulfill the criteria for white coat hypertension is assumed to be low.

NIDDM AND AMBULATORY BP

The influence of changes in metabolic control
Shift from sulfonylurea to insulin in poorly controlled elderly NIDDM patient improved glycemic control but ambulatory BP after one year was unaffected perhaps due to weight gain [35].

Comparison with healthy individuals.
Some discrepancies exist. One study has reported an increase in 24-h systolic (but not diastolic) BP in normoalbuminuric diabetic patients [36]. Two recent studies did not found any difference in 24-h average BP, however the nocturnal reduction of systolic BP was impaired in normoalbuminuric patients [37,38].

If patients (UAE not specified) and healthy subjects were divided into groups with and without hypertension no statistical difference of 24-h BP have been reported [7,39].

The relation to abnormal albuminuria.
No difference in day time or 24-h BP were noticed between normo- and microalbuminuric patients [36,38,40-43]. In contrast ambulatory BP was reported significantly higher in microalbuminuric patients (90 % males, 50 % non-caucasians) than in normoalbuminuric patients (71 % males, 28 % non-caucasians) [44]. In NIDDM both ambulatory and clinic BP correlates with UAE roughly to a similar extent [36,44] although one study using albumin/creatinine ratio reported no correlation [45]. Ambulatory BP is higher in patients with diabetic nephropathy than in normoalbuminuric patients [37,46].

Abnormal diurnal BP pattern (high night BP) are seen in patients with microalbuminuria [38,42,43,46- 49] and overt diabetic nephropathy [37,46,48]. As in IDDM this abnormality seems closely linked to the presence of autonomic neuropathy [37,38,50,51].

The time course of ambulatory BP
In patients receiving standard clinical care including antihypertensive medication, 24-h BP was remarkable stable in both normo- and microalbuminuric patients during an observation period of 4.6 years. Individual changes in both systolic and diastolic 24-h BP were related to changes in UAE [52]. The evolution of UAE did not differ between patients with and without abnormal diurnal BP profile at baseline [52].

Non-dipper: Autonomic neuropathy, diabetic nephropathy and extracellular volume.
Numerous studies in mixed IDDM and NIDDM populations or unclassified diabetic patients have demonstrated a reduction or (in few patients) even a reversal of the normal nocturnal decline of BP [11-13,53-57] in patients with autonomic neuropathy. Also in homogenous NIDDM diabetic patients several studies demonstrates [37,41,50,58] the association between diabetic nephropathy, signs of autonomic neuropathy or both and a blunted diurnal variation of blood pressure. According to two studies increased nocturnal

sympathetic activity (rather than expansion of extracellular volume) seems to be involved in reduced nocturnal BP in NIDDM patients with nephropathy [37,51]. However, a physiological defence against nocturnal volume expansion may explain why a lower night level of aldosteron and a higher level of plasma atrial natriuretic peptide have been reported in "non-dippers", who also had more pronounced signs of autonomic neuropathy than "dippers" [58].

Postprandial hypotension is also a phenomenon observed in patients with autonomic neuropathy [59,60].

The relation to insulin resistance and sodium-lithium countertransport
Ambulatory systolic BP (and clinic systolic BP) correlated in one study with glucose disposal rate, but not with fasting insulin level [61]. However, this relation was not confirmed in another study (S Nielsen personal communication) [40]. No relation has been found between ambulatory BP and sodium-lithium countertransport [44].

The relation to diabetic retinopathy
No studies designed for this purpose exist, one study suggest a relation between "non-dipping" status and retinopathy [52].

IDDM AND AMBULATORY BP

The influence of diabetes duration
Two cross sectional study reports a reduction of the nocturnal BP fall in long term normoalbuminuric diabetic patients [62,63].

The influence of sex
The well known BP difference between healthy males and females seems attenuated in IDDM [63-65].

The influence of short term changes in metabolic control
This question has so far never been addressed by well designed intervention studies employing ambulatory BP. Clinic BP has been reported lower after short term improvement of diabetic control by insulin pumps (24-h insulin dose unchanged) [66]. Intraarterial BP (10-h day time average) was also reduced after improved glycemic control achieved by increasing insulin dose in most patients [67]. No significant change in clinic BP was observed in a study where poor metabolic control was obtained by reducing insulin dose [68].

Recently it has been suggested that intensive insulin therapy by hyperinsulinemia (1.0 U/kg) is associated with high night blood pressure [69]. However, it has convincingly been demonstrated that tight blood glucose control obtained by normal insulin doses (0.6 U/kg) by no means affects the normal nocturnal blood pressure reduction [70].

The influence of smoking and type of day (work day/day-off)
We have compared ambulatory BP in 16 normoalbuminuric smokers and non-smokers without hypertension. Systolic BP was slightly higher (3mmHg day time, 5 mmHg night time) in smokers, but this failed to reach statistical significance [71]. In a larger study encompassing 24 normoalbuminuric smokers and non-smokers diastolic day and night BP was significantly higher (3.9 and 3.5 mmHg respectively) in smokers. In addition a dose response relationship was demonstrated [72]. Notably, this effect of smoking in diabetic individuals contrast the well known finding of a lower night BP in non-diabetic smokers [71,73]. Smoking does not affect the night/day ratio of BP in diabetes [71,72,74].

Day time BP is significantly lower (5 mmHg) on a day off than on a work day [63].

Comparison with healthy individuals
Most studies [75-80], but not all [64,81,82] agree that day time BP is comparable between normoalbuminuric diabetic patients and healthy subjects. Since ambulatory BP is higher in normoalbuminuric females than in healthy females [63,64], the result of a comparison between a diabetic and a control population depends on the sex distribution. Also the majority of investigators found no difference in the diurnal BP profile [75,76,79-82]. In contrast two studies have reported a slightly reduced nocturnal BP fall [64,77] and one study has surprisingly described a much higher night/day ratio of BP in normoalbuminuric patients [78]. Recently ambulatory BP was compared in normoalbuminuric IDDM patients and healthy controls (n=55 in each group) [64] . In contrast to previous comparison [75] (n=34 in each group) a slightly but significantly higher ambulatory BP was observed in diabetic patients. This may be explained by a higher proportion of women (42% vs. 29% in the previous study) and partly by increased statistical power due to the larger number of patients. Ambulatory BP (24h and day) was higher in diabetic women than in control women but no difference (for 24h and day time) was observed between diabetic men and control men. The night dip in BP was similar in diabetic and control women but a reduced night dip was reported for diabetic men compared with control men. Diastolic night dip in BP correlated in the total diabetic population with indices of autonomic neuropathy [64].

With this exceptions, the diversities are minor and may be explained by varying diabetes duration or proportion of males/females. Thus, as a rule normoalbuminuric patients have a 24-h BP profile very similar to healthy control subjects (Fig 27-1).

The relation to abnormal albuminuria
This subject has been reviewed [83]. Ambulatory BP is significantly higher and the diurnal BP pattern is abnormal in consecutively studied patients compared with healthy controls [84]. This largely depends on abnormal albuminuria present in some of the patients [84]. Four studies comparing normo- and microalbuminuric patients as well as healthy controls are summarized in Table 27-1. Ambulatory BP are significantly increased in microalbuminuric as compared with normoalbuminuric patients [75,85-87].

In some studies day time BP were only numerically but not statistically significantly higher in microalbuminuric patients [81,88,89]. This is probably due to lower number of

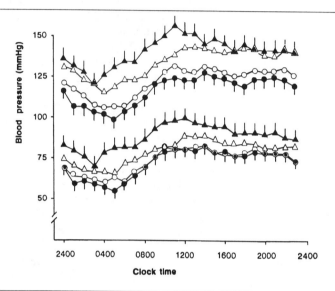

Fig. 27-1. Twenty-four hour profile of mean systolic and diastolic BP for type 1 diabetic patients and healthy controls. Diabetic patients with nephropathy and without antihypertensive treatment (n=13, filled triangles), microalbuminuric patients (n=26, open triangles), normoalbuminuric patients (n=26, open circles) and healthy individuals (n=26, filled circles). From [90] with permission.

microalbuminuric patients in these studies. The night/day ratio of diastolic BP is significantly higher in microalbuminuric patients than in healthy individuals [90] and night/day ratio for normoalbuminuric patients is in between (Fig. 27-2 and Table 27-1). If the comparison between microalbuminuric and normoalbuminuric patients is restricted to patients in good metabolic control and without any signs of autonomic neuropathy day time BP is still elevated in microalbuminuric patients [80]. Ambulatory BP correlates more closely with UAE than clinic BP (Table 27-2). The phenomenon has recently been confirmed [80]. This is probably due to the multiplicity of measurements rather than their quality as true ambulatory values (Fig 27-3).

Ambulatory BP is further increased in patients with overt diabetic nephropathy [90] (Fig 27-1) and the circadian variation of BP is severely disturbed in patients with advanced diabetic nephropathy and antihypertensive medication [90,91] (Fig 27-2).

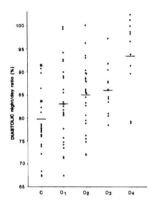

Fig. 27-2. Individual night/day ratio for diastolic BP in healthy individuals and type 1 diabetic patients. C= control subjects (n=26), D_1= normoalbuminuric patients (n=26), D_2= microalbuminuric patients (n=26), D_3= patients with diabetic nephropathy without antihypertensive treatment (n=13), D_4= patients with diabetic nephropathy with antihypertensive treatment. From [90] with permission.

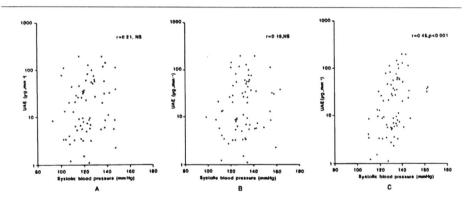

Fig. 27-3 The correlation between overnight urinary albumin excretion (UAE, three collections) and BP in normo- and microalbuminuric type 1 diabetic patients. A) systolic clinic BP measured by sphygmomanometry (average of three values) B) systolic ambulatory BP (average of three) values about 11.00 h) C) day time average of systolic ambulatory BP (average of approximately 48 values). The correlation coefficient (Pearson) and significance level are indicated. Partly from [75] with permission.

Table 27-1. Four studies comparing ambulatory blood pressure in micro- and normoalbuminuric type 1 diabetic patients and healthy control subjects.**(Continue on next page)**

	A Hansen et al [75]			B Moore et al [81]		
	Controls	Normo	Micro	Controls	Normo	Micro
N (male/female)	34	34	34	36	27	11
Sex (male/female	24/10	24/10	24/10	19/17	14/133	5/6
Age (years)	31	31	30	17	18	19
Diabetes duration (yrs)	-	18	18	-	9	14*
HbA1C(%)	5.1	8.3	9.1*	-	12.5	12.7
Body mass Index (kg●m^{-2})	23.1	23.7	23.9	-	-	-
	Three overnight collections			One 24h collection		
UAE (µg●min^{-1})	5.2	5.1	51.7	-	5.3	45.2
Monitor and frequency of measure-ments	Spacelabs 90202 06.00h-24.00h every 20 min 24.00h-06.00h every 60 min			Spacelabs 90202 06.00h-22.00h every 20 min 22.00-06.00h every 60 min		
Definition of day and night periods	Individually recorded periods			Day (06.00h-22.00h) Night (22.00h-06.00)		
BP criteria for inclusion of patients	All patients included (no antihypertensive treatment)			<130/85		
Clinic BP (auscultatory)	119/75	121/77	124/81	-	-	-
Clinic BP (monitor)	125/74	128/74	132/79*	102/54	106/64*	118*/70*
Day time BP	125/77	127/77	136*/82*	117/67	123*/71*	130/76
Night time BP	109/61	112/63	122*/69*	110/59	116*/63*	126*/71*
Night/day ratio(systolic/ diastolic)	0.87/0.80	0.88/0.82	0.90/0.85	0.94/0.88[a]	0.94/0.89[a]	0.97/0.93[a]
Day-night BP difference	16/16	15/14	14/13	7/8[a]	7/8[a]	4/5[a]
24h BP	119/71	122/73	131*/78*	116/66	122*/70*	129/75
Comments	Normoalbuminuric patients individually matched to microalbuminric patients for sex, age and diabetes duration			Glycosulated hemoglobin HbA is presented. Clinic BP is not measured with the same monitor as ambulatory blood pressure		

Values are numbers or mean except for UAE in study A (geomtric mean) and in study C (median). For clarity the level of statistical significance is not indicated more specific and the results of comparison between microalbuminuric patients and healthy controls is not given. *, p<0.05 vesus controls (for normoalbuminuric patients) or versus normoalbuminuric patients (for microalbuminuric patients). [a]; the values are derived from original data without access to statistical analysis.

Table 27-1. Four studies comparing ambulatory blood pressure in micro- and normoalbuminuric type 1 diabetic patients and healthy control subjects.**(Continued from previous page)**

	C Benhamou et al [76]			D Lurbe et al [88]		
	Controls	Normo	Micro	Controls	Normo	Micro
N (male/female)	12	12	12	45	34	11
Sex (male/female)	7/5	7/5	7/5	20/25	-	-
Age (years)	≈31	≈31	31	23	18	24
Diabetes duration (yrs)	-	7	15*	-	5	13*
HbA1C (%)	-	7.3	8.8*	-	-	-
Body mass index (kg•m^{-2})	≈21.5	≈21.5	21.5	22.2	20.1	24.8
	Three overnight collections			Three 24-h collections		
UAE (µg•min^{-1})	-	<15	56	-	4.5	111
Monitor and frequency of measure-ments	Spacelabs 90207 07.00h-17.00h every 15 min 17.00h-07.00h every 30 min			Spacelabs 90207 06.00h-24.00h every 20 min 24.00h-06.00 every 30 min		
Definition of day and night periods	Day (09.00h-19.00h) Night (23.00h-07.00h)			Day (0.8.00h-22.00h) Night(24.00-06.00h)		
BP criteria for inclusion of patients	<140/90			<140/90 or <95 percentile level		
Clinic BP (auscultatory)	118/79	119/78	116/73	121/70	120/69	125/74
Clinic BP (monitor)	-	-	-	-	-	-
Day time BP	116/76	118/78	124/81	117/71	117/71	122/72
Night time BP	100/61	103/65	113*/68	113/60	114/60	121*/69*
Night/day ratio (systolic/diastolic)	0.86/0.80[a]	0.88/0.83[a]	0.91/0.84	0.94/0.83	0.93/0.84	0.97/0.94*
Day-night BP difference	16/15	15/13	11/13	4/11	3/11[a]	1/3
24-h BP	110/71	112/71	119 */75	114/67	116/66	121/71
Comments	Patients were admitted to hospital during the night			No statistical analysis between controls and normoalbuminuric patients have been performed.		

Values are numbers or mean except for UAE in study A (geomtric mean) and in study C (median). For clarity the level of statistical significance is not indicated more specific and the results of comparison between microalbuminuric patients and healthy controls is not given. *, p<0.05 vesus controls (for normoalbuminuric patients) or versus normoalbuminuric patients (for microalbuminuric patients). ; the values are derived from original data without access to statistical analysis.

The transition from normo- to microalbuminuria

In a recent study 40 initially normoalbuminuric patients were reinvestigated with ambulatory BP monitoring and measurement of UAE after a mean period of 3 years [92]. Six patients progressed to microalbuminuria and their baseline UAE (9.7 µg min^{-1}) were statistically significantly higher than baseline UAE in non-progressors (5.5 µg min^{-1}). Importantly, no difference were noticed between 24-h ambulatory BP at baseline in progressors (124/74 mmHg) and non-progressors (124/75 mmHg). However, the rise in UAE even to low microalbuminuria (31.7 µg min^{-1}) were accompanied with an increase in 24-h ambulatory BP (12/5 mmHg) which was statistically higher than the increase in non-progressors (4/2 mmHg). No statistically significant changes were seen if these changes were evaluated from the average of three clinic BP measurements at baseline and at follow up [92]. The diastolic night/day ratio at baseline was significantly higher in progressors (0.88) than in non-progressors (0.81), but no further increase was found in progressors during follow-up and the overlap between the two groups was large.

In a cross sectional study of normoalbuminuric patients the 24-h BP were significantly higher in patients with "high" normal UAE than in patients with "low" normal UAE [93,94]. Similar results have been reported in a study comparing "high" normoalbuminuric patients with healthy individuals [95].

These results support the idea that rise in UAE and ambulatory BP can not be separated even in the very early phase of incipient diabetic nephropathy.

Table 27-2. Correlations between blood pressure and urinary albumin excretion in combined normo- and microalbuminuric type 1 diabetic patients.

	A Hansen et al [75]	B Moore et al [81]	C Benhamou et al [76]	D Lurbe et al [88]
UAE	Three overnight collections	One 24-h collection	Three overnight collections	Three 24-h collections
Correlations:	Normo (n=34) and Micro (n=34)	Normo (n=27) and Micro (n=11)	Normo (n=23) and Micro (n=12)	Normo (n=34) and Micro (n=11)
UAE vs. Clinic BP (auscultatory)	r=0.21, NS (systolic)	-	r=0.01, NS (systolic)	r=0.19, NS (MAP)
UAE vs. Day time BP	r=0.45, p<0.05 (systolic)	-	r=0.17, NS (systolic)	r=0.35, p<0.05(MAP)
UAE vs. Night time BP	r=0.53, p<0.00001 (systolic)	-	r=0.38, p<0.05 (systolic)	r=0.60, p<0.01 (MAP)
UAE vs 24h BP	r=0.49, p<0.0001 (systolic)	R=0.40, p<0.01 (systolic) R=0.60, p<0.01 (diastolic)	r=0.29, NS (systolic)	-

Non-dipper: Autonomic neuropathy, nephropathy and expansion of extracellular volume (ECV)

In IDDM the presence of autonomic neuropathy is clearly associated with impaired reduction of night BP [10,96,97]. Autonomic neuropathy and diabetic nephropathy are closely associated [98-101]. Their relative role for the abnormal diurnal variation in blood pressure is therefore difficult to ascertain. However, the literature gives no examples of a group of IDDM patients with blunted diurnal variation of BP without concomitant signs of autonomic neuropathy either by formal test [96,97] or by increased heart rate [75]. Indeed autonomic dysfunction can be documented even in "high" normoalbuminuric patients if refined test (spectral analysis of heart rate variability) is employed [94]. In contrast an impaired reduction of night BP and increased heart rate is seen in long term diabetic patients who are strictly normoalbuminuric [62,63].

Naturally the question of a possible causative role of autonomic neuropathy for the development of diabetic nephropathy has arisen [102,103]. The link could be a higher night BP which is more readily transmitted to the glomeruli because of renal vasodilation. Alternatively early autonomic dysfunction may just be part of a syndrome indicative of later diabetic complications in patients with suboptimal glycemic control [94,104].

A retrospective study in patients with diabetic nephropathy has described a faster decline of renal function in patients with a "non-dipping" BP profile compared with "dippers" [105]. However there was no baseline or follow-up measurement of ambulatory BP, which was measured at one time point only during a 6 year observation period. Since renal function was already reduced in "non-dippers" at the time when the ambulatory BP measurement was performed it is not possible to postulate a cause/effect relationship.

Expanded ECV has been described even in normoalbuminuric "non-dippers"[106]. Two lines of evidence suggest that homeostasis of ECV is associated with elevated night BP in particular in patients abnormal albuminuria. First   plasma aldosteron is reported significantly lower in "non-dipping" patients with incipient diabetic nephropathy, which could be interpreted as a defence against fluid retention [107]. Second, in patients with overt diabetic nephropathy, elevated nocturnal BP is associated with expansion of ECV. This may reflect the result of a nocturnal shift of fluid from the interstitial to the intravascular space [108]. This view has been challenged by a study which did not find any association between elevated night BP and ECV in IDDM patients with nephropathy [109].

The relation to glomerular filtration rate (GFR)
A negative correlation between ambulatory BP and GFR has been described in microalbuminuric patients [81,110]. Non dippers with microalbuminuria or overt nephropathy seems not to have a reduced GFR [107-109]. One study in normoalbuminuric patients reported a higher night BP and expanded ECV (23 litre) in patients with glomerular hyperfiltration compared with the group with normofiltration (19 litre) [106]. Despite similar methods (Cr EDTA single shot) ECV is found inexplicable high in this latter study [106] compared with the two previously mentioned studies dealing with nephropathy (14 litre) [108,109].

The relation to diabetic retinopathy

Elevated night BP is reported in patients with more advanced signs of diabetic retinopathy. Importantly this association was described in strictly normoalbuminuric patients excluding the confounding effect of diabetic kidney disease [111].

Predisposition to hypertension and diabetic nephropathy

The controversy of predisposition to hypertension and development of diabetic nephropathy has recently been addressed by performing ambulatory BP in parents of IDDM patients with and without diabetic nephropathy [112]. The 24h BP was almost identical among the two group of parents without antihypertensive medication (126/76 vs. 126/74 mmHg respectively, NS) . The frequency of hypertension defined as use of antihypertensive medication or a 24h BP > 135/85 mmHg was significantly higher in parents of patients with nephropathy (57%) than in parents patients without nephropathy (41%).

Relation to pregnancy

Ambulatory BP monitoring has been applied to both non-diabetic [113] (several publications) and diabetic pregnant women with purpose of early identification of patients at risk for developing preeclampsia [114].

AMBULATORY BLOOD PRESSURE AND INTERVENTION STUDIES

Due to the high reproducibility of ambulatory BP compared with clinic measurements it is an ideal tool for intervention studies [26,115]. The 24-h effectiveness of the intervention can be evaluated, the number of patients needed can be reduced without loosing power and small changes in BP, which would be overlooked by traditional measurements, can be recognised. Ambulatory BP has now been used in several intervention studies in diabetes [45,116-131].

So far there have been no reports of an altered circadian BP profile after antihypertensive treatment in diabetic patients. A shift from morning to evening dose of quinapril [132], perindopril [133] or isradipine [134] has reduced night BP in essential hypertension [132,133] and in renal failure [134]. Evening dose may give rise to a higher day time BP and adjustment of the dose may be necessary to achieve a well controlled BP in the day time [133].

AMBULATORY BLOOD PRESSURE AND CARDIAC MASS

An early study did not find any significant differences in either 24-h BP or cardiac mass NIDDM patients and healthy subjects [6]. Later, increased cardiac mass has been reported in diabetic patients (mixed IDDM and NIDDM) with autonomic neuropathy and associated reduced nocturnal decline of BP as compared with patients without autonomic neuropathy [135]. This may be an effect of autonomic dysfunction per se or the higher nocturnal BP. Similar results has been found in NIDDM patients with nephropathy, who have elevated 24h BP and higher night BP than patients with normoalbuminuria [136].

Left ventricular mass (LVM) and day time diastolic BP were found higher in microalbuminuric than in normoalbuminuric IDDM patients [80]. We have found no significant differences in cardiac mass between microalbuminuric IDDM patients with and without a normal reduction of night BP [107]. In an other study LVM did not differ between white coat hypertensive and normotensive NIDDM patients and LVM was lower in dippers compared to non-dippers (no information about UAE) [137]. Ambulatory BP has been employed in studies assessing the impact of different antihypertensive drugs on LVM in diabetes [129-131]

THE RELATION TO CLINIC BP

When studying young professionally active normotensive subjects the clinic BP is in mean 3- 4 mmHg higher than day time averages [75]. This is the opposite of what is normally seen in about 20-25 % of mildly hypertensive non-diabetic subjects (white-coat hypertension) [32,33]. The clinical implication is that BP is underestimated in some microalbuminuric patients with normal clinic BP.

We have found a markedly lower day time (systolic/diastolic) BP (147/ 85 mmHg) than clinic BP (163/95 mmHg) in 102 consecutive NIDDM and IDDM patients referred to ambulatory BP measurement because of repeated clinic BP > 140/90 mmHg [138]. The frequency of white coat hypertension in normoalbuminuric diabetic patients is about 25 % [138,139]. If patients are selected for the presence of organ lesions related to hypertension (diabetic nephropathy) the proportion of white coat hypertension may be reduced [139]. One study reported a much higher frequency of white coat hypertension (41 %) probably due to a shorter observation period before labelling patients as hypertensive and because patients was designated as "true" normotensive on the basis of 24h BP (containing the lower night BP) rather than day time values [140]. Obviously the reported frequency of white coat hypertension also varies with the definition of a normal ambulatory BP [32,33] . A widely used definition requieres repeated clinic BP > 140/90 and a day time value <135/85 mmHg. An extremely high freqency of white coat hypertension (62 %) was reported in a study measuring clinic BP at one occasion only and using the same cutt-off level for establishing the diagnosis of hypertension (clinic mean arterial BP > 100 mmHg) as for identifying those with apparent normal ambulatory BP (day time mean arterial BP < 100 mmHg) [141]. A low frequency (11 %) was reported in NIDDM patients who was categorized as normotensive if day time BP was < 131/86 (women) and < 136/87 (men) [137].   Also in adolescents a very high frequency of white coat hypertension has been disclosed [142].

AMBULATORY BP AND THE DIABETES CLINIC

Several international and national institutions now approve ambulatory BP monitoring in certain clinical circumstances [143, 144, 145]. The important problems about establishing a normal reference for ambulatory BP have recently been reviewed thouroughly [146]. Although large individual differences do exist, a clinic BP of 140/90 roughly corresponds to a day time average of 135/85 mmHg [146]. Even lower cut off limits for a normal day time BP has been suggested 125/80 [144], however the background for this proposal can be questioned indeed [147]. For patients older than 60 years with isolated systolic hypertension the average systolic day time BP is reported much lower (about 20 mmHg) than clinic BP during the placebo run-in phase of the Syst-Eur trial also containing diabetic patients [148]. Since treatment of isolated systolic hypertension (in the Syst-Euro and SHEP trials defined as systolic BP > 160 mmHg) significantly reduces the incidence of cardiovascular events, it is very difficult to suggest a "safe"cut off limit for day time BP in this category of patients. In contrast no difference was noted between clinic and day time systolic BP in a small subset of the SHEP population which underwent ambulatory BP monitoring [149]. This discrepancy between the clinic-day time difference in the Syst-Eur trial and SHEP trial may relate to the fact that the comparison between clinic and day time BP in the SHEP study was performed after 2 to 3 years enrolment in the study, which to some extent may have attenuated the "white coat effect".

The guidelines will doubtless need corrections based on future studies, which ideally should relate ambulatory BP to end organ damage and to clinical events in antihypertensive drug trials.

Three studies in diabetic patients give some information about the level of ambulatory BP, "dipper" or "non-dipper" status and future cardiovascular events [137,148,150]. During a follow-up of 3.2 years the rate of cardiovascular events per 100 patient years was 2.0 in clinic and ambulatory normotensive NIDDM patients (n=29), 2.06 in white coat hypertensive patients (n=12), and 7.06 in ambulatory hypertensive patients (n=94) (p<0.001 versus two other groups). Although the absolute number of events in the three groups were low (three, one and 24 events respectively) the data suggest a benign clinical course of white coat hypertensive patients at least in the short term. Furthermore the study showed a higher event rate in female "non-dippers" versus "dippers" [137]. Importantly the superiority of ambulatory BP (mainly night BP) versus clinic BP as a predictor of cardiovascular risk has recently been documented in two prospective studies with a much larger number of patients [148,150].

The clinical value of large scale implementation of ambulatory BP monitoring has never been investigated. However, it seems wise to hesitate with respect to antihypertensive drug treatment of normoalbuminuric diabetic patients (without any other signs of organ damage) with white coat hypertension. The value of targeting antihypertensive drug regimen towards high night BP is unexplored. At the moment a pragmatic view could be to accept the diagnosis of hypertension if repeated clinic BP > 140/90 and ambulatory day time BP > 135/85 mmHg. If the goal for antihypertensive treatment (in normoalbuminuric patients) is a clinic BP < 130/85 the same levels could be used as a goal for day time BP. The british recommendations of a day time BP goal less than 75 mmHg diastolic is not scientifically based [145].

The guidelines will doubtless need corrections based on future studies, which ideally should relate ambulatory BP to end organ damage and to clinical events in antihypertensive drug trials.

CONCLUSION

Ambulatory BP is increased in NIDDM and IDDM patients with abnormal albuminuria even in the absence of a detectable difference in clinic BP. An association exist in both NIDDM and IDDM patients between impaired reduction of night BP and the two complications, autonomic neuropathy and diabetic nephropathy. This also counts for the very early phases of diabetic nephropathy in IDDM patients. It remains to be eluciated if the abnormal BP variation independtly contributes to development of microalbumimuria or to the progression of diabetic nephropathy, or whether this abnormality is merely a cophenomenon found in patients with poor glycemic control and diabetic complications including autonomic neuropathy [102,103] .

The high reproducibility of ambulatory BP permits registration of small changes in BP which are overlooked by conventional measurement. Large scale longitudinal studies of ambulatory BP and UAE are necessary to characterize the important transition phase from normo- to microalbuminuria. Simultaneous continuos indirect registration of both the sympathovagal balance [150] and BP [151] are perspectives for the future, which probably will add to the understanding of BP variation in diabetes.

Ambulatory BP monitoring is now a well established and valuable procedure [153] also in the diabetes clinic. It seems wise to hesitate with respect to antihypertensive drug treatment in patients with white coat hypertension, if there is no signs of organ damage including microalbuminuria. The number of these patients who ultimately will become hypertensive by ambulatory BP is unknown and careful observation of BP is essential. There is still a need for more secure guidelines for the use of ambulatory BP including the consequences of specifically addressing antihypertensive treatment towards nocturnal hypertension.

REFERENCES

1   Sokolow M, Werdegar D, Kain HK, Hinman AT. Relationship between level of blood pressure measured casually and by portable recorders and severity of complications in essential hypertension. Circulation 1966; 34: 279-298

2   Bevan AT, Honour AJ, Stott FH. Direct arterial pressure recording in unrestricted man. Clin Sci 1969; 36: 329-344

3   Schneider RA, Costiloe JP. Twenty-four hour automatic monitoring of blood pressure and heart rate at work and at home. Am Heart J 1975; 90: 695-702

4   Rubler S, Abenavoli T, Greenblatt HA, Dixon JF, Cieslik CJ. Ambulatory blood pressure monitoring in diabetic males: A method for detecting blood pressure elevations undisclosed by conventional methods. Clin Cardiol 1982; 5: 447-454

5   Osei K. Ambulatory and exercise-induced blood pressure responses in type I diabetic patients and normal subjects. Diabetes Research and Clinical Practice 1987; 3: 125-134

6   Porcellati C, Gatteschi C, Benemio G, Guerrieri M, Boldrini F, Verdecchia P. Analisi ecocardiografica del ventriculo sinistro in pazienti con diabete mellito di tipo II. G Ital Cardiol 1989; 19: 128-135

7   Verdecchia P, Gatteschi C, Benemio G, Porcellati C. Ambulatory blood pressure monitoring in normotensive and hypertensive patients with diabetes (abstract). J Hypertension 1988; 6 (suppl 4): S692-S693

8   Rubler S, Chu DA, Bruzzone CL. Blood pressure and heart rate responses during 24-h ambulatory monitoring and exercise in men with diabetes mellitus. Am J Cardiol 1985; 55: 801-806

9   Guilleminault C, Mondini S, Hayes B. Diabetic autonomic dysfunction, blood pressure and sleep. Ann Neurol 1985; 18: 670-675

10   Reeves RA, Shapiro AP, Thompson ME, Johnsen A-M. Loss of nocturnal decline in blood pressure after cardiac transplantation. Circulation 1986; 73: 401-408

11   Liniger C, Favre L, Adamec R, Pernet A, Assal J-Ph. Profil nyctéméral de la pression artérielle et de la fréquence cardiaque dans la neuropathie diabétique autonome. Schweiz med Wschr 1987; 117: 1949-1953

12   Hornung RS, Mahler RF, Raftery EB. Ambulatory blood pressure and heart rate in diabetic patients: an assessment of autonomic function. Diabetic Med 1989; 6: 579-585

13   Chanudet X, Bauduceau B, Ritz P, Jolibois P, Garcin JM, Larroque P, Gautier D. Neuropathie végétative et régulation tensionelle chez le diabétique. Arch Mal Coer 1989; 82: 1147-1151

14   The National High Blood Pressure Education Program Coordinating Commitee. National High Blood Pressure Education Program Working Group Report on ambulatory blood pressure monitoring. Arch Intern Med 1990; 150: 2270-2280

15   Stewart MJ, Padfield PL. Blood Pressure measurement: an epitaph for the mercury manometer ? Clin Sci 1992; 83: 1-12

16   Purcell HJ, Gibbs SR, Coats AJS, Fox KM. Ambulatory blood pressure monitoring and circadian variation of cardiovascular disease; clinical and research applications. International Journal of Cardiology 1992; 36: 135-149

17   Stewart MJ, Padfield PL. Measurement of blood pressure in the technological age. British Medical Bulletin 1994; 50: 420-442

18   Pickering TG. Blood pressure measurement and detection of hypertension. Lancet 1994; 344: 31-35

19   Staessen JA, Fagard R, Thijs L, Amery A. A consensus view of the technique of ambulatory blood pressure monitoring. Hypertens 1995; [part 1]: 912-918

20   Pickering TG. Recommendations for the use of home (self) and ambulatory blood pressure monitoring. Am J Hypertens 1995; 9: 11

21   Halimi S, Benhamou PY, Mallion JM, Gaudemaris R, Bachelot I. Intérêt de l'enregistrement de la pression artérielle ambulatoire chez les patients diabétiques. Diabete Metab (Paris) 1991; 17: 538-544

22   White WB. Diurnal blood pressure and blood pressure variability in diabetic normotensive and hypertensive subjects. J Hypertension 1992; 10 (suppl 1): S35-S41

23   Hansen KW. How to monitor blood pressure changes in the diabetes clinic: office, home or 24 h-ambulatory blood pressure recordings. In: Mogensen CE, Standl E (eds). Diabetes Forum Series volume IV. Concepts for the ideal diabetes clinic. Berlin, New York: Walter de Gruyter; 1993; pp. 235-248

24   Pinkney JH, Denver AE, Yudkin JS. Ambulatory blood pressure monitoring in diabetes: An analysis of its potential in clinical practice. Cardiovascular risk factors 1997; 7: 175-183

25   Hansen KW, Christiansen JS. Research methodologies for recording blood pressure in diabetic patients. In: Mogensen CE, Standl E (eds). Diabetes Forum Series volume V (part 2). Research methodologies in human diabetes. Berlin, New York: Walter de Gruyter; 1994; pp. 113-124

26 Coats AJS, Radaelli A, Clark SJ, Conway J, Sleight P. The influence of ambulatory blood pressure monitoring on the design and interpretation of trials in hypertension. J Hypertens 1992; 10: 385-391

27 Coats AJS, Clark SJ, Conway J. Analysis of ambulatory blood pressure data. J Hypertens 1991; 9 (suppl 8): S19-S21

28 Germano G, Damiani S, Caparra A, Cassone-Faldetta M, Germano U, Coia F, De Mattia G, Santucci A, Balsano F. Ambulatory blood pressure recording in diabetic patients with abnormal responses to cardiovascular autonomic tests. Acta Diabetol 1992; 28: 221-228

29 Hansen KW, Poulsen PL, Mogensen CE. Ambulatory blood pressure and abnormal albuminuria in type 1 diabetic patients. Kidney Int 1994; 45 (suppl.45): S134-S140 (Correction. Kidney Int 45: 1799-1800, 1994)

30 Verdecchia P, Schillaci G, Guerrieri M, Gatteschi C, Benemio G, Boldrini F, Porcellati C. Circadian blood pressure changes and left ventricular hypertrophy in essential hypertension. Circulation 1990; 81: 528-536

31 Fagard R, Brguljan J, Lutgarde T, Staessen J. Prediction of the actual awake and asleep blood pressure by various methods of 24 h pressure analysis. J Hypertens 1996; 14: 557-563

32 Pickering TG. White coat hypertension. Curr Opin Nephrol Hypertens 1996; 5: 192-198

33 Mancia G, Zanchetti A. White-coat hypertension: misnomers, misconceptions and misunderstandings. What should we do next ?. J Hypertens 1996; 14: 1049-1052

34 Verdecchia P, Schillaci G, Borgioni C, Ciucci A, Zampi I, Gattobigio R, Sacchi N, Porcellati C. White coat hypertension and white coat effect. Similarities and differences. Am J Hypertens 1995; 8: 790-798

35 Tovi J, Theobald H, Engfeldt P. Effect of metabolic control on 24-h ambulatory blood pressure in elderly non-insulin-dependent diabetic patients. J Hum Hypertens 1996; 10: 589-594

36 Schmitz A, Mau Pedersen M, Hansen KW. Blood pressure by 24 h ambulatory recordings in type 2 (non-insulin-dependent) diabetics. Relationship to urinary albumin excretion. Diabete Metab (Paris) 1991; 17: 301-307

37 Nielsen FS, Rossing P, Bang Lia E, Svendsen TL, Gall M-A, Smidt UM, Parving H-H. On the mechanism of blunted nocturnal decline in arterial blood pressure in NIDDM patients with diabetic nephropathy. Diabetes 1995; 44: 783-789

38 Mitchell TH, Nolan B, Henry M, Cronin C, Baker H, Greely G. Microalbuminuria in patients with non-insulin-dependent diabetes mellitus relates to nocturnal systolic blood pressure. Am J Med 1997; 102: 531-535.

39 Fogari R, Zoppi A, Malamani GD, Lazzari P, Destro M, Corradi L. Ambulatory blood pressure monitoring in normotensive and hypertensive type 2 diabetics. Prevalence of impaired diurnal blood pressure patterns. Am J Hypertens 1993; 6: 1-7

40 Nielsen S, Schmitz O, Ørskov H, Mogensen CE. Similar insulin sensivity in NIDDM patients with normo- and microalbuminuria. Diabetes Care 1995; 18: 834-842

41 Jermendy G, Ferenzi J, Hernandez E, Farkas K, Nadas J. Day-night blood pressure variations in normotensive and hypertensive NIDDM patients with asymptomatic autonomic neuropathy. Diabetes Res Clin Pract 1996; 34: 107-114

42 Berrut G, Fabbri P, Bouhanick B, Lalanne P, Guilloteau G, Marre M, Fressinaud P. Loss of nocturnal blood pressure decrease in non-insulin dependent diabetis subjects with microalbuminuria. Arch Mal Coeur 1996; 89: 1041-1044

43 Lindsay RS, Stewart MJ, Nairn IM, Baird JD, Padfield PL. Reduced diurnal variation of blood pressure in non-insulin-dependent diabetic patients with microalbumnuria. J Hum Hypertens 1995; 9: 223-227

44 Pinkney JH, Foyle W-J, Denver AE, Mohamed-Ali V, McKinlay S, Yudkin JS. The relationship of urinary albumin excretion rate to ambulatory blood pressure and erythrocyte sodium-lithium countertransport in NIDDM. Diabetologia 1995; 38: 356-362

45 Waeber B, Weidmann P, Wohler D, Le Bloch Y. Albuminuria in diabetes mellitus. Relation to ambulatory versus office blood pressure and effects of cilazapril. Am J Hypertens 1996; 9: 1220-1227

46 Iwase M, Kaseda S, Iino K, Fukuhura M, Yamamoto M, Fukudome Y, Yoshizumi H, Abe I, Yoshinari M, Fujishima M. Circadian blood pressure variation in non-insulin-dependent diabetes mellitus with diabetic nephropathy. Diabetes Research and Clinical Practice 1994; 26: 43-50

47 Fogari R, Zoppi A, Malamani GD, Lazzari P, Albonico B, Corradi L. Urinary albumin excretion and nocturnal blood pressure in hypertensive patients with type II diabetes. Am J Hyp 1994; 7: 808-813

48 Equiluz-Bruck S, Schnack C, Schernthaner G. Nondipping of nocturnal blood pressure is related to urinary albumin excretion in patients with type 2 diabetes mellitus. Am J Hypertens 1996; 9: 1139-1143

49 Inaba M, Negishi K, Takashi M, Serizawa N, Maruno Y, Takahashi K, Katayama S. Increased night:day blood pressure ratio in microalbuminuric normotensive NIDDM subjects. Diabetes Res Clin Pract 1998; 40: 161-161

50 Nakano S, Uchida K, Kigoshi T, Azukizawa S, Iwasaki R, Kaneko M, Morimoto S. Circadian rhytm of blood pressure in normotensive NIDDM subjects. Its relation to microvascular complications. Diabetes Care 1991; 14: 707-711

51 Nielsen FA, Hansen HP, Jacobsen P, Rossing P, Smidt UM, Christensen NJ, Pevett P, Vivien-Roels B, Parving H-H. Increased sympathetic activity during sleep and nocturnal hypertension in type 2 diabetic patients with diabetic nephropathy. Diabetic Med 1999; 16: 555-562

52 Nielsen S, Schmitz A, Poulsen PL, Hansen KW, Mogensen CE. Albuminuria and 24-h ambulatory blood pressure in normoalbuminuric and microalbuminuric NIDDM patients. Diabetes Care 1995; 18: 1434-1441

53 Chamontin B, Barbe P, Begasse F, Ghisolfi A, Amar J, Louvet JP, Salvador M. Presion artérielle ambulatoire au cours de l'hypertension arterielle avec dysautonomie. Arch Mal Coer 1990; 83: 1103-1106

54 Felici MG, Spallone V, Maillo MR, Gatta R, Civetta E, Frontoni S, Gambardella S, Menzinger G. Twenty-four hours blood pressure and heart rate profiles in diabetics with and without autonomic neuropathy. Funct Neurol 1991; 6: 299-304

55 Liniger C, Favre L, Assal J-Ph. Twenty-four hour blood pressure and heart rate profiles of diabetic patients with abnormal cardiovascular reflexes. Diabetic Med 1991; 8: 420-427

56 Spallone V, Bernardi L, Ricordi L, Soldà P, Maillo MR, Calciati A, Gambardella S, Fratino P, Menzinger G. Relationship between the circadian rhytms of blood pressure and sympathovagal balance in diabetic autonomic neuropathy. Diabetes 1993; 42: 1745-1752

57 Ikeda T, Matsubara T, Sato Y, Sakamoto N. Circadian variation in diabetic patients with autonomic neuropathy. J Hypertens 1993; 11: 581-587

58 Nakano S, Uchida K, Ishii T, Takeuchi M, Azukizawa S, Kigoshi T, Morimoto S. Association of a nocturnal rise in plasma -atrial natriuretic peptide and reversed diurnal rhytm in hospitalized normotensive subjects with non-insulin dependent diabetes mellitus. Eur J Endocrinol 1994; 131: 184-190

59 Sasaki E, Kitaoka H, Ohsawa N. Postprandial hypotension in patients with non-insulin-dependent diabetes mellitus. Diabetes Research and Clinical Practice 1992; 18: 113-121

60   Nakajima S, Otsuka K, Yamanaka T, Omori K, Kubo Y, Toyoshima T, Watanabe Y, Watanabe H. Ambulatory blood pressure and postprandial hypotension. Am Heart J 1992; 124: 1669-1671

61   Pinkney JH, Mohamed-Ali V, Denver AE, Foster C, Sampson MJ, Yudkin JS. Insulin resistance, insulin, proinsulin, and ambulatory blood pressure in type II diabetes. Hypertension 1994; 24: 362-367

62   Rynkiewicz A, Furmanski J, Narkiewicz K, Semetkowska E, Bieniaszewski L, Horoszek-Maziarz S, Krupa-Wojciechowska B. Influence of duration of type 1 (insulin-dependent) diabetes mellitus on 24-h ambulatory blood pressure and heart rate profile (letter). Diabetologia 1993; 36: 577

63   Hansen KW, Poulsen PL, Christiansen JS, Mogensen CE. Determinants of 24-h blood pressure in IDDM patients. Diabetes Care 1995; 18: 529-535

64   van Ittersum FJ, Spek JJ, Praet IJA, Lambert J, Ijzerman RG, Fischer HRA, Nikkels RE, Van Bortel LMAB, Donker AJM, Stehouwer CDA. Ambulatory blood pressure and autonomic function in normoalbuminuric type 1 diabetic patients. Nephrol Dial Transplant 1998; 13: 326-332

65   Donaldson DL, Moore WV, Chonko AM, Shipman JJ, Wiegmann T. Incipient hypertension precedes incipient nephropathy in adolescents and young adults with type I diabetes (abstract). Diabetes 1992; 42 (suppl 1): 97A

66   Mathiesen ER, Hilsted J, Feldt-Rasmussen B, Bonde-Petersen F, Christensen NJ, Parving H-H. The effect of metabolic control on hemodynamics in short-term insulin-dependent diabetic patients. Diabetes 1985; 34: 1301-1305

67   Richards AM, Donelly T, Nicholls MG, Ikram H, Hamilton EJ, Espiner EA. Blood pressure and vasoactive hormones with improved glycemic control in patients with diabetes mellitus. Clin Exp Hypertens [A] 1989; A11:391-406

68   Mathiesen ER, Gall M-A. Hommel E, Skøtt P, Parving H-H. Effects of short term strict metabolic control on kidney function and extracellular volume in incipient diabetic nephropathy. Diabetic Med 1989; 6: 595-600

69   Azar ST, Birbari A. Nocturnal blood pressure elevation in patients with type 1 diabetes receiving intensive insulin therapy compared with that in patients receiving conventional insulin therapy. J Clin Endocrinol Metab 1998; 83: 3190-3193

70   Poulsen PL, Hansen KW, Ebbehøj E, Knudsen ST, Mogensen CE. No deleterious effects of tight blood glucose control on 24-hour ambulatory blood pressure in normoalbuminuric insulin-dependent diabetes mellitus patients. J Clin Endocrinol 2000, 1555-58.

71   Hansen KW, Pedersen MM, Christiansen JS, Mogensen CE. Night blood pressure and cigarette smoking: disparate associations in healthy subjects and diabetic patients. Blood Pressure 1994; 3: 381-388

72   Poulsen PL, Ebbehøj E, Hansen KW, Mogensen CE. Effects of smoking on 24-h ambulatory blood pressure and autonomic function in normoalbuminuric insulin-dependent diabetes mellitus patients. Am J Hypertens 1998; 11: 1093-1099

73   Mikkelsen KL, Wiinberg N, Høegholm A, Christensen HR, Bang LE, Nielsen PE, Svendsen TL, Kampmann JP, Madsen NH, Bentzon MW. Smoking related to 24.h ambulatory blood pressure and heart rate. A study in 352 normotensive danish subjects. Am j Hypertens 1997; 10: 483-491

74   Sinha RN, Patrick AW, Richardson L, MacFarlane IA. Diurnal variation in blood pressure in insulin-dependent diabetic smokers and non-smokers with and without microalbuminuria. Diabetic Med 1997; 14: 291-295.

75   Hansen KW, Christensen CK, Andersen PH, Mau Pedersen M, Christiansen JS, Mogensen CE. Ambulatory blood pressure in microalbuminuric type 1 diabetic patients. Kidney Int 1992; 41: 847-854

76   Benhamou PY, Halimi S, De Gaudemaris R, Boizel R, Pitiot M, Siche JP, Bachelot I, Mallion JM. Early disturbances of ambulatory blood pressure load in normotensive type 1 diabetic patients with microalbuminuria. Diabetes Care 1992; 15: 1614-1619

77   Peters A, Gromeier S, Kohlmann T, Look D, Kerner W. Nocturnal blood pressure elevation is related to adrenomedullary hyperactivity, but not to hyperinsulinemia, in non-obese normoalbuminuric type 1 diabetic patients. J Clin Endocrinol Metab 1996; 81: 507-512

78   Gilbert R, Philips P, Clarke C, Jerums G. Day-night blood pressure variation in normotensive normoalbuminuric type I diabetic subjects. Diabetes Care 1994; 17: 824-827

79   Khan N, Couper J, Dixit M, Couper R. Ambulatory blood pressure and heart rate in adolescents with insulin-dependent diabetes mellitus. Am J Hyp 1994; 7: 937-940

80   Guglielmi MD, Pierdomenico SD, Salvatore L, Romano R, Tascione E, Pupillo M, Porreca E, Imbastaro T, Cuccurullo F, Mezzetti A. Impaired left ventricular diastolic function and vascular postischemic vasodilation associated with microalbuminuria in IDDM patients. Diabetes Care 1995; 18: 353-360

81   Moore WV, Donaldson DL, Chonko AM, Ideus P, Wiegmann TB, Wiegmann. Ambulatory blood pressure in type I diabetes mellitus. Comparison to presence of incipient nephropathy in adolescents and young adults. Diabetes 41; 1992: 1035-1041

82   Sivieri R, Deandrea M, Gai V, Cavallo-Perin P. Circadian blood pressure levels in normotensive normoalbuminuric type 1 diabetic patients. Diabetic Med 1994; 11; 357-361

83   Hansen KW. Ambulatory blood pressure in insulin-dependent diabetes; the relation to stages of diabetic kidney disease. J Diabetes Complications 1996; 10:331-351

84   Wiegmann TB, Herron KG, Chonko AM, Macdougall ML, Moore WV. Recognition og hypertension and abnormal blood pressure burden with ambulatory blood pressure recordings in type I diabetes mellitus. Diabetes 1990; 39: 1556-1560

85   Yip J, Mattock MB, Morocutti A, Sethi M, Trevisan R, Viberti G. Insulin resistance in insulin-dependent diabetic patients with microalbuminuria. Lancet 1993; 342: 883-887

86   Voros P, Lengyel Z, Nagy V, Nemeth C, Rosivall L, Kammerer L. Diurnal blood pressure variation and albuminuria in normotensive patients with insulin-dependent diabetes mellitus. Nephrol Dial Transplant 1998; 13: 2257-2260

87   Sochett EB, Poon I, Balfe W, Daneman D. Ambulatory blood pressure monitoring in insulin-dependent diabetes mellitus with and without microalbuminuria. J Diab Comp 1998; 12;1: 18-23

88   Lurbe A, Redón J, Pascual JM, Tacons J, Alvarez V, Batlle DC. Altered blood pressure during sleep in normotensive subjects with type I diabetes. Hypertension 1993; 21: 227-235

89   Berrut G, Hallab M, Bouhanick B, Chameau A-M, Marre M, Fressinaud Ph. Value of ambulatory blood pressure in type I (insulin-dependent) diabetic patients with incipient diabetic nephropathy. Am J Hyp 1994; 7: 222-227

90   Hansen KW, Mau Pedersen M, Marshall SM, Christiansen JS, Mogensen CE. Circadian variation of blood pressure in patients with diabetic nephropathy. Diabetologia 1992; 35: 1074-1079

91   Torffvit O, Agardh C-D. Day and night variations in ambulatory blood pressure in type 1 diabetes mellitus with nephropathy and autonomic neuropathy. J Intern Med 1993; 233: 131-137

92   Poulsen PL, Hansen KW, Mogensen CE. Ambulatory blood pressure in the transition from normo- to microalbuminuria. A longitudinal study in IDDM patients. Diabetes 1994; 43; 1248-1253

93   Hansen KW, Pedersen MM, Christiansen, Mogensen CE. Diurnal blood pressure variations in normoalbuminuric type 1 diabetic patients. J Int Med 1993; 234: 175-180

94   Poulsen PL, Ebbehøj E, Hansen KW, Mogensen CE. 24-h blood pressure and autonomic function is related to albumin excretion within the normoalbuminuric range in IDDM patients. Diabetologia 1997; 40: 718-725

95   Page SR, Manning G, Ingle AR, Hill P, Millar-Craig MW, Peacock I. Raised ambulatory blood pressure in type 1 diabetes with incipient microalbuminuria. Diabetic Med 1994; 11; 877-882

96   Spallone V, Gambardella S, Maiello MR, Barini A, Frontoni S, Menzinger G. Relationship between autonomic neuropathy, 24-h blood pressure, and nephropathy in normotensive IDDM patients. Diabetes Care 1994; 17: 578-584

97   Monteagudo PT, Nóbrega JC, Cazarini PR, Ferreira SRG, Kohlmann O, Ribeiro AB, Zanella M-T. Altered blood pressure profile, autonomic neuropathy and nephropathy in insulin-dependent diabetic patients. European J of Endocrinology 1996; 135: 683-688.

98   Dyrberg T, Benn J, Sandahl Christiansen J, Hilsted J, Nerup J. Prevalence of diabetic autonomic neuropathy measured by simple bedside test. Diabetologia 1981; 20: 190-194

99   Zander E, Schulz, Heinke P, Grimmberger E, Zander G, Gottschling HD. Importance of cardiovascular autonomic dysfunction in IDDM subjects with diabetic nephropathy. Diabetes Care 1989; 12: 259-264

100   Mølgaard H, Christensen PD, Sørensen KE, Christensen CK, Mogensen CE. Association of 24-h cardiac parasympathetic activity and degree of nephropathy in IDDM patients. Diabetes 1992; 41: 812-817

101   Mølgaard H, Christensen PD, Hermansen K, Sørensen KE, Christensen CK, Mogensen CE. Early recognition of autonomic dysfunction in microalbuminuria: significance for cardiovascular mortality in diabetes mellitus. Diabetologia 1994; 37; 788-796

102   Hansen KW. Diurnal blood pressure profile, autonomic neuropathy and nephropathy in diabetes. European J of Endocrinology 1997; 136: 35-36

103   Poulsen PL, Ebbehøj E, Hansen KW, Mogensen CE. Characteristics and prognosis of normoalbuminuric type 1 diabetic patients. Diabetes Care 1999; 22(suppl.2); B72-5

104   Schernthaner G, Ritz E, Philipp T, Bretzel RG. Night time blood pressure in diabetic patients-the submerged portion of the iceberg? Nephrol Dial Transplant 1999; 14: 1061-1064

105   Farmer CKT, Goldsmith DJA, Quin JD, Dallyn P, Cox J, Kingswood JC, Sharpstone P. Progression of diabetic nephropathy-is diurnal blood pressure rhythm as important as absolute blood pressure level ? Nephrol Dial Transplant 1998; 13: 635-639

106   Pecis M, Azevedo MJ, Gross JL. Glomerular hyperfiltration is associated with blood pressure abnormalities in normotensive normoalbuminuric IDDM patients. Diabetes Care 1997; 20: 1329-1333

107   Hansen KW, Sørensen K, Christensen PD, Pedersen EB, Christiansen JS, Mogensen CE. Night blood pressure: relation to organ lesions in microalbuminuric type 1 diabetic patients. Diabetic Med 1995; 12: 42-45

108   Mulec H, Blohmé G, Kullenberg K, Nyberg G, Bjørck S. Latent overhydration and nocturnal hypertension in diabetic nephropathy. Diabetologia 1995; 38; 216-229

109   Hansen HP, Rossing P, Tarnow L, Nielsen FS, Jensen BR, Parving H-H. Circadian rhythm of arterial blood pressure and albuminuria in diabetic nephropathy. Kidney Int 1996; 50; 579-585

110   Poulsen PL, Juhl B, Ebbehøj E, Klein F, Christiansen C, Mogensen CE. Elevated ambulatory blood pressure in microalbuminuric IDDM patients is inversely associated with renal plasma flow. A compensatory mechanism ? Diabetes Care 1997; 20: 429-432

111   Poulsen PL, Bek T, Ebbehøj E, Hansen KW, Mogensen CE. 24-h ambulatory blood pressure and retinopathy in normoalbuminuric IDDM patients. Diabetologia 1998; 41: 105-110

112   Fagerudd JA, Tarnow L, Jacobsen P, Stenman S, Nielsen FS, Petterson-Fernholm KJ, Grönhagen-Riska C, Parving H-H, Groop P-H. Predisposition to essential hypertension and development of diabetic nephropathy in IDDM patients. Diabetes 1998; 47: 439-444

113   Bellomo G, Narducci PL, Rondoni F, Pastorelli G, Stangoni G, Angeli G, Verdecchia P. Prognostic value of 24-hour blood pressure in pregnancy. JAMA 1999; 282: 1447-1452

114   Flores L, Levy I, Aguilera E, Martinez S, Gomis R, Esmatjes E. Usefulness of ambulatory blood pressure monitoring in pregnant women type 1 diabetes. Diabetes Care 1999; 22: 1507-1501

115   Hansen KW, Schmitz A, Mau Pedersen M. Ambulatory blood pressure measurement in type 2 diabetic patients: Methodological aspects. Diabetic Med 1991; 8: 567-572

116   Mau Pedersen M, Hansen KW, Schmitz A, Sørensen K, Christensen CK, Mogensen CE. Effects of ACE inhibition supplementary to beta blockers and diuretics in early diabetic nephropathy. Kidney Int 1992; 41: 883-890

117   Wiegmann TB, Herron KG, Chonko AM, MacDougall ML, Moore WV. Effect of angiotensin-converting enzyme inhibition on renal function and albuminuria in normotensive type I diabetic patients. Diabetes 1992; 41: 62-67

118   Nielsen FS, Rossing P, Gall M-A, Skøtt P, Smidt UM, Parving H-H. Impact of lisinopril and atenolol on kidney function in hypertensive NIDDM subjects with diabetic nephropathy. Diabetes 1994; 43; 1108-1113

119   Sundaresan P, Lykos D, Daher A, Diamond T, Morris R, Howes LG. Comparative effects of glibenclamide and metformin on ambulatory blood pressure and cardiovascular reactivity in NIDDM. Diabetes Care 1997; 20: 692-697

120   Hansen KW, Klein F, Christensen PD, Sørensen K, Andersen PH, Møller J, Pedersen EB, Christiansen JS, Mogensen CE. Effects of captopril on ambulatory blood pressure, renal and cardiac function in microalbuminuric type 1 diabetic patients. Diabete Metab (Paris) 1994; 20; 485-493

121   Rossing P, Tarnow L, Boelskifte S, Jensen BR, Nielsen FS, Parving H-H. Differences between nisoldipine and lisinopril on glomerular filtration rates and albuminuria in hypertensive IDDM patients with diabetic nephropathy during the first year of treatment. Diabetes 1997; 46: 481-487

122   Rossing P, Hansen BV, Nielsen FS, Myrup B, Holmer G, Parving H-H. Fish oil in diabetic nephropathy. Diabetes Care 1996; 19: 1214-1219

123   Agardh CD, Garcia Puig J, Charbonnel B, Angelkort B, Barnett AH. Greater reduction of urinary albumin excretion in hypertensive type II diabetic patients with incipient nephropathy by lisinopril than by nifedipine. J Hum Hypertens 1996; 10: 185-192

124   Schneider M, Lerch M, Papiri M, Buechel P, Boehlen L, Shaw S, Risen W, Weidmann. Metabolic neutrality of combined varapamil-trandolapril treatment in contrast to beta-blocker-low-dose chlortalidone treatment in hypertensive type 2 diabetes. J Hypertens 1996; 14: 669-677

125   Rasmussen OW, Thomsen C, Hansen KW, Vesterlund M, Winther E, Hermansen K. Effects on blood pressure, glucose and lipid levels of a high-monounsaturated fat diet compared with a high-carbohydrate diet in NIDDM subjects. Diabetes Care 1993; 16: 1565-1571

126   Nielsen S, Hermansen K, Rasmussen OW, Thomsen C, Mogensen CE. Urinary albumin excretion rate and 24-h ambulatory blood pressure in NIDDM with microalbuminuria: effects of a monounsaturated-enriched diet. Diabetologia 1995; 38; 1069-1075

127   Nielsen FS, Rossing P, Gall MA, Smidt UM, Chen JW, Sato A, Parving H-H. Lisinopril improves endothelial dysfunction in hypertensive NIDDM subjects with diabetic nephropathy. Scand J Clin Lab Invest 1997; 57: 427-434

128   Bauduceau B, Genes N, Chamontin B, Vaur L, Renault M, Etienne S, Marre M. Ambulatory blood pressure and urinary albumin excretion in diabetic (non-insulin-dependent and insulin-dependent) hypertensive patients: relationships at baseline and after treatment by the angiotensin converting enzyme inhibitor trandolapril. Am J Hypertens 1998; 11:1065-1073

129   Nielsen FS, Sato A, Ali S, Tarnow L, Smidt UM, Kastrup J, Parving H-H. Beneficial impact of ramipril on left ventricular hypertrophy in normotensive normoalbuminuric NIDDM patients. Diabetes Care 1998; 21: 804-809

130   Tarnow L, Sato A, Ali S, Rossing P, Nielsen FS, Parving H-H. Effects of nisoldipine and lisinopril on left ventricular mass and function in diabetic nephropathy. Diabetes Care 1999; 22: 491-494

131   Gerdts E, Svarstad E, Aanderud S, Myking OL, Lund-Johansen P, Omvik P. Factors influencing reduction in blood pressure and left ventricular mass in hypertensive type-1 diabetic patients using captopril or doxazosin for 6 months. Am J Hypertens 1998; 11: 1178-1187

132   Palatini P, Racioppa A, Raule G, Zaninotto M, Penzo M, Pessina AC. Effect of timing of administration on the plasma ACE inhibitory activity and the antihypertensive effect of quinapril. Clin Pharmacol Ther 1992; 52; 378-383

133   Morgan T, Anderson A, Jones E. The effect on 24h blood pressure control of an angiotensin converting enzyme inhibitor (perindopril) administered in the morning or at night. J Hypertens 1997; 15: 205-211

134   Portaluppi F, Vergnani L, Manfredini R, Uberti ECD, Fersini C. Time-dependent effect of isradipine on the nocturnal hypertension in chronic renal failure. Am J Hyp 1995; 8; 719-726

135   Gambardella S, Frontoni S, Spallone V, Maiello MR, Civetta E, Lanza G, Sandric S, Menzinger G. Increased left ventricular mass in normotensive diabetic patients with autonomic neuropathy. Am J Hyp 1993; 6: 97-102

136   Nielsen FS, Ali S, Rossing P, Bang LE, Svendsen TL, Gall M-A, Smidt UM, Kastrup J, Parving H-H. Left ventricular hypertrophy in non-insulin dependent diabetic patients with and without diabetic nephropathy. Diabetic Med 1997; 538-546

137   Verdecchia P, Porcellati C, Schillaci G, Borgioni, Ciucci A, Gatteschi C, Zampi I, Santucci A, Santucci C, Reboldi G. Ambulatory blood pressure and risk of cardiovascular disease in type II diabetes mellitus. Diab Nutr Metab 1994; 7: 223-231

138   Ebbehøj E, Poulsen PL, Hansen KW, Mogensen CE. White coat effect in diabetes: ambulatory blood pressure in relation to clinic based measurement (abstract). Diabetologia 1997; 40 (suppl 1): A12

139   Nielsen FS, Gæde P, Vedel P, Pedersen O, Parving H-H. White coat hypertension in NIDDM patients with and without incipient and over diabetic nephropathy. Diabetes Care 1997; 20: 859-863

140   Puig JG, Ruilope LM, Ortega R. Antihypertensive treatment efficacy in type II diabetes mellitus. Dissociation between casual and 24-hour ambulatory blood pressure. Hypertension 1995; 26 (part 2): 1093-1099

141   Burgess E, Mather K, Ross S, Josefsberg Z. Office hypertension in Type 2 (non-insulin-dependent) diabetic patients (letter). Diabetologia 1991; 34: 684

142   Holl RW, Pavlovic M, Heinze E, Thon A. Circadian blood pressure during the early course of type 1 diabetes. Analysis of 1,011 ambulatory blood pressure recordings in 354 adolescents and young adults. Diabetes Care 1999; 22: 1151-1157

143   The Joint National Committee on Detection, Evaluation, and Treatment of High Blood Pressure. The sixth report of the joint national committee on detection, evaluation, and treatment of high blood pressure. Arch Intern Med 1997; 157: 2413-2446

144   Guidelines Subcommittee. 1999 World Health Organization-International Society of Hypertension guidelines for the management of hypertension. J Hypertens 1999; 17: 151-183

145   Ramsay LE, Williams B, Johnston GD, MacGregor GA, Poston L, Potter JF, Poulter NR, Russel G. Guidelines for management of hypertension: report of the third working party of the British Hypertension Society. J Hum Hypertens 1999; 13: 569-592

146   O'Brien E, Staessen J. Normotension and hypertension as defined by 24-hour ambulatory blood pressure monitoring. Blood Pressure 1995; 4; 266-282

147   O'Brien E, Staessen JA. What is "hypertension"? Lancet, 1999; 353:1541-1543.

148   Staessen JA, Thijs L, Fagard R, O'Brien E, Clement D, de Leeuw PW, Mancia G, Nachev C, Palatini P, Parati G, Tuomilehto J, Webster J. Predicting cardiovascular risk using conventional vs ambulatory blood pressure in older patients with systolic hypertension. JAMA 1999; 282: 539-546

149   Rutan GH, McDonald RH, Kuller LH. Comparison of ambulatory and clinic blood pressure and heart rate in older persons with isolated systolic hypertension. Am J Hypertens 1992; 5: 880-886

150   Nakano S. Fukuda M, Hotta F, Ito T, Ishii T, Kitazawa M, Nishizawa M, Kigoshi T, Uchida K. Reversed circadian blood pressure rhythm is associated with occurrences of both fatal and nonfatal vascular events in NIDDM subjects. Diabetes 1998; 47: 1501-1506

151   Mølgaard H, Hermansen K. Evaluation of cardiac autonomic neuropathy by heart rate variability. In: Mogensen CE, Standl E (eds). Diabetes Forum Series volume V (part 1). Research methodologies in human diabetes. Berlin, New York: Walter de Gruyter; 1994, pp 219-240

152   Imholz BPM, Langewouters GJ, van Montfrans A, Parati G, van Goudoever J, Wesseling KH, Wieling W, Mancia G. Feasibility of ambulatory, continous 24-hour finger arterial pressure recording. Hypertension 1993; 21: 65-73

153   Staessen JA, Beilin L, Parati G, Waeber B, White W. Task Force IV: Clinical use of ambulatory blood pressure monitoring. Blood Press Monit 1999; 4: 319-331

28.   MICROALBUMINURIA IN YOUNG PATIENTS WITH TYPE 1 DIABETES

Henrik Bindesbøl Mortensen
Pediatric Department, Glostrup Hospital, DK 2600 Glostrup

Diabetic nephropathy is the main cause of the increased morbidity and mortality among patients with Type 1 diabetes [1,2,3]. In recent years, it has been shown that a slightly elevated urinary albumin excretion rate (microalbuminuria) is an early predictor for later development of overt diabetic nephropathy [4,5,6,7] and is associated with elevated arterial blood pressure [8,9,10,11,12]. Based on recent literature, the reported prevalence of microalbuminuria in paediatric populations varies from 4.3 to 20% (Table 28-1). Consequently, microalbuminuria is the first easily identifiable sign of risk of incipient diabetic nephropathy and other vascular complications of the disease. Treatment and intervention consensus guidelines have already been developed for adults [13] and it is equally important to set up a uniform intervention programme for treatment of microalbuminuria in adolescents with Type 1 diabetes.

MEASURING ALBUMIN EXCRETION

There are several different ways of measuring albumin excretion. Timed overnight urine collection was used to assess the prevalence of microalbuminuria in a nation-wide screening for microalbuminuria in Denmark in 1989 [14]. This urine fraction avoids the effect of posture, physical exercise, major blood pressure variations and the acute effect of diet on albuminuria and it is a convenient and practical method for most children. Two samples were taken from each patient, on separate occasions, and if the urinary albumin excretion rate (AER) was over 20 μg min^{-1} in one of the two samples, a third sample was taken to confirm whether the child had elevated albumin excretion – microalbuminuria. This limit was chosen as the lowest AER that is predictive of diabetic nephropathy – on the basis of investigations of the upper 95th percentile for albumin excretion in the control group of 209 healthy children [14]. The AER was determined by an immunoturbidimetric method which on average gave 13% higher results than those measured by radioimmunoassay.

Mogensen C.E. (ed.) THE KIDNEY AND HYPERTENSION IN DIABETES MELLITUS.
Copyright© 2000 by Kluwer Academic Publishers, Boston • Dordrecht • London. All rights reserved.

Various workers have reported upper 95% confidence limits for the different methods of measuring albumin excretion. Rowe et al. [15] established an upper 95% confidence limit for overnight urine of 12.2 μg min^{-1} in normal children, while Davies et al. [16] reported a value related to surface area of 10 μg min^{-1} 1.73m^{-2}. In another study, Gibb et al. [17] estimated the upper 95th centile for overnight albumin excretion rate in healthy children as being 8.2 μg.min^{-1} 1.73m^{-2}.

Table 28-1 The reported prevalence of microalbuminuria in paediatric populations.

Study	Population (n)	Prevalence of microalbuminuria	Age group (yrs)	Duration of diabetes (yrs)	Screening procedure
Mathiesen et al 1986[31]	Clinic (97)	20%	7-18	10	Overnight
Nørgaard et al 1989[32]	Clinic (113)	15%	1-18	9	24-h urine
D'Antonio et al 1989 [33]	Clinic (62)	21%	5.8-20.9	5	24-h urine
Mortensen et al 1990 [14]	Nation-wide (957)	4.3%	2-19	6	Overnight
Joner et al 1992 [34]	Community	12.5%	8-30	10.5	Overnight
Olsen et al 1995 [35]	Nation-wide (339)	9.0%	12-26.9	13.2	overnight

DEFINITION OF MICROALBUMINURIA

Microalbuminuria has been defined using a variety of screening procedures for urine sampling [18-26]:

- Urinary albumin excretion rate (UAE) 20–200 μg/min (overnight urine collection) or 30–300 mg/24 h (24 h urine collection).
- Albumin/creatinine ratio (A/C ratio) 2.5–25 mg/mmol (spot urine) (Europe). Note that a lower limit of 3.5 mg/mmol has been proposed in females because of lower creatinine excretion.
- Albumin/creatinine ratio (A/C ratio) 30–300 mg/g (spot urine). (North America).
- Albumin concentration (AC) 30–300 mg/l (early morning urine).

When screening for microalbuminuria, a spot urine albumin/creatinine ratio or albumin concentration (Micraltest or other bedside test) can be used. However, timed urine collection is more accurate. If the result is positive, microalbuminuria should be confirmed by UAE. Incipient diabetic nephropathy is suspected when microalbuminuria is found in at least two out of three urine samples, preferably within a 1 to 6 month period [13]. The within-individual variation in observations of AER can vary by as much as 40% due to natural fluctuations, and there are several other confounding factors that can affect AER (Table 28-2) [14,27]. Therefore, a minimum of two estimations is necessary per individual to determine the true mean value of urine albumin excretion with reasonable confidence.

Table 28-2 Confounding factors for microalbuminuria.

- Variability in albumin excretion (about 40%)
- Posture or diurnal variation
- Strenuous exercise
- Urinary tract infection
- Acute febrile illness
- Menstrual bleeding
- Vaginal discharge

ALBUMIN EXCRETTION RATE AMONG CHILDREN WITH AND WITHOUT DIABETES

The ranges for AER in urine samples collected overnight in both non-diabetic and diabetic children aged 12 years or less and adolescents from 12 to 19 years are given in Table 28-3. The geometric mean for albumin excretion was significantly higher (p<0.001) in adolescents than in children under 12 years independent of diabetes. There were no significant differences (p>0.05) in albumin excretion rates between the sexes.

Table 28-3 Timed overnight urinary albumin excretion in children and adolescents with and without Type 1 diabetes.

	Children ≤12 years		Adolescents >12-19 years	
	Boys	**Girls**	**Boys**	**Girls**
Normal children				
N	47	30	58	74
AER (μg min $^{-1}$)	1.28x/÷2.75	1.27x/÷1.97	2.73x/÷2.18[a]	2.23x/÷2.14[a]
Diabetic children				
N	154	124	334	297
AER (μg min $^{-1}$)	1.70x/÷2.11	1.72x/÷2.07	2.94x/÷2.38[a]	3.16x/÷2.23[a]
Geomtric mean x/÷ SD factor.				
P<0.001 compared with younger age groups. Boys vs. girls all NS [ref. 14, with permission]				

These findings are consistent with recent results reported on overnight collections of urine [15,16]. In non-diabetic adolescents, the relationship between AER, body surface area and level of maturity was fairly constant, which is in accordance with the results of Gibb et al. [17]. By contrast, in diabetic adolescents, AER was positively correlated with body surface area and age. This correlation was independent of the current HbA_{1c} level, suggesting that specific metabolic changes other than poor blood glucose control might affect AER, particularly in diabetic subjects during the pubertal period. Hypersecretion of growth hormone (GH) as a result of altered feedback drive from reduced insulin-like growth factor I (IGF-1) levels and IGF-1 bioactivity have been demonstrated in adolescents with Type 1 diabetes [28], which may lead to glomerular hyperfiltration [29] and an increased risk of developing microalbuminuria [30].

TYPE 1 DIABETIC CHILDREN WITH ELEVATED ALBUMIN EXCRETION RATE

The prevalence of persistent microalbuminuria was 4.3% in the Danish nation-wide screening study in 1989 (which involved 957 Danish children and adolescents aged 2–19 years with Type 1 diabetes and mean diabetes duration of 6 years) [14]. However, the reported prevalence of microalbuminuria in paediatric populations varies from 4.3 to 20% (see Table 28-1) [14,31,32,33,34,35]. The wide variation in persistent microalbuminuria between these studies may partly be explained by differences in age, diabetes duration, blood glucose control, the populations investigated and the screening procedure. However, a decrease in the incidence of nephropathy in Type 1 diabetes mellitus during the period that these studies were conducted may also have contributed to the variable results [36].

The prevalence of persistent microalbuminuria in different age groups and in groups with different durations of diabetes, from 909 children and adolescents with Type 1 diabetes [14], is shown in figures 28-1 and 28-2. In this study, the prevalence of microalbuminuria in adolescent patients (over 16 years) was 13–14%, which is similar to previous investigations. The occurrence of microalbuminuria is extremely rare before puberty. Two prepubertal children were diagnosed with microalbuminuria in a study by Nørgaard et al. [32], while Joner et al. [34] and Janner et al. [37] each reported one case. In our study [14], two children (both girls) were diagnosed with microalbuminuria, while none were detected in the studies by Mathiesen et al. [31] and Dahlquist et al. [38].

It remains controversial whether diabetes duration *per se* is associated with raised urinary albumin. Some studies have shown a possible association [14,39], while others dispute this [40]. Nonetheless, it seems reasonable that young people should be screened for microalbuminuria regardless of diabetes duration, beginning at the very first stage of puberty [14,37].

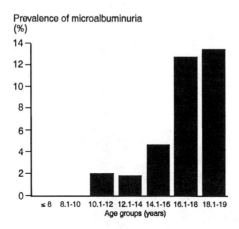

Prevalence of microalbuminuria (%)

Age groups (years)

Figure 28-1   The prevalence of microalbuminuria in different age groups in 909 children and adolescents with type 1 diabetes. [ref. 14, with permission]

OVERNIGHT ALBUMIN EXCRETION RATE AND BLOOD GLUCOSE CONTROL

Several previous reports have suggested a relationship between poor blood glucose control and increased urinary albumin excretion [39,41,42,43]. In our study [14] we found that only females with microalbuminuria had significantly elevated HbA_{1c} values compared with diabetic patients with normoalbuminuria. Blood glucose control tends to be poorer during puberty, particularly in girls, which may be explained by changes in hormonal and/or lifestyle factors [44,45,46,47,48]. In two recent studies [49,50], urinary albumin excretion correlated significantly and independently with prepubertal diabetes duration, prepubertal hyperglycaemia, female sex and poor long-term metabolic control. Thus, good metabolic control should be the goal from the onset of diabetes.   An impaired linear growth observed in females with microalbuminuria may also be associated with long-term poor blood glucose. However, recent studies [51,52] have suggested an association between short stature and diabetic nephropathy, particularly in males. Furthermore, in males who have had diabetes for 10 to 25 years, there is a threefold increase in the prevalence of micro/macroalbuminuria compared with females [53]. The DCCT study [54] demonstrated that improved metabolic control could retard but not prevent the progression of incipient diabetic kidney disease. Recently, Krolewski et al. [55] reported that the risk of microalbuminuria in patients with Type 1 diabetes increases abruptly above an HbA_{1c} level of 8.1%, suggesting that efforts to reduce the frequency of diabetic nephropathy should be focused on the patients with HbA_{1c} values above this threshold.

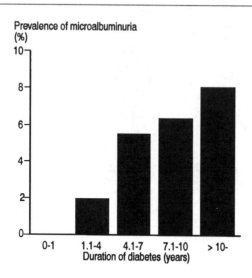

Figure 28-2 The relationship between duration of diabetes and prevalence of microalbuminuria in 909 children and adolescents with type 1 diabetes [ref. 14, with permission]

CLINICAL OUTCOME INDICATORS/TARGETS FOR GLYCAEMIC CONTROL
In view of the importance of good blood glucose control in preventing microvascular complications, we have defined specific outcome indicators to be measured and audited annually:

- 90% of all patients with HbA$_{1c}$ values of 10 % or above should achieve a 1% reduction of this value within a year.
- More than 50% of children aged 0–6 years should have HbA$_{1c}$ values below 9%, or in patients aged 7–18 years, below 8.5%, within at least 2 years and below 8% within 4 years in all age groups.
- The rate of severe hypoglycaemic events (loss of consciousness/seizures) in all our patients should be less than 20/100 patient years.

We use the HbA$_{1c}$ level of 8% as a treatment target in patients aged 7–18 years on the basis of previous evidence [56,57,58,59]. In children under 6 years with Type 1 diabetes, the HbA$_{1c}$ target is a little higher (about 8–9%) because of the greater risk of severe hypoglycaemia [60,61,62,63,64,65], which in this age group may have potentially harmful effects on neuropsychological and intellectual functions in the developing brain [65,66,67,68]. However, we try (carefully) to reduce the HbA$_{1c}$ level to

8% in these children too, if this is achievable without increasing the number of severe hypoglycaemic events.

OVERNIGHT ALBUMIN EXCRETION RATE AND ARTERIAL BLOOD PRESSURE

The normal range for diastolic blood pressure in diabetic boys (Figure 28-3) and girls (Figure 28-4) aged 8 to 18 years with normoalbuminuria was determined in a study of the relationship between blood pressure and urinary albumin excretion in young Danish Type 1 diabetic patients [69]. Figures 28-3 and 28-4 also include data from patients diagnosed with micro- and macroalbuminuria [69]. Ten out of 16 boys with microalbuminuria had diastolic blood pressure above the upper quartile while eight out of 14 girls with microalbuminuria had diastolic blood pressure above this quartile [69]. Three of four boys with macroalbuminuria had diastolic blood pressure below the upper quartile while two of three girls with macroalbuminuria had values above [69]. Overall, 60% of adolescents with microalbuminuria had diastolic blood pressure in the upper quartile for normoalbuminuria [69]. In keeping with this, Kordonouri et al. [70] reported a relationship between diastolic blood pressure and albumin excretion rate in juvenile Type 1 diabetic patients. This excess prevalence of raised blood pressure in Type 1 diabetic patients could, therefore, be explained by the presence of elevated blood pressure in adolescents with micro- and macroalbuminuria [32]

Re-examination of 15 of the adolescents with microalbuminuria, 2 years after identification, revealed that two of these (13%) had developed overt proteinuria during this period. They had initially an overnight albumin excretion rate of 62.0 and 115.7 μg.min[-1], respectively, increasing to 184.4 and 448.3 μg.min[-1], respectively (unpublished data). Gorman et al. [71] showed that microalbuminuria detected in the first decade of disease will persist or progress in the second decade in around two-thirds of patients, while a third of those initially normoalbuminuric will develop microalbuminuria. Thus, without treatment, a marked increase in the progression to overt diabetic nephropathy is seen in many individuals. In a study of young diabetic patients all diagnosed before 15 years of age, Bojestig et al. [72] found no relationship between the level of microalbuminuria at the initial investigation and the development of nephropathy. They conclude that, even in the upper range of AER, excellent glycaemic control seems to be effective in preventing macroalbuminuria and reversing AER to normal.

Altered glomerular haemodynamics with increased glomerular plasma flow and transcapillary pressures are considered key factors in the initiation and progression of diabetic nephropathy [73,74,75,76]. Therapy with an angiotensin converting enzyme (ACE) inhibitor has been shown to lower albumin excretion rate and mean arterial blood pressure in normotensive adolescents [77,78] and adults [79] with Type 1 diabetes and microalbuminuria, in the short term at least. Recently, long-term studies have demonstrated that ACE-inhibition delays progression to diabetic nephropathy in normotensive Type 1 diabetic patients with persistent microalbuminuria [80,81,82,83].

Rudberg et al. 1999 [84] found less progression of early diabetic glomerulopathy in Type 1 diabetic young microalbuminuric patients who were treated with either ACE-inhibitors or beta blockers (for an average of 3 years) than in patients who did not receive antihypertensive treatment and that this effect possibly was due to maintenance of a normal or low blood pressure. Thus, ACE inhibitors have beneficial effects in nephropathy [85], a microvascular complication of Type 1 diabetes that shares many of the risk factors of retinopathy. Interestingly, The EUCLID Study Group [86] recently reported that the ACE inhibitor, lisinopril, both reduced the progression and incidence of retinopathy and that this is not fully accounted for by effects on blood pressure. The EUCLID study investigators suggest that ACE inhibitor therapy should be considered for all patients with Type 1 diabetes who have some degree of retinopathy.

Previous investigations in adults with Type 1 diabetes have shown that, at the time of recognition of microalbuminuria, blood pressure is often within the normal range [87] and tends to increase in parallel with the extent of albuminuria. Only two out of five adolescents with macroalbuminuria had elevated blood pressure in our study of blood pressure and AER (Figures 28-3, 28-4) [69]. This may be a selection bias because two patients with macroalbuminuria were excluded due to antihypertensive treatment. However, shorter duration of diabetes and lower body mass index compared to an adult population could explain the observed discrepancies.

These findings suggest that elevated arterial blood pressure may be related to the increased prevalence of elevated albumin excretion rate observed in adolescents with Type 1 diabetes and it suggests that hypertension plays an important role for the initiation and the progression of diabetic nephropathy in keeping with previous reports [4,7,10]

AT WHAT AGE SHOULD ROUTINE SCREENING FOR MICROALBUMINURIA BEGIN?

Young people should be screened for microalbuminuria regardless of diabetes duration [40] beginning at the very first stage of puberty [37]. Subsequently, annual screening should be carried out particularly if the metabolic control is unsatisfactory or abnormalities are found. Arterial blood pressure should be measured at least annually.

INTERVENTION PROGRAMME FOR TREATMENT OF PERSISTENT MICROALBUMINURIA (20-200 µg/min)

In children with microalbuminuria (>20–200 µg/min) blood glucose control should be improved over a period of 6 months and the status of microalbuminuria should be monitored closely. If microalbuminuria disappears or improves there is no indication for pharmacological intervention. However, if the microalbuminuria deteriorates, whether or not blood glucose control improves and blood pressure is within the normal limits, antihypertensive treatment by an ACE-inhibitor should be instituted.

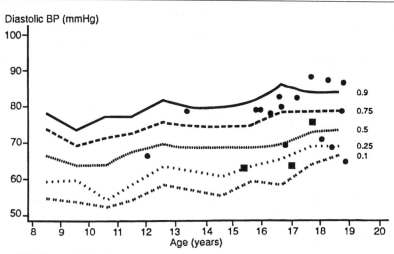

Figure 28-3. Percentile distribution of diastolic blood pressure in 487 boys aged 8 to 18 years with type 1 diabetes. The dots represent diastolic blood pressure for the 16 boys with microalbuminuria, the squares the three boys with macroalbuminuria [ref. 69, with permission].

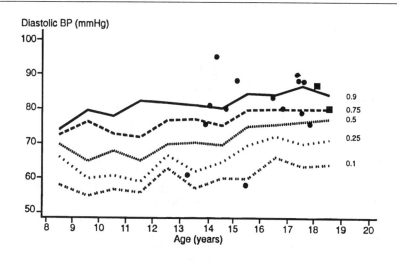

Figure 28-4. Percentile distribution of diastolic blood pressure in 425 girls aged 8 to 18 years with type 1 diabetes. The dots represent diastolic blood pressure of the 14 girls with microalbuminuria, the squares the two girls with macroalbuminuria [69, with permission].

The ACE inhibitors have potential therapeutic advantages over other antihypertensive drugs because they may selectively reduce efferent arteriolar pressures, and thereby glomerular capillary pressures, by lowering angiotensin II levels [88,89]. There has been extensive experience with ACE inhibitor use in children and therapy has been associated with very few side effects at low doses in the presence of normal renal function [78,84,90,91]. However, long-term follow up studies in children are required to evaluate whether intervention at an early stage with ACE inhibitors will prevent or only slow down progression to established diabetic nephropathy [92].

As well as starting ACE inhibitor treatment, the following measures should be taken over a 6-month period:

- Improvement of blood glucose control, HbA_{1c} to below 8.0% (normal HbA_{1c} range 4.3–5.8%).
- Frequent home blood glucose determination (4 times a day) and adjustment of insulin, diet and physical activity according to measured values.
- Monitor the status of microalbuminuria every other month (overnight urine collections).
- Monthly monitoring of arterial blood pressure and comparison of the readings to age appropriate values, if available.
- Discourage smoking and encourage exercise and reduction in overweight.
- Reduce daily protein intake to 1.0 –1.2 g /kg body weight.

Blood pressure should be monitored under standard conditions, after at least 5 min rest, with the adolescent sitting. The measurement should be taken on the right arm with an inflatable cuff size of 140 mm. A diagnosis of hypertension should be based on several readings and home monitored BP values. If 'white coat' hypertension is suspected, 24 h ambulatory BP may be used.

If microalbuminuria disappears or improves, there is no indication for pharmacological intervention. If the status of microalbuminuria deteriorates, even if the blood glucose control improves, the intervention programme for management of microalbuminuria shown in Table 28-4 should be implemented. The target of treatment is to achieve a blood pressure of 120–130/80–85 mmHg or less. The ideal is to achieve a reduction in microalbuminuria of 20–30% per year or at least to stabilise the AER.

PRECAUTIONS WITH ACE-INHIBITOR TREATMENT
It should be noted that treatment with ACE inhibitors should be discontinued in the case of pregnancy and other antihypertensive treatment may be indicated. If serum potassium increases or the patients show sodium retention, low dose diuretic agents should be added.

Table 28-4 Intervention programme for microalbuminuria

Microalbuminuria in normotensive and hypertensive patients	What to monitor
☐ ACE-inhibitor should be initiated (pregnancy contraindication) ☐ Antihypertensive treatment: adolescents > 40 kg, capoten 50 mg, b.d. ☐ Increase the dose gradually from 12.5 mg	☐ Microalbuminuria: 1–3 months using A/C ratio or UAE (depending on the child's ability to comply with the collection method) ☐ Blood pressure: 1–3 months ☐ Serum creatinine: ½ yearly ☐ Serum potassium: ½ yearly ☐ Retinopathy yearly ☐ Neuropathy yearly

CONCLUSION

The prevalence of persistent microalbuminuria was only 4.3% in a study consisting of a large proportion of all Danish children and adolescents with Type 1 diabetes. Elevated AER occurs mainly during the very first stage of puberty, and screening for microalbuminuria is recommended in children at the age of 9, 12, 15 and 18 years at least. However, yearly examinations are recommended if the metabolic control is unsatisfactory or abnormalities are found. Sixty percent of adolescents with microalbuminuria had diastolic blood pressure above the upper quartile for normoalbuminuric patients. Therefore, elevated blood pressure in childhood should lead to careful observation of the blood pressure level in the long term and examination of the urinary albumin excretion rate to prevent development of end-organ damage.

REFERENCES

1.   Dorman JS, Laporte RE, Kuller LH, Cruickshanks KJ, Orchard TJ, Wagener DK, Becker DJ, Cavender DE, Drash AL. The Pittsburgh insulin-dependent diabetes mellitus (IDDM). Morbidity and mortality study. Mortality results. Diabetes 1984;33:271–276.
2.   Borch-Johnsen K, Andersen PK, Deckert T. The effect of proteinuria on relative mortality in Type 1 (insulin dependent) diabetes mellitus. Diabetologia 1985;28:590–596.
3.   Borch-Johnsen K, Kreiner S. Proteinuria: value as predictor of cardiovascular mortality in insulin dependent diabetes mellitus. Br Med J 1987;294:1651–1654.
4.   Mogensen CE, Damsgaard EM, Frøland A, Hansen KW, Nielsen S, Pedersen MM, Schmitz A, Thuesen L, Østerby R. Reduced glomerular filtration rate and cardiovascular damage in diabetes: a key role for abnormal albuminuria. Acta Diabetologia 1992;29:201–213.
5.   Bangstad H-J, Østerby R, Dahl-Jørgensen K, Berg KJ, Hartmann A, Nyberg G, Frahm Bjørn S, Hanssen KF. Early glomerulopathy is present in young, Type 1 (insulin-dependent) diabetic patients with microalbuminuria. Diabetologia 1993;36:523–529.
6.   Ellis EN, Pysher TJ. Renal disease in adolescents with Type 1 diabetes mellitus: A report of the southwest pediatric nephrology study group. Am J Kidney Dis 1993;22:783–790.
7.   Viberti GC. Prognostic significance of microalbuminuria. Am J Hypertens 1994;7:69–72.
8.   Epstein M, Sowers JR. Diabetes mellitus and hypertension. Hypertension 1992;19:403–418.

9. Microalbuminuria Collaborative Study Group, United Kingdom. Risk factors for development of microalbuminuria in insulin dependent diabetic patients: a cohort study. BMJ 1993;306:1235–1239.

10. Mathiesen ER, Rønn B, Storm B, Foght H, Deckert T. The natural course of microalbuminuria in insulin-dependent diabetes: A 10-year prospective study. Diabetic Med 1995;12:482–487.

11. Mangili R, Deferrari G, Di Mario U, Giampietro O, Navalesi R, Nosadini R, Rigamonti G, Spezia R, Crepaldi G, for the Italian Microalbuminuria Study Group. Arterial hypertension and microalbuminuria IDDM: The Italian microalbuminuria study. Diabetologia 1994;-37:1015–1024.

12. Parving H-H. Renoprotection in diabetes: Renoprotection in diabetes: genetic and non-genetic risk factors and treatment. Diabetologia 1998;41:745–759.

13. Mogensen CE, Keane WF, Bennett PH, Jerums G, Parving H-H, Passa P, Steffes MW, Striker GE, Viberti GC. Prevention of diabetic renal disease with special reference to microalbuminuria. Lancet 1995;346:1080-84.

14. Mortensen HB, Marinelli K, Nørgaard K, Main K, Kastrup KW, Ibsen KK et al. A nation-wide cross-sectional study of urinary albumin excretion rate, arterial blood pressure and blood glucose control in Danish children with Type 1 diabetes. Diabetic Med 1990;7:887–897.

15. Rowe DJF, Hayward M, Bagga H, Betts P. Effect of glycaemic control and duration of disease on overnight albumin excretion in diabetic children. BMJ 1984;289:957–959.

16. Davies AG, Postlethwaite RJ, Price DA, Burn JL, Houlton CA, Fielding BA. Urinary albumin excretion in school children. Arch Dis Child 1984;59:625–630.

17. Gibb DM, Dunger D, Levin M, Shah V, Smith C, Barratt TM. Early markers of the renal complications of insulin dependent diabetes mellitus. Arch Dis Child 1989;64:984–991.

18. Mogensen CE, Chachati A, Christensen CK, Close CF, Deckert T, Hommel E, Kastrup J, Lefebvre P, Mathiesen ER, Feldt-Rasmussen B, Schmitz A, Viberti GC. Microalbuminuria: An early marker of renal involvement in diabetes. Uremia Invest 1985–86;9:85–95.

19. Feldt-Rasmussen B, Microalbuminuria and clinical nephropathy in Type 1 (insulin-dependent) diabetes mellitus: Pathophysiological mechanisms and intervention studies. Dan Med Bull 1989;36:405–415.

20. Eshøj O, Feldt-Rasmussen B, Larsen ML, Mogensen EF. Comparison of overnight, morning and 24h urine collections in assessment of diabetic microalbuminuria. Diabetic Med 1987;4:531–533.

21. Viberti GC, Mogensen CE, Passa P, Bilous R, Mangili R. St Vincent declaration, 1994: guidelines for the prevention of diabetic renal failure. In: Mogensen CE, ed. The kidney and hypertension in diabetes mellitus, 2nd ed. Boston/Dordrecht/London: Kluwer, 1994: 515–527.

22. Anon. Prevention of diabetes mellitus: report of a WHO study group. WHO Technical Report Series 844. Geneva: WHO, 1994:55–59

23. Jerums G, Cooper M, Gilbert R, O'Brian R, TaftJ. Microalbuminuria in Diabetes. Med J Aust 1994;161:265–268.

24. Consensus development conference on the diagnosis and management of nephropathy in patients with diabetes mellitus. Diabetes Care 1994;17:1357–1361.

25. Bennett PH, Haffner S, Kasiske BL et al. Screening and management of microalbuminuria in patients with diabetes mellitus: recommendations to the scientific advisory board of the National Kidney Foundation from an ad hoc committee of the council on diabetes mellitus of the National Kidney Foundation. Am J Kidney Dis 1995;25:107–112.

26. Striker GE. Report on a workshop to develop management recommendations for the prevention of progression in chronic renal disease (Bethesda, April, 1994). Nephrol Dial Transplant 1995;10:290–292.

27. Gibb DM, Shah V, Preece M, Barratt TM. Variability of urine albumin excretion in normal and diabetic children. Pediatr Nephrol 1989; 3:414–419.

28. Taylor AM, Dunger DB, Preece MA, Holly JMP, Smith CP, Wass JAH, Patel S, Tate VE. The growth hormone independent insulin-like growth factor-I binding protein BP-28 is associated with serum insulin-like growth factor-I inhibitory bioactivity in adolescent insulin-dependent diabetics. Clin Endocrinol 1990;32: 229–239.

29. Blankestijn PJ, Derkx FHM, Birkenhäger JC, Lamberts SWJ, Mulder P, Verschoor L, Schalekamp MADH, Weber RFA. Glomerular hyperfiltration in insulin-dependent diabetes mellitus is correlated with enhanced growth hormone secretion. J Clin Endocrinol Metab 1993;77:498–502.

30. Chiarelli F, Verrotti A, Morgese G. Glomerular hyperfiltration increases the risk of developing microalbuminuria in diabetic children. Pediatr Nephrol 1995; 9:154–158.

31. Mathiesen ER, Saurbrey N, Hommel E, Parving H.-H. Prevalence of microalbuminuria in children with Type 1 (insulin-dependent) diabetes mellitus. Diabetologia 1986;29:640–643.

32. Nørgaard N, Storm B, Graa M, Feldt-Rasmussen B. Elevated albumin excretion and retinal changes in children with Type 1 diabetes are related to long-term poor blood glucose control. Diabetic Med 1989;6:325–328.

33. D'Antonio JA, Ellis D, Doft BH, Becker DJ, Drash AL, Kuller LH, Orchard TJ. Diabetic complications and glycemic control. The Pittsburgh prospective insulin-dependent diabetes cohort study status report after 5 yr of IDDM. Diabetes Care 1989;12:694–700.

34. Joner G, Brinchmann-Hansen O, Torres CG, Hanssen KF. A nationwide cross-sectional study of retinopathy and microalbuminuria in young Norwegian Type 1 (insulin-dependent) diabetic patients. Diabetologia 1992;35:1049–1054.

35. Olsen BS, Johannesen J, Sjølie AK, Borch-Johnsen K, Hougaard P, Thorsteinsson B, Prammning S, Marinelli K, Mortensen HB and the Danish Study Group of Diabetes in Childhood. Metabolic control and prevalence of microvascular complications in young Danish patients with Type 1 diabetes mellitus. Diabet. Med 1999;16:79–85.

36. Bojestig M, Arnqvist HJ, Hermansson G, Karlberg BE, Ludvigsson J. Declining incidence of nephropathy in insulin-dependent diabetes mellitus. N Engl J Med 1994;330:15–18.

37. Janner M, Eberhard Knill SE, Diem P, Zuppinger KA, Mullis PE. Persistent microalbuminuria in adolescents with Type 1 (insulin-dependent) diabetes mellitus is associated to early rather than late puberty. Eur J Pediatr 1994;153:403–408.

38. Dahlquist G, Rudberg S. The prevalence of microalbuminuria in diabetic children and adolescents and its relation to puberty. Acta Pædiatr Scand 1987;76:795–800.

39. Rudberg S, Ullman E, Dahlquist G. Relationship between early metabolic control and the development of microalbuminuria – a longitudinal study in children with Type 1 (insulin-dependent) diabetes mellitus. Diabetologia 1993;36:1309–1314.

40. Stephenson JM, Fuller JH, the EURODIAB IDDM Complications Study Group and the WHO Multinational Study of Vascular Disease in Diabetes Study Group. Microalbuminuria is not rare before 5 years of IDDM. J Diab Comp 1994;8:166–173.

41.   Bangstad H-J, Østerby R, Dahl-Jørgensen K, Berg KJ, Hartmann A, Hanssen KF. Improvement of blood glucose control in IDDM patients retards the progression of morphological changes in early diabetic nephropathy. Diabetologia 1994;37:483–490.

42.   Powrie JK, Watts GF, Ingham JN, Taub NA, Talmud PJ, Shaw KM. Role of glycaemic control in development of microalbuminuria in patients with insulin dependent diabetes. BMJ 1994;309:1608–1612.

43.   Klein R, Klein BEK, Moss SE, Cruickshanks KJ. Ten-year incidence of gross proteinuria in people with diabetes. Diabetes 1995;44:916–923.

44.   Mortensen HB, Hartling SG, Petersen KE, and the Danish study group of diabetes in childhood. A nation-wide cross-sectional study of glycosylated haemoglobin in Danish children with Type 1 diabetes. Diabetic Med 1988;5:871–876.

45.   Mortensen HB, Villumsen J, Vølund Aa, Petersen KE, Nerup J and The Danish Study Group of Diabetes in Childhood. Relationship between insulin injection regimen and metabolic control in young Danish Type 1 diabetic patients. Diabetic Med 1992;9:834–839.

46.   Mortensen HB, Hougaard P, for the Hvidøre Study Group on Childhood Diabetes. Comparison of metabolic control in a cross-sectional study of 2873 children and adolescents with IDDM from 18 countries. Diabetes Care 1997; 20:714–720.

47.   Mortensen HB, Hougaard P, for the Hvidøre Study Group on Childhood Diabetes. International perspectives in childhood and adolescent diabetes: A review. J Pediatr Endocrinol Metab 1997;10:261–264.

48.   Mortensen HB , Robertson KJ et al., for the Hvidøre Study Group on Childhood Diabetes.Insulin management and metabolic control of Type 1 diabetes in childhood and adolescence in 18 countries. Diabetic Med 1998;15:752–759.

49.   Holl RW, Grabert M, Thon A, Heinze E. Urinary excretion of albumin in adolescents with type 1 diabetes. Persistent versus intermittent microalbuminuria and relationship to duration of diabetes, sex, and metabolic control. Diabetes Care 1999;22:1555–1560.

50.   Schultz CJ, Konopelska-Bamu T, Carroll TA, Stratton I, Gale EAM, Neil A, Dunger D for the Oxford Regional Prospective Study Group. Microalbuminuria prevalence varies with age, sex and puberty in children with type 1 diabetes followed from diagnosis in a longitudinal study. Diabetes Care 1999;22:495–502.

51.   Brenner BM, Chertow GM. Congenital oligonephropathy and the etiology of adult hypertension and progressive renal injury. Am J Kidney Dis 1994;23:171–175.

52.   Rossing P, Tarnow L, Nielsen FS, Boelskifte S, Brenner BM, Parving H-H. Short stature and diabetic nephropathy. BMJ 1995;310:296–297.

53.   Orchard TJ, Dorman JS, Maser RE, Becker DJ, Drash AL, Ellis D, LaPorte RE, Kuller LH. Prevalence of complications in IDDM by sex and duration. Pittsburgh epidemiology of diabetes complications study II. Diabetes 1990;39:1116–1124.

54.   The Diabetes Control and Complications Trial Research Group. The effect of intensive treatment of diabetes on the development and progression of long-term complications in insulin-dependent diabetes mellitus. N Engl J Med 1993;329:977–986.

55.   Krolewski AS, Laffel LBM, Krolewski M, Quinn M, Warram JH. Glycosylated hemoglobin and the risk of microalbuminuria in patients with insulin-dependent diabetes mellitus. N Engl J Med 1995;332:1251–1255.

56.   The Diabetes Control and Complications Trial Research Group. Effect of intensive diabetes treatment on the development and progression of long-term complications in adolescents with insulin-dependent diabetes mellitus. J Pediatr 1994;125:177–188.

57. Danne T, Weber B, Hartmann R, Enders I, Burger W, Hovener G. Long-term glycemic control has a nonlinear association to the frequency of background retinopathy in adolescents with diabetes. Diabetes Care 1994;17:1390–1396.

58. Danne T, Dinesen B, Weber B, Mortensen HB: Threshold of HbA1c for the effect of hypergycaemia on the risk of diabetic micrangiopathy (letter). Diabetes Care 1996;19:183.

59. Lobefalo L, Verrotti A, Della Loggia G, Morgese G, Mastropasqua L, Chiarelli F, Gallenga PE. Diabetic retinopathy in childhood and adolescence. Effects of puberty. Diab Nutr Metab 1997;10:193–197.

60. Davis EA, Keating B, Byrne GC, Russell M, Jones TW. Hypoglycemia: incidence and clinical predictors in a large population-based sample of children and adolescents with IDDM. Diabetes Care 1997;20:22–25.

61. The Diabetes Control and Complications Trial Research Group. Hypoglycemia in the diabetes control and complications trial. Diabetes 1997;46:271–286.

62. Bognetti E, Brunelli A, Meschi F, Viscardi M, Bonfanti R, Chiumello G. Frequency and correlates of severe hypoglycaemia in children and adolescents with diabetes mellitus. Eur J Pediatr 1997:156:589–591.

63. Davis EA, Keating B, Byrne GC, Russell M, Jones TW. Impact of improved glycaemic control on rates of hypoglycaemia in insulin dependent diabetes mellitus. Arch Dis Child 1998;78:111–115.

64. Tupola S, Rajantie J. Documented symptomatic hypoglycemia in children and adolescents using multiple daily insulin injection therapy. Diabetic Med 1998;15:492–496.

65. Rovet JF, Ehrlich RM. The effect of hypoglycemic seizures on cognitive function in children with diabetes: a 7-year prospective study. J Pediatr 1999;134:503–506.

66. Becker DJ, Ryan CM. Intensive diabetes therapy in childhood: Is it achievable? Is it desirable? Is it safe? Editorial. J Pediatr 1999;134:392–394.

67. Hershey T, Bhargva N, Sadler M, White NH, Craft S. Conventional versus intensive diabetes therapy in children with type 1 diabetes. Diabetes Care 1999; 22:1318–1324.

68. Ryan CM. Memory and metabolic control in children (editorial). Diabetes Care 1999;22:1239–1241.

69. Mortensen HB, Hougaard P, Ibsen KK, Parving H-H and The Danish Study Group of Diabetes in Childhood. Relationship between blood pressure and urinary albumin excretion rate in young Danish Type 1 diabetic patients: Comparison to non-diabetic children. Diabetic Med 1994;11:155–161.

70. Kordonouri O, Danne T, Hopfenmüller W, Enders I, Hövener G, Weber B. Lipid profiles and blood pressure: are they risk factors for the development of early background retinopathy and incipient nephropathy in children with insulin-dependent diabetes mellitus. Acta Paediatr 1996;85:43–48.

71. Gorman D, Sochett E, Daneman D. The natural history of microalbuminuria in adolescents with type 1 diabetes. J Pediatr 1999;134:333–337.

72. Bojestig M, Arnqvist HJ, Karlberg BE, Ludvigsson J. Glycemic control and prognosis in Type 1 diabetic patients with microalbuminuria. Diabetes Care 1996; 19:313–317.

73. Mogensen CE. Microalbuminuria as a predictor of clinical diabetic nephropathy. Kidney Int 1987;31:673–689.

74. Mogensen CE, Christensen CK, Christiansen JS, Boyle N, Pederson MM, Schmitz A. Early hyperfiltration and late renal damage in insulin-dependent diabetes. Pediatr Adolesc Endocrinol 1988;17:197–205.

75.   Feldt-Rasmussen B, Mathiesen ER, Deckert T, Giese J, Christensen NJ, Bent-Hansen L, Damkjær Nielsen M. Central role for sodium in the pathogenesis of blood pressure changes independent of angiotensin, aldosterone and catecholamines in Type 1 (insulin-dependent) diabetes mellitus. Diabetologia 1987;30:610–617.

76.   Deckert T, Kofoed-Enevoldsen A, Nørgaard K, Borch-Johnsen K, Feldt-Rasmussen B, Jensen T. Microalbuminuria: implications for micro- and macrovascular disease. Diabetes Care 1992;15:1181–1191.

77.   Cook J, Daneman D, Spino M, Sochett E, Perlman K, Balfe JW. Angiotensin converting enzyme inhibitor therapy to decrease microalbuminuria in normotensive children with insulin-dependent diabetes mellitus. J. Pediatr 1990;117:39–45.

78.   Rudberg S, Aperia A, Freyschuss U, Persson B. Enalapril reduces microalbuminuria in young normotensive Type 1 (insulin-dependent) diabetic patients irrespective of its hypotensive effect. Diabetologia 1990;33:470–476.

79.   Marre M, Chatellier G, Leblanc H, Guyene TT, Menard J, Passa P. Prevention of diabetic nephropathy with enalapril in normotensive diabetics with microalbuminuria. BMJ 1988;297:1092–1095.

80.   Mathiesen ER, Hommel E, Giese J, Parving H-H. Efficacy of captopril in postponing nephropathy in normotensive insulin dependent diabetic patients with microalbuminuria. BMJ 1991;303:81–87.

81.   Hallab M, Gallois Y, Chatellier G, Rohmer V, Fressinaud P, Marre M. Comparison of reduction in microalbuminuria by enalapril and hydrochlorothiazide in normotensive patients with insulin dependent diabetes. BMJ 1993;306:175–182.

82.   Viberti GC, Mogensen CE, Groop LC, Pauls JF, for the European Microalbuminuria Captopril Study Group. Effect of captopril on progression to clinical proteinuria in patients with insulin-dependent diabetes mellitus and microalbuminuria. JAMA 1994;271:275–279.

83.   Breyer JA, Hunsicker LG, Bain RP, Lewis EJ, and The Collaborative Study Group. Angiotensin converting enzyme inhibition in diabetic nephropathy. Kidney Int 1994;45:156–160.

84.   Rudberg S, Østerby R, Bangstad H.-J, Dahlquist G, Persson B. Effect of angiotensin converting enzyme inhibitor or beta blocker on glomerular structural changes in young microalbuminuric patients with type 1 (insulin-dependent) diabetes mellitus. Diabetologia 1999;42:589–595.

85.   The Microalbuminuria Captopril Study Group (Barnes DJ, Cooper M, Gans DJ, Laffel L, Mogensen CE, Viberti GC. Captopril reduces the risk of nephropathy in insulin-dependent diabetic patients with microalbuminuria. Diabetologia 1996; 39:587–593.

86.   Chaturvedi N, Sjolie A-K, Stephenson JM, Abrahamian H, Keipes M, Castellarin A, Rogulja-Pepeonik Z, Fuller JH, and the EUCLID Study Group. Effect of lisinopril on progression of retinopathy in normotensive people with Type 1 diabetes. Lancet 1998;351:28–31.

87.   Mathiesen ER, Rønn B, Jensen T, Storm B, Deckert T. Relation between blood pressure and urinary albumin excretion in development of microalbuminuria. Diabetes 1990;39:245–249.

88.   Zusman RM. Renin- and non-renin-mediated antihypertensive actions of converting enzyme inhibitors. Kidney Int 1984;25:969–83.

89.   Anderson S, Brenner BM. Pathogenesis of diabetic glomerulopathy: Hemodynamic considerations: Diabetes Metab Rev 1988;4:163–177.

90.   Frohlich ED, Cooper RA, Lewis EJ. Review of the overall experience of captopril in hypertension. Arch Intern Med 1984;144:1441–1444.

91.   Mirkin BL, Newman TJ. Efficacy and safety of captopril in the treatment of severe childhood hypertension: report of the International Collaborative Study Group. Pediatrics 1985;75:1091–1100.

92.   Shield JPH. Microalbuminuria and nephropathy in childhood diabetes. Practical Diabetes 1994;11:146–149.

29. EARLY RENAL HYPERFUNCTION AND HYPERTROPHY IN IDDM PATIENTS INCLUDING COMMENTS ON EARLY INTERVENTION

Margrethe Mau Pedersen
Medical Department, Randers Centralsygehus, Randers, Denmark

Diabetic nephropathy is the main cause of reduced survival in insulin-dependent diabetes. Much interest is paid to early alterations in kidney function and structure, since a relationship may exist between such early abnormalities and later development of diabetic nephropathy. A modest increase in urinary albumin excretion, microalbuminuria, has been identified as an early marker of diabetic nephropathy, and therapeutical intervention postponing the onset of overt nephropathy has been introduced. In this chapter the initial renal changes in IDDM, glomerular hyperfunction and renal hypertrophy, will be addressed.

GLOMERULAR HYPERFUNCTION

From the onset of IDDM, kidney function is characterised by elevation of glomerular filtration rate (GFR) and renal plasma flow (RPF) [for recent reviews see 1,2]. Using precise measurements e.g. renal clearance of inulin or iothalamate, it has been found that mean GFR in groups of short-term IDDM patients is increased by 15-25% - to approximately 135-140 ml/min/1.73m^2 during 'usual metabolic control' [3-7]. Before start of insulin treatment, but in the absence of ketoacidosis, glomerular hyperfiltration is even more pronounced, often showing elevations of approximately 40% [8,9]. RPF seems to be elevated synchronously with the increase in GFR, but less pronounced [3,5]. Estimation of RPF from renal clearance of hippuran appears to be a reliable measure also in the diabetic state [10].

During the first one or two decades of diabetes glomerular hyperfunction remains a characteristic feature of kidney function. In cross-sectional studies patients with microalbuminuria - typically developed after 10 to 15 years of diabetes - show more pronounced hyperfiltration than normoalbuminuric patients [7,11]. Until now, however, no prospective studies have described the individual course in GFR during transmission from normo- to microalbuminuria. With further increase in albumin excretion and development of nephropathy, GFR and RPF starts to decline, whereas in patients with

Mogensen, C.E. (ed.), THE KIDNEY AND HYPERTENSION IN DIABETES MELLITUS
Copyright© 2000 by Kluwer Academic Publishers, Boston • Dordrecht • London. All rights reserved.

persistent normoalbuminuria a moderate degree of glomerular hyperfunction persists [12].

Early renal changes in experimental diabetes in some degree parallel the characteristic glomerular hyperfunction in early stages of human diabetes. As described elsewhere in this book, besides hyperperfusion, increased intraglomerular hydraulic pressure is an important factor in hyperfiltration in diabetic animals. In humans the larger increase in GFR than RPF (increased filtration fraction) suggests similar intraglomerular hypertension. However, elevation of the ultrafiltration coefficient due to increased filtration surface, may also offer a mechanism for the increased filtration fraction [13].

RENAL HYPERTROPHY

Kidney volume, estimated from ultrasonic techniques or roentgenographically, like GFR is markedly increased from the debut of diabetes. During initial insulin-treatment, kidney hypertrophy is somewhat reduced. The relative reduction in kidney volume is apparently delayed and smaller than the relative lowering of GFR [14]. The mean size remains elevated by approximately 20-30% during short-term IDDM [5,15-17]. At this stage, kidney volume is strongly correlated to GFR, corresponding to the state in non-diabetic subjects, and in most forms of non-diabetic renal hypertrophy [18]. Later in the course of diabetes this association cannot be found and possibly kidney volume increases further in the microalbuminuric state [19]. Hypertrophy persists also after the onset of overt nephropathy. Morphological studies concerning the initial renal enlargement show glomerular and tubular hypertrophy [20,21]. Subsequent deposition of PAS-positive material in the glomerular tuft and further enlargement of open glomeruli does not play a significant role or the total kidney volume.

DETERMINANTS FOR GLOMERULAR HYPERFUNCTION AND HYPER-TROPHY

The pathophysiological mechanisms behind the increased glomerular filtration rate and renal plasma flow are still unclarified. A number of human and animal intervention studies have suggested a specific importance of one particular substance. In table 29-1 such factors with a possible involvement in glomerular hyperfunction are listed. Many factors, however, may represent normal modulators of kidney function influenced by an abnormal metabolic milieu and changes in fluid homeostasis. Furthermore, many of these factors are interrelated and represent different steps in regulatory mechanisms.

The abnormal carbohydrate metabolism no doubt plays a key-role in development of glomerular hyperfunction. An increase in blood glucose concentration apparently is associated with vasodilation in a number of tissues including the glomerular capillaries [22,23]. Suggested mechanisms for this vasodilation include an osmotic effect on cells lining small vessels [24], an increase in production of kallikrein and endothelium-derived-relaxing-factor (EDRF) [25,26], and increased production of vasodilator prostaglandins [27]. Furthermore, the increased amount of filtered and reabsorbed glucose coupled to increased tubular sodium reabsorption may suppress the tubuloglomerular feedback system and thereby contribute to hyperfiltration [25,28]. In human IDDM the influence of elevated blood glucose on GFR and RPF has been elucidated through intervention studies with glucose administration, through studies with intensified insulin treatment, and through cross-sectional studies analysing correlations between metabolic status and kidney function. In IDDM patients a rise in blood glucose by glucose infusion or an oral glucose load increases GFR and RPF in some studies [29-31]. Results, however, have not been completely uniform [32-34], maybe due to different responses in different subgroups of diabetic patients [33,34]. In studies with intensified insulin treatment, a few days of strict metabolic control has not been found to reduce GFR [35], whereas a reduction in GFR was observed during long-term (2 years) insulin pump treatment [36]. In cross sectional studies a correlation between GFR and HbA_{1c} and between intra-individual variation in blood glucose and in RPF has been reported [37,38,86]. Taken together these studies suggest that the 'acute' glucose level is associated mainly to RPF, whereas long-term metabolic control (e.g. represented by HbA_{1c}) show a closer correlation to GFR. It may be that e.g. biochemical membrane properties are important to the long-term influence of glycemic control of GFR.

Another aspect of hyperglycaemia is enhanced glucose metabolism through the polyol pathway in tissues with insulin-independent glucose uptake. High activity of the enzyme aldose reductase leads to sorbitol accumulation and probably to changes in the redox state. These alterations, which appear to be rather closely linked to depletion of myoinositol [39], have been related to development of late diabetic complications in different tissues and recently also to glomerular hyperfiltration [40-42].

An increase in blood concentration of ketone bodies also accompany fairly well-regulated diabetes and intervention studies have suggested this to be of significance for hyperfiltration and hyperfusion [43]. However, no statistical correlation has been demonstrated between the concentration of ketone bodies and GFR or RPF.

Besides the indirect effect of insulin deficiency on renal hemodynamics through the blood glucose level, it has been suggested that inadequate delivery of insulin to the liver is associated with increased production of renal vasoregulatory factors [44]. In diabetic patients conventional insulin treatment with subcutaneous injections give rise to such portal hypoinsulinaemia, while hyperinsulinaemia is found in the systemic circulation [44]. No influence of insulin per se on GFR and RPF has been found [45].

One consequence of hyperglycaemia and peripheral hyperinsulinaemia appears to be an increase in total exchangeable body sodium and extracellular volume expansion [4,46]. Apart from an influence on the tubuloglomerular feedback system, this condition might induce hyperfiltration through a reflectoric increase in atrial natriuretic peptide (ANP).

ANP has been shown to increase GFR and FF in microalbuminuric IDDM patients [87]. A significant role for ANP in hyperfiltration is also suggested by experimental studies in animals showing marked reductions in GFR during treatment with anti-ANP serum [27,47] or an ANP-receptor antagonist [48]. In our study on intra-individual variation in kidney function [38] an involvement of ANP in the mechanisms behind human diabetic hyperfiltration was indicated by the finding of a close covariation between GFR and ANP (figure 29-1).

Table 29-1. Factors with possible involvement in early diabetic glomerular hyperfunction including suggested intermediary steps.

Metabolic factors:	Blood glucose Long-term glycemic control (HbA$_{1c}$) Activity of polyol pathway Ketone bodies	[bradykinin, EDRF, prosta- glandins]
Hormonal/peptide substances:	GH, IGF-I Glucagon Insulin (peripheral hyperinsulinemia, hepatic insulinpenia) Atrial natriuretic peptide Kallikrein, bradykinin, kinin Catecholamines (abnormal response) Arginine vasopressin C-peptide (lack of)	[prostaglandins] [restraining effect from adenosine] [nitric oxide]
Other vasoactive substances:	Vasodilatory prostaglandins Endothelial derived relaxing factor (EDRF) Nitric oxide	
Dietary factors other than carbohydrates	Protein intake Fat intake Vitamin E	[glucagon, prostaglandins, kallikrein, adenosine, dopamine, nitric oxide] [reduced oxidative stress]
Genetic factors	Angiotensin converting enzyme gene polymorphism	

References : 22-27,29-44,47-54,56-60,64-70, 86-91, 96-97.

Growth hormone (GH) and glucagon have long been known to represent possible mediators of diabetic hyperfiltration. Both hormones induce elevation in GFR when injected (through GH not acutely) [49,50]; increased plasma levels of the hormones may be brought about by the diabetic state, and a statistical correlation between plasma levels and GFR has been reported for both hormones [51]. The influence of GH is apparently indirect - acting through insulin-like growth factor I (IGF-I) [52]. Glucagon seems mainly to be of significance for hyperfiltration in poorly regulated diabetic patients [50].

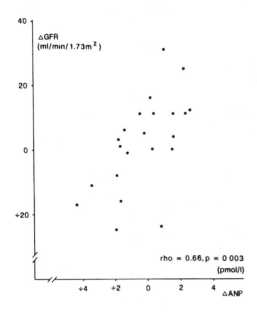

Fig. 29-1 Intra-individual variation in glomerular filtration rate (ΔGFR) in relation to variation in plasma concentration of atrial natriuretic peptide (ΔANP) in 22 patients with IDDM. 0.66 , p=0.003. From Mau Pedersen et al [38, with permission].

Protein intake plays a special role in diabetic hyperfiltration in the sense that it represents a 'iatrogenic' stimulator of GFR. It is well-know that protein meals and infusion of aminoacids increases GFR [53]. Diabetic diets typically have a protein content of approximately 18-20% of total energy intake compared to a protein intake around 14% in non-diabetic (Danish) subjects [54,55]. By lowering protein intake from 19 to 12% we observed a decrease in mean GFR from 146 to 132 ml/min/1.73m^2 in a group of normoalbuminuric IDDM patients [54]. The type of protein ingested seems to be of importance to the magnitude of influence on GFR [56,57] Furthermore, the content of phosphate may be relevant [58].

Lately attention has been paid to a possible beneficial effect of antioxidants, especially vitamin E, on diabetic complications. In early, uncomplicated diabetes, it has been reported that vitamin E reduces glomerular hyperfiltration [88]. However, in this study creatinine clearance from overnight urine collections was used as a measure for GFR. To solve the issue, further investigations with more precise measurements of GFR, will be needed.

Polymorphism in the angiotensin converting enzyme (ACE) gene has been suggested as a genetic factor that may influence the risk of developing nephropathy. It has been found that an insertion/deletion (I/D) polymorphism is important for the plasma ACE level, and that the allele D is associated with high plasma ACE-concentration and with increased risk of developing nephropathy [89]. With respect to glomerular hyperfiltration, no final conclusion on a possible association between the ACE-gene polymorphism and GFR can be drawn from available studies [90-92]. It has been indicated, however, that the genotype may be important by influencing the way renal hemodynamics respond to increases in blood glucose [92]. Thus, in patients with the DD genotype a rise in GFR and RPF has been observed when blood glucose is changed from normo- to hyperglycemia as opposed to findings for the II genotype.

With respect to renal hypertrophy glycemic control is a determinant for kidney volume during the early stage of IDDM, as described above. It is unclarified whether kidney volume may still be modulated by alterations in glycemic control after years of diabetes and during the microalbuminuric state [19,59,60]. Knowledge on other pathogenetic factors in renal hypertrophy in human diabetes is limited. Experimental studies points towards GH/IGF-1 as contributors to very early kidney growth [52] (see also chapter 25), and also a cross-sectional study in human diabetes suggest a role for growth factor in kidney hypertrophy [93]. Furthermore, studies in experimental diabetes indicate that renal hypertrophy is associated with increased activity of the transforming growth factor-beta (TGF-β) system [63, 94,95] and with a depressed protein degradation due to reduced proteinase activity in both glomeruli and tubuli [61,62].

POSSIBLE ROLE OF HYPERFILTRATION AS A RISK MARKER FOR DIABETIC NEPHROPATHY

In certain IDDM patients, glomerular hyperfiltration is especially marked and sustained during many years, and it has been suggested that such hyperfiltration represents a pathogenetic factor for later development of diabetic nephropathy. This suspicion is supported by the apparent analogy between the characteristic early renal hemodynamic changes in human IDDM and in animal models of diabetes. Thus, in experimental diabetes a normalisation of the high GFR or the high intraglomerular hydraulic pressure by pharmacological or dietary means, has attenuated progression of renal disease [71]. In human diabetes retrospective data has suggested that marked hyperfiltration is associated with later nephropathy [12,72]. This finding was later questioned in two follow-up studies [75,76]. However, in a recent prospective study where normoalbuminuric adolescent diabetic patients were followed for 8 years, glomerular hyperfiltration was identified as a strong independent predictor for nephropathy. Other variables (duration of diabetes, albumin excretion rate, blood glucose and HbA$_{1c}$) included in the multiple regression analysis showed no independent association. Also in a group of diabetic children, studied during 10 years, hyperfiltration was found to predict later development of microalbuminuria [74]. In adolescent IDDM patients before the stage of microalbuminuria a new follow-up study (98) has investigated the possibility of an association between hyperfiltration and morphological kidney changes. This biopsy study reported a positive correlation between mesangial ultrastructural changes and the filtration fraction measured repeatedly during years before the biopsy. Available evidence, thus, shows an association between glomerular hyperfiltration and later nephropathy. Whether this association represents a pathogenetic mechanism, however, is still unclarified.

Indirect evidence for a pathogenetic role of abnormal renal hemodynamics is found in the marked slowing of early renal disease observed during antihypertensive treatment. This especially applies for ACE-inhibitors, which are considered to reduce intraglomerular pressure more specifically than other antihypertensives [78]. In a recent pilot study treatment with an ACE-inhibitor reduced both albumin excretion and kidney volume in microalbuminuric, normotensive IDDM patients [79].

Addressing kidney hypertrophy rather than hemodynamic parameters, a recent sonographic study in IDDM patients has indicated that large kidneys may be a morphological marker for later diabetic nephropathy [99].

POSSIBILITIES FOR INTERVENTIONS

An obvious goal for therapeutic intervention is optimizing glycemic control in order to decrease the risk of late complications. Such therapy tend to reduce hyperfiltration. Yet as it appears from above, hyperfiltration *per se* does not constitute an established indication for intervention. It seems rational though, not to prescribe higher protein content in diabetic than in non-diabetic diets to avoid inducing additional hyperfiltration.

Future possibilities for non-glycemic pharmacological intervention include aldose reductase inhibitors, aiming at normalization of the polyol pathway activity [40-42], and treatment with somatostatin analogues [80-82], which may act on GFR through a lowering of GH (or IGF-I) and a suppression of glucagon secretion. Until now these interventions have been tested only in rather short term or small scale studies and the possible long-term benefits awaits further investigations.

Also ACE-inhibitors deserves to be mentioned along with other proposed early interventions. Although these agents have not generally been found to reduce GFR, their ability to reduce the filtration fraction and probably the intraglomerular pressure [83] may prove valuable also before the onset of microalbuminuria [84]. In addition to the hemodynamic effects of ACE-inhibitors, these drugs may also be valuable since they might attenuate growth stimulating effect of ANG II [85].

REFERENCES

1. Mogensen CE. Glomerular hyperfiltration in human diabetes. Diabetes Care 1994; 17: 770-775.
2. Bank N. Mechanisms of diabetic hyperfiltration. Nephrology Forum. Kidney Int 1991; 40: 792-807.
3. Mogensen CE. Glomerular filtration rate and renal plasma flow in short-term and long-term juvenile diabetes mellitus. Scand J Clin Lab Invest 1971; 28: 91-100.
4. Ditzel J, Schwartz M. Abnormally increased glomerular filtration rate in short-term insulin-treated diabetic subjects. Diabetes 1976; 16: 264-267.

5.   Christensen JS, Gammelgaard J, Frandsen M, Parving H-H. Increased kidney size, glomerular filtration rate and renal plasma flow in short-term insulin-dependent diabetics. Diabetologia 1981; 20: 451-456.

6.   Brøchner-Mortensen J, Ditzel J. Glomerular filtration rate and extracellular fluid volume in insulin-dependent patients with diabetes mellitus. Kidney Int 1982; 21: 696-698.

7.   Hansen KW, Mau Pedersen M, Christensen CK, Schmitz A, Christiansen JS, Mogensen CE. Normoalbuminuria ensures no reduction of renal function in type 1 (insulin-dependent) diabetic patients. J Intern Med 1992; 232: 161-167.

8.   Mogensen CE. Kidney function and glomerular permeability to macromolecules in juvenile diabetes. Dan Med Bull 1972; 19: 1-36.

9.   Christiansen JS, Gammelgaard J, Tronier B, Svendsen PA, Parving H-H. Kidney function and size in diabetics before and during initial insulin treatment. Kidney Int 1982; 21: 683-688.

10. Nyberg G, Granerus G, Aurell M. Renal extraction ratios for ^{51}Cr-EDTA, PAH, and glucose in early insulin-dependent diabetic patients. Kidney Int 1982; 21: 706-708.

11. Christensen CK, Mogensen CE. The course of incipient diabetic nephropathy: studies of albumin excretion and blood pressure. Diabetic Med 1985; 2: 97-102.

12. Mogensen CE, Christensen CK. Predicting diabetic nephropathy in insulin-dependent patients. N Engl J Med 1984; 311: 89-93.

13. Ellis EN, Steffes MW, Coetz FC, Sutherland DER, Mauer SM. Glomerular filtration surface in type 1 diabetes mellitus. Kidney Int 1986; 29: 889-894.

14. Christiansen JS, Frandsen M, Parving H-H. The effect of intravenous insulin infusion on kidney function in insulin-dependent diabetes mellitus. Diabetologia 1981; 20: 199-204.

15. Mogensen CE, Andersen MJF. Increased kidney size and glomerular filtration rate in early juvenile diabetes. Diabetes 1973; 22: 706-713.

16. Mogensen CE, Andersen MJF. Increased kidney size and glomerular filtration rate in untreated juvenile diabetes: Normalization by insulin-treatment. Diabetologia 1975; 11: 221-224.

17. Puig JG, Antón FM, Grande C, Pallardo LF, Arnalich F, Gil A, Vázquez JJ, García AM. Relation on kidney size to kidney function in early insulin-dependent diabetes. Diabetologia 1981; 21: 363-367.

18. Schwieger J, Fine LG. Renal hypertrophy, growth factors, and nephropathy in diabetes mellitus. Semin Nephrol 1990; 10: 242-253.

19. Feldt-Rasmussen B, Hegedüs L, Mathiesen ER, Deckert T. Kidney volume in type 1 (insulin-dependent) diabetic patients with normal or increased urinary albumin excretion: effect of long-term improved metabolic control. Scand J Lab Invest 1991; 51: 31-36.

20. Østerby R, Gundersen HJG. Glomerular size and structure in diabetes mellitus: I. Early abnormalities. Diabetologia 1975; 11: 225-229.

21. Seyer-Hansen K, Hansen J, Gundersen HJG. Renal hypertrophy in experimental diabetes: a morphometric study. Diabetologia 1980; 18: 501-505.

22. Mathiesen ER, Hilsted J, Feldt-Rasmussen B, Bonde-Petersen F, Christensen NJ, Parving H-H. The effect of metabolic control on hemodynamics in short-term insulin-dependent diabetic patients. Diabetes 1985; 34: 1301-1305.

23. Wolpert HA, Kinsley BT, Clermont AC, Wald H, Bursell S-E. Hyperglycaemia modulates retinal hemodynamics in IDDM. Diabetes 1993; 42: A489.

24. Gray SD. Effect of hypertonicity on vascular dimensions in skeletal muscle. Microvasc Res 1971; 3: 117-124.

25. Bank N. Mechanisms of diabetic hyperfiltration. Kidney Int 1991; 40: 792-807.

26. Harvey JN, Edmundson AW, Jaffa AA, Martin LL, Mayfield RK. Renal excretion of kallikrein and eicosanoids in patients with Type 1 (insulin-dependent) diabetes mellitus. Relationship to glomerular and tubular function. Diabetologia 1992; 35: 857-862.

27. Perico N, Benigni A, Gabanelli M, Piccinelli A, Rog M, De-Riva C, Remuzzi G. Atrial natriuretide peptide and prostacyclin synergistically mediate hyperfiltration and hyperperfusion of diabetic rats. Diabetes 1992; 41: 533-538.

28. Blantz RC, Peterson OW, Gushwa L, Tucker BJ. Effect of modest hyperglycaemia on tubuloglomerular feedback activity. Kidney Int 1982; 22: S206-S212.

29. Christiansen JS, Christensen CK, Hermansen K, Pedersen EB, Mogensen CE. Enhancement of glomerular filtration rate and renal plasma flow by oral glucose load in well controlled insulin-dependent diabetics. Scand J Clin Lab Invest 1986; 46: 265-272.

30. Christiansen JS, Frandsen M, Parving H-H. Effect of intravenous glucose infusion on renal function in normal man and in insulin-dependent diabetics. Diabetologia 1981; 21: 368-373.

31. Wiseman MJ, Mangili R, Alberetto M, Keen H, Viberti GC. Glomerular response mechanisms to glycemic changes in insulin-dependent diabetics. Kidney Int 1987; 31: 1012-1018.

32. Mogensen CE. Glomerular filtration rate and renal plasma flow in normal and diabetic man during elevation of blood sugar levels. Scand J Clin Lab Invest 1971; 28: 177-182.

33. Marre M, Dubin T, Hallab M, Berrut G, Bouhanick B, Lejeune J-J, Fressinaud P. Different renal response to hyperglycaemia in insulin-dependent diabetics at risk for, or protected against diabetic nephropathy. Diabetes 1993; 42: A423.

34. Skøtt P, Vaag A, Hother-Nielsen O, Andersen P, Bruun NE, Giese J, Beck-Nielsen H, Parving H-H. Effects of hyperglycaemia on kidney function, atrial natriuretic factor and plasma renin in patients with insulin-dependent diabetes mellitus. Scand J Clin Lab Invest 1991; 51: 715-727.

35. Mathiesen ER, Gall M-A, Hommel E, Skøtt P, Parving H-H. Effects of short-term strict metabolic control on kidney function and extracellular fluid volume in incipient diabetic nephropathy. Diabetic Med 1989; 6: 595-600.

36. Christensen CK, Christiansen JS, Schmitz A, Christensen T, Hermansen K, Mogensen CE. Effect of continuous subcutaneous insulin infusion on kidney function and size in IDDM patients - a two years controlled study. J Diabetes and Its Complications 1987; 1: 91-95.

37. Mogensen CE, Christensen CK, Mau Pedersen M, Alberti KGMM, Boye N, Christensen T, Christiansen JS, Flyvbjerg A, Ingerslev J, Schmitz A, Ørskov H. Renal and glycemic determinants of glomerular hyperfiltration in normoalbuminuric diabetics. J Diabetic Compl 1990; 4: 159-165.

38. Mau Pedersen M, Christiansen JS, Pedersen EB, Mogensen CE. Determinants of intra-individual variation in kidney function in normoalbuminuric insulin-dependent diabetic patients: importance of atrial natriuretic peptide and glycemic control. Clin Sci 1992; 83: 445-451.

39. Greene DA, Lattimer SA, Sima AAF. Sorbitol, phosphoinositides, and sodium-potassium-ATPase in the pathogenesis of diabetic complications. N Engl J Med 1987; 316: 599-606.

40. Mau Pedersen M, Christiansen JS, Mogensen CE. Reduction of glomerular hyperfiltration in normoalbuminuric IDDM patients by 6 mo of aldose reductase inhibition. Diabetes 1991; 40: 527-531.

41. Mau Pedersen M, Mogensen CE, Christiansen JS. Reduction of glomerular hyperfunction during short-term aldose reductase inhibition in normoalbuminuric, insulin-dependent diabetic patients. Endocrinol Metab 1995; 2: 55-62.

42.   Passariello N, Sepe J, Marrazzo G, De Cicco A, Peluso A, Pisano MCA, Sgambato S, Tesauro P, D'Onofrio F. Effect of aldose reductase inhibitor (tolrestat) on urinary albumin excretion rate in IDDM subjects with nephropathy. Diabetes Care 1993; 16: 789-795.

43.   Trevisan R, Nosadini R, Fioretto P, Avogaro A, Duner E, Iori E, Valerio A, Doria A, Crepaldi G. Ketone bodies increase glomerular filtration rate in normal man and in patients with type 1 (insulin dependent) diabetes. Diabetologia 1987; 30: 214-221.

44.   Gwinup G, Elias AN. Hypothesis. Insulin is responsible for the vascular complications of diabetes. Med Hypotheses 1991; 34: 1-6.

45.   Christiansen JS, Frandsen M, Parving H-H. The effect of intravenous insulin infusion on kidney function in insulin-dependent diabetes mellitus. Diabetologia 1981; 20: 199-204.

46.   Skøtt P, Hother-Nielsen O, Bruun NE, Giese J, Nielsen MD, Beck-Nielsen H, Parving H-H. Effects of insulin on kidney function and sodium excretion in healthy subjects. Diabetologia 1989; 32: 694-699.

47.   Ortola FV, Ballermann BJ, Anderson S, Mendez RE, Brenner BM. Elevated plasma atrial natriuretic peptide levels in diabetic rats. Potential mediator of hyperfiltration. J Clin Invest 1987; 80: 670-674.

48.   Kikkawa R, Haneda M, Sakamoto K, Koya D, Shikano T, Nakanishi S, Matsuda Y, Shigeta Y. Antagonist for atrial natriuretic peptide receptors ameliorates glomerular hyperfiltration in diabetic rats. Biochem Biophys Res Commun 1993; 193: 700-705.

49.   Christiansen JS, Gammelgaard J, Frandsen M, Ørskov H, Parving H-H. Kidney function and size in normal subjects before and during growth hormone administration for one week. Eur J Clin Invest 1981; 11: 487-490.

50.   Parving H-H, Christiansen JS, Noer I, Tronier B, Mogensen CE. The effect of glucagon infusion on kidney function in short-term insulin-dependent juvenile diabetics. Diabetologia 1980; 19: 350-354.

51.   Hoogenberg K, Dullaart RPF, Freling NJM, Meijer S, Sluiter WJ. Contributory roles of circulatory glucagon and growth hormone to increased renal haemodynamics in type 1 (insulin-dependent) diabetes mellitus. Scand J Clin Lab Invest 1993; 53: 821-828.

52.   Flyvbjerg A. »The role of insulin-like growth factor I in initial renal hypertrophy in experimental diabetes.« In Growth Hormone and Insulin-Like Growth Factor I. Flyvbjerg A, Ørskov H, Alberti KGMM, eds. John Wiley & Sons Ltd., 1993; pp 271-306.

53.   Castellino P, Hunt W, DeFronzo RA. Regulation of renal hemodynamics by plasma amino acid and hormone concentrations. Kidney Int 1987; 32: S-15-S-20.

54.   Mau Pedersen M, Mogensen CE, Schönau Jørgensen F, Møller B, Lykke G, Pedersen O. Renal effects from limitation of high dietary protein in normoalbuminuric diabetic patients. Kidney Int 1989; 36: S-115-S-121.

55.   Mau Pedersen M, Winther E, Mogensen CE. Reducing protein in the diabetic diet. Diabete Metab (Paris) 1990; 16: 454-459.

56.   Jones MG, Lee K, Swaminathan R. The effect of dietary protein on glomerular filtration rate in normal subjects. Clin Nephrol 1987; 27: 71-75.

57.   Pecis M, de Azevedo MJ, Gross JL. Chicken and fish diet reduces glomerular hyperfiltration in IDDM patients. Diabetes Care 1994; 17: 665-672.

58.   Kraus ES, Cheng L, Sikorski I, Spector DA. Effects of phosphorus restriction on renal response to oral and intravenous protein loads in rats. Am J Physiol 1993; 264: F752-F759.

59.   Tuttle KR, Bruto JL, Perusek MC, Lancaster JL, Kopp DT, DeFronzo RA. Effect of strict glycemic control on renal hemodynamic response to amino acids and renal enlargement in insulin-dependent diabetes mellitus. N Engl J Med 1991; 324: 1626-1632.

60. Wisemann MJ, Saunders AJ, Keen H, Viberti GC. Effect of blood glucose control on increased glomerular filtration rate and kidney size in insulin-dependent diabetes. N Engl J Med 1985; 312: 617-621.

61. Shechter P, Boner G, Rabkin R. Tubular cell protein degradation in early diabetic renal hypertrophy. J Am Soc Nephrol 1994; 4: 1582-1587.

62. Schaefer L, Schaefer RM, Ling, Teschner M, Heidland A. Renal proteinases and kidney hypertrophy in experimental diabetes. Diabetologia 1994; 37: 567-571.

63. Shankland SJ, Scholey JW, Ly H, Thai K. Expression of transforming growth factor-ß1 during diabetic renal hypertrophy. Kidney Int 1994; 46: 430-442.

64. Wang YX, Brooks DP. The role of adenosine in glycine-induced glomerular hyperfiltration in rats. J Pharmacol Exp Ther 1992; 263: 1188-1194.

65. Angielski S, Redlak M, Szczepanska KM. Intrarenal adenosine prevents hyperfiltration induced by atrial natriuretic factor. Miner Electrolyte Metab 1990; 16: 57-60.

66. Wang YX, Gellai M, Brooks DP. Dopamine DA1 receptor agonist, fenoldopam, reverses glycine-induced hyperfiltration in rats. Am J Physiol 1992; 262: F1055-F1060.

67. Jaffa AA, Vio CP, Silva RH, Vavrek RJ, Stewart JM, Rust PF, Mayfield RK. Evidence for renal kinins as mediators of amino acid-induced hyperfusion and hyperfiltration in the rat. J Clin Invest 1992; 89: 1460-1468.

68. Friedlander G, Blanchet BF, Nitenberg A, Laborie C, Assan R, Amiel C. Glucagon secretion is essential for aminoacid-induced hyperfiltration in man. Nephrol Dial Transplant 1990; 5: 110-117.

69. Wahren J, Johansson B-L, Wallberg-Henriksson H. Does C-peptide have a physiological role? Diabetologia 1994; 37: Suppl. 2: S99-S107.

70. Bouhanick B, Suraniti S, Berrut G, Bled F, Simard G, Lejeune JJ, Fressinaud P, Marre M. Relationship between fat intake and glomerular filtration rate in normotensive insulin-dependent diabetic patients. Diabete Metab (Paris) 1995; 21: 168-172.

71. Hostetter TH. Diabetic nephropathy. Metabolic versus hemodynamic considerations. Diabetes Care 1992; 15: 1205-1215.

72. Mogensen CE. Early glomerular hyperfiltration in insulin-dependent diabetics and late nephropathy. Scand J Clin Lab Invest 1986; 46: 201-206.

73. Rudberg S, Persson B, Dalqvist G. Increased glomerular filtration rate predicts diabetic nephropathy-results form an 8 year prospective study. Kidney Int 1992; 41: 822-828.

74. Chirelli F, Verrotti A, Morgese G. Glomerular hyperfiltration increases the risk of developing microalbuminuria in diabetic children. Pediatr Nephrol 1995; 9: 154-158.

75. Lervang H-H, Jensen S, Brøchner-Mortensen J, Ditzel J. Does increased glomerular filtration rate or disturbed tubular function early in the course of childhood type 1 diabetes predict the development of nephropathy? Diabetic Med 1992; 9: 635-640.

76. Yip WJ, Jones LS, Wiseman JM, Hill C, Viberti GC. Glomerular hyperfiltration in the prediction of nephropahty in IDDM. Diabetes vol. 45, dec. 1996; 1729-1733.

77. Anderson S. Renal effects of converting enzyme inhibitors in hypertension and diabetes. J Cardiovasc Pharmacol 1990; 15: Suppl. 3: S11-S15.

78. Mau Pedersen M, Christensen CK, Hansen KW, Christiansen JS, Mogensen CE. ACE-inhibition and renoprotection in early diabetic nephropathy. Response to enalapril acutely and in long-term combination with conventional antihypertensive treatment. Clin Invest Med 1991; 14: 642-651.

79. Bakris GL, Slataper R, Vicknair N, Sadler R. ACE inhibitor mediated reductions in renal size and microalbuminuria in normotensive, diabetic subjects. J Diabetic Compl 1994; 8: 2-6.

80.   Mau Pedersen M, Christensen SE, Christiansen JS, Pedersen EB, Mogensen CE, Ørskov H. Acute effects of a somatostatin analogue on kidney function in type i diabetic patients. Diabetic Med 1990; 7: 304-309.

81.   Serri O, Beauregard H, Brazeau P, Abribat T, Lamber J, Harris A, Vachon L. Somatostatin analogue, octreotide, reduces increased glomerular filtration rate and kidney size in insulin-dependent diabetes. JAMA 1991; 265; 888-892.

82.   Jacobs ML, Derkx FH, Stijnen T, Lamberts SW, Weber RF. Effect of long-acting somatostatin analog (Somatolin) on renal hyperfiltration in patients with IDDM. Diabetes Care 1997; 20 (4): 632-636.

83.   Mau Pedersen M, Schmitz A, Pedersen EB, Danielsen H, Christiansen JS. Acute and long-term renal effects of angiotensin converting enzyme inhibition in normotensive, normoalbuminuric insulin-dependent diabetic patients. Diabetic Med 1988; 5: 562-569.

84.   Pecis M, Azevedo JM, Gross LJ. Glomerular Hyperfiltration is associated with blood pressure abnormalities in normotensive normoalbuminuric IDDM patients. Diabetes Care, vol. 20, no. 8, 1997; 1329-1333.

85.   Ichikawa I, Harris RC. Angiotensin actions in the kidney: Renewed insight into the old hormone (Editorial Review). Kidney Int 1991; 40: 583-596.

86.   Soper CP, Barron JL, Hyer SL. Long-term glycaemic control directly correlates with glomerular filtration rate in early Type 1 diabetes mellitus before the onset of microalbuminuria. Diabet Med, 1998; 15: 1012-4.

87.   Jacobs EM, Vervoort G, Branten AJ, Klasen I, Smits P, Wetzels JF. Atrial natriuretic peptide increases albuminuria in type I diabetic patients: evidence for blockade of tubular protein reabsorption. Eur J Clin Invest, 1999; 2: 109-15.

88.   Bursell S-E, Clermont AC, Aiello LP, Aiello LM, Schlossman DK, Feener EP, Laffel L, King GL. High-dose vitamin E supplementation normalizes retinal blood flow and creatinine clearance in patients with type 1 diabetes. Diabetes Care, 1999; 22: 1245-1251.

89.   Fujisawa T, Ikegami H, Kawaguchi Y, Hamada Y, Ueda H, Shintani M, Fukuda M, Ogihara T. Meta-analysis of association of insertion/deletion polymorphism of angiotensin I-converting enzyme gene with diabetic nephropathy and retinopathy. Diabetologia, 1998; 41: 47-53.

90.   Miller JA, Scholey JW, Thaik K, Pei YP. Angiotensin converting enzyme gene polymorphism and renal hemodynamic function in early diabetes. Kidney Int, 1997; 51:119-24.

91.   Bouhanick B, Gallois Y, Hadjadj S, Boux de Casson F, Limal JM, Marre M. Relationship between glomerular hyperfiltration and ACE insertion/deletion polymorphism in type 1 diabetic children and adolescents. Diabetes Care, 1999; 22: 618-22.

92.   Marre M, Bouhanick B, Berrut G, Gallois Y, Le Jeune J-J, Chatellier G, Menard J, Alhenc-Gelas F. Renal changes on hyperglycemia and angiotensin-converting enzyme in type 1 diabetes. Hypertension, 1999; 33: 775-780.

93.   Cummings EA, Sochett EB, Dekker MG, Lawson ML, Daneman D. Contribution of growth hormone and IGF-I to early diabetic nephropathy in type 1 diabetes. Diabetes, 1998; 47: 1341-6.

94.   Wolf G, Ziyadeh FN. Molecular mechanisms of diabetic renal hypertrophy. Kidney Int, 1999; 56: 393-405.

95.   Sharma K, Jin Y, Guo J, Ziyadeh FN. Neutralization of TGF-beta by anti-TGF-beta antibody attenuates kidney hypertrophy and the enhanced extracellular matrix gene expression in STZ-induced diabetic mice.Diabetes, 1996; 45: 522-30.

96.   Bardoux P, Martin H, Ahloulay M, Schmitt F, Bouby N, Trinh-Trang-Tan MM, Bakir L. Vasopressin contributes to hyperfiltration, albuminuria and renal hypertrophy in diabetes mellitus: study in vasopressin-deficient Brattleboro rats. Proc Natl Acad Sci USA, 1999; 96:10397-402.

97.   Forst T, Kunt T, Pfutzner A, Beyer J, Wahren J. New aspects on biological activity of C-peptide in IDDM patients. Exp Clin Endocrinol Diabetes, 1998; 106: 270-6.

98.   Berg UB, Torbjornsdotter TB, Jaremko G, Thalme B. Kidney morphological changes in relation to long-term renal function and metabolic control in adolescents with IDDM. Diabetologia, 1998; 41: 1047-56.

99.   Baumgartl H-J, Sigl G, Banholzer P, Haslbeck M, Standl E. On the prognosis of IDDM patients with large kidneys. Nephrol Dial Transplant, 1998; 13: 630-634.

30.   DIABETES, HYPERTENSION, AND KIDNEY DISEASE IN THE PIMA INDIANS

William C. Knowler, Robert G. Nelson, David J Pettitt[2]
[1]*National Institute of Diabetes and Digestive and Kidney Diseases, Phoenix, Arizona, USA*
[2]*Sansum Medical Research Institute, Santa Barbara, California, USA*

Hypertension and kidney disease are well-known concomitants of both type 1 and type 2 diabetes mellitus. Hypertension, kidney disease, and diabetes are associated with each other, but the associations vary between populations, and the causal interpretations, especially regarding hypertension and diabetic nephropathy, are controversial. The complications of diabetes have been studied extensively among the Pima Indians of Arizona, U.S.A. In this chapter, we describe the epidemiology of diabetic renal disease and its relationship with hypertension in the Pima Indians.

THE PIMA INDIAN DIABETES STUDY
The Pima Indians have the world's highest reported incidence and prevalence of diabetes [1]. Since 1965, this population has participated in a longitudinal epidemiologic study of diabetes and its complications [2]. At each examination, conducted at about two-year intervals, an oral glucose tolerance test was performed and classified according to the World Health Organization criteria [3]. Throughout the study, urine samples with at least a trace of protein on dipstick were assayed for total protein, and the urine protein-to-creatinine ratio was used as an estimate of the protein excretion rate [4]. Since 1982, the urine samples were assayed for albumin, and a urine albumin-to-creatinine ratio was used as an estimate of the urinary albumin excretion rate [5]. Blood pressure was measured at each examination with the subject at rest in the supine position [6].

Renal function was studied in more detail in a subset of non-diabetic and diabetic Pima Indians. These studies include serial measurements of glomerular filtration rate (GFR), renal plasma flow, albumin and IgG excretion, and glomerular capillary permeability to dextran particles of different sizes [7].

The prevalence of diabetes in Pima Indians is almost 13 times as high as in the mostly white population of Rochester, Minnesota [1]. Diabetes occurs in over one-third

Mogensen C.E. (ed.), THE KIDNEY AND HYPERTENSION IN DIABETES MELLITUS.
Copyright© 2000 by Kluwer Academic Publishers, Boston ● Dordrecht ● London. All rights reserved.

of Pima Indians aged 35-44 years and in over 60% of those ≥45 years old [2]. Many cases develop before the age of 25 years. Pima Indians develop only type 2 diabetes [8, 9], and they differ from other populations in that the disease develops at younger ages [1, 2]. Diabetic complications also develop at rates similar to those of other populations. In contrast to populations in which type 2 diabetes usually develops later in life, many Pima Indians have diabetes of sufficient duration for nephropathy to develop.

THE COURSE OF DIABETIC NEPHROPATHY IN PIMA INDIANS

The onset of type 2 diabetes in Pima Indians is characterized, on average, by an elevated GFR and a modest size-selective abnormality of the glomerular capillary wall [10]. Abnormally elevated albuminuria is another characteristic early sign of diabetic nephropathy. In a cross-sectional study of albuminuria in Pima Indians ≥15 years of age, abnormal albuminuria was defined by a urine albumin-to-creatinine ratio ≥ 30 mg/g [5]. Abnormal albuminuria is subdivided by ratios ≥ 30 mg/g and < 300 mg/g, called microalbuminuria, and ratios ≥ 300 mg/g, called macroalbuminuria. Abnormal albuminuria was found in 8% of those with normal glucose tolerance, 15% of those with impaired glucose tolerance, and 47% of those with diabetes [5]. The prevalence was also related to the duration of diabetes, varying from 29% within five years of diagnosis to 86% after 20 years of diabetes. The high prevalence in diabetes and the relationship with diabetes duration indicate that albuminuria is a complication of diabetes, but there is also a substantial prevalence in those with normal or impaired glucose tolerance, indicating that diabetes is not the sole cause of abnormal albuminuria in this population. Abnormal albuminuria is often followed by more serious renal disease. Among diabetic Pimas, the degree of albuminuria over the range of values <300 mg/g predicts the subsequent incidence of overt nephropathy, defined by a protein-to-creatinine ratio ≥1.0 g/g [11].

Among diabetic Pima Indians, the incidence rate of elevated albuminuria (≥30 mg/g) is similar to that previously reported in type 1 diabetes [12]. The incidence of overt diabetic nephropathy, defined by urine protein/creatinine ≥1.0 g/g, is shown in figure 30-1. Incidence rates increased with duration of diabetes, at least until 25 years. Beyond 25 years of diabetes, the incidence rate appears to have stabilized, although the trend with time is uncertain because the standard errors of the rates are high at long durations due to limited observations. Thus it remains uncertain whether beyond a certain duration of diabetes, Pima Indians pass a period of susceptibility to development of nephropathy, as reported after 15-20 years of type 1 diabetes [13, 14].

GFR was measured in Pimas with diabetes of 5 years duration with normal albuminuria (n=20) or with macroalbuminuria (n=34) [15]. At baseline, those with macroalbuminuria had, on average, lower GFR and higher blood pressure. During 48 months of follow-up of 30 of those with macroalbuminuria, the GFR declined by an average of 9 ml/min per year, higher than the rate of decline reported for similar patients with type 1 diabetes. The slope of GFR over time was highly correlated with the increase in urinary albumin or IgG clearance. Dextran sieving studies suggested that the progressive decline in GFR is caused by a decline in average density of glomerular pores, which is accompanied by a widening of the pore size distribution and increased transglomerular passage of plasma proteins.

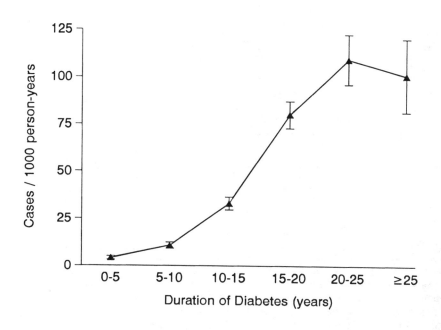

Figure 30-1. Incidence rates of overt nephropathy (urine protein-to-creatinine ratio ≥1.0 g/g) by duration of diabetes in Pima Indians. The rates ±standard errors are shown. Adapted from Kunzelman et al [4].

Figure 30-2 summarizes the degree of albuminuria, expressed as an albumin-to-creatinine ratio, in five groups of subjects followed for up to four years [7]. On average, those with impaired glucose tolerance, newly diagnosed diabetes, or longstanding diabetes with normoalbuminuria (by definition) had normal urine albumin excretion at baseline. There was little change, on average, during follow-up of those in the first two groups. The degree of albuminuria tended to increase, however, in all three groups with long-standing diabetes, whether they had normo-, micro-, or macro-albuminuria at baseline. During this time, GFR increased in persons with impaired glucose tolerance or newly diagnosed diabetes, was relatively stable in those with longstanding diabetes with normo- or micro-albuminuria, and declined in those with macro-albuminuria at baseline (figure 30-2). The major predictor of declining GFR was the degree of albuminuria. By contrast, baseline GFR did not predict change in GFR or in albuminuria. Thus the degree of elevation in albumin excretion is the major predictor of worsening diabetic nephropathy.

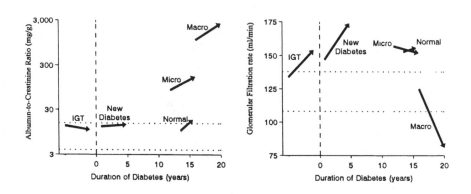

Figure 30-2. Changes in median urinary albumin-to-creatinine ratio (left) and mean glomerular filtration rate (right) from baseline to the end of follow-up in persons with impaired glucose tolerance (IGT), newly diagnosed diabetes, and longstanding diabetes according to baseline albuminuria. Each arrow connects the value at the baseline examination and the value at the end of follow-up. The vertical dashed line indicates the time of diagnosis of diabetes, and the horizontal dotted lines the 25th and 75th percentiles of values in subjects with normal glucose tolerance. Adapted from Nelson et al. [7].

In diabetic persons, the onset of clinical proteinuria, defined by the urinary excretion of at least 500 mg protein per day, heralds a progressive decline of renal function that often leads to end-stage renal disease (ESRD) [16]. Figure 30-3 shows the cumulative incidence of ESRD as a function of the duration of proteinuria in Pima Indians and, using similar definitions of proteinuria, in whites with type 1 [14] or type 2 diabetes [17]. Coronary heart disease is a frequent cause of death in older persons with diabetes, and proteinuria may, in part, account for the lower incidence of ESRD in whites with type 2 diabetes. Due to the relatively young age at onset of diabetes in Pima Indians and their lower death rate from coronary heart disease [18], the cumulative incidence of ESRD in this population more closely resembles that of whites with type 1 diabetes than those with type 2 diabetes.

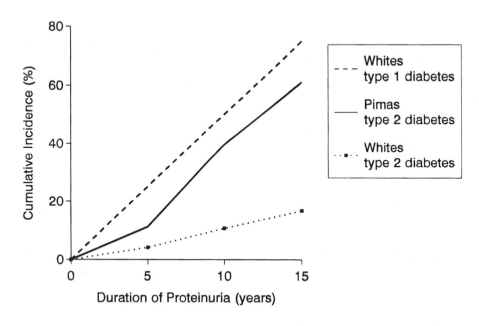

Figure 30-3. Cumulative incidence of end stage renal disease by duration of proteinuria. Adapted from Nelson et al. [16], Krolewski et al. [14], and Humphrey et al. [17].

When expressed as a function of duration of diabetes, the cumulative incidence of ESRD is also nearly identical in the Pimas with type 2 diabetes and the whites with type 1 diabetes [19]. Other studies comparing persons with type 1 diabetes and type 2 diabetes in the same populations have concluded that the duration-specific risk of ESRD is similar in the two types of diabetes [17, 20].

The incidence of ESRD is also very high among other American Indians [reviewed in 21], but diabetes is apparently not responsible for as great a proportion of cases of ESRD in some of the other American Indian tribes. The degree of albuminuria was higher in Pima Indians than in several other American Indian tribes, even when controlled for differences in age, sex, fasting plasma glucose, blood pressure, and fibrinogen [22].

The greater degree of albuminuria in Pima Indians compared with the other American Indian tribes [22], the increased risk of diabetic nephropathy in Pima Indians whose parents have hypertension [23], and the familial aggregation of diabetic nephropathy in this [24] and other populations suggest that susceptibility to diabetic nephropathy may be genetically transmitted, as reviewed in chapters 9 and 10. Further evidence for genetic susceptibility to diabetic nephropathy comes from a genetic linkage study in which 98 diabetic sibling pairs affected with nephropathy were included in a genome-wide scan. A DNA marker on chromosome 7 was tentatively linked to nephropathy (single marker LOD = 2.73, multipoint LOD = 2.04), suggesting that a genetic element in the region of this marker influences susceptibility to diabetic nephropathy [25]. Other factors, including duration of diabetes, blood pressure, level of glycemia, and pharmacologic treatment of diabetes are associated with the development of renal disease in Pima Indians [4, 16, 19]. Risk of diabetic nephropathy is also higher in offspring exposed to diabetes in utero [26] or who were in the lowest or highest extremes of the birth weight distribution [27]; these exposures are also risk factors for diabetes itself [28]. There was no evidence that hantavirus infection, which has been implicated in renal disease in other populations, is involved in diabetic nephropathy in the Pimas [29].

Nearly all of the excess mortality associated with diabetes in this population occurs in persons with clinically detectable proteinuria, and the age-sex-adjusted death rate in diabetic subjects without proteinuria is no greater than the rate in non-diabetic subjects [30]. Thus, proteinuria is a marker not only for diabetic renal disease, but identifies those with diabetes who are at increased risk for a number of macro- and microvascular complications and for death. Similar findings reported in persons with type 1 diabetes suggest a common underlying cause for albuminuria and the other associated diabetic complications, both renal and extrarenal [31].

Autopsy studies indicate that intercapillary glomerular sclerosis, typical of diabetic nephropathy in other ethnic groups, is the predominant renal disease in the Pimas [32], although other glomerular lesions were found in some non-diabetic Pimas [33]. In kidney biopsies from 51 diabetic Pima Indians, total glomerular volume and mesangial volume were positively correlated with stage of diabetic nephropathy. Moreover, clinical nephropathy was associated with thickening of the glomerular basement membrane and a lower number of podocytes per glomerulus [34]. In a 4-year follow-up of the 16 diabetic persons with microalbuminuria, lower podocyte number per glomerulus predicted increasing urinary albumin excretion, suggesting that podocyte injury may play an important role in the development and progression of diabetic nephropathy [35].

RELATIONSHIP OF BLOOD PRESSURE TO DIABETES AND KIDNEY DISEASE

The relationships of blood pressure to glucose tolerance, hyperinsulinemia, and insulin resistance have been examined in many populations. A difficulty in examining these relationships is that many drugs used in treating high blood pressure may also affect insulin resistance or glycemia. Thus, correlations of these variables are difficult to interpret if studies include subjects taking antihypertensive drugs; yet if such subjects are excluded, the associations might be underestimated because of exclusion of those with the most severe hypertension. One approach is to divide blood pressure into two categories, hypertension or not, and include those treated with antihypertensive drugs as hypertensive regardless of their measured blood pressure. Even this approach may not be satisfactory, however, as many diabetic patients are treated with antihypertensive drugs for cardio- or renoprotection rather than because of hypertension, a practice likely to increase in the future in view of evidence of benefit [36, 37].

Blood pressure (or hypertension) is related to glucose tolerance in Pima Indians. The age-sex-adjusted prevalence rates of hypertension (systolic blood pressure ≥ 160 mm Hg, diastolic blood pressure ≥ 95 mm Hg, or receiving antihypertensive drugs) among those with normal glucose tolerance, impaired glucose tolerance, or diabetes were 7%, 13%, and 20%, respectively, an almost three-fold difference [6]. Similarly, as continuous variables, blood pressure and two-hour plasma glucose concentrations were correlated among subjects who were not treated with either antihypertensive or hypoglycemic drugs. This relationship, also observed in other populations, may be explained by hyperinsulinemia, as serum insulin concentrations tend to be higher in persons with impaired glucose tolerance and in some persons with diabetes than in those with normal glucose tolerance. Yet in the Pimas blood pressure has a much stronger correlation with plasma glucose than with serum insulin concentrations, and the partial correlation of blood pressure with fasting insulin, controlled for age, sex, BMI, and glucose, is practically zero [6]. Thus the relationship, at least among the Pimas, is primarily with glucose, and the correlation with insulin may be secondary.

In addition to studies of blood pressure and serum insulin concentrations, the correlation of blood pressure with insulin resistance was assessed by the euglycemic clamp. In a study of three racial groups, among non-diabetic, normotensive subjects not taking any medicines, blood pressure and insulin resistance were correlated only among whites, but not among blacks or Pima Indians [38]. While this study confirmed previous reports of a correlation of blood pressure with insulin resistance in whites, it suggests that such a relationship is race-specific, and hence does not indicate that insulin resistance is an important or consistent cause of hypertension.

Although blood pressure and plasma glucose concentrations are correlated and the prevalence of hypertension is related to 2-hr glucose, even among non-diabetic subjects, hyperglycemia is not the only factor of importance for blood pressure in diabetes. Among adult Pima Indians, urinary albumin-to-creatinine ratios were higher with progressively worse glucose tolerance or longer duration of diabetes, and among diabetic patients were higher in those treated with insulin [39]. Regardless of the degree of hyperglycemia and duration of diabetes, those with hypertension had greater albuminuria. The associations of each of these variables with albuminuria were highly significant, but the causal directions underlying them have not been determined. The relationship of insulin treatment with albuminuria is similar to that of insulin treatment with many complications of diabetes [4 , 5, 18, 40-42] and might reflect more severe diabetes (i.e. those with greater hyperglycemia or more complications have a greater need for insulin treatment).

Blood pressure and kidney disease are clearly related, although the causes of this relationship are not clear and are debated extensively, with some arguing that the elevated blood pressure in diabetes is only secondary to diabetic nephropathy [31, 43], and others that elevated blood pressure is due to a genetic predisposition that contributes to the development of diabetic nephropathy [44, 45]. In the Pima Indians, higher blood pressure *before* the onset of diabetes confers a greater risk of renal disease *after* diabetes develops (figure 30-4), and among the diabetic subjects with normo- or micro-albuminuria, higher blood pressure predicts increasing urinary albumin excretion rates [7]. On the other hand, higher blood pressure does not predict ESRD in diabetic Pima Indians who already have proteinuria [16]. This suggests that blood pressure may contribute to the initiation of diabetic nephropathy [46], but less to its progression once proteinuria has developed [16]. The higher pre-diabetic blood pressure in those destined to have elevated albuminuria after the onset of diabetes may be an early manifestation of an underlying susceptibility to renal disease which develops only in the presence of diabetes. This susceptibility factor for nephropathy may also be a risk factor for diabetes [47].

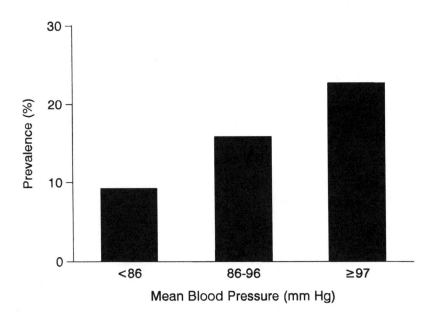

Figure 30-4. Prevalence of elevated albuminuria (urine albumin-to-creatinine ratio ≥100 mg/g) after the diagnosis of diabetes by prediabetic blood pressure. Adapted from Nelson et al. [46].

CONCLUSIONS

Hypertension and kidney disease are common complications of diabetes in the Pima Indians, as they are in other populations, and persons with these conditions have a particularly bad prognosis. Almost all of the excess mortality in diabetic Pimas is associated with nephropathy. The higher prevalence of abnormal albumin excretion in diabetic subjects who had higher blood pressures before the onset of diabetes suggests that the hypertension of diabetes is not entirely secondary to diabetic nephropathy, but that higher blood pressure contributes to this complication.

REFERENCES

1. Knowler WC, Bennett PH, Hamman RF, Miller M: Diabetes incidence and prevalence in Pima Indians: a 19-fold greater incidence than in Rochester, Minnesota. Am J Epidemiol 108:497-505, 1978.
2. Knowler WC, Pettitt DJ, Saad MF, Bennett PH: Diabetes mellitus in the Pima Indians: incidence, risk factors, and pathogenesis. Diabetes/Metabolism Reviews 6:1-27, 1990.
3. Diabetes mellitus: report of a WHO study group. WHO Technical Report Series 727. Geneva, World Health Organization, 1985.
4. Kunzelman CL, Knowler WC, Pettitt DJ, Bennett PH: Incidence of nephropathy in type 2 diabetes mellitus in the Pima Indians. Kidney Int 35:681-687, 1989.
5. Nelson RG, Kunzelman CL, Pettitt DJ, Saad MF, Bennett PH, Knowler WC: Albuminuria in Type 2 (non-insulin-dependent) diabetes mellitus and impaired glucose tolerance in Pima Indians. Diabetologia 32:870-876, 1989.
6. Saad MF, Knowler WC, Pettitt DJ, Nelson RG, Mott DM, Bennett PH: Insulin and hypertension: relationship to obesity and glucose intolerance in Pima Indians. Diabetes 39:1430-1435, 1990.
7. Nelson RG, Bennett PH, Beck GJ, Tan M, Knowler WC, Mitch WE, Hirschman GH, Myers BD, for the Diabetic Renal Disease Study: Development and progression of renal disease in Pima Indians with non-insulin-dependent diabetes mellitus. N Engl J Med 335: 1636-1642, 1996.
8. Knowler WC, Bennett PH, Bottazzo GF, Doniach D: Islet cell antibodies and diabetes mellitus in Pima Indians. Diabetologia 17:161-164, 1979.
9. Dabelea D, Palmer JP, Bennett PH, Pettitt DJ, Knowler WC: Absence of glutamic acid decarboxylase antibodies in Pima Indian children with diabetes mellitus (letter). Diabetologia 42: 1265-1266, 1999.
10. Myers BD, Nelson RG, Williams GW, Bennett PH, Hardy SA, Berg RL, Loon N, Knowler WC, Mitch WE: Glomerular function in Pima Indians with non-insulin-dependent diabetes mellitus of recent onset. J Clin Invest 88:524-530, 1991.
11. Nelson RG, Knowler WC, Pettitt DJ, Saad MF, Charles MA, Bennett PH: Assessment of risk of overt nephropathy in diabetic patients from albumin excretion in untimed urine specimens. Arch Int Med 151:1761-1765, 1991.
12. Nelson RG, Knowler WC, Pettitt DJ, Hanson RL, Bennett PH: Incidence and determinants of elevated urinary albumin excretion in Pima Indians with NIDDM. Diabetes Care 18:182-187, 1995.
13. Andersen AR, Christiansen JS, Andersen JK, Kreiner S, Deckert T: Diabetic nephropathy in Type 1 (insulin-dependent) diabetes: an epidemiological study. Diabetologia 25:496-501, 1983.
14. Krolewski AS, Warram JH, Cristlieb AR, Busick EJ, Kahn C: The changing natural history of nephropathy in Type 1 diabetes. Am J Med 78:785-793, 1985.

15.   Myers BD, Nelson RG, Tan M, Beck GJ, Bennett PH, Knowler WC, Blouch K, Mitch WE: Progression of overt nephropathy in non-insulin-dependent diabetes. Kidney Int 47:1781-1789, 1995.

16.   Nelson RG, Knowler WC, McCance DR, Sievers ML, Pettitt DJ, Charles MA, Hanson RL, Liu QZ, Bennett PH: Determinants of end-stage renal disease in Pima Indians with type 2 (non-insulin-dependent) diabetes mellitus and proteinuria. Diabetologia 36:1087-1093, 1993.

17.   Humphrey LL, Ballard DJ, Frohnert PP, Chu C-P, O'Fallon WM, Palumbo PJ: Chronic renal failure in non-insulin-dependent diabetes mellitus: a population-based study in Rochester, Minnesota. Ann Intern Med 111:788-796, 1989.

18.   Nelson RG, Sievers ML, Knowler WC, Swinburn BA, Pettitt DJ, Saad MF, Garrison R, Liebow IM, Howard BV, Bennett PH: Low incidence of fatal coronary heart disease in Pima Indians despite high prevalence of non-insulin-dependent diabetes. Circulation 81:987-995, 1990.

19.   Nelson RG, Newman JM, Knowler WC, Sievers ML, Kunzelman CL, Pettitt DJ, Moffett CD, Teutsch SM, Bennett PH: Incidence of end-stage renal disease in Type 2 (non-insulin-dependent) diabetes mellitus in Pima Indians. Diabetologia 31:730-736, 1988.

20.   Hasslacher C, Ritz E, Wahl P, Michael C: Similar risks of nephropathy in patients with type I and type II diabetes mellitus. Nephrol Dial Transplant 4:859-863, 1989.

21.   Nelson RG, Knowler WC, Pettitt DJ, Saad MF, Bennett PH: Diabetic kidney disease in Pima Indians. Diabetes Care 16:335-341, 1993.

22.   Robbins DC, Knowler WC, Lee ET, Yeh J, Go OT, Welty T, Fabsitz R, Howard BV: Regional differences in albuminuria among American Indians: an epidemic of renal disease. Kidney Int 49:557-563, 1996.

23.   Nelson RG, Pettitt DJ, de Courten MP, Hanson RL, Knowler WC, Bennett PH: Parental hypertension and proteinuria in Pima Indians with NIDDM. Diabetologia 39:433-438, 1996.

24.   Pettitt DJ, Saad MF, Bennett PH, Nelson RG, Knowler WC: Familial predisposition to renal disease in two generations of Pima Indians with Type 2 (non-insulin-dependent) diabetes mellitus. Diabetologia 33:438-443, 1990.

25.   Imperatore G, Hanson RL, Pettitt DJ, Kobes S, Bennett PH, Knowler WC, and the Pima Diabetes Genes Group: Sib-pair linkage analysis for susceptibility genes for microvascular complications among Pima Indians with type 2 diabetes mellitus. Diabetes 47: 821-830, 1998.

26.   Nelson RG, Morgenstern H, Bennett PH: Intrauterine diabetes exposure and the risk of renal disease in diabetic Pima Indians. Diabetes 47: 1489-1493, 1998.

27.   Nelson RG, Morgenstern H, Bennett PH: Birth weight and renal disease in Pima Indians with type 2 diabetes mellitus. Am J Epidemiol 148: 650-656, 1998.

28.   Dabelea D, Hanson RL, Bennett PH, Roumain J, Knowler WC, Pettitt DJ: Increasing prevalence of type II diabetes in American Indian children. Diabetologia 41: 904-910, 1998.

29.   de Courten MP, Ksiazek TG, Rollin PE, Kahn AS, Daily PJ, Knowler WC: Sero-prevalence study of hantavirus antibodies in Pima Indians with renal disease. J Infectious Dis 171:762-763, 1995.

30.   Nelson RG, Pettitt DJ, Carraher MJ, Baird HR, Knowler WC: Effect of proteinuria on mortality in NIDDM. Diabetes 37:1499-1504, 1988.

31.   Deckert T, Feldt-Rasmussen B, Borch-Johnsen K, Jensen T, Kofoed-Enevoldsen A: Albuminuria reflects widespread vascular damage. The Steno hypothesis. Diabetologia 32:219-226, 1989.

32. Kamenetzky SA, Bennett PH, Dippe SE, Miller M, LeCompte PM: A clinical and histologic study of diabetic nephropathy in the Pima Indians. Diabetes 23:61-68, 1974.

33. Schmidt K, Pesce C, Liu Q, Nelson RG, Bennett PH, Karnitschnig H, Striker LJ, Striker GE: Large glomerular size in Pima Indians: lack of change with diabetic nephropathy. J Am Soc Nephrol 3:229-235, 1992.

34. Pagtalunan ME, Miller PL, Jumping-Eagle S, Nelson RG, Myers BD, Rennke HG, Coplon NS, Sun L, Meyer TW: Podocyte loss and progressive glomerular injury in type II diabetes. J Clin Invest 99: 342-348, 1997.

35. Meyer TW, Bennett PH, Nelson RG: Podocyte number predicts long-trem urinary albumin excretion in Pima Indians with type II diabetes and microalbuminuria. Diabetologia 42: 1341-1344, 1999.

36. UK Prospective Diabetes Study (UKPDS) Group: Efficacy of atenolol and captopril in reducing risk of macrovascular and microvascular compliations in type 2 diabetes: UKPDS 39. Br Med J 317: 713-720, 1998.

37. Heart Outcomes Prevention Evaluation (HOPE) Study Investigators: Effects of remipril on cariovascular and microvascular outcomes in people with diabetes mellitus: results of the HOPE study and MICRO-HOPE substudy. Lancet 355: 253-259, 2000.

38. Saad MF, Lillioja S, Nyomba BL, Castillo C, Ferraro R, DeGregoria M, Ravussin E, Knowler WC, Bennett PH, Howard BV, Bogardus C: Racial differences in the relation between blood pressure and insulin resistance. N Engl J Med 324:733-739, 1991.

39. Knowler WC, Nelson RG, Pettitt DJ: Diabetes, hypertension, and kidney disease in the Pima Indians compared with other populations. In Mogensen CE, ed: The Kidney and Hypertension in Diabetes Mellitus, 2nd ed., Kluwer Academic Publishers, Boston, 1994, pp. 53-62.

40. Knowler WC, Bennett PH, Ballintine EJ: Increased incidence of retinopathy in diabetics with elevated blood pressure: a six-year followup study in Pima Indians. N Eng J Med 302:645-650, 1980.

41. Liu QZ, Knowler WC, Nelson RG, Saad MF, Charles MA, Liebow IM, Bennett PH, Pettitt DJ: Insulin treatment, endogenous insulin concentration, and ECG abnormalities in diabetic Pima Indians: cross-sectional and prospective analyses. Diabetes 41:1141-1150, 1992.

42. Nagi DK, Pettitt DJ, Bennett PH, Klein R, Knowler WC: Diabetic retinopathy assessed by fundus photography in Pima Indians with impaired glucose tolerance and non-insulin-dependent diabetes mellitus. Diabetic Med 14: 449-456, 1997.

43. Mathiesen ER, Rønn B, Jensen T, Storm B, Deckert T: Relationship between blood pressure and urinary albumin excretion in development of microalbuminuria. Diabetes 39:245-249, 1990.

44. Viberti CG, Keen H, Wiseman MJ: Raised arterial pressure in parents of proteinuric insulin-dependent diabetics. Br Med J 295:551-517, 1987.

45. Krolewski AS, Canessa M, Warram JH, Laffel LMB, Christlieb AR, Knowler WC, Rand LI: Predisposition to hypertension and susceptibility to renal disease in insulin-dependent diabetes mellitus. N Engl J Med 318:140-145, 1988.

46. Nelson RG, Pettitt DJ, Baird HR, Charles MA, Liu QZ, Bennett PH, Knowler WC: Prediabetic blood pressure predicts urinary albumin excretion after the onset of type 2 (non-insulin-dependent) diabetes mellitus in Pima Indians. Diabetologia 36:998-1001, 1993.

47. McCance DR, Hanson RL, Pettitt DJ, Jacobsson LTH, Bennett PH, Bishop DT, Knowler WC: Diabetic nephropathy: a risk factor for diabetes in offspring. Diabetologia 38:221-226, 1995.

31. AUTOREGULATION OF GLOMERULAR FILTRATION RATE IN PATIENTS WITH DIABETES

Per K. Christensen and Hans-Henrik Parving
Steno Diabetes Center, 2820 Gentofte, Denmark.

INTRODUCTION

The close relationship between elevated blood pressure and diabetic nephropathy are documented both in Type 1 and Type 2 diabetic patients. Approximately 75-85% of diabetic patients with nephropathy are hypertensive [1-3].

Arterial blood pressure and albuminuria are strong predictors for a faster decline in glomerular filtration rate (GFR). Conversely, antihypertensive treatment reduces the rate of decline in GFR and postponed ESRD in patients with diabetic nephropathy [4-11].

Antihypertensive treatment induces a faster initial and slower subsequent decline in GFR, in hypertensive Type 1 and Type 2 diabetic patients with incipient or overt diabetic nephropathy [7,12,13]. This biphasic phenomenon may be due to a functional (haemodynamic) effect of antihypertensive treatment and/or impaired autoregulation of GFR in patients with diabetic nephropathy [14,15].

AUTOREGULATION OF THE NORMAL KIDNEY

The ability of the kidney to maintain constancy of GFR over a wide range of renal perfusion pressures is termed autoregulation fig 31-1. Experimental studies suggests that autoregulation of GFR is due to autoregulation of two of the main GFR determinants, i.e. renal plasma flow and glomerular capillary pressure [16,17].

Mechanisms

In the normal kidney, autoregulatory mechanisms are efficiently controlling and stabilising GFR by changes in the renal vascular resistance.

The three major mechanisms involved in renal autoregulation are: myogenic factors intrinsic to the pre- and postglomerular arterioles, the tubuloglomerular feedback (TGF)

Mogensen C.E. (ed.), THE KIDNEY AND HYPERTENSION IN DIABETES MELLITUS.
Copyright© 2000 by Kluwer Academic Publishers, Boston ● Dordrecht ● London. All rights reserved.

mechanism, and various vasoactive hormones produced in and out side the kidney acting on the smooth muscle cells in the arterioles.

The myogenic response
The myogenic mechanism is probably the most important component of renal autoregulation and refers to the active contraction of vascular smooth muscle elicited by an increased in intravascular pressure. An increase in wall tension, e.g. caused by increased arterial blood pressure, leads to an activation of the vascular smooth muscle cells and a decrease in vascular diameter and wall tension. The myogenic response probably represents one of the principle means by which many organs and tissue autoregulate blood flow.

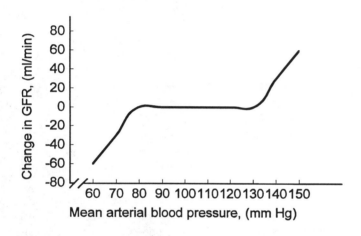

Fig. 31-1 Change in glomerular filtration rate (GFR) induced by change in mean arterial blood pressure in the normal kidney

Tubuloglomerular feedback
The structural basis for the TGF is located in the juxtaglomerular apparatus, where the contact between the thick ascending limb of Henle and the vascular pole of the glomerulus are located.

It is thought that macula dense is a sensor, which is able to send a signal to the afferent and efferent arteriole, which leads to a change in the wall tension in the arterioles, when the flow and/or pressure and/or NaCl concentration and/or osmolality in the thick ascending limb of Henle change [17].

Intra- extrarenale vasoactive hormones

Even though studies indicate that vasodilating and vasoconstricting intrarenal hormones such as prostaglandin's and hormones in the renin-angiotensin system contribute to auto-regulation of GFR [18-22], information is as yet inconclusive [21,23,24].

Extrarenal hormones e.g. ephedrine and norephedrine may be involved in autoregulation of GFR, but studies have shown that autoregulation capacity is normal in denervated and isolated kidneys [24]. Consequently the impact of the above mention sympathetic hormones on autoregulation is of minor importance.

Regardless of the precise mechanisms, the arteriole ability to change the diameter is the key to autoregulation of GFR when perfusion pressure change. Autoregulation of flow requires that resistance increase or decrease parallel to changes in perfusion pressure. If efferent arteriolar resistance declined significantly when perfusion pressure is reduced, glomerular capillary pressure and GFR would also fall. Consequently, it is the afferent arteriole which plays a pivotal role in regulating glomerular capillary pressure, renal plasma flow and consequently GFR [17,25-29].

STRUCTURAL CHANGES THAT MAY IMPAIR AUTOREGULATION OF GFR

The most characteristic glomerular lesion in patients with incipient or overt nephropathy is mesangial expansion. Biopsies from patients with hypertension and/or diabetic nephropathy have furthermore revealed arteriolar hyalinosis [18,19]. Arteriolar hyalinosis may impair the afferent arteriole capacity to constrict, and can thereby lead to enhanced transmission of the systemic pressure into the glomerular capillary network, and lead to glomerular hypertension [30-32]. This haemodynamic alteration is associated with increase wall tension causing distension of the elastic glomerulus. Studies have shown that mechanical stretch of vascular smooth muscle cells, vascular endothelial cells and mesangial cells leads to an overproduction of extracellular matrix [33,34]. Mesangial expansion is closely associated with renal function in diabetic nephropathy [35]. This relationship probably results from the expanding mesangium compromising the structure of contiguous glomerular capillaries and from a reduction in filtration surface, which may per se lead to increased intraglomerular pressure, and creating a vicious circle.

However, impaired autoregulation have been demonstrated in remnant kidney models in rats and in humans with non-diabetic nephropathies in the absence of arteriolar hyalinosis [22,36-38]. Consequently, autoregulation can be impaired before structural changes are detectable and thereby contribute to the progression of nephropathy, by creating glomrular hypertension [39].

AUTOREGULATION IN STREPTOZOTOCIN DIABETIC RATS

Several studies in streptozotocin diabetic rats have demonstrated impaired autoregulation of renal plasma flow early in the cause of experimental diabetes [29,40,41], and thus before structural lesion in the arterioles are detectable.

Improved glycaemic control normalise the autoregulation response to changes in renal perfusion pressure [40].

No human data has yet evaluated the functional impact of varying glycaemic control on this important servo-mechanism.

IMPAIRED AUTOREGULATION OF GFR IN PATIENTS WITH DIABETIC NEPHROPATHY

Originally, we evaluated the autoregulation of GFR in Type 1 diabetic patients with and without diabetic nephropathy [42]. Clonidine was used as the blood pressure lowering drug, because clonidine has no direct pharmacological effects on the renal vessels [43-45] and no peripheral sympathetic inhibition. Furthermore, intravenous injection of clonidine to normo- and hypertensive non-diabetic subjects induces no significant change in renal plasma flow and GFR [42,43,45]. Our study demonstrated impaired autoregulation of GFR in long-term Type 1 diabetic patients with diabetic nephropathy, while the reduction in arterial blood pressure had no impact on GFR in short-term normoalbuminuric Type 1 diabetic patients and in the non-diabetic control group. The reduction in arterial blood pressure induced a reduction in albuminuria in the Type 1 diabetic patients with nephropathy, suggesting diminished glomerular capillary hydraulic pressure.

Later we examined the effect of acute lowering of arterial blood pressure upon GFR in 26 hypertensive Type 2 diabetic patients with nephropathy (n=14) and without (n=12) nephropathy [46]. The individual response to acute lowering of arterial blood pressure in the two groups is shown in fig 31-2. This study extended the findings from Type 1 diabetic patients to Type 2 diabetic patients.

Furthermore we have investigated the autoregulation of GFR in non-diabetic patients with nephropathy using the same methods as mention in the above studies [38]. That study also suggested that albuminuric non-diabetic patients with different nephropathies suffer from impaired autoregulation of GFR. The main results from the above mention 3 studies [38] are shown in fig. 31-3.

CONSEQUENCES OF DEFECTIVE AUTOREGULATION

The impaired myogenic response to pressure changes in patients with nephropathy can lead to enhanced down stream transmission of the systemic pressure into the glomerular capillary network, and glomerular hypertension [30-32]. This haemodynamic alteration is associated with increase in proteinuria and acceleration of glomerulosclerosis [16].

Studies in the 5/6 renal ablation models have revealed that glomerular transmission of hypertension plays a predominant role in the pathogenesis of progressive glomerular injury and proteinuria [47]. Furthermore these animal studies stress the critical importance of autoregulatory mechanism in such transmission and suggest that antihypertensive agents, such as short acting nifedipine may adversely effect autoregulatory ability and thereby enhance pressure transmission.

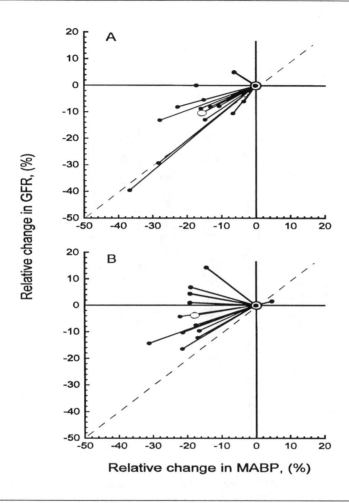

Fig. 31-2 Relative change in glomerular filtration rate (GFR) (percentage change of control GFR) and relative change in MABP (percentage change of control MABP) induced by intravenous injection of clonidine. (A). Fourteen Type 2 diabetic patients with nephropathy (●) *Mean response* (○). (B) Twelve Type 2 diabetic patients with normoalbuminuria (●), *Mean response* (○).
[From Christensen PK, Hansen HP, Parving H-H: Impaired autoregulation of GFR in hypertensive non-insulin dependent diabetic patients. Kidney Int, 1997; 52: 1369-1374. Reprinted with permission].

Unfortunately, we completely lack information on the impact of vasoactive drugs including blood pressure lowering agents on renal autoregulation or for that matter autoregulation in various tissues and organs in diabetic patients.

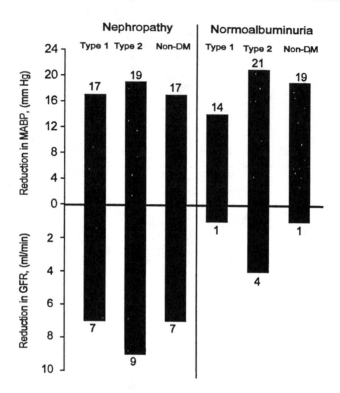

Fig 31-3. Reduction in mean arterial blood pressure (MABP) and glomerular filtration rate (GFR) induced by intravenous injection of clonidine in Type 1 and Type 2 diabetic patients with or without nephropathy, and in non-diabetic (Non-DM) subjects with or without nephropathy.
[From Christensen PK, Hommel E, Clausen P, Feldt-Rasmussen B, Parving H-H: Impaired autoregulation of the glomerular filtration rate in patients with non-diabetic nephropathies. Kidney Int, 1999; 56: 1517-1523. Reprinted by permission].

It has been shown that initiation of antihypertensive treatment induces a faster initial and a slower sustained decline in GFR in diabetic and non-diabetic patients with nephropathy [12,48,49]. Impaired autoregulation of GFR may in part explain the initial decline in GFR and the long-term beneficial effect of aggressive antihypertensive treatment on albuminuria and progression of diabetic and non-diabetic nephropathies.

The clinical significance of impaired autoregulation of GFR in hypertensive diabetic patients with nephropathy is lack or diminished protection against hyper- or hypoperfusion induced by alteration in blood pressure. In other words, there is increased vulnerability to hypertension or ischemic injuries of glomerular capillaries in diabetic patients with nephropathy.

REFERENCES

1.   Mogensen CE, Christensen CK: Predicting diabetic nephropathy in insulin-dependent patients. N Engl J Med 311:89-93, 1984
2.   Andersen AR, Christiansen JS, Andersen JK, Kreiner S, Deckert T: Diabetic nephropathy in Type 1 (insulin-dependent) diabetes: an epidemiological study. Diabetologia 25:496-501, 1983
3.   Tarnow L, Rossing P, Gall M-A, Nielsen FS, Parving H-H: Prevalence of arterial hypertension in diabetic patients before and after the JNC-V. Diabetes Care 17 (11):1247-1251, 1994
4.   Rossing P, Hommel E, Smidt UM, Parving H-H: Impact of arterial blood pressure and albuminuria on the progression of diabetic nephropathy in IDDM patients. Diabetes 42:715-719, 1993
5.   Parving H-H, Smidt UM, Hommel E, Mathiesen ER, Rossing P, Nielsen FS, Gall M-A: Effective Antihypertensive Treatment Postpones Renal Insufficiency in Diabetic Nephropathy. Am J Kidney Dis 22:188-195, 1993
6.   Parving H-H, Rossing P, Hommel E, Smidt UM: Angiotensin converting enzyme inhibition in diabetic nephropathy: ten years experience. Am J Kidney Dis 26:99-107, 1995
7.   Björck S, Mulec H, Johnsen SA, Nordén G, Aurell M: Renal protective effect of enalapril in diabetic nephropathy. Br Med J 304:339-343, 1992
8.   Breyer JA, Bain P, Evans JK, Nahman NS, Lewis E, Cooper ME, McGill JB, Berl T, The Collaborative Study Group: Predictors of the progression of renal insufficiency in patients with insulin-dependent diabetes and overt diabetic nephropathy. Kidney Int 50:1651-1658, 1996
9.   Walker WG, Hermann J, Murphy RP, Russell RP: Prospective study of the impact of hypertension upon kidney function in diabetes mellitus. Nephron 55(suppl 1):21-26, 1990
10.   Yokoyama H, Tomonaga O, Hirayama M, Ishii A, Takeda M, Babazono T, Ujihara U, Takahashi C, Omori Y: Predictors of the progression of diabetic nephropathy and the beneficial effect of angiotensin-converting enzyme inhibitors in NIDDM patients. Diabetologia 40:405-411, 1997
11.   Peterson JC, Adler S, Burkart JM, Green T, Herbert LA, Hunsicker LG, King AJ, Klahr S, Massry SG, Seifter JL: Blood pressure control, proteinuria, and the progression of renal disease. The modification of diet in renal disease study. Ann Intern Med 123:754-762, 1995
12.   Parving H-H, Andersen AR, Smidt UM, Hommel E, Mathiesen ER, Svendsen PA: Effect of antihypertensive treatment on kidney function in diabetic nephropathy. Br Med J 294:1443-1447, 1987

13. Lebovitz HE, Wiegmann TB, Cnaan A, Shahinfar S, Sica D, Broadstone V, Schwartz SL, Mengel MC, Segal R, Versaggi JA, Bolten WK: Renal protective effects of enalapril in hypertensive NIDDM: Role of baseline albuminuria. Kidney Int 45 (suppl. 45):S150-S155, 1994

14. Hansen HP, Rossing P, Tarnow L, Nielsen FS, Jensen BR, Parving H-H:Increased glomerular filtration rate after withdrawal of long-term antihypertensive treatment in diabetic nephropathy. Kidney Int 47:1726-1731, 1995

15. Hansen HP, Nielsen FS, Rossing P, Jacobsen P, Jensen BR, Parving H-H: Kidney function after withdrawal of long-term antihypertensive treatment in diabetic nephropathy. Kidney Int 52:S49-S53, 1997

16. Anderson S: Relevance of single nephron studies to human glomerular function. Kidney Int 45:384-389, 1994

17. Maddox DA, Brenner BM: Glomerular ultrafiltration, in The Kidney, edited by BRENNER BM, Philidelphia, Saunders, 1996, p. 286

18. Dustin P: Arteriolar hyalinosis. Int Rev Exp Pathol 1:73-138, 1962

19. Østerby R, Gall M-A, Schmitz A, Nielsen FS, Nyberg G, Parving H-H: Glomerular structure and function in proteinuric Type 2 (non-insulin-dependent) diabetic patients. Diabetologia 36:1064-1070, 1993

20. Wang X, Aukland K, Iversen BM: Acute effects of angiotensin II receptor antagonist on autoregulation of zonal glomerular filtration rate in renovascular hypertensive rats. Kidney Blood Pressure Research 20:225-232, 1997

21. Iversen BM, Kvam FI, Mørkrid L, Sekse I, Ofstad J: Effect of cyclooxygenase inhibition on renal blood flow autoregulation in SHR. Am J Physiol 32:F534-F539, 1992

22. Pelayo JC, Westcott JY: Impaired autoregulation of glomerular capillary hydrostatic pressure in the rat remnant nephron. J Clin Invest 88:101-105, 1991

23. Iversen BM, Kvam FI, Matre K, Ofstad J: Resetting of renal blood autoregulation during acute blood pressure reduction in hypertensive rats. Am J Physiol 44:R343-R349, 1998

24. Dworkin LD, Brenner BM: The renal circulations, in The Kidney, edited by BRENNER BM, Philadelphia, Saunders, 1996, p. 247

25. Lush DJ, Fray JCS: Steady-state autoregulation of renal blood flow: a myogenic model. Am J Physiol 247:R89-R99, 1984

26. Aukland K, Oeien AH: Renal autoregulation: models combining tubuloglomerular feedback and myogenic response. Am J Physiol 252:F768-F783, 1987

27. Hayashi K, Epstein M, Loutzenhiser R: Determinants of the renal actions of atrial natriuretic peptide (ANP): lack of effect of ANP on pressure-induced vasocontriction. Circ Res 67:1-10, 1990

28. Hayashi K, Epstein M, Loutzenhiser R: Pressure-induced vasocontriction of renal microvessels in normotensive and hypertensive rats: studies in the isolated perfused hydronephrotic kidney. Circ Res 65:1475-1484, 1989

29. Hayashi K, Epstein M, Loutzenhiser R , Forster H: Impaired myogenic responsiveness of the afferent arteriole in streptozotocin-induced diabetic rats: Role of eicosanoid derangements. J Am Soc Nephrol 2:1578-1586, 1992

30. Hill GS, Heptinstall RH: Steorid-induced hypertension in the rat. Am J Pathol 52:1-39, 1968

31. Zatz R, Dunn BR, Meyer TW, Anderson S, Rennke HG, Brenner BM: Prevention of diabetic glomerulopathy by pharmacological amelioration of glomerular capillary hypertension. J Clin Invest 77:1925-1930, 1986

32.   Iversen BM, Ofstad J: Loss of renal blood flow autoregulation in chronic glomeru-lonephritic rats. Am J Physiol 254:F284-F290, 1988

33.   Riser BL, Cortes P, Zhao X, Bernstein J, Dumler F, Narins RG: Intraglomerular pressure and mesangial stretchning stimulate extracellular matrix formation in the rat. J Clin Invest 90:1932-1943, 1992

34.   Kollros PR, Bates SR, Mathews MB, Horwitz AL, Glagov S: Cyclic AMP inhibits in-creased collagen production by cyclically stretched smooth muscle cells. Lab Invest 56:410-417, 1987

35.   Mauer SM: Structural-functional correlations of diabetic nephropathy. Kidney Int 45:612-622, 1994

36.   Griffin KA, Picken MM, Bidani AK: Method of renal mass reduction is a critical modula-tor of subsequent hypertension and glomerular injury. J Am Soc Nephrol 4:2023-2031, 1994

37.   Bidani AK, Schwartz M, Lewis E: Renal autoregulation and vulnerability to hypertensive injury in remnant kidney. Am J Physiol 252:F1003-F1010, 1987

38.   Christensen PK, Hommel E, Clausen P, Feldt-Rasmussen B, Parving H-H: Impaired auto-regulation of the glomerular filtration rate in patients with nondiabetic nephropathies. Kidney Int 56:1517-1523, 1999

39.   Hostetter TH, Rennke HG, Brenner BM: The case for intrarenal hypertension in the initia-tion and progression of diabetic and other glomerulopathies. Am J Med 72:375-380, 1982

40.   Hashimoto Y, Ideura Y, Yoshimura A, Koshikawa S: Autoregulation of renal blood flow in streptozocin-induced diabetic rats. Diabetes 38:1109-1113, 1989

41.   Tolins JP, Shultz PJ, Raij L, Brown DM, Mauer M: Abnormal renal hemodynamic re-sponse to reduced renal perfusion pressure in diabetic rats: role of NO. Am J Physiol 265:F866-F895, 1993

42.   Parving H-H, Kastrup J, Smidt Um, Andersen AR, Feldt-Rasmussen B, Christiansen JS: Impaired autoregulation of glomerular filtration rate in Type 1 (insulin-dependent) dia-betic patients with nephropathy. Diabetologia 27:547-552, 1984

43.   Brod J, Horbach L, Just H, Rosenthal J, Nicolescu R: Acute effects of clonidine on central and peripheral haemodynamics and plasma renin activity. Eur J Clin Pharm 4:107-114, 1972

44.   Onesti G, Bock KD, Heimsoth V, Kim KE, Merguet P: Clonidine: a new antihypertensive agent. Am J Cardiol 28:74-83, 1971

45.   Onesti G, Schwartz AB, Kim KE, Pas-Martinez V, Swartz C: Antihypertensive effect of clonidine. Circ Res 28:53-69, 1971

46.   Christensen PK, Hansen HP, Parving H-H: Impaired autoregulation of GFR in hyperten-sive non-insulin dependent diabetic patients. Kidney Int 52:1369-1374, 1997

47.   Griffin KA, Picken MM, Bidani AK: Deleterious effects of calcium channel blockade on pressure transmission and glomerular injury in rat remnant kidneys. J Clin Invest 96:793-800, 1995

48.   Apperloo AJ, De Zeeuw D, De Jong PE: A short-term antihypertensive treatment-induced fall in glomerular filtration rate predicts long-term stability of renal function. Kidney Int 51:793-797, 1997

49.   Klahr S: The modification of diet in renal disease study. N Engl J Med 320:864-866, 1989

32.   ACE INHIBITION, ANGIOTENSIN II RECEPTOR BLOCKADE, AND DIABETIC NEPHROPATHY

Norman K. Hollenberg, M.D., Ph.D.
Departments of Medicine and Radiology, Brigham and Women's Hospital, Boston.

Only a large, rigorous randomized double-blind assessment of a therapeutic candidate compared to the appropriate alternative can prove therapeutic efficacy. One such trial assessed the effect of captopril in patients with insulin-dependent diabetes mellitus (IDDM) who were at risk of nephropathy [1] with results that were sufficiently impressive that the use of captopril quickly became a professional necessity supported by public policy. Moreover, multiple lines of evidence accumulated over a decade suggested that this useful feature of captopril was a class action, extending to all ACE inhibitors [2,3]. In the case of the angiotensin II (Ang II) AT_1 receptor blockers (AT_1 antagonists), we are fortunate in having very early in the development of these agents two ongoing major, high quality trials in patients with NIDDM who are at risk of nephropathy -- one involving Irbesartan, the other involving Losartan. Unfortunately, the outcome of these trials is unlikely to be available to us until the coming millennium, and this chapter is due well before!

The issue of the pharmacologic mechanisms by which ACE inhibitors retard the progression of nephropathy lies at the center of any discussion on whether or not AT_1 antagonists will match their efficacy. Ichikawa, an authority on the renin system and the kidney, marshalled multiple lines of evidence to indicate that much of the salutary actions of ACE inhibitors did not involve Ang II formation, but rather alternative pathways [4]. In a recent editorial, I countered with an alternative view [5] to indicate that the AT_1 receptor blockers held promise beyond what ACE inhibition can offer. What were the arguments?

Ichikawa based his analysis on a range of considerations, the majority of which seem to favor ACE inhibition as these considerations suggest that angiotensin is not important [4]. ACE inhibitors can influence alternative pathways that might, in turn, influence extracellular matrix protein degradation and the rate of development of glomerulosclerosis. Macrophage infiltration is also ACE inhibitor responsive. Blocking the AT1 receptor opens the short feedback loop, thereby leading to renin release and increased Ang II formation. With the AT1 receptor blocked, this sequence could lead to unopposed activation of the AT2 receptor -- with unknown but potentially negative consequences. All of these considerations, Ichikawa believed, favor ACE inhibition over Ang II AT1 antagonist action. Perhaps the most important consideration in Ichikawa's analysis involved glomerular hemodynamics, especially glomerular capillary pressure: that much of the ACE inhibitor dependent improvement in natural history might reflect the salutary effect of ACE inhibition on glomerular capillary pressure via bradykinin-mediated efferent arteriolar dilatation.

Thus, the kininase action of ACE inhibitors is considered to be crucial, and the reduction in Ang II formation is less important -- or even irrelevant. Conversely, one can make an equally compelling argument for potential efficacy of Ang II antagonists, based on more effective blockade of the renin system [5,6].

Much of the most important data reviewed above were obtained in vitro or in small animal models. If studies in rats never predicted responses in humans, we would probably never do studies in rats -- or at least would not read them. If studies in rats always predicted what would happen in humans, we could not justify studies in humans. Is this an area in which there might be important species differences? I addressed that issue specifically in a recent editorial on ACE inhibition and the kidney [6]. To isolate species differences one has to apply an essentially identical protocol to multiple species. There are species differences. As one example, bradykinin antagonists blunted the renovasodilator response to ACE inhibitors in the dog and in the rat, but not in the rabbit. In accord, an Ang II antagonist blunted ACE inhibitor induced renal vasodilation in the rat and dog very little, but blocked it completely in the rabbit. ACE inhibition increased prostaglandin release in rat and canine kidneys, but not that of the rabbit. In an elegant study Roman, et al [7] showed that in the rat it was medullary perfusion that was especially kinin dependent. Thus, apparent species differences may be primarily anatomical, reflecting the relative contribution of medullary perfusion to total renal blood flow: In this feature humans resemble the rabbit far more than they do the rat or dog [6]. Whatever the explanation one clear message emerges: We cannot extrapolate from studies in a limited range of species, especially the rat, to control mechanisms in humans, even in health and much less so when disease is superimposed.

What of information on the control of the renal circulation in humans, and the mechanisms by which ACE inhibition might influence the renal circulation? Although there are limitations in the approaches that can be employed in humans, several lines of evidence provide an answer. The striking influence of salt intake on the renal vasodilator response to ACE inhibition was recognized early, and supports a dominant role for the Ang II mechanism. This observation is necessary but is not sufficient. More recently, comparative pharmacology has strengthened that conclusion substantially. If the renal vasodilatation induced by ACE inhibitors in humans included a substantial component due to bradykinin, prostaglandins, or nitric oxide, one would anticipate that the renal vasodilator response to renin inhibitors would be substantially less. To our surprise the renal vasodilator response to a renin inhibitor, enalkiren, exceeded expectations from early experience with ACE inhibitors [6]. To address this issue, we performed a range of follow-up studies. To ascertain whether the observation represented an idiosyncracy associated with one renin inhibitor, we studied a second --

with an identical result. Because of the notorious risk of employing historic controls, we performed a study in which patients received an ACE inhibitor, a renin inhibitor, or vehicle during the same week. This study was coded and double blind. To avoid an idiosyncracy associated with one ACE inhibitor, we employed three, each at the top of the dose response curve. The findings all provided support for a surprising but unambiguous conclusion. Despite the fact that our original premise on the kinin contribution to the renal response to ACE inhibition supported by a wealth of information in animal studies, the renovasodilator response to renin inhibition -- in the neighborhood of 140 ml/min/1.73m^2 -- was substantially larger than the response to ACE inhibition, in the 90-100 ml/min/1.73 m^2 range.

Although the fundamentals of pharmacology would favor as the explanation more effective pharmacological interruption of the renin system at the rate-limiting step, there is an alternative interpretation. As the two renin inhibitors were structurally related, it is possible that they shared a renovasodilator action through a mechanism unrelated to a reduction in Ang II formation. If, indeed, the renin inhibitors operated via the renin cascade, one would anticipate a similar or larger renovasodilator response to Ang II antagonists, in studies performed in the same way. This is precisely what we found. In studies performed with an identical model, protocol and technique, two Ang II antagonists induced a renovasodilator response that matched, or exceeded slightly the response to renin inhibition in healthy humans on a low salt diet [8,9]. From this observation we would draw several conclusions. The renal hemodynamic response to ACE inhibition has underestimated, systematically, the magnitude of the contribution of Ang II to renovascular tone when the renin system is activated. The effectiveness of renin inhibition suggests that this response represents interruption of primarily renin-dependent, additional non-ACE-dependent pathways. In healthy humans, there might be a small contribution from proteolytic pathways that bypass both renin and ACE.

The percentage of non-ACE-dependent AngII generation in the kidney varies with conditions. The 30-40% estimate was based on studies performed on a low-salt diet, to activate the renin-angiotensin system. In an, as yet unreported, extension of that study, we compared the responses to captopril and to candesartan in healthy subjects who were studied when in balance on a high-salt diet, to suppress the renin-angiotensin system. As anticipated, the response to captopril was reduced sharply to about 20 mL/min/1.73m$_2$. The response to candesartan was also reduced, but it still exceeded 70 mL/min/1.73 m^2. Under these conditions, which mimick most of our lives, over ninety percent of the AngII generation was non-ACE dependent.

In disease, on the other hand, alternative pathways may provide a more substantial contribution [9].

PLASMA-RENIN ACTIVITY, RENAL TISSUE RENIN AND DIABETES:
What evidence is there from studies on the state of the renin system and the contribution of Ang II to renal vascular tone to suggest that angiotensin might be involved in the pathogenesis? When studies on the circulating renin system were first undertaken, the goal was to ascertain whether the hypertension that frequently complicates the course of

diabetes could be attributed to the renin system [10]. An unanticipated suppression of the renin system was found in many patients, especially in those with diabetic nephropathy, an observation that has been repeated frequently [11,13]. The low renin state has typically been attributed to organic sclerotic changes in the arteriolar and glomerular region, possibly accentuated by volume expansion and autonomic neuropathy. Several lines of evidence suggest a more interesting, more complex and immediately relevant alteration in the renal tissue renin system in this process. In animal models, multiple studies have shown that renal tissue renin levels, and the message supporting renin production are normal or increased, even in animal models in which PRA is reduced [14,16]. In patients with NIDDM in whom renal function was intact and who were free of evidence of nephropathy, we found an unanticipated abnormality in the control of renin release. In these patients in whom plasma renin activity was normal on challenge with a low salt diet and posture, there was evidence of renin system autonomy [17]. On a low salt diet, renin system activation appeared to be normal and intact as PRA rose normally, and the renal vasodilator response to ACE inhibition with enalapril was identical to normal. Conversely, when the patients received a high salt diet, despite the fact that they showed more positive sodium balance, PRA suppressed less well in patients with NIDDM than in age-matched normal subjects. Moreover, the renal vasodilator response to enalapril on a high salt diet in NIDDM exceeded substantially the response in normal subjects, in whom ACE inhibitor-induced renal vasodilatation is minimal.

This vasodilator response in NIDDM was attributable to Ang II based on indirect evidence. At baseline, the renal vascular response to Ang II was already blunted in NIDDM, in keeping with renin system activation. If the renal vasodilator response to enalapril had reflected kinin production, and consequent prostaglandin synthesis or nitric oxide release we would have anticipated further blunting of the response to Ang II. Conversely, if the renal vasodilator response reflected a reduction in Ang II production, we would have anticipated enhancement of the renal vascular response. The dramatic enhancement of responses to Ang II that occurred favored an ACE inhibitor action primarily reflecting reduced Ang II formation.

This indirect evidence is supported further by more recent studies with the Ang II antagonist, Irbesartan [9]. In patients with NIDDM and nephropathy in whom the renin system response to restriction of sodium intake was blunted, the renal vasodilator response to Irbesartan was enhanced, exceeding the response to normal substantially over a range of doses. PRA, suppressed at baseline in the patients with diabetes, responded to the Ang II antagonist with a progressive rise that eventually matched normal. These observations suggest that measures of PRA can be misleading, providing little insight into the state of the intrarenal renin system. Activation of this system in diabetes, perhaps in part due to the effects of hyperglycemia [18] could contribute to pathogenesis.

To pursue that possibility, we assessed the influence of hyperglycemia on renal control mechanisms in healthy volunteers, in protocols similar to that employed for assessing non-ACE-dependent pathways. Each volunteer participated in three study days, all performed on a high salt diet. On one study day, they received a glucose infusion. On a second study day, they received captopril. On a third study day, they received both [19]. As anticipated, hyperglycemia induced a sharp increase in renal plasma flow, of about 80 ml/min/1.73m^2. Captopril alone in studies on a high salt diet, induced little or no renal vasodilator response. On the other hand, when captopril was added to the hyperemic state created by glucose infusion, the result was a dramatic accentuation of the renal vasodilator response to captopril -- to a level exceeding 120 ml/min/1.73m^2. PRA did not change during gluocse infusion, but the renal vascular response to AngII was blunted sharply. Treatment with captopril enhanced the renal vascular response to AngII, suggesting that intrarenal activation of the renin system participated. In an as yet unreported follow-up to that study, we have shown in an identical protocol that the renal vasodilator response to eprosartan is accentuated sharply. Clearly, hyperglycemia, per se, can activate the intrarenal renin system.

The final conclusion is that therapeutic trials with Ang II antagonists offer far more promise than did ACE inhibitors, despite the gloomy predictions. They are more effective blockers.

REFERENCES:

1. Lewis EJ, Hunsicker LG, Bain RP, and Rohde RD: The effect of angiotensin-converting enzyme inhibition on diabetic nephropathy. N Engl J Med 1993;329:1456-1462.
2. Kasiske BL, Kalil RSN, Ma JZ, Liao M, and Keane WF: Effect of therapy on the kidney in patients with diabetes: A meta-regression analysis. Ann Intern Med 1993;118:129-138.
3. Hollenberg NK and Raij L. Angiotensin-converting enzyme inhibition and renal protection. An assessment of implications for therapy. Arch Intern Med 1993;153:2426-2435.
4. Ichikawa I. Will Ang II A1 be renoprotective in humans? Kidney Intern 1996;50:684-692.
5. Hollenberg NK. ACE inhibitors, AT1 receptor blockers, and the kidney. E. Ritz (Ed) Nephrol Dial Transplant 1997;12:381-383.
6. Hollenberg NK and Fisher NK. Renal circulation and blockade of the renin-angiotensin system. Is angiotensin-converting enzyme inhibition the last word? Hypertension 1995; 26:602-609.
7. Roman RJ, Kaldunski ML, Scicli AG, and Carretero OA. Influence of kinins and angiotensin II on the regulation of papillary blood flow. Am J Physiol 1988;255:F690-F698.
8. Price D, DeOliveira J, Fisher N, and Hollenberg N. Contribution of Ang II to renal hemodynamics in healthy men: the renal vascular response to eprosartan, an Ang II antagonist. ASN Program Abstract #A1688 from 29th Annual Meeting in New Orleans, Nov. 3-6. J Am Soc Nephrol 1996;7:1587.
9. Price D, Porter LE, DeOliveira J, Fisher N, Gordon M, Laffel L, Williams G, and Hollenberg N. The paradox of the low-renin state: hormonal and renal responses to an Ang II antagonist, Irbesartan, in diabetic nephropathy. J Am Soc Nephrol, 1999; 10: 2382-91.
10. Christlieb AR, Kaldany A, and D'Elia JA. Plasma renin activity and hypertension in diabetes mellitus. Diabetes 1976;25:969-974.
11. Bjorck S. The renin-angiotensin system in diabetes mellitus: a physiological and therapeutic study. Scand J Urol Nephrol Suppl 1990;126:1-50.

12.   Lush DJ, King JA, and Fray JCS. Pathophysiology of low renin syndromes: sites of renal renin secretory impairment and prorenin overexpression. Kid International 1993;43:983-999.

13.   Weidmann P, Ferrari P, and Shaw SG. Renin in Diabetes Mellitus. In: The Renin-Angiotensin System. In: JIS Robertson and MG Nicholls (Ed). Raven Press Ltd., New York, 1991. Chapter 75. pp. 75.1-75.26.

14.   Rosenberg ME, Smith LJ, Correa-Rotter R, and Hostetter TH. The paradox of the renin-angiotensin system in chronic renal disease. Kid Internat 1994;45:403-410.

15.   Kikkawa R, Kitamura E, Fujiwara Y, Haneda M, and Shigeta Y. Biphasic alteration of renin-angiotensin-aldosterone system in streptozotocin-diabetic rats. Renal Physiol 1986;9:187-192.

16.   Anderson S, Jung FF, and Ingelfinger JR. Renal renin-angiotensin system in diabetes: functional immunohistochemical, and molecular biological correlations. Am J Physiol 1993;265:F477-F486.

17.   De'Oliveira JM, Price DA, Fisher NDL, Allan DR, McKnight JA, Williams GH, and Hollenberg NK. Autonomy of the renin system in type II diabetes mellitus: Dietary sodium and renal hemodynamic responses to ACE inhibition. Kidney International 1997;52:771-777.

18.   Miller JA, Floras JS, Zinman B, Skorecki KL, and Logan AG. Effect of hyperglycemia on arterial pressure, plasma renin activity and renal function in early diabetes. Clin Sci 1996;90:189-195.

19.   Osei SY, Price DA, Fisher NDL, Porter LE, Laffel LMB, and Hollenberg NK. Hyperglycemia and angiotensin-mediated control of the renal circulation in healthy humans. Hypertension 1999;3:559-564.

33. THE CONCEPT OF INCIPIENT DIABETIC NEPHROPATHY AND EFFECT OF EARLY ANTIHYPERTENSIVE INTERVENTION

Michel Marre[+], Samy Hadjadj[++], Béatrice Bouhanick[+++]
Diabetes Departments, [+]Hôpital Bichat, Paris; [++]Centre Hospitalier Universitaire, Poitiers; [+++]Centre Hospitalier Universitaire, Angers - France

INTRODUCTION

Diabetic nephropathy is the main cause for premature death among type 1, insulin-dependent diabetic subjects [1]. To date, aggressive antihypertensive treatment is the main intervention along with better metabolic control able to improve prognosis of these patients [2]. The term diabetic nephropathy designates glomerular injury attributable to diabetes [3]. As in all glomerular diseases, its diagnosis is based upon three functional abnormalities: proteinuria (mainly, albuminuria), elevated blood pressure, and reduced glomerular filtration rate. Technical improvements lead to early detection of glomerular dysfunction in type 1, insulin-dependent diabetic subjects: the first ones were sensitive assays for urinary albumin measurement [4, 5]; also sensitive techniques to detect glomerular hyperfiltration early in the course of diabetic renal disease, and only recently automatic blood pressure monitoring to detect minimal blood pressure changes [6, 7]. The concept of incipient diabetic nephropathy was validated by 4 follow-up studies of patients whose urinary albumin was measured serially with sensitive techniques [8-11]. These studies indicated that minimal increases in Urinary Albumin Excretion (UAE) (called microalbuminuria) can have a prognostic value. Therefore, the concept of incipient diabetic nephropathy is based upon the premise that persistent microalbuminuria can already indicate initial glomerular injury, and not only glomerular dysfunction as discussed elsewhere

DESCRIPTION AND NATIONAL HISTORY OF INCIPIENT DIABETIC NEPHROPATHY

Description :

Mogensen C.E. (ed.), THE KIDNEY AND HYPERTENSION IN DIABETES MELLITUS.
Copyright© 2000 by Kluwer Academic Publishers, Boston ● Dordrecht ● London. *All rights reserved.*

UAE

By definition, UAE is elevated in the microalbuminuria range. Although UAE values predictive for diabetic nephropathy varied from 15 to 70 µg/min among the four pilot studies [8 - 11], a consensus was proposed to define microalbuminuria as UAE ranging 30-300 mg/24 h, or 20-200 µg/min, 2 - 3 times over 1 - 6 month period [12]. The Steno group proposed to subdivide into micro- microalbuminuria (30-99 mg/24 h) and macro-microalbuminuria (100-300 mg/24 h), because the prognosis was poorer for the latter than for the former values [13]. However, these differential prognostic values were not confirmed on an individual basis [14, 15].

Blood Pressure

The mean blood pressure values of subjects with incipient diabetic nephropathy are higher than those of healthy controls, or of diabetic subjects with normal UAE, but lower than those of subjects with established diabetic nephropathy. There is a good correlation between blood pressure and UAE values. However, diagnosis of incipient diabetic nephropathy cannot be based upon cut-off values for blood pressure, because of large inter-group overlaps. Only the upper limit for blood pressure values can be fixed, namely those defining permanent hypertension: e.g. 140/90 mmHg or more, and/or concurrent hypertensive treatment. This upper limit has practical implications to delineate different causes for microalbuminuria: microalbuminuria with permanent hypertension indicates severe hypertension, but not incipient diabetic nephropathy, and regression lines between blood presure and UAE are not superimposable for one case and for the other [16].

Automatic devices can improve blood pressure recording precision, but probably not sensitivity to classify subjects with incipient diabetic nephropathy [17]. Nocturnal recordings can ameliorate sensitivity [6, 7, 17], because a reduction in nocturnal blood pressure decline is characteristic of high blood pressure secondary to glomerular disease [18].

In summary, blood pressure values are not in the permanent hypertension range during incipient diabetic nephropathy; they must be recorded precisely and uniformly for follow-up purposes.

Glomerular Filtration Rate

In incipient diabetic nephropathy, GFR can be normal, or elevated, but rarely below normal values. The prognostic significance of glomerular hyperfiltration is discussed in chapter 29. However, it is not clear by which UAE values within the microalbuminuria range GFR starts declining in normotensive diabetic individuals. Mogensen and Christensen proposed that the initially positive relationship between UAE and GFR values becomes negative for UAE ranges above 30-50 µg/min [11]. In figure 33-1, we traced a parabolic regression line between individual UAE and GFR values obtained in 84 type 1, insulin-dependent diabetic subjects without antihypertensive treatment. The calculated top of the line was found for UAE 34 mg/24 h and GFR 130 ml/min/1.73 m^2. Hence, it is possible that glomerular filtration surface is reducing from the lowest UAE values within microalbuminuria, eventhough GFR values are in the normal, or supra-normal ranges. This biphasic relationship between UAE and GFR suggests that the phenomenon observed by Starling [19] on heart muscles is applicable to changes in glomerular function of type 1, insulin-dependent diabetic subjects. This analogy in modelization can have a physical basis, as mesangial cells are of muscular origin.

NATURAL COURSE OF INCIPIENT DIABETIC NEPHROPATHY

Incidence of diabetic nephropathy
Incidence of persistent microalbuminuria in normotensive type 1, insulin-dependent diabetic subjects was studied by several groups [20, 21] over 4 to 7 year-periods. It approximates 1 - 2 % cases/year. The main risk factor for microalbuminuria onset is diabetes duration, which is 5 years minimally. It was recently outlined that subjects with microalbuminuria and long diabetes duration may display a better prognosis than those with diabetes duration shorter than 15-17 years [22]. However, this result must be interpreted cautiously, because the slope of UAE progression can vary widely from one individual to another, and because early interventions can alter the course of the disease, especially with ACEIs. glycaemic control is of paramount importance to prognose microalbuminuria: subjects with HbA1c below 7.5 % have a low risk for microalbuminuria [20, 21]. Recently, Krolewski et al proposed from follow-up observations that type 1, insulin-dependent diabetic subjects with normoalbuminuria and HbA1c level below 8.1 % would have a minimal risk for progression towards microalbuminuria [23]. Accordingly, results from the DCCT indicated that optimized insulin treatment reduced risk for microalbuminuria onset by 21-52 % [24].
Genetic factors can affect risk for incipient or established diabetic nephropathy. This is discussed in chapter 10.

Duration of incipient diabetic nephropathy
Duration of incipient diabetic nephropathy is not determined precisely from large group follow-up. Some studies indicate a 5-15 year duration [13]. Nonetheless, indicence of established diabetic nephropathy may be high: in control groups of clinical trials performed in normotensive subjects with microalbuminuria, it ranged between 8 and 30 % cases /year [14, 15, 26, 27].

EFFECT OF EARLY ANTIHYPERTENSIVE INTERVENTION IN INCIPIENT DIABETIC NEPHROPATHY

Rationale
There is a proportional increase of UAE and of blood pressure during the course of diabetic nephropathy from the incipient stage [28]. Follow-up studies indicated that early, aggressive antihypertensive treatment reduces effectively both albuminuria and the rate of GFR decline in patients with established diabetic nephropathy [29, 30]. These

were pragmatical studies, in which classical antihypertensive drugs were used, e.g. the beta-blocker metoprolol. Then, Christensen and Mogensen reported a six-year follow-up of 6 patients with incipient diabetic nephropathy before and during metoprolol treatment [31]. UAE was reduced, and GFR maintained unchanged with metoprolol. Taken together, these studies [29, 30, 31] supported the concept that reducing blood pressure is an effective mean to reduce microalbuminuria and protect GFR in incipient diabetic nephropathy. However, clinical and experimental data supported that increased UAE results from increased glomerular capillary pressure, which is determined not only by systemic blood pressure, but also by pre. / post glomerular vasoconstriction / dilation [32]. This latter determinant is strongly regulated by the activity of the renin-angiotensin-aldosterone system.

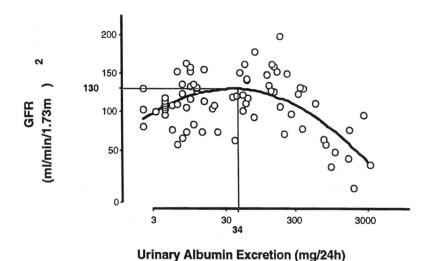

Urinary Albumin Excretion (mg/24h)

Fig. 33-1. Observed relationship between UAE (the mean of 3 consecutive 24-hour urine collections) and GFR (^{51}Cr-EDTA plasma disapperance technique) values measured in 84 consecutive type 1, insulin-dependent diabetic subjects without antihypertensive treatment: r=0.576; p=0.0001; GFR (ml/min/1.73 m^2)=70+78 (SD16) log UAE (mg/24h) – 26 (4) [log UAE]^2 – Calculated top of parabolic curve was UAE = 34 mg/24h and GFR = 130 ml/min/1.73 m^2

Beta-blockers can modify glomerular hæmodynamics, because they reduce renin secretion, in addition to their actions on cardiac output and blood pressure [33]. In the above mentioned studies [29, 30, 31], changes in glomerular hæmodynamics were not studied in relation to those of renin secretion.

Conversely, experimental studies to reduce glomerular capillary hypertension of diabetic rats with ACEI lead to prevention of albuminuria and glomerulosclerosis [34], but systolic blood pressure was lower on ACEI than on placebo. Similarly, we set-up a double-blind, placebo-controlled trial demonstrating prevention, or post-pone of diabetic nephropathy with enalapril in normotensive diabetic subjects with microalbuminuria [14]. However, blood pressure was reduced by enalapril compared to placebo, which made interpretation of this trial difficult, since reducing blood pressure reduces UAE in hypertensive subjects [35].

Thus, confusion rose from these two types of observations, because alterations in systemic blood pressure and in glomerular hæmodynamics were not controlled simultaneously with changes in activity of the renin angiotensin system. Anderson et al demonstrated later on that ACEI efficacy to prevent albuminuria in diabetic rats was due to both hypotension and reduction of intra-glomerular capillary pressure [36]. In a double-blind, double-dummy, one year parallel trial comparing enalapril to hydrochlorothiazide (two drugs with similar hypotensive effects but symmetrical actions on angiotensin II production) to reduce UAE of normotensive type 1, insulin-dependent subjects with microalbuminuria, we demonstrated that reducing systemic blood pressure reduces UAE in the long-term only if the renin-angiotensin system effectiveness is simultaneously blocked [37].

Eligibility for antihypertensive treatment in incipient diabetic nephropathy
Should subjects with incipient diabetic nephropathy be assigned to antihypertensive treatment on the basis of UAE, or of blood pressure values ? Certainly on the basis of a persistent microalbuminuria, because definition of incipient diabetic nephropathy is based on this biological abnormality. Second, microalbuminuria is probably an early sign of, rather than a factor predictive for diabetic nephropathy [38]. In this connection, UAE > 20 µg/min (or 30 mg/24 h) is clearly abnormal : more than fifty per cent of healthy subjects excrete less than 5 mg/24 h [39]. Also, GFR can start declining from the lowest range of microalbuminuria, as illustrated in Fig. 33-1. Finally, UAE reduction can be obtained independently of blood pressure reduction, as detailed below.

Evidence for a superiority of ACEIs over other available hypotensive drugs to reduce UAE in incipient diabetic nephropathy
Several studies indicated that microalbuminuria of normotensive type 1, insulin-dependent diabetic subjects could be reduced by ACEIs, while blood pressure was not modified significantly [15, 40]. We reported in a short-term, double-blind study that small doses of ramipril can reduce microalbuminuria as effectively as hypotensive doses. This UAE reduction was obtained independently of blood pressure reduction, but it was related to the degree of ACE inhibition and to changes in filtration fraction [41]. Comparison of enalapril to hydrochlorothiazide to reduce microalbuminuria of

normotensive type 1, insulin-dependent diabetic subjects lead to similar conclusions: both drugs were not different for their hypotensive effects, but only enalapril reduced microalbuminuria; UAE changes were related to those of filtration fraction, not to those of blood pressure [37]. Thus, dose-response curves for the renal and the hypotensive effects of ACEIs may not be superimposable. A meta-regression analysis supports a preferential role for ACEIs to reduce UAE and to protect GFR of diabetic subjects [42]. The Melbourne Diabetic Nephropathy Study Group could not find a difference between the effect of a dihydropyridine and ACEI on UAE changes [43], but this apparently negative result was probably due to a lack of study's power. Conversely a recent Italian study reported a small difference on UAE progression between the ACEI and the calcium-antagonist nifedipine in diabetic subjects with microalbuminuria [44].

Long-term evolution of GFR in type 1, insulin-dependent diabetic subjects given ACEIs from incipient diabetic nephropathy

Certainly GFR preservation is the only clinically significant outcome for intervention studies in diabetic nephropathy. Microalbuminuria is a surrogate end-point. As outlined above, GFR is normal or still supra-normal during incipient diabetic nephropathy, and GFR reduction is minimal at time of clinical proteinuria onset (See Mogensen, Chapter 2]. Also, clinical trials comparing captopril or enalapril to placebo or to metoprolol showed that GFR degradation was reduced by about 50 % with ACEIs in type 1, insulin-dependent diabetic subjects with clinical proteinuria [45, 46]. The clinical usefulness of ACEIs given from microalbuminuria stage was therefore questionable for type 1, insulin-dependent diabetic subjects with incipient nephropathy. Indeed, GFR evolution was not different between patients on captopril and those on placebo in 2 to 4 year clinical trials [15, 26]. Only a marginal difference was found by our group in a one-year trial comparing enalapril to placebo [14]. In a recent two-year trial, Laffel et al reported that creatinine clearance was maintained by captopril compared to placebo in type 1, insulin-dependent diabetic normotensive patients with microalbuminuria [27], and this was confirmed in a recent combined analysis of the two multicenter trials performed with captopril versus placebo for two years [47]. The median GFR slope was -6.4 ml/min/1.73 m^2/year in the placebo - treated patients. These data must be interpreted with caution for methodological reasons, because GFR was estimated from creatinine clearances and because, baseline GFR values were markedly low (80 ml/min/1.73m^2) in the American trial; second, creatinine clearance can be altered by changes in tubular function provoked by renal vasodilators like ACEIs. However, we found a comparable GFR decline in a recent 4-year follow-up study comparing two treatment strategies with enalapril. Patients' GFR were estimated with the ^{125}I-Iodothalamate constant infusion technique. Those normotensive type 1, insulin-dependent diabetic patients with microalbuminuria given enalapril from microalbuminuria identification kept their GFR unchanged (including those with initial hyperfiltration), while those given enalapril only if they progressed to macroalbuminuria reduced their GFR by 0.62 ml/min/1.73m^2/month. At follow-up, 6 of the 11 patients assigned to late enalapril treatment displayed GFR values < 100 ml/min/1.73m^2 (the lower limit of normal values) [48]. Taken together, these recent studies indicate that GFR degradation slope is nearly as high in patients with incipient as in patients with established nephropathy. These longitudinal results fit with the parabolic figure of the relationship between GFR and UAE shown above, and described firstly by Mogensen and Christensen in 1984 [11]. Thus, treatment with ACEIs in proteinuric type 1, insulin-dependent diabetic subjects may be too late to protect their GFR [45]. These results support the current recommendation that ACEIs must be given from microalbuminuria identification in normotensive type 1, insulin-dependent diabetic patients [49]. A recent extension [50] of an earlier study by Mathiesen [15] documents also preservation of GFR by ACEIs.

Unanswered questions on the use of ACEIs for diabetic patients with microalbuminuria
First, the above-mentioned data deal with normotensive type 1, insulin-dependent diabetic patients with microalbuminuria. The specific value of ACEIs vs conventional antihypertensive treatment is not demonstrated for kidney function of patients with essential hypertension [51], and this condition can be associated with insulin-dependent diabetes sometimes.

Second, longer-term follow-up studies are required to ascertain if cardiovascular morbidity/mortality is reduced by early ACEIs treatment in these relatively young patients, in addition to the benefit obtained for kidney function.

Third, it not known which are the long-term side-effect attached to the use of ACEIs in young patients [52]. Pharmacovigilant studies are required in this respect.

Fourth, the promising data obtained in type 1, insulin-dependent diabetic patients cannot be applied to type 2, non-insulin-dependent diabetic patients. Only one study reported a benefit for kidney function of normotensive type 2, non-insulin-dependent diabetic patients with microalbuminuria attributable to enalapril compared to placebo [53, 54]. However, the type 2, non-insulin-dependent diabetic patients in this study [53, 54] were relatively young and thin compared to those commonly encountered in clinical practice. Although such patients are identifiable and may share renal prognosis similar to type 1, insulin-dependent diabetic patients [14], such results cannot be applied to the vast majority of type 2, non-insulin-dependent diabetic patients. Most of them are obese, with hypertension and mixed dyslipidæmia, and the prognostic value of microalbuminuria deals with cardiovascular events in these patients[55]. A multifactorial intervention in type 2 diabetes patients with microalbuminuria was published [56] showing a benefit on the progression to proteinuria. However, the blood pressure was significantly lower in the intervention group, and it is not clear whether the observed benefit was attributable solely to the systematic use of ACEIs, or also to other therapeutic interventions in the intensive treatment group [56]. To date, no trial has established a clinical benefit from the preferential use of ACEIs in these patients.

Preventive treatment in normoalbuminuric patient would be interesting but requires long-term intervention [40].

ACKNOWLEDGMENTS
We thank Mrs Line GODIVEAU and Isabelle GOULEAU for their excellent secretarial assistance.

REFERENCES

1   Andersen AR., Christiansen JS, Andersen JK., Kreiner S, Deckert T. Diabetic nephropathy in type 1 (insulin-dependent) diabetes : an epidemiological study Diabetologia, 1983, 2 : 496-501

2   Mathiesen ER., Borch-Johnsen K., Jensen DV, Deckert T. Improved survival in patients with diabetic nephropathy Diabetologia, 1989, 32 : 884-886

3   Deckert T., Poulsen JE, Larsen M. Prognosis of diabetics with diabetes onset before the age of thirty-one. I-Survival, causes of death and complications Diabetologia, 1978, 14 : 363-370

4   Keen H., Chlouverakis C. An immunoassay method for urinary albumin at low concentrations. Lancet, 1963, ii, 913

5   Miles DM, Mogensen CE, Gundersen HJG. Radioimmunoassay for urinary albumin using a single antibody Scand. J. Clin. Lab. Invest., 1970, 25 : 5-11

6   Benhamou PY, Halimi S., De Gaudemaris R., Boizel R, Pitiot M, Siche JP, BACHELOT I, Mallion JM. Early disturbances of ambulatory blood pressure in normotensive type 1 diabetic patients with microalbuminuria Diabetes Care, 1992, 15 : 1614-1619

7   Hansen KW, Mau Pedersen M, Marshall SM, Christiansen JS, Mogensen CE. Circadian variation of blood pressure in patients with diabetic nephropathy Diabetologia, 1992, 35 : 1074-1079

8   Viberti RC, Hill RD, Jarret RJ, Argyropoulos A, Hahmud U, Keen M. Microalbuminuria as a predictor of clinical nephropathy in insulin dependent diabetes mellitus Lancet, 1982, i, 1430-1432

9   Parving H-H, Oxenboll B, Svendsen PAA, Christiansen JS, Andersen AR. Early detection of patients at risk of developing diabetic nephropathy. A longitudinal study of urinary albumin excretion Acta Endocrinologica, 1982, 100, 550-555

10   Mathiesen ER, Enboll B., Johansen K. Svendsen PAA., Deckert T Incipient nephropathy in type 1 (insulin-dependent) diabetes. Diabetologia, 1984, 26 : 406-410

11   Mogensen CE, Christensen CK. Predicting diabetic nephropathy in insulin-dependent patients N. Engl. J. Med., 1984, 311 : 89-93

12   Mogensen CE., Chachati A, Christensen CK. et al. Microalbuminuria: an early marker of renal involvement in diabetes Uremia Investigation, 1985-86, 9 : 85 - 95

13   Feldt-Rasmussen B., Mathiesen E.R., Jensen T., Lauritzen T., Deckert T. Effect of improved metabolic control on loss of kidney function in type I (insulin-dependent) diabetic patients : an update of the Steno studies. Diabetologia, 1991, 34 : 164-170

14   Marre M, Chatellier G, Leblanc H, Guyenne TT, Menard J, Passa P. Prevention of diabetic nephropathy with enalapril in normotensive diabetics with microalbuminuria B.M.J., 1988, 297 : 1092-1095

15   Mathiesen ER, Hommel E, Giese J, Parving H-H. Efficacy of captopril in postponing nephropathy in normotensive insulin dependent diabetic patients with microalbuminuria B.M.J., 1991, 303 : 81-87

16   Christensen CK, Krusell LR, Mogensen CE. Increased blood pressure in diabetes : essential hypertension or diabetic nephropathy ?Scand. J. Clin. Lab. Invest., 1987, 47 : 363-370

17   Berrut G, Hallab M., Bouhanick B, Chameau AM., Marre M., Fressinaud Ph. Value of ambulatory blood pressure monitoring in type 1 (insulin-dependent) diabetic patients with incipient diabetic nephropathy Am. J. Hypertension, 1994, 7 : 222-227

18   Middeke M., Schrader J. Nocturnal blood pressure in normotensive subjects and those with while coat, primary, and secondary hypertension B.M.J., 1994, 308 : 630-632

19   Starling EH. Physiological factors involved in the causation of dropsy Lancet, 1896, (1) : 1405

20   Mathiesen ER, Ronn B, Jensen T, Storm B, Deckert T. The relationship between blood pressure and urinary albumin excretion in the development of microalbuminuria Diabetes, 1990, 39 : 245-249

21   Microalbuminuria Collaborative Study Group, Predictors of the development of microalbuminuria in patients with type 1 diabetes mellitus: a seven year prospective study. Diabet. Med, 1999; 16: 918-25.

22   Forsblom CM, Groop PH, Ekstrand A, Groop LC. Predictive value of microalbuminuria in insulin-dependent diabetes of long duration. B.M.J., 1992 ; 305 : 1051-1053

23   Krolewski AS, Laffel LM, Krolewski M, Quinn M, Warram JH. Glycosylated hemoglobin and the risk of microalbuminuria in patients with insulin-dependent diabetes mellitus. N. Engl. J. Med, 1995, 332 : 1251-1255

24   The Diabetes Control and Complications Trial Research Group. The effect of intensive treatment of diabetes on the development and progression of long-term complications in insulin-dependent diabetes mellitus. N. Engl. J. Med., 1993 ; 329 : 977-986

25   Feldt-Rasmussen B, Mathiesen ER, Deckert T.Effect of two years of strict metabolic control on progression of incipient nephropathy in insulin-dependent diabetes. Lancet, 1986, ii : 1300-1304

26   Viberti GC, Mogensen CE., Groop LC, Pauls JF., for the European Microalbuminuria Study Group. Effect of Captopril on progression to clinical proteinuria in patients with insulin-dependent diabetes mellitus and microalbuminuria. J.A.M.A., 1994, 271 : 275-279

27   Laffel LBM., McGill JB, Gans DJ., on behalf of the North American Microalbuminuria Study Group : The beneficial effect of angiotensin converting enzyme inhibition with captopril on diabetic nephropathy in normotensive IDDM patients with microalbuminuria. Am. J. Med., 1995, 99 : 497-504

28   Mogensen CE, Osterby R, Hansen KW, Damsgaard EM Blood pressure elevation versus abnormal albuminuria in the genesis and prediction of renal disease in diabetes. Diabetes Care, 1992, 15 : 1192-1204

29   Mogensen CE. Long-term antihypertensive treatment inhibiting progression of diabetic nephropathy B.M.J., 1982, 285 : 685-688

30   Parving H-H., Andersen AR, Smidt UM, Svendsen PAA. Early aggressive antihypertensive treatment reduces the rate of decline in kidney function in diabetic nephropathy. Lancet, 1983, i : 1175-1179

31   Christensen CK, Mogensen CE. Effect of antihypertensive treatment on progression of incipient diabetic nephropathy. Hypertension, 1985, 7 (suppl II) : 109 - 113

32   Brenner BM, Humes HD. Mechanisms of glomerular ultrafiltration. N. Engl. J. Med., 1977, 297, 148-154

33   Keeton T, Campbell WB.The pharmacological alterations of renin release Pharmacol. Rev., 1980 ; 32 : 81-227

34   Zatz R, Meyer TW, Rennke HG, Brenner BM. Predominance of hemodynamic rather than metabolic factors in the pathogenesis of diabetic glomerulopathy Proc. Natl. Acad. Sci., U.S.A., 1985 ; 82 : 5963-5967

35   Parving H-H, Jensen HA, Mogensen CE., Evrin PE. Increased urinary albumin excretion rate in benign essential hypertension Lancet, 1974, i ; 15 : 1190-1192

36   Anderson S., Rennke H.G., Garcia D.L., Brenner B.M. Short and long term effects of antihypertensive therapy in the diabetic rat. Kidney Int., 1989, 36 : 526-536

37   Hallab M, Gallois Y, Chatellier G, Rohmer V, Fressinaud Ph, Marre M. Comparison of reduction in microalbuminuria by enalapril and hydrochlorothiazide in normotensive patients with insulin dependent diabetes. B.M.J., 1993, 306 : 175-182

38   Mogensen CE. Prediction of clinical diabetic nephropathy in IDDM patients : alternatives to microalbuminuria ?Diabetes, 1990, 39 : 761-767

39   Marre M, Claudel JP, Ciret P, Luis N, Suarez L, Passa P. Laser immunonephelometry for routine quantification of urinary albumin excretion Clin. Chem., 1987, 33 : 209-213

40   The Euclid Study Group Randomized placebo-controlled trial of lisinopril in normotensive patients with insulin-dependent diabetes and normoalbuminuria or microalbuminuri. Lancet, 1997, 349: 1787-1792

41   Marre M., Hallab M., Billiard A., Le Jeune J.J., Bled F., Girault A., Fressinaud P. Small doses of ramipril to reduce microalbuminuria in diabetic patients with incipient nephropathy independently of blood pressure changes J. Cardiovasc. Pharmacol., 1991, 18 : S165-8

42   Kasiske BL, Kalil RS, Ma JZ, Liao M, Keane WF. Effect of antihypertensive therapy on the kidney in patients with diabetes : a meta-regression analysis. Ann. Int. Med., 1993, 118 : 129-138

43   Melbourne Diabetic Nephropathy Study Group. Comparison between perindopril and nifedipine in hypertensive and normotensive diabetic patients with microalbuminuria. B.M.J., 1991, 302 : 210-216

44   Crepaldi G, Carta Q, Deferrari G, Mangili R, Navalesi R, Santeusanio F, Spalluto A., Vanasia A, Marco-Villa G, Nosadini R., The Italian Microalbuminuria Study Group in IDDM. Effects of Lisinopril and Nifedipine on the Progression to Overt Albuminuria in IDDM patients with Incipient Nephropathy and Normal Blood Pressure. Diabetes Care, 1998, 21: 104-110

45   Björk S, Mulec H, Johnsen SA, Nyberg G, Aurell M. Renal protective effect of enalapril in diabetic nephropathy. B.M.J., 1992, 304 : 339-343

46   Lewis EJ, Hunsicker LG, Bain RP, Rohde RD., for the Collaborative Study Group. The effect of angiotensin-converting-enzyme inhibition on diabetic nephropathy N. Engl. J. Med., 1993, 329 : 1456-1462

47   The microalbuminuria Captopril Study Group. Captopril reduces the risk of nephropathy in insulin-dependent diabetic patients with microalbuminuria. Diabetologia, 1996, 39: 587-593

48   Marre M, Fabbri P, Bouhanick B, Berrut G, LeJeune JJ. BLED F. Long-term follow-up of the glomerular filtration rate in normotensive type 1 diabetic subjects with microalbuminuria during angiotensin 1 converting enzyme inhibition. Nephrol. Dial. Transplant., 1998, 13: 1065-1066

49   American Diabetes Association. Diabetic Nephropathy. Diabetes Care, 1998, 21 (suppl. 1): 50-53

50   Mathiesen ER, Hommel E, Hansen HP, Smidt UM, Parving H-H. Randomised controlled trial of long term efficacy of captopril on preservation of kidney function in normotensive patients with insulin dependent diabetes and microalbuminuria. BMJ, 1999, 319: 24-25

51   Erley CM, Haefele U, Heyne N, Braun N, Risler T. Microalbuminuria in essential hypertension; reduction by different antihypertensive drugs. Hypertension, 1993, 21: 810-815

52 Azizi M, Rousseau A, Ezan E, Guyene TT, Michelet S, Grognet JM, Lenfant M, Corvol P, Menard J. Acute angiotensin-converting enzyme inhibition increases the plasma level of the natural stem cell regulator N-acetyl-seryl-aspartyl-lysyl-proline. J. Clin. Invest., 1996, 97 : 839-844

53 Ravid M, Savin H, Jutrin I, Bental T, Katz B., Lishner M.Long-term stabilizing effect of angiotensin converting enzyme inhibition on plasma creatinine and proteinuria in normotensive type II diabetic patients. Ann. Intern. Med., 1993, 118 : 577-581

54 Ravid M, Lang R, Rachmanil R, Lishner M. Long-term renoprotective effect of angiotensin-converting enzyme inhibition in non-insulin-dependent diabetes mellitus. A 7-year follow-up study Arch. Int. Med., 1996, 156 : 286-289

55 Mogensen CE. Microalbuminuria predicts clinical proteinuria and early mortality in maturity-onset diabetes N. Engl. J. Med., 1984, 310 : 356-60

56 Gaede P, Vedel P, Parving H-H, Pedersen O. Intensified multifactorial intervention in patients with type 2 diabetes mellitus and microalbuminuria : the Steno type 2 randomised study. The Lancet, 1999, 353: 617-622

34. REVERSIBILITY OF DIABETIC NEPHROPATHY LESIONS: A NEW CONCEPT

Paola Fioretto and Michael Mauer
Department of Medical and Surgical Sciences and Center of the National Research Council for the Study of Aging, University of Padova, Italy;
Department of Pediatrics, University of Minnesota, Minneapolis, MN, USA;

IMPROVED METABOLIC CONTROL AND PREVENTION OF DIABETIC NEPHROPATHY

The early lesions of diabetic glomerulopathy can be slowed or prevented by improved metabolic control [1, 2]. Little is known, however, regarding the potential for reversal of established structural changes. Unfortunately by the time renal functional abnormalities become manifest in diabetic patients, renal structural lesions are quite advanced [3]. At these late stages current treatments may slow but usually cannot arrest progression towards end-stage renal disease (ESRD) [4]. However, only a minority of patients with diabetes develop ESRD and, since early predictors of risk are unavailable or imprecise, it may not be reasonable to treat all patients aggressively. Thus, it is important to examine the possibility that certain renal structural changes may be reversible once functional changes are manifest.

The DCCT demonstrated a reduced incidence of microalbuminuria in patients with type 1 diabetes receiving intensified insulin therapy as compared with standard treatment [5]. Similar findings have been reported in type 2 diabetes by the UKPDS [6]. In a randomized controlled study intensive therapy resulted in less accumulation of mesangial matrix over 5 yrs in patients who had received renal allografts [2] and, in another study, in patients with their own kidneys there was reduced glomerular basement membrane thickening over 18 to 24 months during intensified insulin treatment [7]. Moreover, successful pancreas transplantation performed 2 to 4 yrs after kidney transplantation was associated, 4 to 6 yrs later, with less mesangial expansion than in diabetic patients after kidney transplantation alone [1].

EXTRACELLULAR MATRIX ACCUMULATION

Diabetic nephropathy (DN) is a disease resulting mainly from the accumulation of extracellular matrix (ECM) in the mesangium, glomerular (GBM) and tubular (TBM) basement membranes, and interstitium [3, 8-12]. ECM accumulation in DN largely represents increased quantities of the normal site specific ECM components. These include the α3 and α4 type IV collagen chains and laminins in the GBM and α1 and α2 chains of types IV and VI collagen, laminins, and fibronectin in mesangial matrix [13]. Interstitial (types I and III) collagens are absent from the glomerulus throughout most of the natural history of DN, becoming evident only in the final stages [13].

In normal subjects mesangial fractional volume and GBM width do not change between ages 16 and 60 yrs, this representing a remarkable constancy in adult life in the balance of glomerular ECM production and removal [14]. In contrast in diabetes there is a progressive accumulation in ECM in all renal compartments; whether this is due to increased production, decreased removal, or both is currently still unknown.

Regardless of the pathway(s) whereby the balance between ECM production and removal is altered in DN, if reversal of lesions is possible, it needs to operate by switching renal cellular function towards excess of removal of ECM.

ARE DIABETIC NEPHROPATHY LESIONS REVERSIBLE?
Islet transplantation in diabetic rats results in rapid reversal of established mesangial matrix and cell expansion but not of GBM thickening [15]. A more recent study suggested that glomerular lesions are reversible after shorter but not longer durations of diabetes in rats [16] but previous studies have shown that reversal also occurs in rats with long-standing diabetes and well-established diabetic glomerulopathy [17]. However, lesions in rats do not entirely parallel those seen in man.

In diabetic patients the possibility of reversal of DN can be adequately addressed by studying the recipients of pancreas transplantation (PTx) alone. We have studied 13 of these PTx recipients and found that, despite five yrs of normoglycemia, there was no amelioration of the established DN lesions [18]. In fact, GBM width was abnormal before PTx and was unchanged after 5 years; mesangial fractional volume [Vv(Mes/glom)] increased in these 13 patients, due to a decrease in glomerular volume (GV), while the total mesangial volume per glomerulus (TM) remained unchanged. Both GV and Vv(Mes/glom), and thus TM, increased over 5 years in a group of persistently diabetic patients. Thus, the mesangium stopped expanding in the PTx recipients but continued in the untreated patients [18]. Nevertheless the disappointing conclusion of this study was that diabetic glomerulopathy lesions were not ameliorated nor reversed by 5 yrs of normoglycemia.

Effects of longer-term normoglycemia: evidence for reversibility
Of the original cohort of 13 PTx recipients 8 were available for studies after 10 yrs of normoglycemia [19]. Of the remaining patients, 2 underwent kidney transplant 6 and 8 yrs after PTx, 2 lost graft function and required insulin therapy, and 1 deferred having the 10-yr studies performed. In the 8 available patients renal function tests and kidney biopsies were performed before and at 2, 5, and 10 yrs after PTx. At the time of PTx these patients were 33±3 (mean±SD) yrs old, had a duration of diabetes of 22±5 yrs and an HbA1c of 8.7±1.5%. The data on renal function in these patients are complex to

interpret, given the effects of cyclosporine on glomerular filtration rate (GFR) and albuminuria. Indeed there was a significant correlation between the changes in GFR and cyclosporine (CSA) dose and blood levels in these patients, especially in the first yr, as we described elsewhere [20]. The results on renal structure are easier to interpret. As discussed above, there was no beneficial effect on glomerular structure at 5 yrs post PTx; in contrast we observed obvious reversal of diabetic glomerulopathy lesions in all 8 patients, with glomerular and tubular morphometric parameters returning into the normal range in several instances. GBM and TBM width, unchanged at 5-yrs, decreased at 10-yr follow-up. The values at 10 yrs fell into the normal range in several patients, and in the remaining patients were approaching normal. Mesangial fractional volume and mesangial matrix fractional volume increased from baseline to 5 yrs but were lower at 10 yrs than at baseline or 5 yrs. Mean glomerular volume decreased from baseline to 5 yrs and was stable thereafter. Total mesangial and total mesangial matrix volumes per glomerulus were consequently unchanged at 5 yrs and markedly decreased at 10 yrs. Light microscopic observations revealed a remarkable remodelling of glomerular architecture in these patients, including the total disappearance of Kimmelstiel-Wilson nodular lesions and reopening of glomerular capillaries, previously compressed by mesangial expansion. Thus this study provides clear evidence that diabetic glomerular and tubular lesions are reversible in humans.

The improvement in kidney structure in the patients reported here is more likely due to prolonged normoglycemia than to immunosuppressive treatment since lesions of diabetes develop in the renal allograft at rates similar to those seen in native kidneys. The reasons for the long delay in reversal of diabetic nephropathy lesions are unknown. It can be hypothesized that renal cells have developed "memory" for the diabetic state [21], or that ECM molecules are heavily glycosylated and thus more resistant to proteolysis until replaced by less glycosylated molecules [22]. Nevertheless, the long time necessary for these diabetic lesions to disappear is consistent with their slow development [3, 8, 10, 12]. In fact diabetic renal lesions develop and progress from onset of diabetes over at least one decade before they can cause any functional abnormality [23]. Regardless of the mechanisms involved, at some point after PTx, ECM removal begins to exceed ECM production. This is abnormal since, as noted, renal ECM production and removal remain in near perfect balance during adult life [14]. If balance had been reestablished, the renal lesions would have remained stable, but this was not the case. In simplest terms, glomerular and tubular cells can "sense" that their ECM environment is abnormal and can alter their behaviour towards ECM removal and architectural remodeling.

As mentioned above, all PTx recipients were receiving CSA as part of their immunosuppressive regimen, and CSA is known to be nephrotoxic [24, 25]. As we have previously reported [20], there was indeed an increase in interstitial lesions and in the proportion of atrophic tubules at 5 yrs post PTx in these patients related to CSA treatment. Preliminary results suggest that at 10 yrs, when the CSA dose has substantially been reduced compared to the first yr, the interstitial lesions ameliorate returning to the degree observed pre-PTx [26]. Thus also the interstitium is capable of remodelling and healing upon reduction of CSA dose.

CONCLUSIONS

This study provides clear evidence that diabetic glomerular and tubular lesions in humans are reversible. This beneficial effect on renal structure was obtained with prolonged normoglycemia, and whether improved metabolic control or antihypertensive treatment might result in similar effects remains to be demonstrated. A recent study [27] described that angiotensin converting enzyme inhibitors and beta-blockers were similarly able to halt progression of the early lesions of diabetic glomerulopathy during a follow-up of 36-48 months in young type 1 diabetic patients with microalbuminuria; however, also in the untreated group several important parameters of glomerulopathy remained unchanged. Nevertheless, there was no evidence for reversal of lesions in the treated patients.

It is our view that all the therapeutic claims need to be accompanied by evidence of amelioration of the specific lesions of diabetic nephropathy before any given treatment can be accepted capable of reversing diabetic renal injury.

Despite the encouraging results of the studies summarized in this review, PTx cannot currently be considered a primary treatment for diabetic nephropathy. Recent studies have shown improved survival in type 1 diabetic recipients of simultaneous pancreas and kidney transplantation compared to kidney transplantation alone [28, 29]. Until similar data are available in recipients of PTx alone, this treatment should be reserved to those patients whose quality of life becomes unacceptable because of the metabolic instability of their diabetes. Nevertheless, regardless of the implications in terms of indications for PTx alone, these studies indicate that diabetic renal lesions are not only preventable, but reversible. This concept calls for further studies aimed at understanding the cellular and molecular mechanisms involved in the reversal and healing processes. The understanding of these processes could lead to new directions in the treatment of diabetic nephropathy.

REFERENCES

1. Bilous RW, Mauer SM, Sutherland DER, Najarian JS, Goetz FC, Steffes MW. The effects of pancreas transplantation on the glomerular structure of renal allografts in patients with insulin-dependent diabetes. N Engl J Med 1989; 321: 80-85.
2. Barbosa J, Steffes MW, Connet J, Venkateswara RK, Mauer SM. Effects of glycemic control on early diabetic renal lesions. JAMA 1994; 272: 600-606.
3. Mauer SM, Steffes MW, Ellis EN, Sutherland DER, Brown DM, Goetz FC: Structural-functional relationships in diabetic nephropathy. J Clin Invest 1984; 74: 1143-1155.
4. Lewis EJ, Hunsicker LG, Bain RP, Rhode RD. The effect of angiotensin-converting enzyme inhibition on diabetic nephropathy. N Engl J Med 1993; 329: 1456-1462.
5. DCCT Research Group. The effect of intensive treatment of diabetes on the development and progression of long-term complications in insulin-dependent diabetes mellitus. N Engl J Med 1993; 329: 977-986.
6. UKPDS Group. Intensive blood-glucose control with sulphonylureas or insulin compared with conventional treatment and risk of complications in patients with type 2 diabetes. Lancet 1998; 352: 837-853.

7.   Bangstad HJ, Østerby R, Dahl-Jørgensen K, Berg KJ, Hartmann A, Hanssen K F. Improvement of blood glucose control in IDDM patients retards progression of morphological changes in early diabetic nephropathy. Diabetologia 1994; 37: 483-490.

8.   Fioretto P, Steffes MW, Mauer SM. Glomerular structure in non-proteinuric insulin-dependent diabetic patients with various levels of albuminuria. Diabetes 1994; 43: 1358-1364.

9.   Østerby R. Early phases in the development of diabetic glomerulopathy. Acta Med Scand 1975; 475: 1-84.

10.   Mauer M, Mogensen CE, Friedman EA. Diabetic nephropathy. In Diseases of the Kidney, 5th edn. Edited by Schrier RW, Gottschalk CW. Boston: Little, Brown & Co. 1996: 2019-2062.

11.   Brito PL, Fioretto P, Drummond K, Kim Y, Steffes MW, Basgen JM, Sisson-Ross S, Mauer M. Proximal tubular basement membrane width in insulin-dependent diabetes mellitus. Kidney Int 1998; 53: 754-761.

12.   Steffes MW, Bilous RW, Sutherland DER, Mauer SM. Cell and matrix components of the glomerular mesangium in type I diabetes. Diabetes 1992; 41: 679-684.

13.   Zhu D, Kim Y, Steffes MW, Groppoli TJ, Butkowski RJ, Mauer SM. Glomerular distribution of type IV collagen in diabetes by high resolution quantitative immunochemistry. Kidney Int 1994; 45: 425-433.

14.   Steffes MW, Barbosa J, Basgen JM, Sutherland DER, Najarian JS, Mauer SM. Quantitative glomerular morphology of the normal human kidney. Lab Invest 1983; 49: 82-86.

15.   Steffes MW, Brown DM, Basgen JM, Mauer SM. Amelioration of mesangial volume and surface alterations following islet transplantation in diabetic rats. Diabetes 1980; 29: 509-515.

16.   Pugliese G, Pricci F, Pesce C, Romeo G, Lenti E, Caltabiano V, Vetri M, Purrello F, Di Mario U. Early, but not advanced, glomerulopathy is reversed by pancreatic islet transplants in experimental diabetic rats: Correlation with glomerular extracellular matrix mRNA levels. Diabetes 1997; 46: 1198-1206.

17.   Orloff MJ, Yamanaka N, Greenleaf GE, Huang Y-T, Huang D-G, Leng X-S. Reversal of mesangial enlargement in rats with long-standing diabetes by whole pancreas transplantation. Diabetes 1986; 35: 347-354.

18.   Fioretto P, Mauer SM, Bilous RW, Goetz FC, Sutherland DER, Steffes MW. Effects of pancreas transplantation on glomerular structure in insulin-dependent diabetic patients with their own kidneys. Lancet 1993; 342: 1193-1196.

19.   Fioretto P, Steffes MW, Sutherland DER, Goetz FC, Mauer M. Reversal of lesions of diabetic nephropathy after pancreas transplantation. N Engl J Med 1998; 339: 69-75.

20.   Fioretto P, Steffes MW, Mihach MJ, Strøm EH, Sutherland DER, Mauer M. Cyclosporine associated lesions in native kidneys of diabetic pancreas transplant recipients. Kidney Int 1995; 48: 489-495.

21.   Roys S, Sala R, Cagliero E. Lorenzi M. Overexpression of fibronectin induced by diabetes or high glucose: phenomenon with a memory. Proc Nat Acad Sci USA 1990; 87: 404-408.

22.   Brownlee M, Cerami A, Vlassara H. Advanced glycosylation end products in tissue and the biochemical basis of diabetic complications. N Engl J Med 1988; 318: 1315-1322.

23.   Krolewski AS, Warram JH, Christleb AR, Busick EJ, Kahn CR. The changing natural history of nephropathy in type I diabetes. Am J Med 1985; 78: 785-794.

24.   Myers BD, Sibley R, Newton L, et al. The long-term course of cyclosporine-associated chronic nephropathy. Kidney Int 1988; 33: 590-600.

25. Feutren G, Mihatsch MJ. Risk factors for cyclosporine induced nephropathy in patients with autoimmune diseases. N Engl J Med 1992; 326: 1654-1660.

26. Fioretto P, Steffes MW, Sutherland DER, Mauer M. Reversal of Cyclosporin associated interstitial changes in diabetic patients after long-term pancreas transplantation. JASN 1999; 10: 586A (abs).

27. Rudberg S, Østerby R, Bangstad HJ, Dahlquist G, Persson B. Effect of angiotensin converting enzyme inhibitor or beta blocker on glomerular structural changes in young microalbuminuric patients with type 1 diabetes mellitus. Diabetologia 1999; 42: 589-595.

28. Smets YFC, Westendorp RGJ, van der Pijl JW, de Charro FT, Ringers J, de Fijter JW, Lemkes HHPJ. Effects of simultaneous pancreas-kidney transplantation on mortality of patients with type 1 diabetes mellitus and end-stage renal disease. Lancet 1999; 353: 1915-1919.

29. Tyden G, Bolinder J, Solders G, Brattstrom C, Tibell A, Groth CG. Improved survival in patients with insulin-dependent diabetes mellitus and end-stage diabetic nephropathy 10 years after combined pancreas and kidney transplantation. Transplantation 1999; 67: 645-648.

35. ANTIHYPERTENSIVE TREATMENT IN NIDDM, WITH SPECIAL REFERENCE TO ABNORMAL ALBUMINURIA

Mark E. Cooper, Paul G. McNally and Geoffrey Boner
Department of Medicine, University of Melbourne, Austin & Repatriation Medical Centre (Repatriation Campus) West Heidelberg Australia and Leicester Royal Infirmary NHS Trust, Leicester, UK

The deleterious effects of systemic blood pressure on glomerular structure were reported more than twenty years ago in a patient with NIDDM and unilateral renal artery stenosis, in which characteristic nodular diabetic glomerulosclerosis was present in the non-ischaemic kidney only [1]. To date the impact of antihypertensive therapy on renal injury in NIDDM has received less attention than in IDDM. This is despite the cumulative incidence of persistent proteinuria and microalbuminuria in NIDDM subjects being comparable in frequency to IDDM subjects of similar duration [2, 3]. The clinical relevance of these figures is reflected by statistics which now show that over 50% of patients entering renal replacement programs have NIDDM [4-7]. Furthermore, in NIDDM the relationship between nephropathy and hypertension is more complex than in IDDM, since hypertension is not necessarily linked to the presence of renal disease, and often precedes the diagnosis of diabetes.

This review focuses on the role of antihypertensive agents in NIDDM subjects with abnormal albuminuria (microalbuminuria and macroalbuminuria), the significance of albuminuria in NIDDM and the consequences of treatment with these agents.

USE OF ANTIHYPERTENSIVE AGENTS IN NIDDM SUBJECTS WITH ESTABLISHED DIABETIC NEPHROPATHY (TABLE 35-1)

The impact of angiotensin converting enzyme inhibitors (ACEI), calcium channel blockers (CCB) and conventional antihypertensive agents on renal function has been evaluated in both normotensive and hypertensive NIDDM subjects with persistent proteinuria and variable degrees of renal impairment [8-23]. In hypertensive NIDDM subjects with persistent proteinuria studied for periods of at least 6 months, ACEI [8, 11, 22] and certain CCB [11, 22] reduced albuminuria. Parving's group has reported a disparity in effects on albuminuria and renal function [13]. Whereas lisinopril was more

Mogensen C.E. (ed.), THE KIDNEY AND HYPERTENSION IN DIABETES MELLITUS.
Copyright© 2000 by Kluwer Academic Publishers, Boston • Dordrecht • London. All rights reserved

effective than atenolol in reducing albuminuria, both agents were similar in efficacy in terms of rate of decline in GFR. A number of studies have confirmed that ACE inhibitors are superior to other antihypertensive agents including the dihydropyridine CCB including nifedipine [14, 16, 20] and nitrendipine [15] as well as the vasodilator, hydralazine [18], in reducing albuminuria in hypertensive NIDDM subjects with macroproteinuria. More recent studies have now included comparisons with AII antagonists [23]. In the recently reported study by Fogari et al which compared ramipril to nitrendipine, ACE inhibition was associated with an earlier and greater reduction in albuminuria than that observed with the CCB [15].

There have been significant differences in the effect on albuminuria obtained with various CCB, which has been attributed by Bakris and coworkers to the particular class of CCB [11, 19]. Bakris [11] initially demonstrated in hypertensive, nephrotic NIDDM subjects that diltiazem, a benzothiazepine CCB, had a comparable response to lisinopril in decreasing albuminuria. This author has also reported an anti-proteinuric effect with the CCB, verapamil [17]. In contrast, nifedipine, a dihydropyridine CCB, given for 6 weeks to 14 hypertensive NIDDM patients with baseline renal impairment, precipitated an increase in albuminuria and a deterioration in renal function, despite equivalent blood pressure reduction to diltiazem [24]. A similar lack of efficacy of the dihydropyridine class of CCB has been reported by other groups [14, 16]. In a study in African American NIDDM subjects with hypertension and macroproteinuria, isradipine was associated with an increase in proteinuria whereas captopril reduced proteinuria [21]. The role of alpha blockers in these patients has not been as well documented. Nevertheless, Rachmani et al in a cross-over study which included predominantly macroproteinuric but also microalbuminuric NIDDM subjects, the alpha blocker doxazosin tended to reduce albuminuria although possibly to a lesser extent than the ACEI, cilazapril [25].

Slataper et al have reported in a randomized parallel group study comparing diltiazem, lisinopril and conventional therapy (atenolol and frusemide) in hypertensive NIDDM subjects with marked albuminuria (> 2.5 g/24 hours) and renal insufficiency (creatinine clearance < 70 ml/min/1.73 m^2) [19] that after 18 months of therapy the rate of decline of glomerular filtration rate was attenuated with either diltiazem or lisinopril when compared to the conventional therapy group despite comparable blood pressure reduction [19]. The beneficial changes on glomerular filtration rate were paralleled by changes in albuminuria with significant reductions in the diltiazem and lisinopril groups, but no change in the conventionally treated group.

More recently, Bakris et al have reported the findings of 2 studies in hypertensive NIDDM subjects with overt proteinuria followed for at least 4 years [9, 10]. In both studies, the beta blocker atenolol was associated with a more rapid decline in GFR and less efficacy in terms of reduction in albuminuria than the non-dihydropyridine CCBs, verapamil and diltiazem [9, 10] or the ACEI, lisinopril [10].

THE USE OF ANTIHYPERTENSIVE AGENTS IN HYPERTENSIVE NIDDM WITH NORMOALBUMINURIA AND MICROALBUMINURIA (TABLE 35-2)

The use of antihypertensive therapy in NIDDM subjects with hypertension and microalbuminuria has been evaluated by an increasing number of investigators over the last decade [14, 26-34]. Gambardella and coworkers [26] showed that indapamide 2.5 mg daily did not alter albuminuria or glomerular filtration rate over a 24 month period in hypertensive normoalbuminuric patients despite a significant reduction in blood pressure. In contrast, in the microalbuminuric patients indapamide reduced albuminuria after 6 months and this effect was sustained at 36 months [26]. A double blind study compared captopril with conventional therapy (metoprolol and hydrochlorothiazide) in normoalbuminuric and microalbuminuric hypertensive NIDDM subjects over a 3 year period [27]. Both regimens reduced blood pressure without altering albuminuria in the normoalbuminuric NIDDM subjects. However, their findings in hypertensive NIDDM patients with microalbuminuria indicated that despite a comparable reduction in blood pressure, only the ACEI induced a persistent decline in albuminuria during the 36 months of therapy.

Although these findings suggested that the ACEI conferred a beneficial renoprotective effect long-term, these data are potentially biased by the fact that the conventionally treated group had a lower baseline glomerular filtration rate than the captopril treated group (87 versus 99 ml/min) and hence, possibly a greater potential to progress to macroalbuminuria. Also, the lack of a placebo group makes it difficult to determine if the effects of the conventional treatment could still represent a beneficial effect.

Schnack et al have recently reported that ramipril ± felodipine stabilised albuminuria. By contrast, atenolol ± diuretic treatment was associated with an increase in urinary albumin excretion [34]. Furthermore, the ramipril treated group had stable renal function whereas the group receiving beta blockers had a decline in GFR. A reduction in albuminuria by ACE inhibition has also been observed by a number of other investigators [14, 30-33, 35].

In the Melbourne Diabetic Nephropathy Study, nifedipine was shown to produce a similar response to perindopril in decreasing albuminuria over 12 months in the NIDDM subjects with microalbuminuria [28]. It has been reported by Chan et al that the ACEI, enalapril, was more effective than nifedipine over a median of 5 years in reducing albuminuria in a group of hypertensive microalbuminuric subjects [14]. Several studies have been reported which have compared calcium channel blockade with ACE inhibition in hypertensive microalbuminuric NIDDM subjects [30, 32, 33]. In a study over 3 years, in a relatively small number of subjects, amlodipine was as effective as the ACEI, cilazapril in reducing albuminuria with both treatment groups having similar declines in renal function [32]. Similar efficacy between enalapril and amlodipine in 50 hypertensive NIDDM subjects with microalbuminuria has recently been reported by Fogari et al [35]. However, in a much larger multi-centre study of over 300 subjects, the ACEI, lisinopril, reduced albuminuria over 12 months whereas nifedipine failed to significantly influence urinary albumin excretion [33].

Table 35-1. The effect of antihypertensive agents on albuminuria, renal function and blood pressure in hypertensive NIDDM subjects with established nephropathy

Agent	Duration	n	AER(%)*	GFR	BP	Reference
Captopril	6 months	9	↓(-62)	→	↓	Stornello et al [8]
Lisinopril (L)	5 years	18	↓(-25)	↓	↓	Bakris et al [9]
Atenolol		16	→	↓↓	↓	
V or Diltiazem		16	↓(-18)	↓	↓	
Verapamil	>4 years	18	↓(-60)	↓	↓	Bakris et al [10]
Atenolol		16	↓(-20)	↓↓	↓	
Diltiazem	18 weeks	8	↓(-38)	→	↓	Bakris [11]
Lisinopril			↓(-43)	→	↓	
Captopril	6 months	12	→	→	↓	Valvo et al [12]
Lisinopril	12 months	16	↓(-45)	↓	↓	Nielsen et al [13]
Atenolol		19	→	↓	↓	
Enalapril	5 years	11	→	→	↓	Chan et al [14]
Nifedipine		14	→	↓	↓	
Ramipril	2 years	26	↓(-32)	→	↓	Fogari et al [15]
Nitrendipine		25	↓(-19)	→	↓	
Enalapril	12 months	18	↓(-87)	→	↓	Ferder et al [16]
Nifendipine		12	→	→	↓	
Lisinopril	12 months	8	↓(-59)	↓	↓	Bakris et al [17]
Verapamil		8	↓(-50)	↓	↓	
L+V		8	↓(-78)	↓	↓	
G+H		6	→	↓	↓	
Captopril	18 months	24	↓(-27)	→	↓	Liou et al [18]
Hydralazine		18	→		↓	
Lisinopril	18 months	10	↓(-42)	→	↓	Slataper et al [19]
Diltiazem		10	↓(-45)	→	↓	
Frus & Atenolol		10	↓	↓	↓	
Captopril	6 months	10	↓(-50)	↓	↓	Romero et al [20]
Nifedipine		10	→(+18)	→	↓	
V	12 months	14	↓(-30)	→	↓	Bakris et al [22]
Trandolapril (T)		12	↓(-35)	→	↓	
T + V		11	↓(-63)	→	↓	
Irbesartan	12 weeks	24	↓(-8.5)	→	↓	Pohl et al [23]
Amlodipine		23	↑(+20)	↓	↓	

AER, Albumin excretion rate. GFR, glomerular filtration rate. BP, Blood pressure. V, Verapamil, Frus, Frusemide. G+H, Guanfacine + Hydrochlorothiazide. * In some of these studies proteinuria rather than AER was measured.

THE USE OF ANTIHYPERTENSIVE AGENTS IN NORMOTENSIVE NIDDM WITH MICROALBUMUNURIA (TABLE 35-2)

The possibility that early therapy will postpone or retard progression of renal injury in diabetes has led to the use of antihypertensive agents in normotensive subjects. Albuminuria was reduced in a group of normotensive NIDDM patients with microalbuminuria treated with captopril over a 6 month period, whereas the untreated group had no change in albuminuria [36]. In the Melbourne study [28] there was no change in albuminuria after 12 months treatment with either nifedipine or perindopril in normotensive microalbuminuric patients, despite a small but significant reduction in blood pressure (4 mmHg). Nonetheless, on stopping therapy at 12 months a dramatic increase in albuminuria was detected in the NIDDM but not in the IDDM subjects (Figure 35-1), which was independent of mode of treatment [37].

The inability of either agent to reduce albuminuria in the normotensive cohort coupled with the rapid rise after stopping therapy needs to be considered in the setting of the natural history of microalbuminuria. Albuminuria would be anticipated to rise by an average rise of 20 to 50 per cent if left untreated for 12 months in microalbuminuric NIDDM subjects. This phenomenon of a rapid rise in albuminuria was not as clearly apparent in the IDDM patients and may indicate a difference in the underlying etiology and pathogenesis of albuminuria in NIDDM as compared to IDDM. It is possible that there are differences in the sensitivity to structural damage incurred from blood pressure between IDDM and NIDDM.

The first long-term (5 years) placebo controlled double blind randomized study to evaluate the effect of an antihypertensive agent in normotensive microalbuminuric NIDDM with normal renal function (as assessed by a serum creatinine < 123 μmol/l) was reported by Ravid et al [38]. During the first year of treatment albuminuria decreased in the enalapril treated group from an initial mean of 143 mg/24 hours to a mean of 122 mg/24 hours. Thereafter, a small but steady increase in albuminuria occurred in the enalapril treated patients to 140 mg/24 hours after 5 years

Conversely, in the placebo treated patients a gradual increase in albuminuria occurred form a baseline of 123 to 310 mg/24 hours over the 5 years. Albuminuria exceeded 300 mg/24 hours in only 6/49 (12.2%) of the enalapril group compared to 19/45 (42.2%) of the placebo treated group. Renal function remained unchanged in the enalapril group during the first 2 years of follow up, but from the third year a small but non-significant decrease was evident, in the order of 1% after 5 years, in contrast to 13% in the placebo treated group. Although the assessment of renal function (assessed by the reciprocal of serum creatinine) was rather crude this is the first long-term study to demonstrate both an antiproteinuric effect of an ACEI in normotensive NIDDM patients with microalbuminuria and preservation of renal function. A follow up report after 7 years of treatment has confirmed a renoprotective effect of ACE inhibition in this cohort [41].

Table 35-2. The effect of anithypertensive agents on albumuninuria, renal function and blood pressure in NIDDM with normo-and microalbuminuria

Patients	Agent	Duration of study	n	Δ in AER (%)	Δ in GFR	Δ in BP	Reference
Normo	Enalapril (E)	5 years	18	→	→	↓	Chan et al [14]
HT	Nifedipine (N)		25	→	→	↓	
Micro	Enalapril		21	↓(-13)	→	↓	
HT	Nifedipine		13	↑(+13)	→	↓	
Micro HT	Indapamide	36 mths	10	↓(-64)	→	↓	Gambardella et al [26]
Normo	Captopril	36 mths	25	→	→	↓	Lacourcière et al [27]
HT	M or HCTZ		28	→	→	↓	
Micro	Captopril		9	↓(-65)	→	↓	
HT	M or HCTZ		12	→	→	↓	
Micro	Nifedipine	12 mths	13	→	→	→	MDNSG [28]
NT	Perindopril		11	→	→	→	
Micro	E + N	48 mths	11	↓(-42)	→	↓	Sano et al [29]
HT	Nifedipine		13	↑(+29)	→	↓	
	Enalapril		12	↓(-47)	→	↓	
Micro NT	Untreated		12	→	→	→	
Micro	Enalapril	12 mths	8	↓(-28)	↑	↓	Ruggenenti et al [30]
HT	Nitrendipine		8	↓(-17)	↑	↓	
Micro	Ramipril (R)	6 mths	54	↓(-27)	N/D	↓	Trevisan et al [31]
HT+NT	Placebo		54	↑(+28)	N/D	→	
Micro	Cilazipril	3 years	9	↓(-27)	↓	↓	Velussi et al [32]
HT	Amlodipine		9	↓(-31)	↓	↓	
Micro	Lisinopril	12 mths	156	↓(-37)	→	↓	Agardh et al [33]
HT	Nifedipine		158	→	→	↓	
Micro	R ± Felodipine	12 mths	46	→	→	↓	Schnack et al [34]
HT	A± HCTZ		45	↑	↓	↓	
Micro	Captopril	6 mths	13	↓(-36)	→	↓	Romero et al [36]
NT	Untreated		13	→	→	→	
Micro	Enalapril	5 years	49	→	→	→	Ravid et al [38]
NT	Placebo		45	↑(+152)	↓	→	
Micro	Enalapril	5 years	52	↓(-64)	→	→	Ahmad et al [39]
NT	Placebo		51	↑(+60)	→	→	

Normo, Normoalbuminuria. Micro, Microalbuminuria. HT, Hypertensive. NT, Normotensive. N/D, not done. AER, Albumin excretion rate. GFR, glomerular filtration rate. BP, Blood pressure. HCTZ, hydrochlorothiazide. M, metoprolol. A, atenolol.

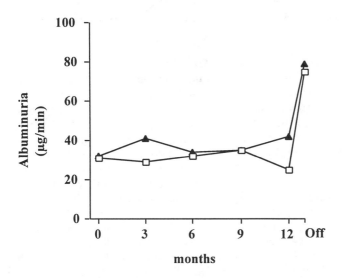

Figure 35-1. Effects of perindopril (□, n=11) or nifedipine (▲, n=13) on albuminuria (geometric means) over 12 months of treatment and after 1 month off treatment (Off) in normotensive microalbuminuric NIDDM patients from the Melbourne Diabetic Nephropathy Study, adapted from [40].

Sano et al have observed in a 4 year study that enalapril treatment reduced albuminuria whereas placebo treatment was associated with no change in albuminuria in a group of normotensive, microalbuminuric NIDDM patients [29]. Similar effects on albuminuria have been observed in a 6 month study by an Italian multi-centre group using the ACEI, ramipril [31].

Ahmad et al have reported similar effects on albuminuria after 5 years of ACEI therapy in a group of Indian normotensive NIDDM subjects with microalbuminuria [39]. Enalapril treatment was associated with a reduction in albuminuria whereas in the placebo group there was a progressive rise in urinary albumin excretion. Of particular interest was the finding that these effects were observed in the absence of a discernible difference in blood pressure between the two groups. Whether these effects of ACE inhibitors in normotensive patients will also be observed with other antihypertensive agents such as CCBs is the subject of a new placebo controlled study by the Melbourne Diabetic Nephropathy Study Group [42].

The exciting results obtained with antihypertensive drugs including ACE inhibitors in hypertensive and macroalbuminuric diabetic subjects stimulated investigators to explore the possible role of these agents in the prevention of diabetic nephropathy. Ravid et al have recently reported that treatment with enalapril for 6 years in a group of normotensive, normoalbuminuric NIDDM subjects was associated with a retardation in the increase in AER and in the decrease in renal function [43].

THE ROLE OF ANGIOTENSIN II RECEPTOR ANTAGONISTS

Although most studies involving agents which interrupt the renin-angiotensin system have used ACE inhibitors, the advent of angiotensin II (AII) receptor antagonists such as losartan provides a more specific approach to inhibit the actions of AII without influencing other hormonal systems such as bradykinin [44]. As yet, it is not clear if this new class will confer similar renal protection to ACE inhibitors [45]. Recently, several small studies have been performed in hypertensive and diabetic patients [46, 47]. In a study of elderly Chinese hypertensive subjects, some of whom had diabetes, losartan reduced albuminuria whereas the calcium channel blocker, felodipine, was ineffective [46]. A similar finding has been suggested from a preliminary analysis of a multi-centre study in European NIDDM subjects comparing amlodipine to losartan [47]. The AII antagonist, losartan but not amlodipine reduced albuminuria. Pohl et al have compared amlodipine to irbesartan in a 12 week study in hypertensive macroalbuminuric NIDDM subjects. Despite a similar decrease in blood pressure, treatment with irbesartan resulted in a decrease whereas amlodipine was associated with an increase in proteinuria [23]. The relevance of these findings are now being explored with several large clinical trials in progress to assess the renoprotective effects of AII receptor antagonists in NIDDM patients with macroproteinuria. (Table 35-3). The primary end-points of the 2 studies are similar to that previously used in a similarly designed study in IDDM subjects with nephropathy [48], i.e a composite end-point of doubling of serum creatinine, renal transplantation, dialysis and all-cause death. Secondary end-points of the 2 studies will include cardiovascular events

Table 35-3

Trial	Inclusion criteria	Drug Protocol	N	Duration
IDNT [49]	NIDDM Hypertension Macroproteinuria	Irbesartan Placebo Amlodipine	1650	Minimum 2 yrs
RENAAL [50]	NIDDM Macroproteinuria (UA/C > 300mg/g)	Losartan vs placebo (all agents except ACEi or AIIRA)	1500	Mean duration 4.5 yrs

ROLE OF COMBINATION THERAPY

It has been proposed that the combination of a calcium antagonist with a converting enzyme inhibitor should result in a greater reduction in urinary protein excretion and slowed morphological progression of nephropathy [51]. Bakris et al have compared the renal hemodynamic and antiproteinuric effects of a calcium antagonist, verapamil, and an ACEI, lisinopril, alone and in combination in three groups of non-insulin dependent diabetic subjects with documented nephrotic range proteinuria, hypertension, and renal insufficiency [17]. Patients treated with the combination of a calcium antagonist and an ACEI manifested the greatest reduction in albuminuria. In addition, the decline in GFR was the lowest in this group. Similar findings are suggested by another study performed in microalbuminuric subjects using the combination of verapamil and cilazapril [52]. Sano et al have shown that the addition of enalapril to nifedipine conferred an additional effect in decreasing albuminuria in a group of microalbuminuric NIDDM subjects [29]. Bakris et al have suggested that the combination of verapamil and trandolapril, administered in a fixed dose combination, is more effective at reducing proteinuria than either drug alone, despite similar effects on blood pressure [22, 53]. Similar findings have also been reported by Fogari et al who have shown that benazepril plus amlodipine tended to be more effective than benazepril alone in reducing albuminuria in microalbuminuric, hypertensive NIDDM patients [54]. Rachmani et al have explored the combination of cilazapril and doxazosin and shown this regimen to be effective at reducing blood pressure and albuminuria [25]. The above findings with combination therapy provide an exciting approach for optimizing antihypertensive therapy in diabetic patients with renal disease. Indeed, the recent criteria for blood pressure control in diabetes as proposed by JNC-VI [55] and WHO-ISH [56] will require the use of multiple antihypertensive agents.

Recently, it has been postulated that more effective blockade of the renin-angiotensin system by combining an ACE inhibitor with an AII antagonist may be a useful approach for reducing blood pressure and albuminuria in hypertensive, microalbuminuric type II diabetic patients. Indeed, in the CALM study, preliminary analysis suggests that the combination of lisinopril and candesartan is superior to monotherapy in decreasing blood pressure and possibly urinary albumin excretion in such a population [57]

THE USE OF ANTIHYPERTENSIVE AGENTS IN PATIENTS WITH NIDDM.

The choice of an antihypertensive agent in the management of abnormal albuminuria in NIDDM depends not only on its potential renoprotective effect but must take into consideration other factors which could be deleterious to the patient. Microalbuminuria in the NIDDM patient is more closely linked to subsequent death from cardiovascular disease than from nephropathy [58]. Therefore, it is important that any antihypertensive intervention in the NIDDM patient with abnormal albuminuria does not exacerbate existing hypertriglyceridaemia or further reduce HDL-cholesterol, lipid abnormalities associated with NIDDM [59]. Furthermore, reduced sensitivity to insulin after administration of thiazides and various beta-blockers may be detrimental [60]. However, more recent studies suggest that low dose diuretics do not have deleterious effects on plasma glucose or lipid levels [61]. In contrast, improved insulin sensitivity is seen after captopril [60] and doxazocin [62] and minimal or neutral effects are observed with CCB [63]. Also, in contrast to beta-blockers and thiazide diuretics, neither CCB nor ACEI affect glucose tolerance deleteriously [63]. The effects of the AII receptor antagonists such as losartan have not been as extensively studied but they appear to have either no effect [64] or a beneficial effect on insulin sensitivity [65].

WHICH AGENT TO USE?

The limited evidence so far published on the effects of antihypertensive agents in NIDDM with abnormal albuminuria concur with findings in IDDM [66]. Both ACEI and CCB may possess beneficial effects over and above simple blood pressure control, although in most studies the small numbers of subjects included may have introduced a Type II statistical error.   Several meta-analyses of trials involving patients with either IDDM or NIDDM have demonstrated the salutary effects of ACEI on proteinuria and renal function compared to other classes of antihypertensive agent, whether or not the patients had IDDM or NIDDM, hypertension, normoalbuminuria, microalbuminuria or macroproteinuria [67,68]. These analyses have suggested that ACE inhibitors have an ability to reduce proteinuria independent of their hypotensive effects. However, a recent update of one of these meta-analyses has suggested that at maximal hypotensive doses no significant difference was observed in the anti-proteinuric effects of ACE inhibitors and other antihypertensive drugs [69].

ANTIHYPERTENSIVE THERAPY IN NIDDM: MORE THAN JUST REDUCING ALBUMINURIA

Microalbuminuria predicts not only nephropathy in NIDDM subjects but also is a strong predictor of all-cause mortality, particularly from cardiovascular diseases [58]. Therefore, the effects of these antihypertensive agents must include assessment of cardiovascular endpoints.   In the ABCD study it was suggested that ACE inhibitor therapy was superior to dihydropyridine CCBs in conferring vascular protection [70]. Similar findings were reported from the FACET study which suggested that fosinopril was associated with less cardiovascular events than amlodipine [71]. If ACE inhibitors confer cardioprotective effects which are not as clearly evident with dihydropyridine CCBs remains an area of intense investigation. It is more likely that the ACE inhibitors are conferring an additional beneficial effect rather than the CCBs having a deleterious effect on cardiovascular events in this population. For example, in the Syst-EUR study, a subgroup analysis of the diabetic cohort with systolic hypertension revealed a beneficial effect of nitrendipine on cardiovascular outcomes [72]. In the HOT study which involved randomisation of subjects to 3 different target blood pressures with a felodipine based regimen, analysis of the diabetic subgroup showed that the lowest blood pressure target group had the lowest incidence of cardiovascular morbidity and mortality [73]. This would suggest that blood pressure reduction *per se* is a major determinant of cardioprotection in this diabetic population.   However, it must be appreciated that the group randomized to the lowest blood pressure group had the highest prevalence of concomitant antihypertensive agents, including ACE inhibitors and beta-blockers, which may have conferred additional cardioprotection. In the recently published CAPPP study, within the diabetic subgroup, captopril appeared to be superior to the diuretic/beta blocker regimen despite similar blood pressure reduction [74]. There was an approximately 40% decrease in the primary end-point, fatal and non-fatal myocardial infarction and stroke and other cardiovascular deaths with captopril compared to diuretic/beta blocker therapy. In the UKPDS blood pressure reduction was clearly shown to reduce vascular events [75]. Further analysis revealed no difference between the group treated with captopril or atenolol [76]. However, in this study there was a very high level of non-compliance (20-40%) and over 60% of subjects were on 2 or more drugs. Currently there a number of large studies in progress which are further addressing this issue [77-79].

The importance of ACE inhibitors in conferring macrovascular in addition to renal protection has recently been demonstrated in the HOPE study. In the diabetic subgroup, despite ramipril treatment reducing blood pressure by only 2/1 mmHg, there was a 25% decrease in cardiovascular death, myocardial infarction and stroke and a 24% decrease in total mortality[80].

ALBUMINURIA AND RENAL STRUCTURE IN NIDDM

Although the principal endpoint in evaluating the influence of an antihypertensive agent on renal function in diabetes is its ability to alter the progression of the disease, it is clear that abnormally elevated albuminuria is also associated with progressive renal injury [81]. Although many of the short-term trials that have been performed in subjects with NIDDM only document a reduction in albuminuria in the absence of a change in glomerular filtration rate, longterm studies in IDDM subjects suggest that the severity of proteinuria also correlates with the rate of progression of renal disease [82]. A similar link between the level of albuminuria and decline in renal function has been reported in a study of hypertensive NIDDM patients [83]. Nonetheless, studies involving renal structural assessment are warranted to more accurately determine the response to antihypertensive agents. Fioretto et al have investigated the underlying pathology which occurs in NIDDM patients with various stages of nephropathy [84]. There appears to be a marked variation in the degree of glomerulosclerosis and tubulointerstitial fibrosis in this population with only about one third having the typical histology of diabetic nephropathy. Recently it has been demonstrated in a small study that the ACEI, perindopril, can attenuate the development of renal injury and in particular tubulointerstitial expansion [85].

Finally, although the focus of treatment of NIDDM subjects with early and overt renal disease has been on antihypertensive therapy one cannot ignore the role of glycaemic control. In natural history studies, it has been shown that glycaemic control is a major determinant of the rate of progression of albuminuria, not only in IDDM but also in NIDDM subjects [86]. Furthermore, a recent study in Japanese NIDDM subjects has shown that intensified insulin therapy over a 6 year period prevented the progression of diabetic microvascular complications including nephropathy [87]. These findings are similar to those reported from the DCCT study performed in IDDM subjects [88]. The recent findings from the UKPDs confirm a pivotal role for glycaemic control in the progression of vascular complications including nephropathy [89]. Ravid et al have shown in a cross-sectional analysis of recently diagnosed NIDDM patients that multiple factors are involved in the increase in albuminuria and the decrease in renal function [90]. These include glycated hemoglobin, mean blood pressure and total cholesterol. Indeed, the recent Steno 2 study has emphasized in a group of type II diabetic patients with microalbuminuria, the role of multifactorial intervention including not only intensified glycemic control and blood pressure reduction, but also other treatments, including lipid lowering drugs, exercise, cessation of smoking, aspirin and antioxidants [91].

REFERNCES

1. Berkman J, Rifkin H.   Unilateral nodular diabetic glomerulosclerosis (Kimmelstiel-Wilson). Report of a case. Metabolism Clin Exp 1973; 22: 715-722.
2. Nelson RG, Knowler WC, McCance DR, Sievers ML, Pettitt DJ, Charles MA, Hanson RL, Liu QZ, Bennett PH. Determinants of end-stage renal disease in Pima Indians with type 2 (non-insulin-dependent) diabetes mellitus and proteinuria. Diabetologia 1993; 36: 1087-93.
3. Ritz E, Stefanski A. Diabetic nephropathy in type II diabetes. Am J Kidney Dis 1996; 27: 167-194.
4. Grenfell A, Bewick M, Snowden S, Watkins PJ, Parsons V. Renal replacement for diabetic patients: experience at King's College Hospital 1980-1989. Q J Med 1992; 85: 861-74.
5. Excerpts from the United States Renal Data System. 1998 Annual Data Report. Chapter II Incidence and prevalence of ESRD. Am J Kidney Dis 1998; 32 (Suppl 1): S39-S49.
6. Pugh JA, Medina RA, Cornell JC, Basu S. NIDDM is the major cause of diabetic end-stage renal disease. More evidence from a tri-ethnic community. Diabetes 1995; 44: 1375-80.
7. Cowie CC. Diabetic renal disease: racial and ethnic differences from an epidemiologic perspective. Transplant Proc 1993; 25: 2426-30.
8. Stornello M, Valvo E, Vasques E, Leone S, Scapellato L. Systemic and renal effects of chronic angiotensin converting enzyme inhibition with captopril in hypertensive diabetic patients. J Hypertension 1989; 7 (suppl 7): S65-S67.
9. Bakris GL, Copley JB, Vicknair N, Sadler R, Leurgans S. Calcium channel blockers versus other antihypertensive therapies on progression of NIDDM associated nephropathy. Kidney International 1996; 50: 1641-1650.
10. Bakris GL, Mangrum A, Copley JB, Vicknair N, Sadler R. Effect of calcium channel or beta-blockade on the progression of diabetic nephropathy in African Americans. Hypertension 1997; 29: 744-750.
11. Bakris GL. Effects of diltiazem or lisinopril on massive proteinuria associated with diabetes mellitus. Ann Intern Med 1990; 112: 707-708.
12. Valvo EV, Bedogna V, Casagrande P, Antiga L, Zamboni M, Bommartini F, Oldrizzi L, Rugiu C, Maschio G. Captopril in patients with type II diabetes and renal insufficiency: systemic and renal hemodynamic alterations. Am J Med 1988; 85: 344-348.

13. Nielsen FS, Rossing P, Gall MA, Skott P, Smidt UM, Parving HH. Impact of lisinopril and atenolol on kidney function in hypertensive NIDDM subjects with diabetic nephropathy. Diabetes 1994; 43: 1108-13.

14. Chan JCN, Ko GTC, Leung DHY, Cheung RCK, Cheung MYF, So WY, Swaminathan R, Nicholls MG, Critchley J, Cockram CS. Long-term effects of angiotensin-converting enzyme inhibition and metabolic control in hypertensive type 2 diabetic patients. Kidney Int, 2000; 57: 590-600.

15. Fogari R, Zoppi A, Corradi L, Mugellini A, Lazzari P, Preti P, Lusardi P. Long-term effects of ramipril and nitrendipine on albuminuria in hypertensive patients with type II diabetes and impaired renal function. J Hum Hypertens 1999; 13: 47-53.

16. Ferder L, Daccordi H, Martello M, Panzalis M, Inserra F. Angiotensin converting enzyme inhibitors versus calcium antagonists in the treatment of diabetic hypertensive patients. Hypertension 1992; 19: II237-42.

17. Bakris GL, Barnhill BW, Sadler R. Treatment of arterial hypertension in diabetic humans: importance of therapeutic selection. Kidney Inter 1992; 41: 912-9.

18. Liou HH, Huang TP, Campese VM. Effect of long-term therapy with captopril on proteinuria and renal function in patients with non-insulin-dependent diabetes and with non-diabetic renal diseases. Nephron 1995; 69: 41-8.

19. Slataper R, Vicknair N, Sadler R, Bakris GL. Comparative effects of different antihypertensive treatments on progression of diabetic renal disease. Arch Intern Med 1993; 153: 973-80.

20. Romero R, Salinas I, Lucas A, Teixido J, Audi L, Sanmarti A. Comparative effects of captopril versus nifedipine on proteinuria and renal function of type 2 diabetic patients. Diabetes Res Clin Pract 1992; 17: 191-8.

21. Guasch A, Parham M, Zayas CF, Campbell O, Nzerue C, Macon E. Contrasting effects of calcium channel blockade versus converting enzyme inhibition on proteinuria in african americans with non-insulin-dependent diabetes mellitus and nephropathy. Journal of the American Society of Nephrology 1997; 8: 793-798.

22. Bakris GL, Weir MR, Dequattro V, McMahon FG. Effects of an ACE inhibitor calcium antagonist combination on proteinuria in diabetic nephropathy. Kidney International 1998; 54: 1283-1289.

23. Pohl M, Cooper M, Ulrey J, Pauls J, Rohde R. Safety and efficacy of irbesartan in hypertensive patients with type II diabetes and proteinuria. Am J Hypertens 1997; 10: 105A.

24. Demarie BK, Bakris GL. Effects of different calcium antagonists on proteinuria assocaited with diabetes mellitus. Ann Intern Med 1990; 113: 987-988.

25. Rachmani R, Levi Z, Slavachevsky I, Half-Onn E, Ravid M. Effect of an alpha-adrenergic blocker, and ACE inhibitor and hydrochlorothiazide on blood pressure and on renal function in type 2 diabetic patients with hypertension and albuminuria. A randomized cross- over study. Nephron 1998; 80: 175-82.

26. Gambardella S, Frontoni S, Lala A, Felici MG, Spallone V, Scoppola A, Jacoangeli F, Menzinger G. Regression of microalbuminuria in type II diabetic, hypertensive patients after long-term indapamide treatment. Am Heart J 1991; 122: 1232-8.

27. Lacourciere Y, Nadeau A, Poirier L, Tancrede G. Captopril or conventional therapy in hypertensive type II diabetics. Three-year analysis. Hypertension 1993; 21: 786-94.

28. Melbourne Diabetic Nephropathy Study Group. Comparison between perindopril and nifedipine in hypertensive and normotensive diabetic patients with microalbuminuria. Br Med J 1991; 302: 210-6.

29. Sano T, Kawamura T, Matsumae H, Sasaki H, Nakayama M, Hara T, Matsuo S, Hotta N, Sakamoto N. Effects of long-term enalapril treatment on persistent micro-albuminuria in well-controlled hypertensive and normotensive NIDDM patients. Diabetes Care 1994; 17: 420-4.

30. Ruggenenti P, Mosconi L, Bianchi L, Cortesi L, Campana M, Pagani G, Mecca G, Remuzzi G. Long-term treatment with either enalapril or nitrendipine stabilizes albuminuria and increases glomerular filtration rate in non-insulin-dependent diabetic patients. American Journal of Kidney Diseases 1994; 24: 753-761.

31. Trevisan R, Tiengo A. Effect of low-dose ramipril on microalbuminuria in normotensive or mild hypertensive non-insulin-dependent diabetic patients. North-East Italy Microalbuminuria Study Group. Am J Hypertens 1995; 8: 876-83.

32. Velussi M, Brocco E, Frogato F, Zolli M, Muollo B, Maioli M, Carraro A, Tonolo G, Fresu P, Cernigoi AM, Fioretto P, Nosadini R. Effects of cilazapril and amlodipine on kidney function in hypertensive NIDDM patients. Diabetes 1996; 45: 216-222.

33. Agardh CD, Garcia Puig J, Charbonnel B, Angelkort B, Barnett AH. Greater reduction of urinary albumin excretion in hypertensive type II diabetic patients with incipient nephropathy by lisinopril than by nifedipine. J Hum Hypertens 1996; 10: 185-92.

34. Schnack C, Hoffmann W, Hopmeier P, Schernthaner G. Renal and metabolic effects of 1-year treatment with ramipril or atenolol in niddm patients with microalbuminuria. Diabetologia 1996; 39: 1611-1616.

35. Fogari R, Zoppi A, Malamani GD, Lusardi P, Destro M, Corradi L. Effects of amlodipine vs enalapril on microalbuminuria in hypertensive patients with type II diabetes. Clinical Drug Investigation 1997; 13: 42-49.

36. Romero R, Salinas I, Lucas A, Abad E, Reverter JL, Johnston S, Sanmarti A. Renal function changes in microalbuminuric normotensive type II diabetic patients treated with angiotensin-converting enzyme inhibitors. Diabetes Care 1993; 16: 597-600.

37. Jerums G, Allen TJ, Tsalamandris C, Cooper ME, Melbourne Diabetic Nephropathy Study Group. Angiotensin Converting Enzyme inhibition and Calcium Channel Blockade in incipient diabetic nephropathy. Kidney Int 1992; 41: 904-911.

38. Ravid M, Savin H, Jutrin I, Bental T, Katz B, Lishner M. Long-term stabilizing effect of angiotensin-converting enzyme inhibition on plasma creatinine and on proteinuria in normotensive type II diabetic patients. Ann Intern Med 1993; 118: 577-81.

39. Ahmad J, Siddiqui MA, Ahmad H. Effective postponement of diabetic nephropathy with enalapril in normotensive type 2 diabetic patients with microalbuminuria. Diabetes Care 1997; 20: 1576-1581.

40. Cooper ME, Doyle AE. The management of diabetic proteinuria. Which antihypertensive agent? Drugs Aging 1992; 2: 301-9.

41. Ravid M, Lang R, Rachmani R, Lishner M. Long-term renoprotective effect of angiotensin-converting enzyme inhibition in non-insulin-dependent diabetes mellitus. A 7-year follow-up study. Arch Intern Med 1996; 156: 286-9.

42. Melbourne Diabetic Nephropathy Study Group, Cooper ME, Allen T, Jerums G, DeLuise M, Alford F, Doyle AE. Effects of different antihypertensive agents on normotensive microalbuminuric type I and type II diabetic patients. Proc XIIth International Congress of Nephrology 1993; Jerusalem: 424.

43. Ravid M, Brosh D, Levi Z, Bardayan Y, Ravid D, Rachmani R. Use of enalapril to attenuate decline in renal function in normotensive, normoalbuminuric patients with type 2 diabetes mellitus - a randomized, controlled trial. Annals of Internal Medicine 1998; 128: 982-8.

44. Johnston CI. Angiotensin receptor antagonists: focus on losartan. Lancet 1995; 346: 1403-7.

45. Ichikawa I, Madias NE, Harrington JT, King AS, Singh A, Levey AS. Will angiotensin II receptor antagonists be renoprotective in humans? Kidney International 1996; 50: 684-692.

46. Chan JCN, Critchley J, Tomlinson B, Chan TYK, Cockram CS. Antihypertensive and anti-albuminuric effects of losartan potassium and felodipine in chinese elderly hypertensive patients with or without non-insulin-dependent diabetes mellitus. American Journal of Nephrology 1997; 17: 72-80.

47. Os I. Losartan vs. amlodipine in hypertensive patients with NIDDM. . Proc 15th International Congress of Nephrology Symposium 'Emerging therapeutic intervention with AII antagonism in diabetic nephropathy'; 1997.

48. Lewis EJ, Hunsicker LG, Bain RP, Rohde RD. The effect of angiotensin converting enzyme inhibition on diabetic nephropathy. N Engl J Med 1993; 329: 1456-62.

49. Rodby RA. Antihypertensive treatment in nephropathy of type II diabetes: role of the pharmacological blockade of the renin-angiotensin system. Nephrol Dial Transplant 1997; 12: 1095-6.

50. Brenner B, Shahinfar S, for the RENAAL Investigators. Reduction of endpoints in NIDDM with the angiotensin II antagonist losartan. Proc XVth International Congress of Nephrology 1999; : 163 (abstract 648).

51. Brown SA, Walton CL, Crawford P, Bakris GL. Long-term effects of antihypertensive regimens on renal hemodynamics and proteinuria. Kidney Int 1993; 43: 1210-8.

52. Fioretto P, Frigato F, Velussi M, Riva F, Muollo B, Carraro A, Brocco E, Cipollina MR, Abaterusso C, Trevisan M, Crepaldi G, Nosadini R. Effects of angiotensin converting enzyme inhibitors and calcium antagonists on atrial natriuretic peptide release and action and on albumin excretion rate in hypertensive insulin-dependent diabetic patients. Am J Hypertens 1992; 5: 837-46.

53. Bakris G, Weir M, De Quattro V, Rosendorff C, McMahon G. Renal effects of a long acting ACE inhibitor, trandolapril (T) or nondihydropyridine calcium blocker, verapamil (V) or in a fixed dose combination in diabetic nephropathy: A randomized double blind placebo controlled multicenter study. Nephrology 1997; 3 (Suppl 1): S271.

54. Fogari R, Zoppi A, Mugellini A, Lusardi P, Destro M, Corradi L. Effect of benazepril plus amlodipine vs benazepril alone on urinary albumin excretion in hypertensive patients with type ii diabetes and microalbuminuria. Clinical Drug Investigation 1997; 13: 50-55.

55. Joint National Committee on Prevention, Detection, Evaluation, and Treatment of High Blood Pressure. The sixth report of the Joint National Committee on Prevention, Detection, Evaluation, and Treatment of High Blood Pressure. Arch Intern Med 1997; 157: 2413-2445.

56. Guidelines Subcommittee. 1999 World Health Organization - International Society of Hypertension guidelines for the management of hypertension. J Hypertens 1999; 17: 151-183.

57. Mogensen CE, Cooper ME. Unpublished data, 1999.

58. Mogensen CE. Microalbuminuria predicts clinical proteinuria and early mortality in maturity-onset diabetes. N Engl J Med 1984; 310: 356-60.

59. Garber AJ, Vinik AI, Crespin SR. Detection and management of lipid disorders in diabetic patients. A commentary for clinicians. Diabetes Care 1992; 15: 1068-74.

60. Lind L, Pollare T, Berne C, Lithell H. Long-term metabolic effects of antihypertensive drugs. Am Heart J 1994; 128: 1177-83.

61.   Harper R, Ennis CN, Heaney AP, Sheridan B, Gormley M, Atkinson AB, Johnston GD, Bell PM. A comparison of the effects of low- and conventional-dose thiazide diuretic on insulin action in hypertensive patients with NIDDM. Diabetologia 1995; 38: 853-9.

62.   Giordano M, Matsuda M, Sanders L, Canessa ML, DeFronzo RA. Effects of angiotensin-converting enzyme inhibitors, Ca2+ channel antagonists, and alpha-adrenergic blockers on glucose and lipid metabolism in NIDDM patients with hypertension. Diabetes 1995; 44: 665-71.

63.   Stein P, Black H. Drug treatment of hypertension in patients with diabetes mellitus. Diabetes Care 1991; 14: 425-448.

64.   Laakso M, Karjalainen L, Lempiainenkuosa P. Effects of losartan on insulin sensitivity in hypertensive subjects. Hypertension 1996; 28: 392-396.

65.   Moan A, Hoieggen A, Nordby G, Eide IK, Kjeldsen SE. Effects of losartan on insulin sensitivity in severe hypertension - connections through sympathetic nervous system activity. Journal of Human Hypertension 1995; 9: 50.

66.   Mathiesen ER, Hommel E, Giese J, Parving H-H. Efficacy of captopril in postponing nephropathy in normotensive insulin dependent diabetic patients with microalbuminuria. Br Med J 1991; 303: 81-7.

67.   Kasiske BL, Kalil RS, Ma JZ, Liao M, Keane WF. Effect of antihypertensive therapy on the kidney in patients with diabetes: a meta-regression analysis. Ann Intern Med 1993; 118: 129-38.

68.   Bohlen L, de Courten M, Weidmann P. Comparative study of the effect of ACE-inhibitors and other antihypertensive agents on proteinuria in diabetic patients. Am J Hypertens 1994; 7: 84s-92s.

69.   Weidmann P, Schneider M, Bohlen L. Therapeutic efficacy of different antihypertensive drugs in human diabetic nephropathy: an updated meta-analysis. Nephrol Dial Transpl 1995; 10(suppl): 39-45.

70.   Estacio RO, Jeffers BW, Hiatt WR, Biggerstaff SL, Gifford N, Schrier RW. The effect of nisoldipine as compared with enalapril on cardiovascular outcomes in patients with non-insulin-dependent diabetes and hypertension. N Engl J Med 1998; 338: 645-652.

71.   Tatti P, Pahor M, Byington RP, DiMauro P, Guarisco R, Strollo G, Strollo F. Outcome results of the Fosinopril versus Amlodipine Cardiovascular Events randomised Trial (FACET) in patients with hypertension and non-insulin dependent diabetes mellitus. Diabetes Care 1998; 21: 597-603.

72.   Tuomilehto J, Rastenyte D, Birkenhager WH, et al. Effects of calcium-channel blockade in older patients with diabetes and systolic hypertension. New England Journal of Medicine 1999; 340: 677-684.

73.   Hansson L, Zanchetti A, Carruthers SG, Dahlof B, Elmfeldt D, Julius S, Ménard J, Rahn KH, Wedel H, Westerling S, for the HOT Study Group. Effects of intensive blood-pressure lowering and low-dose aspirin in patients with hypertension: principal results of the Hypertension Optimal treatment (HOT) randomised trial. Lancet 1998; 351: 1755-62.

74.   Hansson L, Lindholm LH, Niskanen L, Lanke J, Hedner T, Niklason A, Luomanmaki K, Dahlof B, de Faire U, Morlin C, Karlberg BE, Wester PO, Bjorck JE. Effect of angiotensin-converting-enzyme inhibition compared with conventional therapy on cardiovascular morbidity and mortality in hypertension: the Captopril Prevention Project (CAPPP) randomised trial. Lancet 1999; 353: 611-616.

75.   UK Prospective Diabetes Study (UKPDS) Group. Tight blood pressure control and risk of macrovascular and microvascular complications in type 2 diabetes - UKPDS 38. British Medical Journal 1998; 317: 703-713.

76. UK Prospective Diabetes Study (UKPDS) Group. Efficacy of atenolol and captopril in reducing risk of macrovascular and microvascular complications in type 2 diabetes - UKPDS 39. British Medical Journal 1998; 317: 713-720.

77. Passa P, Chatellier G. The Diab-HYCAR study. Diabetologia 1996; 39: 1662-1667.

78. Gerstein HC, Bosch J, Pogue J, Taylor DW, Zinman B, Yusuf S. Rationale and design of a large study to evaluate the renal and cardiovascular effects of an ACE inhibitor and vitamin E in high-risk patients with diabetes. The MICRO-HOPE Study. Microalbuminuria, cardiovascular, and renal outcomes. Heart Outcomes Prevention Evaluation. Diabetes Care 1996; 19: 1225-8.

79. Davis BR, Cutler JA, Gordon DJ, Furberg CD, Wright JT, Cushman WC, Grimm RH, Larosa J, Whelton PK, Perry HM, Alderman MH, Ford CE, Oparil S, Francis C, Proschan M, Pressel S, Black HR, Hawkins CM. Rationale and design for the antihypertensive and lipid lowering treatment to prevent heart attack trial (ALLHAT). American Journal of Hypertension 1996; 9: 342-360.

80. The Heart Outcomes Prevention Evaluation (HOPE) Study Investigators. Effects of Ramipril on cardiovascular and microvascular outcomes in people with diabetes mellitus: results of the HOPE study and MICRO-HOPE substudy. Lancet, 2000; 355: 253-259.

81. Remuzzi G, Bertani T. Is glomerulosclerosis a consequence of altered glomerular permeability to macromolecules? Kidney Int 1990; 38: 384-394.

82. Rossing P, Hommel E, Smidt UM, Parving HH. Impact of arterial blood pressure and albuminuria on the progression of diabetic nephropathy in IDDM patients. Diabetes 1993; 42: 715-9.

83. Lebovitz HE, Wiegmann TB, Cnaan A, Shahinfar S, Sica DA, Broadstone V, Schwartz SL, Mengel MC, Segal R, Versaggi JA, et al. Renal protective effects of enalapril in hypertensive NIDDM: role of baseline albuminuria. Kidney Int Suppl 1994; 45: S150-5.

84. Fioretto P, Stehouwer CD, Mauer M, Chiesura-Corona M, Brocco E, Carraro A, Bortoloso E, van Hinsbergh VW, Crepaldi G, Nosadini R. Heterogeneous nature of microalbuminuria in NIDDM: studies of endothelial function and renal structure. Diabetologia 1998; 41: 233-6.

85. Cordonnier DJ, Pinel N, Barro C, Maynard M, Zaoui P, Halimi S, de Ligny BH, Reznic Y, Simon D, Bilous RW. Expansion of cortical interstitium is limited by converting enzyme inhibition in type 2 diabetic patients with glomerulosclerosis. The Diabiopsies Group. J Am Soc Nephrol 1999; 10: 1253-63.

86. Gilbert RE, Tsalamandris C, Bach L, Panagiotopoulos S, O'Brien RC, Allen TJ, Goodall I, Young V, Seeman E, Murray RML, Cooper ME, Jerums G. Glycemic control and the rate of progression of early diabetic kidney disease: a nine year longitudinal study. Kidney Int 1993; 44: 855-859.

87. Ohkubo Y, Kishikawa H, Araki E, Miyata T, Isami S, Motoyoshi S, Kojima Y, Furyoshi N, Shichiri M. Intensive insulin therapy prevents the progression of diabetic microvascular complications in Japanese patients with non-insulin-dependent diabetes mellitus: a randomized prospective 6-year study. Diabetes Res Clin Pract 1995; 28: 103-117.

88. Diabetes Control and Complications Trial Research Group. The effect of intensive treatment on the development and progression of long-term complications in insulin-dependent diabetes mellitus. N Engl J Med 1993; 329: 977-86.

89.   UK Prospective Diabetes Study (UKPDS) Group. Intensive blood-glucose control with sulphonylureas or insulin compared with conventional treatment and risk of complications in patients with type 2 diabetes (UKPDS 33). Lancet 1998; 352: 837-53.

90.   Ravid M, Brosh D, Ravid-Safran D, Levy Z, Rachmani R.   Main risk factors for nephropathy in type 2 diabetes mellitus are plasma cholesterol levels, mean blood pressure, and hyperglycemia. Arch Intern Med 1998; 158: 998-1004.

91.   Gaede P, Vedel P, Parving HH, Pedersen O. Intensified multifactorial intervention in patients with type 2 diabetes mellitus and microalbuminuria: the Steno type 2 randomised study. Lancet 1999; 353: 617-622.

ADDENDUM REGARDING RENOVASCULAR HYPERTENSION AND RENAL ARTERY STENOSIS (especially NIDDM)

Co-author: Bryan Williams

Since diabetes is associated with accelerated atherosclerosis, it has been presumed that it is a state of increased prevalence of renal artery stenosis (RAS). This is of clinical relevance since ACE inhibitors, which can precipitate renal failure in the setting of bilateral RAS [1], are widely used in diabetic patients for nephropathy, heart failure and hypertension. Autopsy studies have suggested that RAS may be increased in diabetic patients [2] but it is likely that the pathologically detected stenoses are not functionally significant.

Only a few studies have been performed to screen for RAS in hypertensive diabetic patients. Ritchie et al have reported in a cross-sectional study of hypertensive NIDDM subjects that RAS is commonly detected [3].   However, more detailed functional studies performed by this group suggested that the RAS was haemodynamically insignificant and unlikely to be a significant cause of hypertension in the majority of patients. In a recent study by Parving et al [personal communication] in patients with NIDDM and overt nephropathy who had a mean age of 60 years, no clinical evidence of RAS was noted during treatment with an ACE inhibitor or beta blocker.

At present, there are no specific recommendations from any of the appropriate societies with respect to screening for RAS in diabetic patients. Since there is no convincing evidence to suggest that diabetic patients with hypertension have a much higher prevalence of RAS than non-diabetic, hypertensive patients we recommend that the presence of diabetes *per se* is not a justification for routine screening for RAS. Nevertheless, there are clearly clinical features which are associated with an increased prevalence of RAS. RAS is more common with aging male gender, history of smoking, in those subjects with evidence of peripheral and coronary vascular disease and in those subjects with hypertension refractory to treatment [4, 5]. This patient profile should alert the clinician to the possibility of RAS. Where a strong clinical suspicion of RAS exists, it would be prudent to investigate the patient prior to commencing ACE inhibitor therapy [6, 7]. These investigations might include renal ultrasound and renal artery doppler studies or functional studies such as renal isotopic scanning, depending on local expertise. Renal angiography is usually reserved for confirmation of the diagnosis in those in whom intervention is being contemplated. In the vast majority of diabetic patients however, these investigations are not warranted prior to the prescription of ACE inhibitor therapy. Prior to, and within a week of commencing ACE inhibitors, serum creatinine and potassium should be measured to determine whether there has been an acute deterioration in renal function secondary to bilateral RAS [1]. This often occurs rapidly after the introduction of ACE inhibitors and is usually reversible if detected immediately. An acute deterioration in renal function after commencing ACE inhibition does not necessarily imply the presence of RAS as this clinical scenario often occurs in the setting of volume depletion, particularly with concurrent diuretic therapy. It is suggested that at this stage similar caution is exerted with the introduction of angiotensin II receptor antagonists such as losartan to diabetic patients [8].

In conclusion, an appropriate level of clinical vigilance and simple clinical assessment of hypertensive diabetic patients should identify most of those at risk of RAS and allow the safe use of agents which interrupt the renin-angiotensin system such as ACE inhibitors and AII antagonists in diabetic patients.

REFERENCES

1. Hricik DE, Browning PJ, Kopelman R, Goomo WE, Madias NE, Dzau VJ. Captopril induced functional renal insufficiency in patients with bilateral renal-artery stenoses or renal-artery stenosis in a solitary kidney. N Engl J Med 1983; 308: 373-376.

2. Sawicki PT, Kaiser S, Heinernann L, Frenzel H, Berger M. Prevalence of renal artery stenosis in diabetes mellitus--an autopsy study. J Intem Med 1991; 229: 489-92.

3. Ritchie CM, MeGrath E, Hadden DR, Weaver JA, Kennedy L. Renal artery stenosis in hypertensive diabetic patients. Diab Med 1988; 5: 265-267.

4. Jean WJ, al Bitar I, Zwicke DL, Port SC, Schmidt DH, Bajwa TK. High incidence of renal artery stenosis in patients with coronary artery disease. Cathet Cardiovasc Diagn 1994; 32: 8-10.

5. Isaksson H, Danielsson Nt Rosenhamer G, Konarski Svensson JC, Ostergren J. Characteristics of patients resistant to antihypertensive drug therapy. J Intem Med 199 1; 229: 421-6.

6. Robinson ACJ, Kong C, Henzen C, Pacy P, Chong P, Gedroyc W, Elkeles RS, Robison S. Magnetic resonance angiography and renal artery stenosis in hypertensive patients with type 2 diabetes (Abstract). Diabetologia, 1996; 39 suppl. 1:A36

7. Courreges JP, Bacha J, Maraoui M, Taurines H, Paris F, Aboud E. Renal artery stenosis prevalence in non-insulin dependent diabetes (NIDDM) and hypertension. (Abstract) Diabetologia, 1995; suppl. 1: A269.

8. Johnston CI. Angiotensin receptor antagonists: focus on losartan. Lancet, 1995; 346: 1403-7.

36.   THE COURSE OF INCIPIENT AND OVERT DIABETIC NEPHROPATHY: THE PERSPECTIVE OF MORE OPTIMAL TREATMENT

Bo Feldt-Rasmussen
Medical Department P, Rigshospitalet, Copenhagen, Denmark

The long-term objective of treatment of diabetes mellitus is prevention of late complications. Through the years it has been a widely accepted hypothesis that development of microvascular as well as macrovascular complications should be, at least in part, due to the lack of good glycemic control. This hypothesis has been unduly hard to prove but results from a number of small scaled intervention studies and the result of the larger scaled American Diabetes Control and Complication Trial (DCCT) some years ago decisively documented, that development and progression of diabetic complications is closely associated with poor glycemic control in Type 1 diabetic patients. More recently with the result of the United Kingdom Prospective Diabetes Study (UKPDS) it has been shown that glycaemic control plays an important role also in Type 2 diabetic patients. The design and outcome of a number of these studies will be presented and discussed in this chapter as will the practical consequences of this newly gained knowledge.

THE CONCEPT OF MICROALBUMINURIA

Much of our present knowledge has been obtained because it is possible in a very early stage to identify patients at risk of clinical diabetic nephropathy as recently reviewed in a number of dissertations and elsewhere [1-6]. The proteinuria of clinical diabetic nephropathy is classically defined as a total urinary protein excretion of 0.5 g per 24 h or more, equivalent to a urinary albumin excretion rate (UAER) of approximately 300 mg/24h or 200 µg/min. It has been documented that a UAER raised above a certain lower level is a good predictor of the development of clinical diabetic nephropathy. Patients at high risk of diabetic nephropathy have a UAER above the normal range but below that of clinical nephropathy. In 1986 a general consensus was made stating that this range of microalbuminuria should be defined as a UAER between 30 to 300 mg/24 h (20 to 200 µg/min) in a 24h or a short term, timed urine collection [7]. At early onset of nephropathy (UAER just above 300 mg/24 h) when the GFR is mainly within the normal range, an annual decline in GFR of approximately 3 to 4 ml/min can be demonstrated. Furthermore patients with microalbuminuria share a number of cardiovascular risk factors with patients with nephropathy [1-7]. In fact, microalbuminuria is a strong and independent risk factor of cardiovascular morbidity and mortality in Type 1 and Type 2 diabetic patients as well as in healthy controls as reviewed in a previous chapter in this book (chapter 13). Therefore the variations of the UAER have been an important end-point to study in many of the recent studies of effects of glycemic control in diabetes.

EFFECT OF IMPROVED GLYCEMIC CONTROL IN TYPE 1 DIABETES

The Scandinavian Experience
Following the introduction of intensified insulin treatment regimens with multiple injections or continuous subcutaneous infusion of short-acting insulins, it became possible to establish and maintain a long-term improvement of the glycemic control. On this basis a number of prospective randomized studies of the effect of improved glycemic control on development and progression of late diabetic complications were initiated as recently reviewed [8,9]. Among the early but smaller scaled studies including from 36 to 91 patients, three Scandinavian studies will be briefly summarized.

In the Steno studies 1 and 2, a total of 70 patients with Type 1 diabetes had been included and randomized to either unchanged conventional insulin treatment or to intensified treatment using portable insulin infusion pumps [10-12].

The long-term glycemic control given as the mean of all HbA_{1c} readings during the entire follow up period had been significantly improved in the insulin infusion groups during the 5 to 8 years of follow-up:

HbA_{1c} at entry - HbA_{1c} mean of all; (insulin infusion group vs control group), (%)) Steno I: 2.0±0.6 versus 0.7±1.2; Steno 2: 1.8±1.2 versus 0.4±1.3 (p<0.01). In Steno I with the longest follow-up, the decline rate of glomerular filtration rate was reduced from -3.7 (-5.4 to -2.0) (mean, 95% confidence interval) to - 1.0 (-2.1 to -0.1) ml/min/1.73m^2 (p<0.05). More patients had progressed to clinical nephropathy during conventiona l insulin treatment than in the insulin infusion groups. Also among the 19 patients with an initial UAER in the high range from 100 to 300 mg/24h, a significant treatment effect was observed. Thus clinical nephropathy (10/10 versus 2/9, p<0.01) and arterial hypertension (7/10 vs 1/9, p<0.01) were diagnosed more often in the the the conventional treatment group.

In the Oslo study [13-15] 45 Type 1 diabetic patients had been included. In general the patients had less severe microangiopathy than the patients of the Steno Studies. After four years of continuous subcutaneous insulin infusion, UAER was reduced from 26±3 (SEM) to 16±5 mg/24h (2p<0.01). No change was observed in the conventional treatment group: 21±4 to 22±6 mg/24h. After 4 years the randomization had been broken. The follow up after 7 years analyzed the patients according to their long-term glycemic level in terms of 7 year mean HbA_1 values [14]. None of the patients received antihypertensive treatment and the protein intake had been unchanged. The patients increasing their UAER by more than 300 mg/24h had significantly higher HbA_1 values during the 7 years of study. The diastolic blood pressure was unchanged in patients with a mean $HbA_1<10\%$, but increased slightly in patients with $HbA_1 >10\%$ (NS). The changes in glomerular filtration rates were not associated to the glycemic control, but the changes had only been minor in the study groups with a mean change of -1.1 ml/min/year or less [14].

In the Stockholm Study [16,17,18] all the patients had to have a poor glycaemic control at entry. The control was improved by means of intensified treatment regimens without the use of insulin infusion pumps. Ninety-five patients had been included and randomized to an unchanged regimen (n=51) or intensified treatment (n=44). They all had non-proliferative retinopathy and a normal s-creatinine and had been followed for 5 years or more. Antihypertensive treatment was added if needed but was not accounted for in the paper [16]. Eight in the control group developed diabetic nephropathy in contrast to none in the intensified treatment group (p<0.05). The changes in UAER was related to the mean HbA_{1c} levels in a dose-related manner. Manifest nephropathy after 3 years was seen almost exclusively in patients with HbA_{1c} levels above 9%. The glomerular filtration rate decreased by a mean of 7 ml/min during three years of study with no differences between the groups (intensified treatment group: 122±3 to 115±3 ml/min, p<0.05).

In a ten-year follow-up, endothelial function was measured as flow-mediated dilation of the right brachial artery. Also the carotid arteries were scanned for plaques, intima-media thickness was measured and arterial wall stiffness was calculated [18]. Patients with lower HbA_{1C} generally had better endothelial function and less stiff arteries [18].

A meta regression analysis of the results from 16 prospective randomized studies including the Scandinavian studies was performed [8]. In these studies, the mean reduction of HbA_{1c} had been 1.45% (as an example, a reduction of HbA_{1c} from 9.2% to 7.8%). After more than two years of intensified therapy the risk of retinopathy progression was lower (odds ratio 0.49 (95% confidence interval 0.28-0.85, p=0.011). The risk of nephropathy progression was also decreased significantly (odds ratio 0.34 (0.20-0.58, p<0.001). The incidence of severe hypoglycemia was increased by 9.1 episodes per 100 patient years in the intensively treated patients. The incidence of diabetic ketoacidoses increased by 12.6 episodes per 100 patient years (95 confidence interval 8.7-16.5) in the patients treated with continuous subcutaneous insulin infusion.

The Diabetes Control and Complication Trial (DCCT). The American Experience
The DCCT study was a multicenter study performed in the period 1983 to 1993 [19-21]. A follow-up 4 years after the original paper was published in January 2000 [22]. The study comprised 1441 Type 1 diabetic patients of whom only 19 patients dropped out. They had been randomized to either conventional insulin treatment with 1 to 2 daily insulin injections or to intensified treatment with more than 3 daily injections. This group also had to measure blood-glucose 4 times a day (and the adherence to this regimen had been documented). If so wished they could choose to be treated with portable insulin infusion pumps.

The aims were:
1.   To study if intensified treatment can prevent development of retinopathy (primary intervention of complications, 726 patients).
2.   To study if intensified treatment can delay or stop the progression of retinopathy (secondary prevention of complications, 715 patients).
      Other indicators of diabetic complications as for instance the UAER and blood pressure were carefully monitored as well.

The main results were:
The mean HbA$_{1c}$ at baseline had been 8.8 and 9.0% in the study groups. In the intensified treatment group the mean HbA$_{1c}$ was maintained at about 7.0% throughout the study i.e. for a mean of 6.5 years. The upper reference level of HbA$_{1c}$ was 6.05%. Only 5% of the patients on intensified treatment were consistently treated to a level below or equal to that level.

      Intensified treatment had reduced the risk of developing the first microaneurism by 27% (95% confidence interval; 11-40) (primary intervention) and of developing moderate retinopathy by 76% (62-85) (secondary intervention). In the secondary intervention study, the risk of progression to severe non-proliferative - or proliferative retinopathy had been reduced by 47% (14-67). A positive correlation between HbA$_{1c}$ and development of retinopathy was observed (Figure 36-1). This was taken by the authors to indicate that any reduction of HbA$_{1c}$ should reduce the risk of retinopathy. The figure may to my mind however also be taken as an indication of the existence of a cut off point of HbA$_{1c}$ of about 7.5% below which very little extra protection against complications can be obtained.

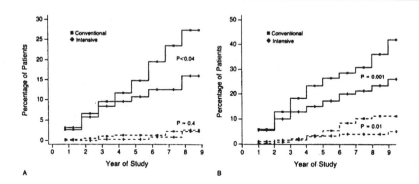

Figure 36-1 Cumulative incidence of urinary albumin excretion ≥ 300 mg per 24 hours (dashed line) and ≥40 mg per 24 hours (solid line) in patients with IDDM receiving intensive or conventional therapy. In the primary-prevention cohort (Panel A), intensive therapy reduced the adjusted mean risk of microalbuminuria by 34% (P<0.04). In the secondary-intervention cohort (Panel B), patients with urinary albumin excretion of ≥ 40 mg per 24 hours at baseline were excluded from the analysis of the development of microalbuminuria. Intensive therapy reduced the adjusted mean risk of albuminuria by 56% (P=0.01) and the risk of microalbuminuria by 43% (P=0.001), as compared with conventional therapy

In the intensified treatment groups, the risk of *developing* microalbuminuria (UAER >40 mg/24h) were reduced by 39% (21-52) and for *developing* clinical nephropathy (UAER >300 mg/24h), by 54% (19-74). A recent sub-analysis of 73 patients with microalbuminuria at entry showed no difference in the rate of *progression* to clinical albuminuria which occurred in eight patients in each group [20].

The risk reductions of development and progression of neuropathy was 60 % (38-74).

The most serious side-effects of intensified treatment had been the risk of severe hypoglycaemia which had been increased by a factor 3.5. An inverse correlation between HbA$_{1c}$ and severe hypoglycaemia was observed (figure 36-2). The risk of ketoacidoses were similar in the groups, 1.8 versus 2.0 cases per 100 patient year respectively.

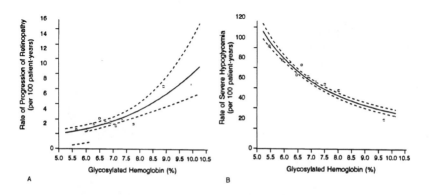

Figure 36-2. Risk of sustained progression of retinopathy (panel A) and rate of severe hypoglycaemia (panel B) in the patients receiving intensive therapy, according to their mean glycosylated haemoglobin values during the trial. In panel A, the glycosylated haemoglobin values used were the mean of the values obtained every six months. In panel B, the mean of the monthly values was used. Squares indicate the crude rates within deciles of the mean glycosylated haemoglobin values during the trial; each square corresponds to more than 400 patient-years. The solid lines are regression lines estimated as a function of the log of the mean glycosylated haemoglobin value in panel A and the log of the lines are regression lines estimated as a function of the log of the mean glycosylated haemoglobin value in panel A, and the log of the glycosylated haemoglobin value in panel B; the dashed lines are 95 per cent confidence intervals.

At the end of the DCCT the patients in the conventional therapy group were offered intensive therapy and the care of all patients was transferred to their own physicians. During the fourth year after DCCT retinopathy was evaluated on the basis of centrally graded fundus photographs in 1,208 patients [22]. Nephropathy was evaluated on the basis of urine specimens obtained from 1,302 patients approximately half of whom were from each treatment group. The difference in the median glycosylated hemoglobin narrowed during follow-up (median during last four years, 8,2% and 7,9% respectively; $p < 0,001$). Nevertheless, the proportion of patients with an increase in urinary albumin excretion was significantly lower in the group of patients who were originally randomized to intensive therapy and the reduction in the risk of progressive retinopathy was significant as well (odds reduction, 72% to 87%; $p < 0,01$). There are two major points to be made. First the risk reduction resulting from intensive therapy seems to persist for at least four years despite increase in hyperglycemia. Second, except for the Steno II Study [11, 12] it has been unduly hard to demonstrate effects of improved glycemic control on the progression of nephropathy. With these new data it is an established fact that there is such an effect!

In another publication it was shown that also in the DCCT study, intensive glycemic control had extended the time of demonstrable islet function [21].

Microalbuminuria collaborative study group. The UK Experience
From 1984 to 1993 in the UK a randomized controlled multicentre study of intensive versus conventional therapy was performed [23]. Seventy patients with Type 1 diabetes and microalbuminuria in the range of 30 µg/min-200 µg/min (overnight urine) were included and followed for a medium of 5 years (2-8 years). Mean HbA$_1$ which initially was similar (10.3% vs, 9.8%) fell significantly in the intensive therapy group only. The difference was maintained for three years with an absolute difference of about 1% between the groups. It could be questioned whether this small improvement of the glycaemic control is sufficient to rule out effects of improved control. Progression to clinical proteinuria occurred in six patients in each group. The Study Group concluded: Arterial blood pressure rather than glycated haemoglobin concentration seems to be the main predictor of progression of microalbuminuria.

The experience from normoglycaemic reentry following pancreas transplantation.
The pancreas transplantation programmes have improved their outcome substantially. As of today more than 10.000 transplantations have been performed. The one year patient survival is now 95 % and the one year graft survival is higher than 82% [24]. There is an overall agreement that this transplantation should mainly be offered to patients having received or is simultaneously receiving a kidney transplant, since the heavy immuno suppression needed in most cases would outweigh the potential benefits of single pancreas transplantations. Furthermore the results are by far the best when performing simultaneous kidney and pancreas transplantations. A reluctance against pancreas transplantations may change since it has recently been shown that among the survivors substantial morphological changes in the glomerular structure were almost normalized 10 years after successful pancreas transplantation [25].

EFFECT OF IMPROVED GLYCAEMIC CONTROL IN TYPE 2 DIABETES

The United Kingdom Prospective Diabetes Study (UKPDS)
The United Kingdom Prospective Diabetes Study (UKPDS) started in 1977. The UKPDS was designed to establish whether, in patients with type 2 diabetes, intensive

blood glucose control reduced the risk of macrovascular or microvascular complications and whether any particular therapy was advantageous [26, 27]. Newly diagnosed patients with type 2 diabetes (n=3,867) and with a median age of 54 years were included. Fasting plasma glucose concentration had to be between 6,1 to 15,0 mmol/l. Patients were randomized to a conventionally treated group or an intensified treatment group. The intensive treatment policy was sulphonylureas or insulin and amongst obese patients, metformin. The aim in the intensive group was FPG< 6 mmol/l. In the conventional group the aim was the best achievable FPG with diet alone. Drugs were added only if there were hyperglycemic symptoms or FPG>15 mmol/l. Over ten years hemoglobin A1c (HbA1c) was 7,0 (6,2-8,2) in the intensive group compared with 7,9% (6,9-8,8) in the conventional group - an 11% reduction. There was no difference in HbA1c among agents in the intensive group. The primary outcome measures were three aggregate endpoints: Any diabetes related endpoints, diabetes related death and all cause mortality. Compared with the conventional group the risk in the intensive group was 12% lower (95% CI (1-21), p=0,029) for any diabetes related end point; The risk reduction was not significant for the other two aggregate endpoints; it was 10% lower (11 - 27, p=0,34) for any diabetes related death (NS) and 6% lower (10 - 20, p= 0,44) for all cause mortality (NS). Most of the risk reduction in the "any diabetes related aggregate end point" was due to a 25% risk reduction ((7-40), p=0,0099) in the microvascular end points including the need for retinal fotocoagulation. There was no difference for any of the aggregate end points between the four intensive agents (chlorprobamide, glibenclamide, metformin or insulin). Moreover, most patients in the intensive group were eventually treated with combination therapy. Thus, improved glycemic control seems to be the principal factor. The only macrovascular endpoint that tended to show a risk reduction in the main analysis was myocardial infarction (16% risk reduction, (p=0,052)). In the metformin subgroup analysis in the UKPDS, however, there were significant risk reductions in diabetes related death (risk reduction 42%, p=0,017). Any diabetes related endpoint (risk reduction 32%, p=0,017) any diabetes related endpoints (risk reduction 32%, p=0,0023) and myocardial infarction (risk reduction 39%, p=0,01). More hypoglycemic episodes were observed in the intensive group and weight gain was significantly higher in the intensive group (mean 2,9 kg) than in the conventional group (p< 0,001). Patients assigned insulin had an even greater gain in weight (4,0 kg) than those assigned to chlorprobamide (2,6kg) or glibenclamide (1,7kg). Despite these weight gains intensified treatment was beyond any doubt worthwhile.

A major observation of the UKPDS was that antihypertensive treatment was of great importance in preventing progression of microangiopathic as well as macroangiopathic disease. The combined effect of antihypertensive treatment and intensified glycemic control has been shown to be much more substantial than the additive effect of each of these measures. These results combining treatment modalities have been presented at meetings but have not as yet been published.

Similar results have been presented in a Japanese study [28].

Multifactorial intervention studies.
The Steno type 2 Study [29]. In this study 160 type 2 diabetic patients 40-65 years of age and with microalbuminuria were included. They were randomized to conventional treatment or intensive treatment. The latter meant behavioural modification (diet, exercise, smoking, etc). Intensive polypharmacy (ACE-inhibition, insulin and oral anti-diabetic treatment towards an HbA1c below 6,5%, treatment with statins towards a fasting total cholesterol below 5,0, HDL-cholesterol above 1,1 and fasting triglyceride below 1,7, vitamin C/E and acetylic salicylic acid. After 3,8 years of study fewer patients in the intervention group had progressed to nephropathy (OR=0,27, p= 0,01), there was less progression in retinopathy (OR=0,45, p=0,04) and there was less progression of autonomic neuropathy (OR=0,31, p=0,01) compared to the control group.

INTENSIFIED INSULIN TREATMENT. PRACTICAL GUIDELINES
In Type 1 as well as Type 2 diabetes the key to risk reduction is to achieve meticulous glycaemic control. In both the UKPDS and the DCCT, the relationship between glycaemic exposure and the risk of complications was evident across the range of HbA1c, and without evidence of a threshold. Therefore the appropriate goals should be a HbA1c below 7% and a fasting plasma glucose below 6.7 mmol/l.

Since there is a progressive loss of beta-cell function in Type 2 diabetes, many patients on top of dietary treatment will require combinations of oral agents and then insulin therapy. A growing number of classes of pharmacological agents are available including the secretagogues (sulphunylureas and repaglinide), insulin sensitizers (biguanides and thiazolidinediones) and alpha glucosidase inhibitors. It is however important that a multifactorial approach to the treatment of the patients is taken. The treatment should be designed to deal with also hypertension, dyslipidaemia and should include also behavioural modifications whenever appropriate (diet, exercise, smoking etc). In Type 1 diabetes the intensified treatment regimens operates with at least three important principles

First, frequent or continuous administration of fast-acting insulins and little or no (infusion pumps) use of intermediate or long-acting insulins. The advantages of this is (a) small differences between the administered and absorbed amounts of insulin over 24 h, (b) post-prandial insulin peaks and (c) a stable overnight insulin level (at least when administered by insulin infusion pumps).

Second, frequent blood glucose readings before meals and bedtime, making it possible to adjust the injected amount of insulin, not only according to experience (size and character of meal, physical exercise etc.) but also according to actual glycemic level. For this purpose, the development of new glucose monitors, transcutaneous or subcutaneous, are in progress.

Third, educational programmes making possible all the above.

Practical guidelines for optimal B-glucose levels during intensified insulin treatment are presented in table 36-1.

Table 36-1. Target of B-glucose levels during intensified treatment regimens

Fasting	4-7 mmol/l
Post-prandial	5-10 mmol/l
Avoid values below	3 mmol/l
Avoid values above	10 mmol/l

CONCLUSION

The development of all late diabetic complications are closely associated with the quality of long-term glycemic control, and improving the control significantly reduces the risk of complications. Progression of established lesions may benefit from improved glycemic control [25]. Optimizing glycaemic control and other treatment modalities after myocardial infarction is also an important new area for improving the prognosis of patients with diabetes mellitus [30]. The most recent studies of effect of multifactorial intervention has lead to the conclusion that optimising treatment of hyperglycaemia, blood-pressure and dyslipidaemia has to be given an equal priority in the pharmacological treatment aiming at reducing development of macroangiopathy

REFERENCES

1.   Rosenstock J, Raskin P. Early diabetic nephropathy: Assessment and potential therapeutic interventions. Diabetes Care 1986; 9: 529-545.
2.   Symposium on diabetic nephropathy. Kidney Int 1992; 41: 717-729.
3.   Feldt-Rasmussen B. Microalbuminuria and clinical nephropathy in Type 1 (insulin-dependent). diabetes mellitus: Pathophysiological mechanisms and intervention studies (Thesis). Dan Med Bull 1989; 36: 405-415.
4.   Jensen T. Albuminuria-a marker of renal and general vascular disease in IDDM (Thesis). Dan Med Bull 1991; 38: 134-144.
5.   Mathiesen ER. Prevention of diabetic nephropathy: Microalbuminuria and perspectives for intervention in insulin-dependent diabetes (Thesis). Dan Med Bull 1993; 40: 273-285.
6.   Christensen CK. The pre-proteinuric phase of diabetic nephropathy (Thesis). Dan Med Bull 1991; 38: 145-159.
7.   Mogensen CE, Chacati A, Christensen CK, Close CF, Deckert T, Hommel E, Kastrup J, Lefebre P, Mathiesen ER, Feldt-Rasmussen B, Schmitz A, Viberti GC. Microalbuminuria: An early marker of of renal involvement in diabetes. Uremia Invest 1986; 9: 85-95.
8.   Wang PH, Lau J, Chalmers TC. Meta-analysis of effects of intensive blood-glucose control on late complications of Type 1 diabetes. Lancet 1993; 341: 1306-1309.
9.   Hanssen KF, Dahl-Jørgensen K, Lauritzen T, Feldt-Rasmussen B, Brinchmann-Hansen O, Deckert T. Diabetic control and microvascular complications: The near-normoglycaemic experience. Diabetologia 1986; 29: 677-684.
10.   Lauritzen T, Frost-Larsen K, Larsen HW, Deckert T, Steno Study Group. Two years experience with continuous subcutaneous insulin infusion in relation to retinopathy and neuropathy. Diabetes 1985; 34 suppl 3: 74-79.
11.   Feldt-Rasmussen B, Mathiesen ER, Deckert T. Effect of 2 years of   strict metabolic control on progression of incipient nephropathy in insulin-dependent diabetes. Lancet 1986; i: 1300-1304.

12.   Feldt-Rasmussen B, Mathiesen ER, Jensen T, Lauritzen T, Deckert T. Effect of improved metabolic control on loss of kidney function in insulin-dependent diabetic patients. Diabetologia 1991; 34: 164-170.

13.   Dahl-Jørgensen K, Hanssen KF, Kierulf P, Bjøro T, Sandvik L, Aagenaess Ø. Reduction of urinary albumin excretion after 4 years of continuous subcutaneous insulin infusion in insulin-dependent diabetes mellitus. Acta Endocrinol 1988; 117: 19-25.

14.   Dahl-Lørgensen K, Bjøro T, Kierulf P, Sandvik L, Bangstad HJ, Hanssen KF. The effect of long-term stict glycemic control on kidney function in insulin-dependent diabetes mellitus: seven years result from the Oslo Study. Kidney Int 1992; 41; 920-923.

15.   Bangstad H-J, Østerby R, Dahl-Jørgensen K, et al. Early glomerulopathy is present in young Type 1 (insulin-dependent) diabetic patients with microalbuminuria. Diabetologia 1993; 36: 523-529.

16.   Reichard P, Berglund B, Britz A, Cars I, Nilsson BY, Rosenqvist U. Intensified conventional insulin treatment retards the microvascular complications of insulin-dependent diabetes mellitus (IDDM). The Stockholm Diabetes Intervention Study after five years. J Int Med 1991; 230: 101-108.

17.   Reichard P, Nilsson BY, Rosenqvist U. The effect of long-term intensified insulin treatment on the development of microvascular complications of diabetes mellitus. N Engl J Med 1993; 329: 304-309.

18.   Jensen-Urstadt KJ, Reichard PG, Rosfors JS, Lindblad JS, Lindblad LEL, Jensen-Urstadt MT. Early atherosclerosis is retarded by improved long-term blood glucose control in patients with IDDM. Diabetes 1996; 45: 1253-1258.

19.   The Diabetes Control an Complication Trial Research Group. The effect of intensive treatment of diabetes on the development and progression of long-term complications in insulin-dependent diabetes mellitus. N Engl J Med 1993; 329: 977-986.

20.   Diabetes Control and Complications (DCCT) Research Group. Effect of intensive therapy on the development and progression of diabetic nephropathy in the diabetes control and complications trial. Kidney Int 1995; 42: 1703-1720.

21.   Steffes M, Tamburlane W, Becker D, Palmer J, Cleary P for the DCCT research group. The effect of intensive diabetes treatment on residual beta cell function in the Diabetes Control and Complications Trial (DCCT) Abstract. Diabetes 1996; 46 suppl. 2: 18A.

22.   The Diabetes Control and Complications Trial/Epidemiology of Diabetes Interventions and Complications Research Group. Retinopathy and nephropathy in patients with type 1 diabetes four years after a trial of intensive therapy. N Engl J Med, 2000; 342: 381-89.

23.   Microalbuminuria Collaborative Study Group, United Kingdom. Intensive therapy and progression to clinical albuminuria in patients with insulin dependent diabetes mellitus and microalbuminuria. BMJ 1995; 311: 973-977.

24.   White SA, Nicholson ML, London NJM. Vascularized pancreas allotransplantation - clinical indications and outcome. Diabetic Medicine 1999; 16: 533-543.

25.   Fioretto P, Steffes MW, Sutherland DER, Goetz FC, Mauer M. Reversal of lesions of diabetic nephropathy after pancreas transplantation. N Engl J Med 1998; 339: 69-75.

26.   Anonymous. Intensive blood-glucose control with sulphonylureas or insulin compared with conventional treatment and risk of complications in patients with type 2 diabetes (UKPDS 33). UK Prospective Diabetes Study (UKPDS) Group. Lancet 1998; 352: 837-853.

27.   Anonymous. Effect of intensive blood-glucose control with metformin on complications in overweight patients with type 2 diabetes (UKPDS 34). UK Prospective Diabetes Study (UKPDS) Group. Lancet 1998; 352: 854-865.

28. Okhubo Y, Kishikawa H, Araki E, Miyata T, Isami S, Motoyoshi S, Kojima Y, Furuyoshi N, Shichiri M. Intensive insulin therapy prevents the progression of diabetic microvascular complications in Japanese patients with non-insulin-dependent diabetes mellitus: a randomized prospective 6-year study. Diabetes Res. Clin. Pract. 1995; 28: 103-117.

29. Gaede P, Vedel P, Parving HH, Pedersen O. Intensified multifactorial intervention in patients with type 2 diabetes mellitus and microalbuminuria: the Steno type 2 randomized study. Lancet 1999; 353: 617-622.

30. Malmberg K, Rydén L, Efendic S, Herlitz J, Nicol P, Waldenström A, Wedel H, Welin L on behalf of the Digami Study Group. Randomized trial of insulin-glucose infusion followed by subcutaneous insulin treatment in diabetic patients with acute myocardial infarction (DIGAMI study): Effects on mortality at 1 year. JACC 1995; 26: 57-65.

37.   NON-GLYCAEMIC INTERVENTION IN DIABETIC NEPHROPATHY: THE ROLE OF DIETARY PROTEIN INTAKE

James D. Walker
Department of Diabetes, Royal Infirmary of Edinburgh, Edinburgh,Scotland

By the time clinical diabetic nephropathy is diagnosed by persistent proteinuria and a declining glomerular filtration rate (GFR), treatment options to preserve renal function are limited. Improving glycaemic control at this stage of the disease process is difficult and has little influence on the rate of decline of the GFR [1-3] whereas treatment of a raised blood pressure (BP) is more efficacious [4-8]. Dietary protein restriction has long been known to influence renal function [9] and numerous studies have tested the effect of dietary protein restriction in various renal diseases [10]. Additionally in animal models of chronic renal failure dietary protein restriction lessens proteinuria, mesangial expansion and glomerulosclerosis and preserves GFR [11-14]. This chapter discusses the influence of dietary protein on renal function and examines the effects of the therapeutic manoeuvre of restricting dietary protein in diabetic nephropathy.

DIETARY PROTEIN AND RENAL FUNCTION

Normal humans
Vegans who eat less total protein than omnivores (0.95 vs. 1.29 g/kg/day) and 100% of their protein intake is the form of vegetable protein, have glomerular filtration rates that are 11% lower than matched omnivores [15]. In addition, urinary albumin excretion and blood pressure levels are lower [15]. A similar effect of diet on blood pressure is seen after a 6 week period of a lacto-ovo-vegetarian diet in healthy habitually omnivorous subjects independent of changes in weight and sodium or potassium intake [16]. In normal humans consuming a usual diet GFR increases by 7-18% and urinary albumin excretion by 100-300% in response to a meat meal of 80 g of protein as lean cooked beef [17,18]. In contrast a 3 week period of low-protein diet (LPD) (43 g/day) causes a 14% reduction in baseline GFR, a 9% reduction in renal plasma flow (RPF) and a 50%

reduction in the urinary albumin excretion rate [17].

In diabetic patients
Normoalbuminuric insulin-dependent patients completing 3 weeks of LPD (45 g/day) had a reduction in GFR with no difference in RPF and thus a reduction in filtration fraction (FF) (FF=GFR/RPF) [19]. This contrasts to the effect of LPD on FF in non-diabetics [17]. Glycaemic control and blood pressure levels were unchanged while the fractional clearance of albumin was lower on LPD. A larger study involving 35 normoalbuminuric insulin-dependent diabetic patients investigated the response to a 100 g/1.73 m^2 protein load in the form of a meat meal [18]. The area under the glomerular filtration rate curve rose more in normals than in the diabetic patients by a factor of 3.8. The impaired response of glomerular filtration rate to the meat meal in the diabetic patients was not due to differences in absorption of the meal since plasma levels of branched-chain amino acids were not different between normals and diabetics. Possible mechanisms of the differing responses included glucagon-mediated increases in the vasodilatory prostaglandins, prostaglandin E_2 and 6-keto prostaglandin $F_{1\alpha}$, which were impaired in diabetics.

A similar study employing a cross-over design tested the renal effects of 10 days of a diet of 0.9 g/kg/day or 1.9 g/kg/day of dietary protein. GFR and FF were lower on the diet containing the lesser amount of protein with a more marked fall in GFR in those patients with glomerular hyperfiltration (GFR >127 ml/min) [20].

At the stage of microalbuminuria a reduction in GFR, urinary albumin excretion rate and fractional clearance of albumin was seen after 3 weeks of a low-protein diet (47 g/day) [21]. These changes were independent of changes in glycaemia or blood pressure. In insulin-dependent diabetic patients with diabetic nephropathy 3 weeks of LPD was associated with an improvement in glomerular permselectivity while no differences were seen in renal haemodynamics (GFR, RPF, and FF) between the two diet periods [22,23]. The reabsorption rate of B_2 microglobulin was similar in both diet periods, suggesting that tubular function was not influenced by the different diets.

Thus in both normals and diabetic subjects with microalbuminuria and glomerular hyperfiltration, short-term dietary protein restriction leads to a reduction in albuminuria and GFR whereas in diabetic patients with proteinuria although urinary protein loss is diminished in the short-term, this intervention has no effects on renal haemodynamics.

MEDIATORS OF RENAL EFFECTS OF DIETARY PROTEIN
In order to define some of the determinants of the change in glomerular filtration rate in response to different dietary protein intakes, Krishna and colleagues administered a 1 g of protein/kg body weight as beef steak, to 9 healthy males [24]. The renal haemodynamic studies were repeated on three separate occasions after pretreatment with

either placebo, indomethacin (to inhibit renal prostaglandin synthesis) or enalapril (to inhibit angiotensin II synthesis). Following placebo GFR increased by 29% with an accompanying increase in RPF and a fall in renal vascular resistance (RVR). Pretreatment with indomethacin attenuated the rise in the GFR (12% rise) whereas treatment with enalapril was not different to placebo. Urinary excretion rates of prostaglandin E_2 fell significantly in the indomethacin group, levels of plasma renin activity were increased in the enalapril group while plasma noradrenaline and adrenaline were unchanged in all groups. From these data it appears that the protein-mediated elevation in glomerular filtration is in part associated with prostaglandin levels. In diabetic patients the attenuated glucagon response to a protein challenge may mediate the reduced prostaglandin effect [18].

The effects of similar amounts of animal and vegetable protein ingestion on renal haemodynamics were investigated in a short-term study of 10 normal males [25]. GFR, RPF and the fractional clearance of albumin were all lower on the vegetable protein diet while renal vascular resistance (RVR) was higher compared to the animals protein diet. In a separate experiment, seven normal subjects were given an 80 g protein load of animal protein (lean cooked beef) and subsequently 80 g of diluted soya powder (vegetable protein). While an elevation in GFR and RPF and a reduction in RVR was seen after animal protein no changes occurred after soya. The incremental glucagon area was greater for meat than soya and whereas the vasodilatory prostaglandin 6-keto PGF $_{1\alpha}$ rose significantly after the animal protein, it did not change after soya challenge. From these data, it appears that the same quantity of vegetable protein causes different renal effects compared to animal protein, and that this difference is associated with a smaller glucagon and vasodilatory prostaglandin response. These hormonal mediators have been also implicated from a study in which infusion of somatostatin diminished the renal response to amino-acid infusion [26].

Elevated levels of plasma renin activity on high protein diets have been observed in man and experimental animals [22,27]. This difference could not be explained in terms of differences in sodium or potassium intakes, which were identical between the two diets. As prostaglandins are known to mediate renin release [27,28] the elevated levels of prostaglandins may have caused the elevated renin levels. Although there were no changes in mean arterial pressure between the two diet periods the elevated renin levels may have resulted in increased levels of angiotensin II to cause constriction of both the afferent and efferent glomerular arterioles. The role of angiotensin II in the physiological and pathophysiological response to low-protein feeding may be important since in the rat captopril reverses the reduced GFR and RPF and increased renal vascular resistance seen with LPD [29].

Other mediators in addition to glucagon, prostaglandin and the renin/angiotensin/ aldosterone system may be involved in the renal response to dietary protein. Recently increased levels of mRNA for PDGF-A and -B chains and TGF-ß genes have been shown to correlate with glomerulosclerosis in a rat model [30]. Low-protein feeding reduced the prevalence of glomerulosclerosis and attenuated the abnormally high expression of the PDGF-A and -B and TGF-ß genes. These data suggest that growth factors may play a role in the development of glomerulosclerosis and can be modulated by LPD.

LONG-TERM CLINICAL STUDIES OF LOW-PROTEIN DIETS IN PATIENTS WITH DIABETIC NEPHROPATHY

Some studies designed to test the effects of a diet restricted in protein in insulin dependent patients with diabetic nephropathy have used creatinine clearance or the reciprocal of the serum creatinine to assess renal function (table 37-1). This is not an accurate or precise measure of GFR compared to isotopic clearance methods, such as the plasma clearance of ^{51}Cr EDTA, which give nearly identical values to insulin clearances. In addition changes in the creatine pool and creatinine intake seen in low-protein diet studies further render such measurements unreliable for the assessment of GFR [31-35].

Study designs have varied. Evanoff used patients as their own control [36]. After a 12 month observation period a LPD of 0.6 g/kg/day was instituted and, using creatinine clearance and the reciprocal of the serum creatinine to assess renal functional response, 11 patients were studied for 2 years [35]. The period of LPD was associated with a slowing in the rate of decline of the reciprocal of the serum creatinine and no change in the creatinine clearance levels during the 2 years of study. However, 9 of the 11 patients had antihypertensive agents initiated during the study and systolic blood pressure levels fell significantly. No attempts were made to correct for the substantial fall in systolic blood pressure (about 20 mmHg) and it is therefore difficult to separate the effects of the blood pressure reduction from those of LPD making interpretation of the effects of LPD in this study difficult. Using the same study design Barsotti followed 8 patients with more severe renal impairment for 16 months on a normal protein diet (NPD) (1.2 to 1.4 g/kg/day) and then instituted a more restrictive protein prescription of 0.25 to 0.35 g/kg/day with essential amino acid supplementation for a mean duration of 17 months [37]. Urinary urea and urinary protein levels fell during the diet, body weight, triceps skin thickness, mid-arm muscle circumference and plasma albumin levels were unchanged and insulin requirements fell despite an increase in the carbohydrate intake. The rate of decline of creatinine clearance was slowed on LPD in a heterogeneous manner.

A 6 month controlled study involving 7 patients in a LPD and 9 in a control group revealed no changes in creatinine clearance but a reduction in urinary albumin excretion on LPD [38]. The majority of patients in both groups had serum creatinine levels that were within the normal range indicating well preserved renal function and thus it was not surprising that no change in creatinine clearances were observed in this short-term study. A more recent study employing the same study design with 11 patients in each group, with more impairment of GFR, demonstrated that during a six month follow-up LPD stabilised the decline in GFR and reduced the degree of proteinuria from 2.15 to 1.13 g/day [39]. Importantly, GFR was measured isotopically and blood pressure was similar in both the NPD and LPD patients.

A larger controlled trial that employed an isotopic clearance method for measurement of GFR demonstrated a significant reduction in the rate of decline of GFR after 37 months on a low-protein diet (0.72 g/kg/day) compared to a control group on a normal protein diet (1.08 g/kg/day) for this period [40]. Blood pressure was lower in the group on the low-protein diet but when included as an independent variable in a stepwise regression analysis with change in glomerular filtration rate as the dependent variable, it was found to exert no significant effect. Interestingly, the rate of decline of GFR was only significantly different between the patients on the two diets when those with initial glomerular filtration rates above 45 ml/min were considered. This may be taken to suggest that dietary intervention should be introduced early in the course of diabetic nephropathy before significant reductions in glomerular filtration rate occur. There was no indication that the LPD had any nutritional adverse effect. Serum cholesterol and triglyceride levels were increased during the LPD period but the changes failed to reach statistical significance.

The only other prospective study employing an isotopic clearance method to assess GFR investigated the effect of LPD in 19 insulin-dependent diabetic patients with nephropathy. Patients were followed for 29 months on NPD (1.11 g/kg/day) and subsequently for 33 months on LPD (0.66 g/kg/day). GFR decline was slowed by an average of 0.47 ml/min/month (figure 37-1) and the rise in albuminuria halted independent of changes in glycaemia or blood pressure [41]. The effect of LPD on the decline in GFR was heterogeneous with 10 of the 19 patients exhibiting a significant slowing yet in the remaining 9 the rate was either non-significantly slower or in some cases faster. No identified factors separated the responders from the non-responders. This study quantitated and emphasised the heterogeneity of the GFR response with has also been observed in a trial of antihypertensive therapy in patients with diabetic nephropathy [5].

A prospective study investigated the effects of 0.8g/kg/day in a large number of patients with type 2 diabetes with normoalbuminuria or low level microalbuminuria [58]. Mean age was 64 years and the change in albuminuria the primary outcome measure. The reduction in protein intake on the low protein diet was small at 6 months and even smaller at 12 months with the majority of studied patients being unable to comply with the dietary regimen. Despite this albuminuria was 15% lower at 1 year after adjusting for changes in diastolic pressure and occurred in both normoalbuminuric and microalbuminuric patients.

A recently published meta-analysis of the effect of dietary protein restriction on the progression of renal disease has included patients with diabetic nephropathy [42]. The studies identified for the meta-analysis included 4 presently summarised in table 37-1 [37,38,40,41] and a study involving microalbuminuric patients [44]. The relative risk for progression of renal disease in insulin-dependent diabetic patients on a low-protein diet was 0.56 (95% confidence intervals 0.40 to 0.77). A reduced relative risk was also seen in cases of non-diabetic renal disease treated with a low-protein diet [42]. The validity of this metanalysis has recently been questioned by Parving [43].

A Cochrane review on protein restriction in diabetic renal disease, including 4 of the studies summarised in table 37-1. [37-40] and the study of microalbuminuric patients by Dullaart et al [44], also concluded that lower protein intake slows the progression of diabetic nephropathy towards renal failure [59].

PROBLEMS WITH LOW-PROTEIN DIETS
Two main problems are associated with the prescription of a LPD namely protein/calorie malnutrition and compliance [44,47]. Protein intakes below 0.6 g/kg/day have been associated with protein malnutrition [45,46] and the aim of a LPD should be reduce protein intake to a non-harmful yet achievable level by the majority of patients. Despite increased carbohydrate intake, necessary to compensate for the calorie reduction caused by a reduction in dietary protein, energy intake has been reported to fall and a small degree of weight loss occur on LPD in some studies [37,41]. However, stable or increased serum albumin levels and no change in mid-arm muscle circumference are reassuring parameters and suggest that the levels of protein reduction in reported studies are not associated with muscle loss and protein malnutrition [40,41].

Compliance is a prerequisite for this form of treatment and 3 recent studies, two involving patients with diabetes and microalbuminuria, have demonstrated how difficult this is to achieve [44,47,58]. Locatelli, in a large study, prescribed a LPD of 0.6 g/kg/day yet the achieved level of protein intake was 0.83 g/kg/day [47] - not a low-protein diet. In patients with diabetes and microalbuminuria only 7 of 14 patients achieved the prescribed protein reduction of <0.8 g/kg/day during a 2 year study [44]. The reasons for the poor level of compliance in this study may include the lack of concern of the patients about their renal condition at this early stage of renal disease.

Compliance with, or more correctly adherence to, a low protein diet has recently been debated following the publication of a study investigating the effect of a LPD on the progression of chronic renal failure in children [48] in which the protein content of LPD was greater than 25% of the WHO recommended amount [49]. Thus whether such a trial can analyse the effect of a LPD on the progression of chronic renal failure is open to question [50]. Secondary analysis [51] of the Modification of Diet in Renal Disease study [52] demonstrates a close correlation between achieved protein intake and the rate of decline of the GFR suggesting that if the intervention is correctly adhered to the achieved results are more promising.

Table 37-1. Clinical studies of low protein diet in insulin-dependent patients with diabetic nephropathy.

AUT-HOR/ YEAR	STUDY DESIGN	DIATARY PRES-CRIPTION	DIE-TARY ASSESS-MENT	GFR ASSESS-MENT	DURA-TION OF LPD	OUTCOME
Raal, 1994	Random-ised controlled, 22 pts	0.8 g/kg/day in pts 1.6 g/kg/day in controls		Plasma clearance of ^{51}Cr EDTA	6 months	Decrease in TUP in LPD group GFR fell at 1.3 ml/min/mo in NPD group. No change in LPD group
Zeller, 1991	Random-ised controlled, 68 pts	0.72 g/kg/day in pts 1.08 g/kg/day in controls	Weighed food records Urinary urea nitrogen	Iothalamate clearances	37 months	Iothalamate clearances 0.26 ml/min/mo in pts. 1.01 ml/min/mo in controls MBP 102 in pts., 105 in controls
Walker, 1989	Self control 19 pts	1.1 g/kg/day on NPD→ 0.66g/kg/day on LPD	Weighed food records Urinary urea nitrogen	Plasma clearance of ^{51}Cr EDTA	29 months on NPD 33 months on LPD	GFR 0.61 ml/min/mo on NPD, 0.14 ml/min/mo on LPD MBP 106 on NPD, 102 on LPD
Evanoff, 1989	Self controls 11 pts	1.2 g/kg/day on NPD→ 0.95g/kg/day on LPD	Dietary recall urinary urea nitrogen	Creatinine clearance 1/serum creatinine	24 months	Δl/serum creatinine -0.18/yr on NPD -0.03/yr on LPD Systolic BP 147 LPD vs. 126 NPD
Barsotti, 1988	Self controls 8 pts	1.3 g/kg/day on NPD 0.3g/kg/day on LPD (supplemented with essential amino- and ketoacids)	Urinary urea nitrogen	Creatinine clearance	17 months	Decrease in TUP Increase in TPP Rate of decline in CrCl on NPD 1.38 ml/min/mo on LPD 0.03 ml/min/mo
Ciava-rella, 1987	Random-ised controlled 16 pts	0.71 g/kg/day in pts. 1.44 g/kg/day in controls	Diatary interview Blood urea nitrogen Urinary urea nitrogen	Creatinine clearance	4.5 months	Decrease in AER in LPD group

AER=Urinary albumin excretion rate; TUP=Urinary total protein excretion rate; LPD=Low protein diet; CrCl=Creatinine clearance; NPD=Normal protein diet; TPP=Total plasma protein level; Δ=Delta (change in); All blood pressure values are in mmHg; MBP=Mean blood pressure

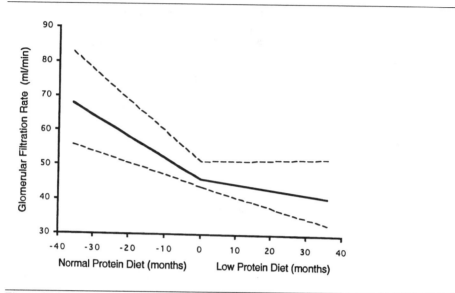

Figure 37-1. GFR decline (mean-solid line and 95% confidence intervals – dashed lines) in 19 insulin-dependent diabetic patients with nephropathy on a normal and subsequently a low protein diet [Data taken from ref. 41].

BLOOD PRESSURE TREATMENT AND DIETARY PROTEIN RESTRICTION IN DIABETIC NEPHROPATHY

No study has tested the effects of blood pressure reduction **and** dietary protein restriction in diabetic nephropathy. In non-diabetic renal disease evidence for an additive effect is provided by a short-term study of 17 patients in whom addition of enalapril to a LPD resulted in a further decrease in proteinuria and a reversal of some acute renal haemodynamic changes associated with LPD [53]. In diabetic patients with nephropathy, the 2 clinical trials that used isotopic clearances to assess GFR found that the small reduction in mean blood pressure on LPD exerted a very small effect on the change in GFR [40,41]. In these studies mean blood pressure was only 4 mmHg lower on LPD [40,41]. This contrasts with the 12 mmHg fall in mean blood pressure caused by antihypertensive treatment in the study reported by Parving [5]. The achieved mean blood pressure level in the LPD studies was 102 mmHg a level similar to the level of 99 mmHg achieved in the study reported by Parving [5]. The reduction in the rate of GFR decline associated with LPD is similar to that seen with treatment of hypertension. However, as levels of mean blood pressure on NPD were considerably lower than the untreated blood pressures levels of Parving's patients (106 vs. 112 mmHg) the further slowing of GFR decline on LPD argues for an additional effect of this therapeutic manoeuvre.

DIETARY SALT AND DIABETIC NEPHROPATHY

Surprisingly few studies have investigated the relationship between dietary salt and diabetic nephropathy given the extensive literature on salt and blood pressure in the general population and particularly the relationship in the renal patient [54]. One controlled study of 16 IDDM patients with nephropathy and mild renal impairment compared blood pressure and renal responses during a 4 week period during which subjects consumed 92 or 199 mmol of sodium a day [55]. No differences were observed between the two groups in term of blood pressure or renal parameters. This lack of difference may have been due to the small number of subjects studied, the relatively short duration of the study or the fact that GFR was well preserved in the individuals studied.

Dietary sodium intake tends to fall when patients are placed on a LPD. In one study with IDDM mean urinary sodium excretion fell significantly from 178 on a usual protein diet to 143 mmol/day on a LPD [41]. Thus the prescription of a LPD will in itself cause a reduction in salt intake.

In clinical practice all patients with diabetes are assessed by dietician and a part of this assessment details the dietary salt intake and advice is given when indicated. In those with significant renal functional impairment the advice on dietary sodium restriction will be more specific.

CONCLUSIONS AND IMPLICATIONS

There is now enough evidence to strongly support the hypothesis that a reduction in the dietary intake of protein retards the rate of decline of renal functional loss in cases of established diabetic nephropathy in patients with insulin-dependent diabetes mellitus, but generally more work needs to be done [56]. Subjecting a patient to this dietary regime should not be undertaken lightly and needs full co-operation of the patient and full involvement of a nutritionist experienced in this field. GFR response to LPD appears to be heterogeneous thus making it is vital to assess whether an individual is benefiting from the intervention. Patients who remain heavily proteinuric (>6 g/day) despite adequate blood pressure control and treatment with an angiotensin-converting enzyme inhibitor should be strongly considered for LPD therapy. It would thus be prudent for such patients to have a run-in period on their usual diet and therapy with 3 isotopic measurement of GFR to establish a baseline rate of decline against which the response to LPD can be compared. Protein restriction of 0.6 g/kg/day appears to have no untoward nutritional effect. Interestingly nutritional intake of protein continue to be generally high among diabetic patients [57], and patients with microalbuminuria and macroalbuminuria consume even more total protein and animal protein than those with normoalbuminuria [57,60].

REFERENCES

1.   Bending JJ, Pickup JC, Viberti GC, Keen H. Glycaemic control in diabetic nephropathy. BMJ 1984; 288: 1187-1191.
2.   Bending JJ, Viberti GC, Watkins PJ, Keen H. Intermittent clinical proteinuria and renal function in diabetes: evolution and the effect of glycaemic control. BMJ 1986; 292: 83-86.
3.   Viberti GC, Bilous RW, Mackintosh D, Bending JJ, Keen H. Long term correction of hyperglycaemia and progression of renal failure in insulin-dependent diabetes. BMJ 1983; 286: 598-602.
4.   Mogensen CE. Long-term antihypertensive treatment inhibiting progression of diabetic nephropathy. BMJ 1982; 285: 685-688.
5.   Parving H-H, Andersen AR, Smidt UM, Hommel E, Mathiesen ER, Svendsen PA. Effect of antihypertensive treatment on kidney function in diabetic nephropathy. BMJ 1987; 294: 1443-1447.
6.   Björck S, Mulec H, Johnsen SA, Nyberg G, Aurell M. Contrasting effects of enalapril and metoprolol on proteinuria in diabetic nephropathy. BMJ 1990; 300: 904-907.
7.   Björck S, Mulec H, Johnsen SA, Nordén G, Aurell M. Renal protective effect of enalapril in diabetic nephropathy. BMJ 1992; 304: 339-343.
8.   Mogensen CE. Angiotensin converting enzyme inhibitors and diabetic nephropathy. Their effects on proteinuria may be independent of their effects on blood pressure. BMJ 1992; 304: 327-328.
9.   Folin P. Laws governing the chemical composition of urine. Am J Physiol 1905; 13: 66.
10.   Fouque D, Laville M, Boisell JP, Chifflet R, Labeeuw M, Zech PY. Controlled low protein diets in chronic renal insufficiency: meta-analysis. BMJ 1992; 304: 216-220.
11.   Nath KA, Kren SA, Hostetter TH. Dietary protein restriction in established renal injury in the rat. J Clin Invest 1986; 78: 1199-1205.
12.   Hostetter TH, Meyer TW, Rennke HG, Brenner BM. Chronic effects of dietary protein in the rat with intact and reduced renal mass. Kidney Int 1986; 30: 509-517.
13.   El Nahas AM, Paraskevakou H, Zoob S, Rees AJ, Evans DJ. Effect of dietary protein restriction on the development of renal failure after subtotal nephrectomy in rats. Clin Sci 1983; 65: 399-406.
14.   Mauer SM, Steffes MW, Azar S, Brown DM. Effect of dietary protein content in streptozotocin-diabetic rats. Kidney Int 1989; 35: 48-59.
15.   Wiseman MJ, Hunt R, Goodwin A, Gross JL, Keen H, Viberti GC. Dietary composition and renal function in healthy subjects. Nephron 1987; 46: 37-42.
16.   Rouse IL, Armstrong BK, Beilin LJ, Vandongen R. Blood pressure-lowering effect of a vegetarian diet: controlled trial in normotensive subjects. Lancet 1983; i: 5-10.
17.   Viberti GC, Bognetti E, Wiseman MJ, Dodds R, Gross JL, Keen H. Effect of protein-restricted diet on renal response to a meat meal in humans. Am J Physiol 1987; 253: F388-F393.

18. Fioretto P, Trevisan R, Valerio A, et al. Imparied renal response to a meat meal in insulin-dependent diabetes: role of glucagon and prostaglandins. Am J Physiol 1990; 258: F675-F683.

19. Wiseman MJ, Bognetti E, Dodds R, Keen H, Viberti GC. Changes in renal function in response to protein restricted diet in type I (insulin-dependent) diabetic patients. Diabetologia 1987; 30: 154-159.

20. Rudberg S, Dahlquist G, Aperia A, Persson B. Reduction of protein intake decreases glomerular filtration rate in young Type 1 (insulin-dependent) diabetic patients mainly in hyperfiltering patients. Diabetologia 1988; 31: 878-883.

21. Cohen D, Dodds R, Viberti GC. Effect of protein restriction in insulin dependent diabetics at risk of nephropathy. BMJ 1987; 294: 795-798.

22. Rosenberg ME, Swanson JE, Thomas BL, Hostetter TH. Glomerular and hormonal responses to dietary protein intake in human renal disease. Am J Physiol 1987; 253: F1083-F1090.

23. Bending JJ, Dodds RA, Keen H, Viberti GC. Renal response to restricted protein intake in diabetic nephropathy. Diabetes 1988; 37: 1641-1646.

24. Krishna GP, Newell G, Miller E, Heeger P, Smith R, Polansky M, Kapoor S, Hoeldtke R. Protein-induced glomerular hyperfiltration: role of hormonal factors. Kidney Int 1988; 33: 578-583.

25. Kontessis P, Jones SL, Dodds RA, et al. Renal, metabolic and hormonal responses to ingestion of animal and vegetable proteins. Kidney Int 1990; 38: 136-144.

26. Castellino P, Giordano C, Perna A, DeFronzo RA. Effects of plasma amino acid and hormonal levels on renal hemodynamics in humans. Am J Physiol 1988; 247: F444-F449.

27. Paller MS, Hostetter TH. Dietary protein increases plasma renin and reduces pressor reactivity to angiotensin II. Am J Physiol 1986; 251: F34-F39.

28. Oates JA, Whorton AR, Gerkens JF, Branch RA, Hollifield JW, Frolich JC. The participation of prostaglandins in the control of renin release. Fed Proc 1979; 38: 72-74.

29. Fernandez-Repollet E, Tapia E, Martinez-Maldonado M. Effects of angiotensin-converting enzyme inhibition on altered renal hemodynamics induced by low protein diet in the rat. J Clin Invest 1987; 80: 1045-1049.

30. Fukui M, Nakamura T, Ebihara I, Nagaoka I, Tomino Y, Koide H. Low-protein diet attenuates increased gene expression of platelet-derived growth factor and transforming growth factor-ß in experimental glomerulosclerosis. J Lab Clin Med 1993; 121: 224-234.

31. Perrone RD, Madias NE, Levey AS. Serum creatinine as an index of renal function: new insights into old concepts. Clin Chem 1992; 38: 1933-1953.

32. Crim MC, Calloway DH, Margen S. Creatinine metabolism in man: creatine and creatinine excretions with creatine feeding. J Nutr 1975; 105: 428-438.

33. Crim MC, Calloway DH, Margen S. Creatinine metabolism in men: creatine pool size and turnover in relation to creatine intake. J Nutr 1976; 106: 371-381.

34. Shemesh O, Globetz M, Kriss JP, Meyers BD. Limitations of creatinine as a filtration marker in glomerulopathic patients. Kidney Int 1985; 28: 30-38.

35. Walker JD, Dodds RA, Bending JJ, Viberti GC. Monitoring kidney function in diabetic nephropathy. Diabetologia 1995; 38: 252.

36. Evanoff G, Thompson C, Brown J, Weinman E. Prolonged dietary protein restriction in diabetic nephropathy. Arch Intern Med 1989; 149: 1129-1133.

37.   Barsotti G, Ciardella F, Morelli E, Cupitsti A, Mantovanelli A, Giovenetti S. Nutritional treatment of renal failure in Type 1 diabetic nephropathy. Clin Nephrol 1988; 29: 280-287.

38.   Ciavarella A, Di Mizio GF, Stefoni S, Borgniino L, Vannini P. Reduced albuminuria after dietary protein restriction in insulin-dependent diabetic patients with clinical nephropathy. Diabetes Care 1987; 10: 407-413.

39.   Raal FJ, Kalk WJ, Lawson M, Esser JD, Buys R, Fourie L, Panz VR. Effect of moderate dietary protein restriction on the progression of overt diabetic nephropathy: a 6-mo prospective study. Am J Clin Nutr 1994; 60: 579-585.

40.   Zeller K, Whittaker E, Sullivan L, Raskin P, Jacobson HR. Effect of restricting dietary protein on renal failure in patients with insulin-dependent diabetes mellitus. N Engl J Med 1991; 324: 78-84.

41.   Walker JD, Bending JJ, Dodds RA, Mattock MB, Murrells TJ, Keen H, Viberti GC. Restriction of dietary protein and progression of renal failure in diabetic nephropathy. Lancet 1989; ii: 1411-1414.

42.   Pedrini MT, Levey AS, Lau J, Chalmers TC, Wang PH. The effect of dietary protein restriction on the progression of diabetic and non-diabetic renal disease: a meta-analysis. Ann Intern Med 1996; 124: 627-632.

43.   Parving H-H. Effects of dietary protein in renal disease (letter). Ann Intern Med 1997; 126: 330-331.

44.   Dullaart RPF, Van Doormaal JJ, Beusekamp BJ, Sluitter WJ, Meijer S. Long-term effects of protein-restricted diet on albuminuria and renal function in IDDM patients without clinical nephropathy and hypertension. Diabetes Care 1993; 16: 483-492.

45.   Lucas PA, Meadows JH, Roberts DE, Coles GA. The risks and benefits of a low protein-essential amino acid-keto acid diet. Kidney Int 1986; 29: 995-1003.

46.   Goodship THJ, Mitch WE. Nutritional approaches to preserving renal function. Adv Intern Med 1988; 33: 37-56.

47.   Locatelli F, Alberti D, Graziani G, Buccianti G, Redaelli B, Giangrande A. Prospective, randomized, multicentre trial of effect of protein restriction on progression of chronic renal insufficiency. Lancet 1991; 337: 1299-1304.

48.   Wingen AM, Fabian-Bach C, Schaefer F, Mehls O. Randomised multicentre study of a low-protein diet on the progression of chronic renal failure in children. Lancet 1997; 349: 1117-1123.

49.   Ledermann S, Shaw V, Trompeter R. Low-protein diet on the progression of chronic renal failure (letter) Lancet 1997; 350:146.

50.   Locatelli F. Low-protein diet on the progression of chronic renal failure (letter). Lancet 1997; 350:145.

51.   Levey AS, Adler S, Caggiula AW et al. Effects of dietary protein restriction on the progression of advanced renal disease in the modification of diet in renal disease study. Am J Kidney Dis. 1996; 27: 652-663.

52.   Klahr S, Levey AS, Beck GJ et al. The effects of dietary protein restriction and blood pressure control on the progression of chronic renal disease. N Engl J Med 1994; 330: 877-884.

53.   Ruilope LM, Casal MC, Praga M, et al. Additive antiproteinuric effect of converting enzyme inhibition and a low protein intake. J Am Soc Nephrol 1992; 3: 1307-1311.

54.   Ritz E, Matthias S. What you should know about blood pressure in renal disease. Proc R Coll Physicians Edinb. 1997; 27: 449-462.

55. Mulhauser I, Prange K, Sawicki PT, Bender R, Dworschak A, Berger M. Effects of dietary sodium on blood pressure in IDDM patients with nephropathy. Diabetologia 1996; 39: 212-219.

56. Maschio G. Low-protein diet and progression of renal disease: an endless story. Nephrol Dial Transplant 1995; 10: 1797-1800.

57. Toeller M, Klischan A, Heitkamp G, Schumacher W, Milne R, Buyken A, Karamanos B, Gries FA and the EURODIAB IDDM Complications Study Group. Nutritional intake of 2868 IDDM patients from 30 centres in Europe. Diabetologia 1996; 39: 929-939.

58. Pijls LT, de Vries H, Donker AJ, van Eijk JT. The effect of protein restriction on albuminuria in patiens with type 2 diabetes mellitus: a randomised trial. Nephrol Dial Transplant 1999, 14:1445-53.

59. Waugh NR, Robertson AM. Protein restriction in diabetic renal disease. In: Williams R, Nicolucci A, Krans HMJ, Ramirez G (eds). Diabetes module of the Cochrane database of systematic reviews (updated 1 September 1997). The Cochrane library. The Cochrane Collaboration, Issue 4, Oxford, 1997.

60. Toeller M, Buyken A, Heitkamp G, Bramswig S, Mann J, Milne R, Gries FA, Keen H. Protein intake and urinary albumin excretion rate in the EURODIAB IDDM Complications study. Diabetologia 1997; 40: 1219-26.

38.   DIABETIC NEPHROPATHY AND PREGNANCY

John L. Kitzmiller, MD, and C. Andrew Combs, MD, Ph.D
Division of Maternal-Fetal Medicine, Good Samaritan Hospital, San Jose, California, USA

The potential problems of diabetic nephropathy and pregnancy require the anticipation of preconception care. Every clinician who cares for adolescent and adult diabetic women has an obligation to recognise that these women may become pregnant, that most of the risks to mother and offspring are related to poor glycemic control, and that the risks may be reduced through special programs that achieve meticulous metabolic balance before conception and throughout pregnancy.

With diabetic nephropathy (DN), as with diabetes in general, in recent years the most common cause of perinatal morbidity and mortality is major congenital malformations [1]. A major advance is the demonstration that most malformations can be prevented by institution of strict metabolic control before conception in women with DN [2-4]. Every diabetic woman should have instruction in contraception [5,6] and should be intensively treated or referred to a specialized center when pregnancy is considered. The encouragement by diabetes care practitioners is a major factor in preventing unplanned pregnancies [7, 8].

In the past, women with DN were generally advised to avoid pregnancy because there was a low probability of a healthy infant and a chance that nephropathy would worsen. Although advances in obstetrical and neonatal care have improved the outlook, nephropathy in pregnancy still presents a challenging situation requiring coordination between the patient, obstetrician, perinatologist, diabetologist, nephrologist, ophthalmologist, neonatologist, nurse-educator, dietitian, social worker, and other personnel. As reviewed in this chapter, women with nephropathy remain at high risk for many pregnancy complications in addition to congenital malformations, including superimposed preeclampsia or accelerated hypertension, preterm delivery, fetal growth restriction, and cesarean delivery. Good glycemic balance and control of hypertension are necessary to reduce these complications and to slow the expected decline in renal function during and after pregnancy.

EVALUATION BEFORE CONCEPTION

An outline of preconception management of women with established diabetes is included in table 38-1. Evaluation for diabetic microvascular disease and hypertension are critical. Creatinine clearance (CrCl) as an estimate of GFR, and the degree of microalbuminuria (incipient DN, 30-299 mg/24 hrs)[9] or clinical total proteinuria (overt DN, >300 mg/24 hrs albumin, >500 mg/24 hrs total protein)[9] should be quantified, preferably with a 24-hour specimen [10,11,12]. If nephropathy is diagnosed, the patient should be thoroughly counselled regarding possible complications of pregnancy and her own probability of reduced life expectancy. She must then decide whether to attempt pregnancy.

Table 38-1 Management of diabetic nephropathy before and during pregnancy

At all times
Prevent hyperglycaemia
Control hypertension
Low protein diet
Restrict exercise

Prior to pregnancy
Measure renal function
Ophthalmologic exam
Cardiovascular evaluation
 (history, exam, EKG)
Thyroid evaluation
Hepatitis B surface antigen
Serologic testing for syphilis
Counseling and education

First prenatal visit
Measure renal function
Ophthalmologic exam
sonogram for dating

Second trimester
Measure renal function (12, 24 weeks)
Maternal serum alphafetoprotein (15-18 weeks)
Detailed sonogram with fetal echocardiogram (18-20 weeks)

Third trimester
Monthly sonogram
Weekly nonstress test (26 weeks)
Ophthalmologic exam
Measure renal function (36 weeks)
Delivery planning

Antihypertensive therapy is indicated for most patients with microalbuminuria or overt nephropathy. Agents should be used which are safe in early pregnancy. Angiotensin converting-enzyme (ACE) inhibitors are contraindicated during pregnancy because they may be teratogenic [13] and are associated with neonatal renal failure [14, 15]. This is unfortunate because there are extensive data, reviewed elsewhere in this volume, indicating that ACE-inhibitors retard the development and progression of nephropathy. The hypothesis that use of ACE-inhibitors in the preconception period will also decrease complications in the subsequent pregnancy [16] should be tested in controlled trials in women with excellent glycemic control. In a study of 8 women with presumed DN, Jovanovic found that normoglycemia achieved by early pregnancy also resulted in stable renal function and low complication rates [17]. Diltiazem and other calcium-entry blockers are probably best avoided during the first trimester since some data indicate an association with fetal limb defects [18]. Agents believed to be relatively safe for pregnancy include alpha-methyldopa, prazocin, clonidine, and beta-adrenergic antagonists.

Ophthalmologic examination is especially important for women with nephropathy because most also have diabetic retinopathy. Rapid normalization of blood glucose may cause worsening of retinopathy [19]. With background or proliferative retinopathy, allow a few months to normalize blood glucose before pregnancy. Proliferative retinopathy should be in remission or laser-treated before pregnancy. In women with background retinopathy at the beginning of pregnancy, there is a 6-10 % risk of development of neovascularization during gestation [20, 21].

The association of DN with cardiovascular disease [22] gives concern in evaluating patients for pregnancy, since there has been a high mortality in diabetic women with coronary artery disease [23]. There are no cross-sectional or prospective studies of the coronary vessels in diabetic women preparing for pregnancy. However, Manske et al found little coronary disease among diabetic patients <45 years old with end-stage renal disease if diabetes duration was less than 25 years, and there were no ST-T wave changes on ECG [24]. Therefore, pregnancy should be safe if these conditions are met. Otherwise, coronary angiography should be considered, since maternal-foetal outcome after coronary artery bypass grafts has been good [25].

Glycemic control is achieved with a meal plan, monitoring the food intake and blood glucose levels, and intensive insulin therapy. The diet prescription for pregnancy is 25-35 kcal/kg ideal body weight. With nephropathy, protein intake should be restricted, but 60 g/day is probably required for foetal development. The preferred insulin regimen includes a mix of short and intermediate-acting human insulins or continuous subcutaneous insulin infusion therapy. The optimal doses and timing are determined by self-monitored capillary blood glucose determinations before and after each meal. The targets for capillary blood glucose control before and during pregnancy are premeal values of 3.9-5.6 mM (70-100 mg/dL) and peak postprandial values of 5.6-7.2 mM (100-129 mg/dL) [1].

COURSE OF NEPHROPATHY DURING PREGNANCY

GFR rises by 40-80% in normal pregnancy, as reflected by increasing creatinine clearance and decreasing serum creatinine [26]. With diabetic nephropathy, however, the normal rise in CrCl is seen in only about one-third of patients, as summarized in table 38-2 [17,27,28]. In another one-third, CrCl actually decreases, probably reflecting the underlying natural progression of nephropathy or accelerating hypertension. Jovanovic found that prevention of hyperglycaemia and hypertension allowed a normal rise in CrCl during pregnancy in 8 diabetic women with sub-par values prior to conception [17]. On the other hand, Biesenbach et al observed that mean CrCl declined by 16% during the first two trimesters in 7 proteinuric diabetic women with subnormal CrCl prior to pregnancy (37-73 ml/min/1.73m2), in spite of intensified glycemic control and anthypertensive therapy during pregnancy [29].

Table 38-2

Changes in creatinine clearance in 44 women with diabetic nephopathy with measurements in both first and third trimester of pregnancy[a]

CrCl	First trimester n(%)	Third trimester Increased >25%	Stable	Decreased>15%
>90 ml/min	14 (32%)	3 (21%)	5 (36%)	6 (43%)
60-89 ml/min	20 (45.5%)	9 (45%)	6 (30%)	5 (25%)
<60 ml/min	10 (22.5%)	2 (20%)	6 (60%)	2 (20%)
Total	44 (100%)	14 (32%)	17 (39%)	13 (29%)

Data stratified by CrCl in first trimester: normal, moderate reduction, and severe reduction. Data pooled from Kitzmiller et al [27], Jovanovic and Jovanovic [17], and Reece et al [28].

An increase in kidney volume can be measured by ultrasound in pregnancies in normal controls [30] and in insulin-dependent diabetic women [31]. In the latter group the expansion occurs in spite of strict glycaemic control, and the increase correlates with CrCl but not with albuminuria, BP levels, or with the placental hormone hPL. Renal expansion is less in pregnant women with diabetic nephropathy, but renal volume did not decline as expected 4 months postpartum in this group in one study [31]. Interestingly, development of persistent microalbuminuria was most likely in the group of diabetic women with normoalbuminuria and relatively small renal volumes in early pregnancy.

The excretion of albumin increases slightly in normal pregnancy [32-34], while total urinary protein excretion increases by 40-200%, albeit to <300 mg/24hrs [35,36], presumably due to increased GFR and decreased tubular reabsorption (table 38-3) [12,36,37]. Therefore the charge- and pore size-specific glomerular barrier to filtration of albumin seems to remain intact. In diabetic women without microalbuminuria in early pregnancy, urinary albumin excretion increases slightly in the second trimester and sometimes greatly in the third trimester, while urinary total protein excretion can rise to >300 mg/24hrs [38-41]. Of course, some cases of this proteinuria may be explained by mild preeclampsia, which always clouds the view of changes in renal function in pregnant diabetic women. With microalbuminuria before pregnancy in diabetic women, the increase in albumin and total protein excretion during gestation is even greater (table 38-3) [42-44]. (Many [42,44-47] but not all investigators [48, 49] have observed that diabetic microalbuminuria in early pregnancy predicts a risk of superimposed preeclampsia of 35-60%). These gestational changes in total proteinuria mean that most clinical studies of DN in pregnancy have probably included women with undetected microalbuminuria prior to conception who happened to progress to mild macroproteinuria (400-600 mg total protein/24hrs) in early pregnancy, and thus were inappropriately counted as patients with mild DN. With definite clinical diabetic nephropathy diagnosed prior to pregnancy, albuminuria and total proteinuria often increases dramatically during gestation, even without associated hypertension, frequently exceeding 10 g/day in the third trimester. Though some of this increase may reflect the underlying progression of nephropathy, protein excretion usually subsides after delivery [27-29].

Table 38-3
Proteinuria before, during and after normal and type 1 diabetic pregnancies without clinical nephropathy.

	Before	3rd trimester	4*-6**mo PP
11 nl controls *			
ur alb (mg/d)	9	12	13
ur total prot (mg/d)	117*	262	174
7 normoalb type 1**			
ur alb	12	71	13
ur total prot	73	417	96
7 microalb type 1**			
ur alb	80	478	114
ur total prot	233	2350	239

* Roberts et al: Am J Physiol 270:F338, 1996; UAE 9 mg/d 12 mo PP
TPE 177 "" "" """"
** Biesenbach, Zasgornik: Br Med J 299:366, 1989

Maternal characteristics identified in early pregnancy in 225 cases of DN reported in 1981-1996 include ~50% frequencies of proliferative retinopathy (PDR), anemia, and hypertension. There were 45% of cases with reduced CrCl (<80 ml/min), and 15% with serum creatinine (Cr) >134uM (table 38-4) [17, 27,28, 50-57]. Minimal proteinuria (<1 gm total protein/24 hrs before 20 weeks gestation) was detected in many of the women, so these cases are suspected not to be "true" DN, therefore the frequencies of anemia, hypertension, PDR, and impaired glomerular filtration probably should be higher. Of 146 diabetic women with >1 gm total protein/24 hrs in early pregnancy, 57 had impaired renal function at that stage of gestation (Cr>134 uM or CrCl <80 ml/min), and 37% showed a further decline of >15% during later pregnancy. Subsequent series of pregnant women with DN reported since 1996 by Biesenbach [29] and Reece [58] show similar proportions of these complications.

Table 38-4
Course of renal parameters during and after pregnancy in women with diabetic nephropathy. Data pooled from references 27,28, 52-57

	Hypertension	Ur Prot > 5 gm/d	Decr CrCl Incr Cr	Renal Failure	Death
Early preg	42%	9%	34%	0	0
Late preg	71%	26%	26%	0	0
Follow-up	60%	17%	43%	23%**	5.6%

* 195 women x 1-10 yrs, median 2.6 yrs

Diabetic nephropathy can progress to end-stage renal disease during pregnancy, although this is unusual. Of 195 women followed after pregnancy and summarized in table 38-4, none progressed to end-stage disease during pregnancy. There is some experience with both haemodialysis and peritoneal dialysis in pregnancy [59, 60]. Complications of dialysis include preeclampsia, placental abruption and stillbirth. The latter two are related to large shifts in extravascular volume and may be less common with peritoneal dialysis [59]. Because of the high complication rate, pregnancy is probably contraindicated if the serum creatinine is above 177 uM or creatinine clearance is below 50 ml/min, at least until renal transplantation can be performed.

EFFECT OF PREGNANCY ON THE NATURAL HISTORY OF DN
For years, there has been a hypothetical concern that the physiologic hyperfiltration of pregnancy might damage the glomeruli and accelerate the postpartum progression of diabetic nephropathy to end-stage renal disease. However, the few data available that directly address this hypothesis do not support it. Three studies assessed renal function after pregnancy in women with nephropathy [27,55,61]. All three found that creatinine clearance declined an average of about 10 ml/min per year, no different than the average rate in men and women with diabetic nephropathy without pregnancy [62].

In the pooled series of 195 women experiencing pregnancies with DN and having renal function assessed 1-10 years afterwards, 23% were in renal failure and 5.6% had died (table 38-4). Not surprisingly, the frequency of progression to renal failure after pregnancy was 49% in the group of women with impaired renal function in early pregnancy, compared to 7% if Cr was <134 uM or CrCl was >80 ml/min in early gestation (table 38-5) [17, 27,28,50-57]. This risk prediction based on pre- or early pregnancy CrCl was also observed in the recent study of Biesenbach, and he speculated that inadequate antihypertensive therapy may contribute to this [29]. Other approaches have been used to examine the question of whether experiencing pregnancy hastens the progression of diabetic nephropathy. With impaired renal function, the speed of progression to end-stage disease is little or no different whether a pregnancy is terminated in the first trimester or carried into the third trimester [27]. Miodovnik observed that increasing parity did not increase the risk of renal failure after pregnancy [55], and the EURODIAB type 1 complications survey found that parity did not increase the incidence of micro- or macroalbuminuria [63]. Purdy et al thought that 5 of 11 women with DN and moderate renal insufficiency had an accelerated rate of decline in renal function during pregnancy, but in follow-up for a mean of 2 years postpartum the group of 11 had slightly less decline in inverse Cr than 11 similar patients without pregnancy [56]. Mackie and colleagues [57] and Kaaja et al [64] also found no evidence for accelerated decline of renal function after pregnancy compared to non-pregnant patients. Therefore the medical practice of discouraging pregnancy in women with DN with mild-to-moderate impairment of renal function based on presumed increased risks of renal failure has no basis on published experience.

Table 38-5
Course of diabetic nephropathy during and after pregnancy comparing patients with preserved vs impaired renal function in early pregnancy. Data pooled from references 27,28,52,53,54 . Note the limited number of cases with severe azotemia in early pregnancy.

| | Initial renal function | | Cr |
	Preserved	Impaired*	>177
Number	70	57	(6)
Decline during pregnancy	12 (17%)	21 (37%)	(1)
Renal failure after preg**	4 of 57 (7%)	37 of 55 (49%)	(3)
Died	2 (3.5%)	5 (9.1%)	(0)

* Cr >100 uM, CrCl < 80 ml/min
** 1-10 yrs.

DIABETIC NEPHROPATHY AND PERINATAL OUTCOME
In spite of the dramatic improvements in perinatal outcome over the last 25 years in pregnancies of diabetic women [65], complications remain more frequent when DN is present. Examining the pooled results of the 13 clinical series published in 1981-96 (table 38-6) [16,17,27,28,50-57,66], of 265 infants born to women with DN, nearly 2/3 were preterm deliveries prior to 37 weeks gestation, 72.5% were delivered by caesarean section, and respiratory distress syndrome was diagnosed in 24.5% of liveborn infants.

Foetal growth restriction was noted in 14.3%, and the major correlates of small size for dates were the degree of maternal hypertension and impaired renal function [27,28,53]. Major congenital malformations were diagnosed in 7.55% of the 265 infants. The frequencies of these perinatal complication were similar in 90 pregnancies reported in 1981-88 compared to 175 reported in 1992-96 (table 38-6), and in the subsequent report of Reece et al [58]. Perinatal mortality rates were 5.55/1000 and 34.3/1000 in the earlier and latter group, respectively. Overall, 95.8% of infants survived to leave the neonatal intensive care unit.

It must be noted that these clinical results may be somewhat worse in women with "true" clinical DN, since at least 16% of the pooled cases probably had only microalbuminuria prior to pregnancy, because they were included in the DN series based on <1 gm/day total protein excretion in the first trimester. Limiting the analysis of perinatal mortality to 223 cases with >1 gm/day total urinary protein excretion in the first trimester, perinatal mortality rates were 54.8/1000 in 1982-88 compared to 71.4/1000 in 1992-96 (table 38-6). Major congenital malformations and severe foetal growth restriction were responsible for most of the perinatal deaths.

Table 38-6
Diabetic nephropathy and perinatal outcome in two eras in which perinatal technology was utilized. Data pooled from references 17,27,28,50-57.

Year of report	1981-88	1992-96
Infants	90	275
Perinatal survival	94.4%	96.6%
Foetal growth restriction	13.3%	14.9%
Preterm delivery	57.8%	64.6%
Caesarean delivery	68.9%	74.3%
Respiratory distress syndrome	25.6%	24.2%
Major congenital malformations	7.8%	7.7%

The relationship of perinatal morbidity to the severity of diabetic nephropathy is illustrated in table 38-7. Selecting out cases from the pooled series with sufficient detail for analysis [27, 28, 52, 53], 19 women had >1 gm/day total urinary protein with preserved renal function in early pregnancy, compared to 41 proteinuric diabetic women with CrCl <80 ml/min. or serum Cr >134 uM. Not surprisingly, the latter group had much higher rates of foetal growth restriction, preeclampsia, foetal distress causing delivery, and serious prematurity (table 38-7). These data can be used for counselling women with DN prior to pregnancy.

Superimposed preeclampsia is a leading cause of prematurity in women with diabetes [67, 68] and DN [27, 28, 52, 53, 69]. The condition is suspected when there is an increase in blood pressure and proteinuria in the third trimester. With preexisting nephropathy, it may not be possible to clinically distinguish "true" preeclampsia from a "simple" worsening of hypertension and proteinuria. The distinction is important because the former is best treated by delivery whereas the latter is treated with bed rest and antihypertensive agents. Edema and hyperuricemia are common in patients with renal disease and therefore are not useful in the differential diagnosis. Occasionally, thrombocytopenia or elevated transaminases are found and these support a diagnosis of superimposed preeclampsia. As a practical matter, it is generally necessary to observe the patient at hospital bed rest, with or without antihypertensive therapy. Hypoalbuminemia commonly results from excessive proteinuria and leads to generalized edema. Serious edema can be treated with diuretics. It is controversial whether albumin infusions are beneficial or useless. The decision to deliver the infant must balance the gestational age, the severity of the maternal condition, and indicators of foetal well-being.

Table 38-7
Perinatal outcome related to renal status in early pregnancy in women with diabetic nephropathy. Data combined from cases reported in references 27,28,52,53.

		Initial Renal Function	
	Prot 0.3-0.9gm/d	Preserved	Impaired*
Number	18	19	41
Fetal growth restriction	1 (6%)	1 (5%)	11 (27%)
Preeclampsia	2 (11%)	4 (21%)	15 (37%)
Fetal distress	1 (6%)	4 (21%)	12 (29%)
Fetal death	1	1	1
Deliv 24-33 w	4 (22%)	5 (26%)	18 (38%)
Uncomplicated	10 (56%)	6 (32%)	9 (24%)
*Cr >1.2 or CrC1 <80 ml/min			

Maternal anemia results from both decreased erythropoietin production by damaged glomeruli and the physiologic hemodilution of pregnancy. The degree of anemia is related to the severity of nephropathy as reflected in lower creatinine clearance and is not usually associated with abnormal iron studies [27]. Exogenous erythropoietin can be considered to treat anemia unresponsive to iron and folate replacement [70-72].

As noted, foetal growth delay is related to maternal hypertension. Serial sonography is indicated to evaluate foetal growth. In addition, foetal heart rate monitoring or biophysical assessment should be employed because growth restriction or foetal hyperglycemia-hypoxia-acidosis [73] is frequently associated with evidence of foetal distress. For women with clinical DN, begin weekly nonstress testing at 26 weeks' gestation and twice-weekly testing at 34 weeks, earlier if there is growth delay. Vaginal delivery is preferred if there is no evidence of foetal distress and no obstetric contraindication. However, as noted in table 38-6, there was a remarkably high caesarean rate with DN, the reasons for which are not entirely elucidated.

PREGNANCY AFTER RENAL TRANSPLANTATION

Ogburn et al. compiled the experience of nine diabetic women from several centers who had pregnancy after renal transplantation for DN [74]. All were managed with prednisone and azathioprine. No transplant rejections occurred during pregnancy. Complications were frequent, including preeclampsia in six, fetal distress in six, and preterm delivery in all. Armenti and the US Transplant Pregnancy Registry reported 28 pregnancies in diabetic renal transplant recipients [75]. Rejection was observed in 4% and graft dysfunction in 11%. Preeclampsia was diagnosed in 17% although 59% had hypertension - 47% of the infants had neonatal complications. Combined kidney-pancreas transplants prior to pregnancy have been reported several times [76, 77], and Armenti and colleagues also reported 12 pregnancies after combined transplants [75]. In this group 25% had preeclampsia while 83% were hypertensive. Two-thirds of these gravidas were treated for some type of infections. Barrou et al reviewed 19 cases of pregnancy after simultaneous pancreas-kidney transplants reported to the International Pancreas Transplant Registry [78]. There were 19 live births with average birth weight 2150 + 680 gm and two major congenital malformations. Only one pancreas graft and one kidney graft were lost after pregnancy in two different recipients.

Beyond these studies, there has been hypothetical concern that pregnancy may adversely affect renal graft survival. However, two recent studies with long-term follow-up found no difference in graft survival or function between women who became pregnant and matched controls who did not [79, 80].

REFERENCES

1. Kitzmiller JL, Buchanan TA, Kjos S, et al. Pre-conception care of diabetes, congenital malformations, and spontaneous abortions. Technical review. Diab Care 1996; 19:514-41
2. Fuhrmann K, Reiher H, Semmler K, Glockner E. The effect of intensified conventional insulin therapy before and during pregnancy on the malformation rate in offspring of diabetic mothers. Exp Clin Endocrinol 1984; 83: 173-7.
3. Damm P, Molsted-Pedersen L. Significant decrease in congenital malformations in newborn infants of an unselected population of diabetic women. Am J Obst Gynec 1989; 161:1163-7
4. Kitzmiller JL, Gavin LA, Gin GD, et al. Preconception care of diabetes. Glycemic control prevents congenital anomalies. JAMA 1991; 265: 731-6.
5. StJames PJ, Younger MD, Hamilton BD, Waisbren SE. Unplanned pregnancies in diabetic women. Diab Care 1993; 16:1572-8
6. Kjos SL. Contraception in diabetic women. Obst Gynecol Clinics North Amer 1996; 23:243-57
7. Janz NK, Herman WH, Becker MP, et al. Diabetes and pregnancy: factors associated with seeking pre-conception care. Diab Care 1995; 18: 157-65.
8. Holing E, Beyer CS. Why don't women with diabetes plan their pregnancies? Diab 1997; 46, Suppl 1: 15A.
9. Mogensen CE, Chachati A, Christensen CK et al. Microalbuminuria: an early marker for renal involvement in diabetes. Uremia Invest 1985-86; 9:85-95.
10. Combs CA, Wheeler BC, Kitzmiller JL. Urinary protein/creatinine ratio before and during pregnancy in women with diabetes mellitus. Am J Obstet Gynecol 1991; 165: 920-923.

11. Stehouwer CDA, Fischer HRA, Hackeng WHL, et al. Diurnal variation in urinary protein excretion in diabetic nephropathy. Nephrol Dial Transplant 1991; 6: 238-243.
12. Quadri KHM, Bernardini J, Greenberg MD, et al. Assessment of renal function during pregnancy using a random urine protein to creatinine ratio and Cockcroft-Gault ratio. Amer J Kid Dis 1994; 24:416-20.
13. Piper JM, Ray WA, Rosa FW. Pregnancy outcome following exposure to angiotensin-converting enzyme inhibitors. Obst Gynec 1992; 80: 429-32.
14. Rosa FW, Bosco LA, Graham CF, et al. Neonatal anuria with maternal angiotensin-converting enzyme inhibition. Obst Gynec 1989; 74:371.
15. Hanssens M, Keirse MJNC, Vankelecom F, Van Assche FA. Fetal and neonatal effects of treatment with angiotensin-converting enzyme inhibitors in pregnancy. Obstet Gynecol 1991; 78: 128-135.
16. Hod M, van Dijk DJ, Karp M, et al. Diabetic nephropathy and pregnancy: the effect of ACE inhibitors prior to pregnancy on maternal outcome. Neph Dial Transpl 1995; 10: 2328-33
17. Jovanovic R, Jovanovic L. Obstetric management when normoglycemia is maintained in diabetic pregnant women with vascular compromise. Am J Obstet Gynecol 1984; 149: 617-623.
18. Magee LA, Conover B, Schick B, et al. Exposure to calcium channel blockers in human pregnancy: a prospective, controlled, multicentre cohort study. Teratol 1994; 49:372-6.
19. Brinchmann-Hansen O, Dahl-Jørgensen K, Hanssen KF, et al. Effects of intensified insulin treatment on various lesions of diabetic retinopathy. Am J Ophthalmol 1985; 100: 644-9
20. Klein BEK, Moss SE, Klein R. Effect of pregnancy on progression of diabetic retinopathy. Diab Care 1990;13:34-40.
21. Chew EY, Mills JL, Metzger BE, et al. The diabetes and early pregnancy study. Metabolic control and progression of retinopathy. Diab Care 1995;18:631-7.
22. Jensen T, Borch-Johnson K, Kofoed-Enevoldsen A, Deckert T. Coronary heart disease in young type 1 (insulin dependent) diabetic patients with and without diabetic nephropathy: incidence and risk factors. Diabetologia 1987; 30: 144-8.
23. Reece EA, Egan JFX, Coustan DR, et al. Coronary artery disease in diabetic pregnancies. Amer J Obst Gynec 1986; 154: 150-1.
24. Manske CL, Thomas W, Wang Y, Wilson RF. Screening diabetic transplant candidates for coronary artery disease: identification of a low risk subgroup. Kidney Intl 1993; 44: 617-21
25. Salomon NW, Page US, Okies JE, et al. Diabetes mellitus and coronary artery bypass: short term risk and long term prognosis. J Thorac Cardiovasc Surg 1983; 85: 264-8.
26. Krutzen E, Olofsson P, Back SE, Nilsson-Ehle P. Glomerular filtration rate in pregnancy: a study in normal subjects and in patients with hypertension, preeclampsia and diabetes. Scand J Clin Lab Invest 1992; 52: 387-392.
27. Kitzmiller JL, Brown ER, Phillippe M, et al. Diabetic nephropathy and perinatal outcome. Am J Obstet Gynecol 1981; 141: 741-751.
28. Reece EA, Coustan DR, Hayslett JP, et al. Diabetic nephropathy: pregnancy performance and fetomaternal outcome. Am J Obstet Gynecol 1988; 159: 56-66.
29. Biesenbach G, Grafinger P, Stoger H, Zasgornik J. How pregnancy influences renal function in nephropathic type 1 diabetic women depends on their pre-conception creatinine clearance. J Nephrol. 1999; 12:41-46.
30. Christensen T, Klebe JG, Berthelsen V, Hansen HE. Changes in renal volume during normal pregnancy. Acta Obst Gynec Scand 1989; 68:541-3.

31. Lauszas FF, Klebe JG, Rasmussen OW, et al. Renal growth during pregnancy in insulin-dependent diabetic women. A prospective study of renal volume and clinical variables. Acta Diabetol 1995; 32:225-9.

32. Pedersen EB, Rasmussen AB, Johannsen P, et al. Urinary excretion of albumin, beta-2-microglobulin and light chains in preeclampsia, essential hypertension in pregnancy, and normotensive pregnant and non-pregnant control subjects. Scand J Clin Lab Investig 1981; 41:777-84.

33. Lopez-Espinoza I, Humphreys S, Redman CWG. Urinary albumin excretion in pregnancy. Br J Obst Gynec 1986; 93:176-81.

34. Wright A, Steele P, Bennett JR, et al. The urinary excretion of albumin in normal pregnancy. Br J Obstet Gynaecol 1987; 94: 408-412.

35. Cheung CK, Lao T, Swaminathan R. Urinary excretion of some proteins and enzymes during normal pregnancy. Clin Chem 1989; 35: 1978-1980.

36. Higby K, Suiter CR, Phelps JY, et al. Normal values of urinary albumin and total protein excretion during pregnancy. Am J Obst Gynec 1994; 171: 984-9.

37. Roberts M, Lindheimer MD, Davison JM. Altered glomerular permselectivity to neutral dextrans and heteroporous membrane modeling in human pregnancy. Am J Physiol 1996; 270: F338-43.

38. McCance DR, Traub AI, Harley JMG, et al. Urinary albumin excretion in diabetic pregnancy. Diabetologia 1989; 32:236-9.

39. Biesenbach G, Zasgornik J. Incidence of transient nephrotic syndrome during pregnancy in diabetic women with and without pre-existing microalbuminuria. Br Med J 1989; 299: 366-7.

40. MacRury SM, Pinion S, Quin JD, et al. Blood rheology and albumin excretion in diabetic pregnancy. Diabetic Med 1995; 12: 51-5.

41. Diglas J, Bali C, Simon C, Strassegger-Bohm, Irsigler K. [Renal excretion of albumin during pregnancy and after birth in type 1 diabetic patients compared to metabolically healthy women]. [article in German]. Acta Med Austriaca 1997; 24:170-174.

42. Winocour PH, Taylor RJ. Early alterations in renal function in insulin-dependent diabetic pregnancies and their importance in predicting preeclamptic toxaemia. Diabetes Res 1989; 10: 159-164.

43. Biesenbach G, Zasgornik J, Stoger H, et al. Abnormal increases in urinary albumin excretion during pregnancy in IDDM women with preexisting albuminuria. Diabetologia 1994; 37: 905-10.

44. Combs CA, Rosenn B, Kitzmiller JL, et al. Early-pregnancy proteinuria in diabetes related to preeclampsia. Obstet Gynecol 1993; 82: 802-807.

45. Bar J, Hod M, Erman A, et al. Microalbuminuria as an early predictor of hypertensive complications in pregnant women at high risk. Am J Kidney Dis 1996; 28: 220-5.

46. Das V, Bhargava T, Das SK, Pandey S. Microalbuminuria: a predictor of pregnancy-induced hypertension. Br J Obst Gynec 1996; 103: 928-30.

47. Ekbom P and the Copenhagen Pre-eclampsia in Diabetic Pregnancy Study Group. Pre-pregnancy microalbuminuria predicts pre-eclampsia in insulin-dependent diabetes mellitus. Lancet 1999; 353:377.

48. Konstantin-Hansen KF, Hesseldahl H, Moller Pedersen S. Microalbuminuria as a predictor of preeclampsia. Acta Obst Gynec Scand 1992; 71: 341-6.

49. Mogensen CE, Klebe JG. Microalbuminuria and diabetic pregnancy, in Mogensen, CE (ed.) The Kidney and Hypertension in Diabetes Mellitus. Fourth Edition. 1998 by Kluwer Academic Publishers, Boston/Dordrecht/London, 455-462

50. Dicker D, Feldberg, Peleg, et al. Pregnancy complicated by diabetic nephropathy. J Perin Med 1986; 14: 299-306.

51. Grenfell A, Brudenell JM, Doddridge MC, Watkins PJ. Pregnancy in diabetic women who have proteinuria. Quart J Med 1986; 59: 379-386

52. Biesenbach G, Stoger H, Zasgornik J. Influence of pregnancy on progression of diabetic nephropathy and subsequent requirement of renal replacement therapy in female type I diabetic patients with impaired renal function. Nephrol Dial Transplant 1992; 7: 105-109.

53. Kimmerle R, Zass R-P, Cupisti S, et al. Pregnancies in women with diabetic nephropathy: long-term outcome for mother and child. Diabetologia 1995; 38: 227-235.

54. Gordon M, Landon MB, Samuels P, et al. Perinatal outcome and long-term follow-associated with modern managment of diabetic nephropathy. Obstet Gynecol 1996; 87: 401-409.

55. Miodovnik M, Rosenn BM, Khoury JC, et al. Does pregnancy increase the risk for development and progression of diabetic nephropathy? Am J Obst Gynecol 1996:174:1180-91.

56. Purdy LP, Hantsch CE, Molitsch ME, et al. Effect of pregnancy on renal function in patients with moderate-to-severe diabetic renal insufficiency. Diab Care 1996; 19: 1067-74

57. Mackie ADR, Doddridge MC, Gamsu HR, et al. Outcome of pregnancy in patients with insulin-dependent diabetes mellitus and nephropathy with moderate renal impairment. Diabetic Med 1996; 13: 90-96.

58. Reece EA, Leguizamon G, Homko C. Stringent controls in diabetic nephropathy associated with optimization of pregnancy outcomes. J Mat-Fetal Med 1998; 7:213-216.

59. Yasin SY, Bey Doun SN. Hemodialysis in pregnancy. Obst Gynec Surv 1988; 43: 655-68.

60. Hou S. Pregnancy in women requiring dialysis for renal failure. Am J Kidney Dis 1987; 9: 368-375.

61. Reece EA, Winn HN, Hayslett JP, et al. Does pregnancy alter the rate of progression of diabetic nephropathy? Am J Perinat 1990; 7: 193-7.

62. Mogensen CE. Progression of nephropathy in long-term diabetics with proteinuria and effect of initial antihypertensive treatment. Scand J Clin Lab Invest 1976; 36: 383-7.

63. Chaturvedi N, Stephenson JM, Fuller JH, et al. The relationship between pregnancy and long-term maternal complications in the EURODIAB IDDM complications study. Diabetic Med 1995; 12: 494-9.

64. Kaaja R, Sjoberg L, Hellstedt T, et al. Long-term effects of pregnancy on diabetic complications. Diabetic Med 1996; 13: 165-9.

65. Kitzmiller JL. Sweet success with diabetes. The development of insulin therapy and glycemic control for pregnancy. Diab Care 1993; 16 (Suppl 3): 107-21.

66. Holley JL, Bernardini J, Quadri KHM, et al. Pregnancy outcomes in a prospective matched control study of pregnancy and renal disease. Clinical Nephrol 1996; 45:77-82.

67. Greene MF, Hare JW, Krache M, et al. Prematurity among insulin-requiring diabetic gravid women. Am J Obst Gynec 1989; 161: 106-11.

68. Garner PR, D'Alton ME, Dudley DK, et al. Preeclampsia in diabetic pregnancies. Am J Obst Gynec 1990; 163: 505-8.

69. Hopp H, Vollert W, Ebert A, Weitzel H, Glockner E, Jahrig D. [Diabetic retinopathy and nephropathy û complications during pregnancy and delivery]. [article in German]. Geburtsh. U. Frauenheilk. 1995; 55:275-279.

70. Yankowitz J, Piraino B, Laifer A, et al. Use of erythroitin in pregnancies complicated by severe anemia of renal failure. Obst Gynecol. 1992; 80:485-488.

71. Hou S, Orlowski J, Pahl M, et al. Pregnancy in women with end-stage renal disease: treatment of anemia and premature labor. Am J Kidney Dis 1993; 21: 16-22.

72. Braga J, Marques R, Branco A, et al. Maternal and perinatal implications of the use of human recombinant erythroitin. Acta Obst Gynecol Scand 1996; 75:449-453.

73. Salvesen DR, Higueras MT, Brudenell M, et al. Doppler velocimetry and fetal heart studies in nephropathic diabetics. Am J Obst Gynec 1992; 167: 1297-1303.

74. Ogburn PL, Jr, Kitzmiller JL, Hare JW, et al. Pregnancy following renal transplantation in class T diabetes mellitus. JAMA 1986; 225: 911-5.

75. Armenti VT, McGrory CH, Cater J, et al. The national transplantation registry: comparison between pregnancy outcomes in diabetic cyclosporine-treated female kidney recipients and CyA-treated female pancreas-kidney recipients. Transpl Proc 1997; 29: 669-70.

76. Skannal DG, Miodovnik M, Dungy-Poythress LJ, First MR. Successful pregnancy after combined renal-pancreas transplantation: a case report and literature review. Am J Perinatol 1996; 13: 383-7.

77. Karaitis LK, Nankivell BJ, Lawrence S, et al. Successful obstetric outcome after simultaneous pancreas and kidney transplantation. Med J Aust 1999; 170:368-370.

78. Barrou BM, Gruessner AC, Sutherland DE, Gruessner RW. Pregnancy after pancreas transplantation in the cyclosporine era: report from the International Pancreas Transplant Registry. Transplantation 1998:65:524-527.

79. Davison JM. The effect of pregnancy on kidney function in renal allograft recipients. Kidney Int 1985; 27: 74-9.

80. First MR, Combs CA, Weiskittel P, Miodovnik M. Lack of effect of pregnancy on renal allograft survival or function. Transplantation 1995; 59: 472-6.

39. EVOLUTION WORLDWIDE OF RENAL REPLACEMENT THERAPY IN DIABETES

Rudy Bilous
Audrey Collins Teaching Unit, Education Centre, South Cleveland Hospital, Marton Road, MIDDLESBROUGH, UK, TS4 3BW

The numbers of patients entering renal replacement therapy (RRT) with diabetic nephropathy as their primary disease continues to rise world-wide, although there is some suggestion that the rate of increase may be declining in the USA [1]. However, long term survival of patients on RRT remains much less good for diabetic compared to non-diabetic recipients [2], although short term (one year) mortality adjusted for age has declined from 40.4 to 23.2 per 100 patient years in the decade 1986-96 in the USA [3].

It must be remembered that much of these data are extracted from registers of patients who have been accepted onto RRT programmes, they are therefore an underestimate of the true prevalence of renal failure in diabetes as many patients will not survive until end stage renal disease (ESRD). Secondly, some registers are much less comprehensive, with ascertainment rates as low as 55% of patient questionnaires in Europe [2]. Finally, methods of reporting differ between registers. The USRDS data retrieval only begins after patients have survived 90 days of RRT [4] whereas data from Europe and Japan relate to entry onto RRT[2,5].

Nonetheless, reported differences and contrasts in the incidence and outcome between countries raise intriguing questions about both the pathophysiology of diabetic nephropathy and optimum management of ESRD in diabetes [6,7]. The following areas will be covered in turn:-

1. Evolution of acceptance of diabetic patients onto RRT.
2. Impact of age, type of diabetes and ethnicity of subject population.
3. Mode and outcome of RRT used to treat diabetic patients.
4. Suggested management strategies.

Since the last edition, there have been more reports from countries on acceptance and outcomes for diabetic patients on dialysis, and this chapter will be an update incorporating these data.

EVOLUTION OF ACCEPTANCE OF DIABETIC PATIENTS ONTO RRT

The USRDS has shown a year on year increase in the incidence of new diabetic patients entering RRT to 41.8% of the total enrolled in 1997 (33,096 of 79,102 patients) [1]. This represents a rate of 120 per million population (pmp). The annual increase in incidence rates for diabetic ESRD fell from 14% in 1988-92 to 9% in 1992-96, but this rate was still 3 times higher than that recorded for non-diabetic causes. Overall prevalence seems to be showing a decline in the rate of increase from 15% in 1988-92 to 11% in 1992-96; however, in 1982, diabetic patients would comprise only 3% (21pmp) patients on RRT in an average dialysis centre, whereas nationally the figures were 26.1% (188pmp) in 1991 and 33.2% (366pmp) in 1997 [1].

In Japan in 1994, the incidence of diabetes as a cause of RRT requiring haemodialysis (HD), (which represents 92.7% of all RRT), was 31.2% (60pmp) and the prevalence was 18.2% (209pmp) total population, which is more than double the figure for 1984 (8.2%) [5].

In Europe, recent data collection is much less complete than previously [2] and it is hard to draw firm conclusions across frontiers since 1992. However, where the data are confirmed by national registers, it is still possible to detect more recent trends. In 1978 overall prevalence of diabetes as the primary renal disease was 3.8%, compared to 13% in 1989 and 17% (50pmp) in 1992 [8]. These prevalence figures hide a wide range in international and within country incidence rates, however; Austria recording 21pmp, Denmark 14pmp, and the Netherlands 8.5pmp; whereas in the UK the national figure was 6pmp, with one inner city unit in London recording 34pmp in 1993. More recent reports illustrate how the overall figures have grown but emphasise contrast between and within countries. For example, in Germany [9], the total incidence and prevalence of patients entering RRT from all causes of renal failure was 156 and 713pmp in 1998, with diabetes representing 48 and 150pmp respectively. In Catalunya in Spain, the incidence of patients with diabetes entering RRT rose from 8-19.8pmp from 1984-94 [10]. In Madrid there was a similar rise from 10 to 21pmp over the same period, the latest figures are of 32 pmp in 1998 [11]. In France the proportion of diabetic patients entering RRT in 1995-96 was 40% in Alsace but only 13.2% for the rest of the mainland [12]. This apparent and as yet unexplained geographical north east to south west gradient requires further exploratory research.

Reports from Latin America for 1993 [13] and one centre in India for 1996/7 [14] from highly selected populations of patients entering RRT are of 16.9 and 13.8% respectively having diabetic nephropathy. These figures cannot be taken as representative of the overall renal failure population however, because of very variable selection criteria. The latest international comparison shows a range of prevalences of diabetic patients entering RRT from 11.2% in Poland to 42% in the USA (figure 39-1) [15]. The overall message however, is of a continuing and exponential growth in diabetic patients entering RRT, in nearly all countries.

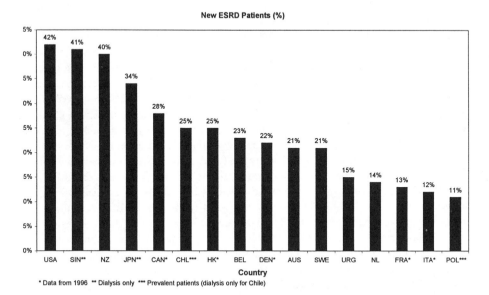

Figure 39-1. Percentage of incident ESRD patients with diabetic nephropathy as a cause. Australia (AUS), New Zealand (NZ), Canada (CAN), Chile (CHL) are prevalent patients and dialysis only. Uruguay (URG), Japan (JPN), and Singapore (SIN) are for dialysis only. Hong Kong (HK) and Poland (POL) are for prevalent patients. All data are from 1997 except from Canada, Denmark, France, Hong Kong and Italy which are from 1996. Figure reproduced from the USRDS Report 1999. With kind permission of the Editor of the American Journal of Kidney Disease (ref 15).

IMPACT OF AGE, TYPE OF DIABETES AND ETHNICITY OF POPULATION

Part of the explanation for the increasing numbers of diabetic patients on RRT has been a relaxation of age limits for entry [2]. Diabetes prevalence increases dramatically with age and one of the major risk factors for the development of nephropathy is duration of disease. Thus it is no surprise that as the average age of acceptance onto RRT for all causes of ESRD has increased from 45.8 years in 1977 to 57.4 years in 1992 in Europe, and the number of new patients commencing RRT over 65 years at acceptance increased from 9 to 37% of the total over the same period of time [2], that the proportion with diabetes has jumped dramatically. In Japan the mean age rose from 49.2 to 57.3 years over the period 1984-94 [5], and in the USA the increase in median age of incidence of ESRD was slightly less dramatic from approximately 62 years in 1988 to 65 years in

1997 [1]. Diabetes remains the commonest single cause of ESRD in those aged over 64 years entering RRT in 1993-7 in the USA (37.3%) [1].

Although the cumulative incidence and rates of development of nephropathy are similar for both types of diabetes [16], a smaller proportion of patients with type 2 enter RRT, probably because of excess cardiovascular mortality prior to developing ESRD [17]. However as there are numerically many more patients with type 2 diabetes, and the treatments for cardiovascular disease become more effective, they represent a greater and growing proportion of the diabetic population on RRT (table 39-1). The reported figures are not totally reliable however, because the assignation of patients by type of diabetes has been shown to be very imprecise, particularly in the EDTA register [18,19]. Using a carefully designed algorithm for the diagnosis of diabetes type, Cowie et al [20] found an increased probability of developing ESRD over a 10 year period of 5.82% in type 1 but only 0.5% in type 2 African American and Europid patients. However there was a suggestion of an increasing incidence in type 2 patients over the decade 1974-83. The proportion of diabetic patients with carefully defined type 2 diabetes on RRT varies from 50-90% in Europid populations world-wide [21]. In the latest USRDS Report, approximately 71% of 143,854 patients registered with diabetic ESRD from 1993-7 were recorded as type 2 (table 39-1) [1].

It is difficult to separate the impact of type of diabetes from ethnic factors. In Japan for example, >90% of patients on RRT have type 2 diabetes [5] but this is a reflection of the remarkably low incidence of type 1 nationally. Many ethnic groups have high prevalences of both type 2 diabetes and nephropathy [22], and countries with minorities with these characteristics will reflect an over preponderence in their RRT population.

For example, in 1993 diabetic Aboriginal patients in Australia and Maori/Pacific Islanders in New Zealand receiving RRT were 85% and 83% type 2 respectively, compared to Europid populations of 48 and 55% in the same countries (table 39-1) [21].

The USRDS reports that incidence of ESRD for all causes in 1997 for African Americans was 873, for Native Americans 586, and for Asian/Pacific Islanders 344 pmp per year, compared to 218 pmp per year for Europids [1]. Analysis of incidence data from 1993-7 has revealed that although Native Americans with diabetic ESRD represented just 2.3% of the total diabetic population receiving RRT, diabetes accounted for 65.1% of all Native Americans registered on the database. The figures for Asian/Pacific Islanders were similarly discrepant at 3.5 and 42.6%; whereas those for African Americans were 28.5 and 39%; and for Europids 63.6 and 40.1% respectively (table 39-1). The incidence rates of treated ESRD for diabetes for the period 1991-3 were 322, 89, 224, and 57 pmp/year for Native Americans, Asian/Pacific Islanders, African Americans and Europid patients respectively [23]. Cowie et al [20] found an increased ratio of probability of developing ESRD in African Americans of 1.62 and 3.93 for type 1 and type 2 diabetes respectively, when compared to Europids.

In the UK there has been a dramatic increase in ESRF in patients from Southern Asia (India, Pakistan, Bangladesh, Sri Lanka) and the West Indies, such that in 1991-2 these patients were accepted onto RRT at a rate of 239 and 220 pmp respectively [24], with diabetes as a major cause in both groups. The reported risk of developing diabetic ESRD is up to fourteen-fold in South Asians compared to Europid patients in Leicester [22]. Interestingly South Asian patients also have an increased risk of approximately five-fold for non-diabetic ESRD [22]. Recently it has been estimated that the proportion of patients from Southern Asia and the Caribbean requiring RRT in the UK will rise from 39 to >50% by the year 2001 [24].

The reasons for the increased incidence of diabetes and its complications in ethnic minorities are not understood and are currently the source of intense controversy, particularly the low birth weight - thrifty phenotype hypothesis [25]. Whatever the cause, the consequence will be rapidly increasing numbers of patients with diabetic ESRD world-wide for the foreseeable future [26].

Table 39-1. Worldwide incidence and prevalence of ESRD in patients with diabetes mellitus.

Country	Popu-lation studied	Year of obser-vation	Prevalence per million pop.		Incidence per million pop.		Type 2 diabetes %	Ref.
			All causes	Diabetes	All causes	Diabetes		
USA	National	1997	1105	366	287	120	71	1
	Europid	1993-7			63%	40%	67	
	Native American				1.5%	65%	81	
	African American				30%	39%	75	
	Asians/ Pacific Islanders				3.2%	43%	80	
Japan	National	1994	1149	209	194	60	>90	5
Europe (EDTA)		1994	312	61	59	10		2
Australia	National	1993	427	33	65	10	64	21
	Europid		374	23	54	7	48	
	Aboriginal		1129	335	338	125	85	
New Zealand	National		406	58	65	20	79	21
	Europid	1993	311	16	37	4	55	
	Maori/ Pacific Islanders		648	273	166	91	83	

MODE OF TREATMENT AND OUTCOME

There is a wide range of preferred RRT options for diabetic ESRD world-wide for reasons that are cultural/religious (eg. low transplantation rates in Japan) [6], financial (eg. higher rates of haemodialysis (HD) in some European countries because of its link to government remuneration), and medical (eg. theoretical advantages of CAPD v. HD) [27]. No randomised control trials have ever been performed, perhaps for obvious reasons, thus it is hard to draw firm conclusions about preferred treatment.

International comparisons of outcome must be made with caution because of differences in acceptance rates onto RRT, patient demographics, socio-economic factors, and national health care legislation [27]. Nonetheless, with these provisos it is still useful to look at different practice and results world-wide.

In the USA in 1997, 17.9% of diabetic patients with ESRD had a functioning transplant (Tx), 72.2% were on HD and 9.1% were on a form of peritoneal dialysis (PD) [28]. For Europe in 1992 the figures were 15%, 68% and 32% respectively, with considerable variation between countries [8]. For example, in the UK in 1991, 50% were on PD, 35% on HD and 15% had a functioning graft. For France and Scandinavia the proportions were <10% and 33% for PD, 65% and 37% for HD, and 25% and 30% for Tx respectively. More recent data from Catalunya report rates of 5.5, 72.8 and 21.6% for PD, HD and Tx with around 50% of those transplanted receiving a combined kidney and pancreas graft [10]. In Japan in 1994, 96% of diabetic patients were on HD and 4% on PD [5].

In most reported series, survival is best in those diabetic patients receiving a kidney transplant [28,10], but this almost certainly reflects a degree of patient selection. In an attempt to overcome this bias, a recent study from the USA compared the survival of patients receiving a kidney during 1991-6, to those who had been accepted onto the transplant programme but who did not receive a graft in the same period. Survival was dramatically better for the transplanted patients, and diabetic subjects were particularly advantaged with an estimated increase in survival of 11 years [29]. Short term survival for diabetic patients has gradually increased in the USA over the decade until 1996 [3] with a reduction of 45% from the death rate of 40.4 per 100 patient years recorded in 1986. Prevalent death rates in 1995 ranged from approximately 75 per 1000 patient years for 15-19 year olds to >300 per 1000 patient years for 60-64 year olds, and >400 per 1000 patient years for >70 year olds. These rates were highest for Europid patients [30]. For non-diabetic patients, the rates were approximately 40, 200, and >300 per 1000 patient for 15-19, 60-64, and >70 year olds respectively.

In the USA during 1993-5 for never transplanted patients aged 20-44 years, the death rate was approximately twice as high in diabetic compared to non-diabetic patients (160.7 v. 83.3 per thousand patient years), but this was five times the rate seen in diabetic subjects with a functioning transplant (31.4 per thousand patient years); and this in turn was almost three times the rate in non-diabetic transplant recipients over the same period (11.9 per thousand patient years). The major cause of death in these diabetic patients was cardiovascular disease (49% for never transplanted, 30% for functioning transplant v. 29% and 22% for non-diabetic patients respectively) (figure 39-2) [30]. The latest registry report confirms a 1.5 fold increase in death rate for all diabetic patients on HD (205 v. 141 per 1000 patient years; diabetic v. non-diabetic), increasing to two fold for those on PD (282 v. 146 per 1000 patient years) [31]. Five year survival rates for diabetic patients are not given separately in these reports.

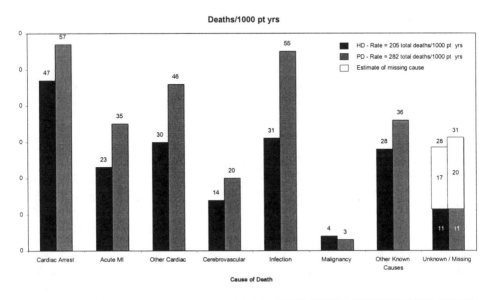

Figure 39-2. Core specific death rates for all diabetic dialysis patients aged 45 to 64 years coded by treatment modality for the years 1995-97. Dialysis patients only. HD = haemodialysis, PD = peritoneal dialysis. Figure reproduced from USRDS 1999 Annual Data Report. Reproduced by kind permission of the Editor of American Journal of Kidney Disease (ref 31).

In Japan, 5 and 10 year survival for diabetic patients on HD from 1983 onwards was 47% and 21% respectively, compared to 71% and 53% for patients with chronic glomerulonephritis [5]. Detailed causes of death are not provided, and the data are not age banded.

For the whole of Europe, the latest information on survival relates to >60 year olds on treatment from 1983-92 [2]. For diabetic patients, five year survival rates were 23% for 60-64 year olds and 18% for 70-74 year olds compared to 56% and 36% for non-diabetic ESRD respectively but the proportion dying from cardiovascular causes was not very different between diabetic and non-diabetic >60 year olds (59 v. 55%) [2]. More recent reports from individual centres in Europe show a wide range of survival rates. In Spain the Catalunya Registry reports a five year survival of 30% for all diabetic patients entering RRT from 1984-94 [10], whilst in Madrid a 54% five year survival is reported in patients registered from 1983-98 [11]. However in Alsace, France, the two year survival in 84 patients admitted to the Dialysis Unit with diabetic nephropathy was only 32% [32].

The survival rates for Japanese patients on HD [34] are better than for Europe [2] and the USA [3] and this may be a reflection of the longer time and consequently more effective dialysis in the Japanese patients [6]. Currently, studies are ongoing to explore this proposition. Longer survival in Japanese patients may also be explained by their lower risk of cardiovascular disease.

Because of the increased rate of cardiovascular death in diabetic patients on all modalities of RRT, some centres are advocating full vascular investigation prior to ESRD with coronary angiography in high risk subjects [35]. These workers have reported improved survival in patients who undergo coronary artery bypass grafting prior to renal transplantation [36].

SUGGESTED MANAGEMENT STRATEGIES

One of the key factors determining outcome of RRT for all patients is clinical status at entry. This is particularly true for diabetic patients in whom there is often considerable co-morbidity. The guidelines for referral suggested by the kidney working group of the St Vincent Declaration include joint assessment by nephrologist and diabetologist once serum creatinine exceeds 200µmol/l [37]. Reports from a German centre and from Alsace suggest that in practice many patients are presenting in established renal failure [32,38]. In addition, specific treatments of proven worth such as angiotensin converting enzyme inhibitor drugs, and good blood pressure control were either absent or inadequate. Moreover no mention is made in these reports of cholesterol lowering therapy, and despite the high prevalence of cardiovascular disease in French patients less than 10% received a beta-blocker and only 25% were on treatment with aspirin [32]. A multiple risk factor intervention strategy has been described by the Steno Hospital in Denmark in microalbuminuric type 2 patients and they provide a model for pre-renal failure care [39] A major priority for all of us looking after diabetic patients with renal complications is to improve our pre-ESRD care in our patients because only then are we likely to see significant improvements in survival.

CONCLUSIONS

Incidence of diabetic ESRD is increasing world-wide, particularly in Southern Asian, Afro-Caribbean, Native American, Hispanic, and Pacific Islander populations. Rates in North American Europid subjects may be slowing down.

Acceptance of diabetic patients onto RRT is consequently increasing with a prevalence of around 366 pmp in the USA in 1997. European rates are much less than this but growing rapidly.

Survival on RRT is less good for diabetic patients who tend to have much higher death rates from cardiovascular disease. Regional and national variations in causes and rates of mortality need further study. Renal transplantation is the recommended option.

Early referral and aggressive management of vascular risk factors and established arterial disease is recommended.

REFERENCES

1. United States Renal Data System 1999 - Annual Data Report. II Incidence and prevalence of ESRD. Am J Kid Dis 1999; 34: suppl 1: S40-50.
2. Valderrabano F, Berthoux F C, Jones E H P, Mehls O. Report on management of renal failure in Europe XXV, 1994. Endstage renal disease and dialysis report. Nephrol Dial Transplant 1996; 11: suppl 1: 2-21.
3. United States Renal Data System 1999 - Annual Data Report. V Patient mortality and survival. Am J Kid Dis 1999; 34: suppl 1: S74-86.
4. United States Renal Data System 1999 - Annual Data Report. XIII Analytical methods. Am J Kid Dis 1999; 34: suppl 1: S152-176.
5. Shinzato T, Nakai S, Akiba T et al. Current status of renal replacement therapy in Japan: results of the annual survey of the Japanese society for dialysis therapy. Nephrol Dial Transplant 1997; 12: 889-898.
6. Valderrabano F. Renal replacement therapy. What are the differences between Japan and Europe? Nephrol Dial Transplant 1996; 11: 2151-2153.
7. United States Renal Data System 1997 - Annual Data Report. XII International comparisons of ESRD therapy. Am J Kid Dis 1997; 30: suppl 1: S187-94.
8. Valderrabano F, Jones E H P, Mallick N P. Report on management of renal failure in Europe XXIV, 1993. Nephrol Dial Transplant 1995; 10: suppl 5. 1-25.
9. Frei U. Schober-Halstenberg and the Quaisi-Niere Task Group. Annual Report of the German Renal Registry 1998. Nephrol Dial Transplant 1999; 14: 1085-1090.
10. Rodriguez J A, Cleries M, Vela E, and Renal Registry Committee. Diabetic patients on renal replacement therapy: Analysis of Catalan Registry Data. Nephrol Dial Transplant 1997; 12: 2501-2509.
11. Perez-Garcia R, Rodriguez Beniteze P, Verde E, Valderrabano F. Increasing of renal replacement therapy (RRT) in diabetic patients in Madrid. Nephrol Dial Transplant 1999; 14: 2525-2527.
12. Cordonnier D G, Halimi S, Zaoui P. Health policies and epidemiology of diabetes among dialysed patients in France. Nephrol Dial Transplant 1999; 14: 2519.
13. Mazzuchi N, Schwedt E, Fernandez J M, Cusumano A N, Ancao M S, Poblete H, Saldana-Arevalo M et al. Latin American Registry of Dialysis and Renal Transplantation: 1993 Annual Dialysis Data Report. Nephrol Dial Transpant 1997; 12: 2521-2527.
14. Rao M, Juneja R, Shirly R B M, Jacob C K. Haemodialysis for endstage renal disease in Southern India – A perspective from a tertiary referral care centre. Nephrol Dial Transplant 1998; 13: 2494-2500.
15. United States Renal Data System 1999 – Annual Data Report. XII International Comparisons of ESRD Therapy. Am J Kid Dis 1999; 34: suppl 1 S144-151.
16. Hasslacher C, Ritz E, Wahl P, Michael C. Similar risks of nephropathy in patients with type I and type II diabetes mellitus. Nephrol Dial Transplant 1989; 4: 859-863.

17. Lippert J, Ritz E, Schwarzbeck A, Schneider P. The rising tide of endstage renal failure from diabetic nephropathy type II - an epidemiological analysis. Nephrol Dial Transplant 1995; 10: 462-467.

18. Catalano C, Postorino M, Kelly P J et al. Diabetes mellitus and renal replacement therapy in Italy: prevalence, main characteristics and complications. Nephrol Dial Transplant 1995; 788-96.

19. Zmirou D, Benhamou P-Y, Cordonnier D, Borgel F, Balducci F, Papoz L, Halimi S. Diabetes mellitus prevalence among dialysed patients in France (UREMIDIAB Study). Nephrol Dial Transplant 1992; 7: 1092-1097.

20. Cowie C C, Port F K, Wolfe R A, Savage P J, Moll P P, Hawthorne V M. Disparities and incidence of diabetic endstage renal disease according to race and type of diabetes. N Engl J Med 1989; 321: 1074-1079.

21. Ritz E, Stefanski A. Diabetic nephropathy in type II diabetes. Am J Kid Dis 1996; 27: 167-194.

22. Buck K, Feehally J. Diabetes and renal failure in Indo-Asians in the UK - A paradigm for the study of disease susceptibility. Nephrol Dial Transplant 1997; 12: 1555-1557.

23. United States Renal Data System 1997 – Annual Data Report. II Incidence and Prevalence of ESRD. Am J Kid Dis 1997; 30: suppl 1 S40-53.

24. Raleigh V S. Diabetes and hypertension in Britain's ethnic minorities: implications for the future of renal services. BMJ 1997; 314: 209-213.

25. Barker D J P, Hales C N, Fall C H D, Osmond C, Phipps K, Clark P M S. Type II (non-insulin dependent) diabetes mellitus, hypertension and hyperlipidaemia (syndrome X); relation to reduced foetal growth. Diabetologia 1993; 36: 62-67.

26. Amos A F, McCarty D J, Zimmet P. The rising global burden of diabetes and its complications: Estimates and projections to the year 2010. Diabetic Medicine 1997; 14: suppl 5: S7-85.

27. Khanna R. Dialysis considerations for diabetic patients. Kidney Int 1993; 43: suppl 40: S 58-64.

28. United States Renal Data System 1999 - Annual Data Report. III Treatment modalities for ESRD patients. Am J Kid Dis 1999; 34: suppl 1 S51-62.

29. Wolfe R A, Ashby V B, Milford E L, Ojo A O, Ettenger R E, Agodoa L Y C, Held P J, Port F K. Comparison of mortality in all patients on dialysis, patients on dialysis awaiting transplantation and recipients of a first cadaveric transplant. N Engl J Med 1999; 341: 1725-30.

30. United States Renal Data System 1997 - Annual Data Report. VI Causes of death. Am J Kid Dis 1997; 30: suppl 1: S107-117.

31. United States Renal Data System 1999 – Annual Data Report. VI Causes of death. Am J Kid Dis 1999; 34: suppl 1 S87-94.

32. Medina R A, Pugh J A, Monterrosa A, Cornell J. Minority advantage in diabetic endstage renal disease survival on haemodialysis: due to different proportions of diabetic type? Am J Kid Dis 1996; 28: 226-234.

33. Chantrel F, Enache I, Bouiller M, Kolb I, Kunz K, Petitjean P, Moulin B, Hannedouche T. Abysmal prognosis of patients with type 2 diabetes entering dialysis. Nephrol Dial Transplant 1999; 14: 129-136.

34. Shinzato T, Nakai S, Akiba T et al. Survival in long term haemodialysis patients: results from the annual survey of the Japanese society for dialysis therapy. Nephrol Dial Transplant 1997; 12: 884-888.

35. Manske C L, Thomas W, Wang Y, Wilson R F. Screening diabetic transplant candidates for coronary artery disease: identification of a low risk sub-group. Kidney Int. 1993; 44: 617-621.

36. Manske C L, Wang Y, Rector T, Wilson R F, White C W. Coronary revascularisation in insulin dependent diabetic patients with chronic renal failure. Lancet 1992; 340: 998-1002.

37. Viberti G C, Mogensen C E, Passa P, Bilous R, Mangili R. St Vincent Declaration, 1994: Guidelines for the prevention of diabetic renal failure. In, The kidney and hypertension in diabetes mellitus, second ed, Mogensen C E ed. Boston, Dordrecht, London: Kluwer Academic Publishers, 1994; pp 515-527.

38. Pommer W, Bressel F, Chen F, Molzahn M. There is room for improvement of pre-terminal care in diabetic patients with endstage renal failure - the epidemiological evidence in Germany. Nephrol. Dial. Transplant 1997; 12: 1318-1320.

39. Gaede P, Vedel P, Parving H-H, Pedersen O. Intensified multi-factorial intervention in patients with type 2 diabetes mellitus and microalbuminuria: the Steno type 2 randomised study. Lancet 1999; 353: 617-22.

40.   HEMODIALYSIS AND CAPD IN TYPE I AND TYPE II DIABETIC PATIENTS WITH ENDSTAGE RENAL FAILURE

Eberhard Ritz and Michael Schömig
Medizinische Klinik, Ruperto Carola University Heidelberg ,Germany

In the early days of hemodialysis, efforts to treat and rehabilitate uremic patients with diabetes were largely unsuccessful [1] until dialysis procedures and particularly volume control had become more effective. Although diabetic patients have a poorer outcome than non-diabetic patients, survival has improved progressively, although long-term survival is still very unsatisfactory, e.g. at 5 years 38% in type I and 5% in type II diabetics in Germany [2], as shown in fig. 40-1. International comparison of survival (table 40-1) shows that survival of diabetics on renal replacement therapy goes in parallel with differences between country of cardiovascular deaths in non-uremic diabetics and in the general population [3]. It is certainly no longer justified, however, to deny admission to renal replacement therapy to any patient because of his or her diabetes [4]. The rising number of admissions of diabetic patients for renal replacement therapy is a medical catastrophe of world-wide dimensions [3]. It will require intense efforts in the predialytic phase to delay progression and to prevent complications, mainly cardiovascular, which later on jeopardise survival on dialysis [5-7].

EPIDEMIOLOGY
In many countries, endstage renal failure in patients with diabetes as a co-morbid condition has meanwhile become the single most important cause of endstage renal failure [3, 8]. This is also true in Europe, where a constant increase in the absolute number and proportion of diabetics entering renal replacement programs has been noted [3, 8, 9], so that in many countries diabetes has become the single most frequent condition associated with uremia [3, 8-10]. In Heidelberg, diabetics accounted for 58% of admissions for renal replacement therapy in 1996 and 90% of these had type II diabetes. The absolute rates of admission differ widely between different countries in Europe and a North-South gradient continues to persist. An increase in admissions of diabetic patients has been uniformly found, however, not only throughout Europe but also throughout the Western world (table 40-2). It is obvious that on an epidemiological basis type 2 diabetes is the main problem [3]. In the past, the renal risk in type II

Mogensen C.E. (ed.), THE KIDNEY AND HYPERTENSION IN DIABETES MELLITUS.
Copyright© 2000 by Kluwer Academic Publishers, Boston • Dordrecht • London. All rights reserved.

diabetes had clearly been underappreciated [5]. Misclassification has occured in many studies, since the use of insulin was commonly equated with type I diabetes. Benhamou [11] noted that the relative proportion of type I diabetics decreased by 50% when patients were re-examined by diabetologists and when C-peptide measurements were performed. While virtually all patients with type I diabetes entering renal replacement programs suffer from diabetic nephropathy, a certain proportion of type II diabetics, in our experience approximately 20% [12] suffer from standard primary renal diseases. Several studies showed pronounced ischemic lesions of the kidney of many patients with type II diabetes, recently also by renal biopsy [13]. By imaging we found small (in contrast to the usually large) kidneys in 21% of type II diabetics [12]. A substantial proportion of patients with type II diabetes go into terminal renal failure following an episode of acute renal failure ("acute on chronic renal failure") mostly after administration of contrast media or non-steroidal antiinflammatory agents, after cardiac events or after septicemic episodes [12, 14]. Late referral continues to be a problem [14, 15] and many patients have insufficient control of risk factors, and no vascular access. In a recent study, 80% of the patients underwent the first session of dialysis under emergency conditions [14] a condition known to adversely affect long-term outcome.

Table 40-1: Comparison of actuarial 5-year survival of non-diabetic and diabetic patients on dialysis treatment (% surviving patients) (Ref. 3)

Country	no diabetes	diabetes
Australia[*]	60	42/27
Japan[**]	64/73	50/40
Taiwan	65	37
Hong Kong	70	20
Lombardy (Italy)	61	28
Catalunya (Spain)	65	30
Germany[*]	-	38/5
USA	35	21

[*] - reported as diabetes type 1/ type 2
[**] - reported as HD/CAPD

SURVIVAL AND CAUSES OF DEATH

According to the recent US Data Report in 1997 [8] the death rate was 270 per 100,000 patient years in diabetics vs. 200 in non-diabetics. The causes of deaths are mostly cardiovascular [16], as shown in table 40-3. Ischemic heart disease is the main cause [17, 18], although other cardiac pathologies, e.g. LV hypertrophy and systolic dysfunction are also more frequent than in non-diabetic patients. Nevertheless in the study of Koch, LV hypertrophy was not predictive of mortality or cardiac death in diabetics [16]. Undoubtedly, the rate of de novo ischemic heart disease is greater in diabetic than non-diabetic patients on renal replacement therapy [17, 18]. Survival of diabetics is roughly similar on hemodialysis and CAPD. While in a European series, a slightly better survival on CAPD was found for elderly patients, specifically elderly diabetics [19]; the US Renal Data System shows somewhat better survival of diabetic patients on hemodialysis compared to CAPD/CCPD [8]. The long-term survival after myocardial infarction is generally poor in dialysed patients, but particularly poor, i.e. 37,7% at one year, in diabetic patients [20]. Septicemia continues to be an important cause of death; it originates usually from foot gangrene and rarely from infected vascular access [16].

Table 40- 2: Incidence of diabetic patients with end-stage renal disease – evolution during the last decade (Ref. 3).

	1984	1994
Austria	7,3	18,0
Catalunya (Spain)	8,0	26,6
Denmark	6,5	16,9
Iceland	0,0	10,0
Lombardia (Italy)	6,5	13,0
Netherlands	4,2	10,4
Norway	6,5[*]	15,4
Sweden	15,3	23,4
Australia	4,0[**]	14,0
New Zealand	6,0[**]	28,0
Japan	23,4[***]	66,0
Taiwan	-	59,0[****]
USA	29,2	107,0[****]

* data for 1997; ** data for 1986 and 1996; *** data for 1986 and 1995; ****data for 1995

Table 40-3: Causes of death in 109 diabetic patients followed prospectively for 57 month (after Ref. 16).

	Type I	Type II
Dead	29 (=40%)	80 (43%)
Cardiovascular death	62%	60 %
myocardial infarction	8/29	12/80
sudden death	7/29	13/80
cardiac other	3/29	17/80
stroke	0/29	6/80
Noncardiovascular death	38%	40%
septicemia	7/29	11/80
cessation of treatment	2/29	8/80
other	2/29	13/80

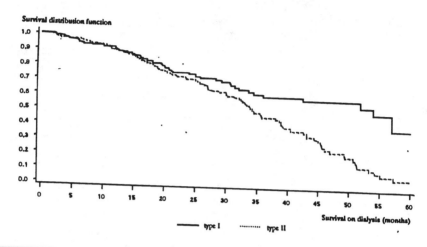

Figure 40-1. Survival of patients with type 1 vs. type 2 diabetes on hemodialysis – results of a prospective study in Germany (ref. 2)

PREDICTORS OF SURVIVAL

It is clearly important to identify the high risk patients in order to target appropriate preventive measures. Cardiac death is strongly predicted by a history of vascular disease, specifically myocardial infarction or angina pectoris [2, 16, 21]. Proliferative retinopathy and polyneuropathy are also predictive, the latter possibly through causing imbalance of autonomic cardiac innervation [16, 22]. Biochemical predictors are lipoprotein concentrations [23], not surprising in view of important compositional diabetes-specific abnormalities with lipoproteins [24]. Low apolipoprotein A concentrations are particularly predictive [2] as are low molecular weight isoforms of Lp(a) [25]. Further predictors are smoking [21, 26] and, interestingly, poor glycemic control (fig. 40-2), both on CAPD [27] and on hemodialysis [28]. It has been claimed that the risk of cardiac events is particularly high in individuals with the DD (deletion) genotype of the ACE gene [29].

METABOLIC CONTROL ON RENAL REPLACEMENT THERAPY

Using the euglycemic clamp technique, De Fronzo documented impaired efficacy of insulin in uremic subjects [30] and this was partially improved by institution of maintenance hemodialysis. This observation suggests that putative dialysable inhibitors of the action of insulin are removed by dialysis. Peptidic inhibitors of non-insulin-mediated glucose uptake have also been identified in the ultrafiltrate of dialysis patients

[31]. In clinical practice, the need for insulin decreases upon institution of maintenance hemodialysis, although complexities arise because of the prolongation of insulin half life in anephric patients and the confounding effects of reduced food intake (anorexia of renal failure) and of refeeding (after commencement of hemodialysis). Most nephrologists prefer to dialyse against glucose (100-200 mg/dl) to achieve better stabilisation of plasma glucose concentrations. This strategy allows the patients to stay on their regular insulin schedules and take their regular meals irrespective of dialysis sessions. Diabetic control is occasionally rendered difficult by diabetic gastroparesis and the tendency of gastric motility to deteriorate acutely during dialysis sessions. Despite all these complexities, efforts to aim at good glycemic control received a strong rationale by the recent observation that glycemia predicts survival [27, 28].

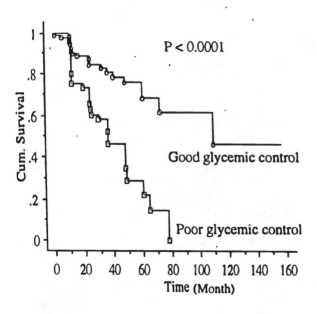

Figure 40-2. Survival of patients on hemodialysis with good vs. poor glycemic control (ref. 27)

DIAEBETIC COMPLICATIONS ON RENAL REPLACEMENT THERAPY
In contrast to previous experience [1], de novo amaurosis has become rare in the diabetic on dialysis. In a series of 200 diabetics entering hemodialysis from 1987-1989, no single case experienced loss of vision in an eye the vision of which had been normal when

entering hemodialysis [16]. With appropriate laser treatment and control of blood pressure, previous concerns about hemorrhagic retinal complications as a result of dialysis-related anticoagulation are no longer justified. Diabetic polyneuropathy, specifically autonomic polyneuropathy with cystopathy, gastroparesis and intestinal dysmotility have emerged as major problems on dialysis.

The observation that polyneuropathy is predictive of cardiac death suggests that imbalanced autonomic innovation of the heart also contributes to arrhythmia and sudden death. This suspicion gains further credence from the observation that 3% of patients dying from myocardial infarction vs. 18% of survivors had been on betablockers, the agents of choice for treating unbalanced autonomic innovation [16]. This has recently led to the postulate that betablockers should be administered more liberally [32]. Ischemic heart disease has emerged as a major threat to the dialysed diabetic. The issue is further compounded by the fact that this complications is often clinically silent. Significant coronary stenosis is found in approximately 40% of diabetics worked up for renal allotransplantation [33]. Conventional cardiovascular risk profiles are not valid predictors in these patients. Although there is no consensus whether routine coronary angiography should be performed in asymptomatic diabetics considered for renal transplantation, the majority of nephrologists go for coronarography, although relatively simple algorithms [34] have been proposed to identify low risk patients. In a small number of patients, Manske et al. [35] documented that survival was superior in diabetic patients with CHD who had surgical intervention than in those who remained on medical therapy. This finding calls for aggressive diagnosis and management. In the future the main problem will be to interfere with development of coronary heart disease in the predialytic phase, since ischemic heart disease is already prevalent when patients enter renal replacement programs and is then often diffuse and difficult to treat even by bypass surgery [5, 6, 15]. It is currently under investigation whether administration of statines effectively reduce this risk [36]. The reocclusion rate after simple PTCA, i.e. without stent and modern antihemostatic intervention, is generally disappointing in patients on renal replacement therapy, i.e. 70% after one year in non-diabetic patients. Diabetic patients consistently do even worse. Longterm patency with bypass surgery appears to be more encouraging [37]. Uncontrolled observations suggest that symptomatic ischemic heart disease is strikingly ameliorated when hemoglobin levels are raised by treatment with recombinant human erythropoietin [38]. Left ventricular hypertrophy and diastolic left ventricular malfunction are early [39] and very common complications which may lead to arrhythmia and circulatory instability during dialysis sessions [40].

Amputation because of neuropathic or ischemic foot lesions is required in approximately 8% of dialysed diabetic patients over three years. Preexisting arteriooclusive disease and a history of smoking are potent predictors. Ischemic foot lesions benefit strikingly from treatment in rhEPO in our experience, although there are reports to the contrary. Interestingly, in transplanted diabetics, the rate of amputation tends to be higher, possibly because of the use of steroids and/or cyclosporin.

It is commonly stated that vascular access is more difficult in diabetics. Venous hypoplasia is very common in elderly female diabetics and in polymorbid patients veins are often thrombosed from preceding i.v. therapy. Amazingly, however, fistula problems in our unit are not more frequent in diabetics compared to non-diabetics. The Achilles heel is usually not venous outflow, but arterial inflow. It is useful to monitor arterial blood flow by Duplex sonography. In case of low peripheral arterial flow, a higher anastomosis in the elbow region is recommended and with this procedure, the patency rates in diabetics was even higher than in non-diabetics, presumably because of endstage arterial flow rates (Konner K, Cologne, personal communication). It is advisable to create the fistula prophylactically once the creatinine clearance is approximately 25 ml/min, since "maturation" of the fistula takes decidedly longer in the diabetic patient.

In the past it has been a point of controversy when dialysis treatment should be started. In the diabetic patient with preterminal renal failure, factors other than glomerular filtration rate, particularly uncontrollable hypervolemia, repeated episodes of pulmonary edema, malnutrition and vomiting from gastroparesis may necessitate earlier start of dialysis treatment than in non-diabetic patients [37].

CONTINUOUS AMBULATORY PERITONEAL DIALYSIS (CAPD)

In the past, CAPD has been proposed as the preferred mode of treatment for the diabetic patient because of some unique benefits, i.e. the slow and sustained ultrafiltration, associated with a relative lack of rapid fluid and electrolyte changes compared to hemodialysis, the better preservation of residual renal function, the possibility to use the intraperitoneal route for insulin administration, the easier control of blood pressure and the absence of the need for vascular access [41]. Indeed, CAPD is the only option in some diabetic patients in whom a functioning vascular access can not be created.

Nevertheless, CAPD has also some drawbacks including loss of protein through the dialysate and nutritional problems secondary to protein loss on the one hand and caloric overload on the other hand, as a consequence of the use of glucose-containing dialysate. This may lead to excessive weight gain, hypertension and potentially accelerated atherosclerosis.

One potential hazard, i.e. greater frequency of peritonitis episodes or infections of the exit site of the peritoneal catheter did not materialize in more recent studies using modern connector and bag systems. For instance Tzamaloukas et al. [42] failed to note a difference between diabetic and non-diabetic patients with regard to peritonitis rate, persistence of peritonitis or relapse of peritonitis. Nevertheless, the death rate was higher in diabetic patients who developed peritonitis episodes.

One potentially attractive feature of CAPD in the diabetic patient is the possibility of intraperitoneal administration of insulin, since there are similarities between the absorption kinetics of intraperitoneally administered insulin and the normal secretion of insulin by islet cells via the portal system. Intraperitoneally administered insulin is absorbed by diffusion across the visceral peritoneum into the portal venous circulation and cleared by the liver during first pass. Insulin absorption is continuous, thus simulating physiological insulin secretion [43]. It has been claimed that peritoneal delivery of insulin causes less hypoglycemic episodes [44] and fewer glycemic excursions during the day. This opinion is not universally shared by all nephrologists and as a result intraperitoneal administration is not universally used. One potential threat, i.e. an increased rate of peritonitis, has not been confirmed by the National CAPD Registry [45], where indeed those patients on a combination of s.c. and i.p. insulin had the lowest peritonitis rates. The consistency of absorption of i.p. administered insulin is somewhat problematic because of substantial insulin losses, i.e. binding to and retention on the dialysis bags and tubing [46] and possible degradation by insulinases in the peritoneum [47]. In contrast to previous opinion, recent studies [48] failed to show a beneficial effect on dyslipidemia. Furthermore autopsy examination showed subcapsular liver steatosis which was not associated, however, with hepatic abnormalities ante mortem [49]. This interesting finding may be due to the high local concentrations of insulin to which the most superficial layers of hepatocytes are exposed.

An important consideration is the glucose and calory load. On average, the CAPD patient absorbs 100-150 g of glucose daily. While on CAPD treatment he is exposed annually to an impressive 3-7 tons of fluid with 50-175 kg pure glucose.

The effort to avoid the glucose load has spurred the search for alternative osmotic agents. So far, neither glycerol-containing solutions [50] nor aminoacid-containing solutions [51] have been adopted for routine use, but high molecular polymers such as icodextrin with the potential to remove fluid via colloid osmotic pressure, have been used successfully to increase ultrafiltration rates in patients on CAPD [52]. Its use in diabetic patients has not been studied specifically, however.

The high glucose concentrations in the CAPD fluid cause a number of clinical problems, e.g. infusion pain, chemical peritonitis and decay of ultrafiltration rates with time. This can be traced to chemically identified degradation products, particularly methylglyoxal, glyoxal, formaldehyde and particularly 3-deoxyglucosone. These compounds are oxydants and are very potent in non-enzymatically cross-linking proteins to form advanced glycation endproducts. They are generated during heat sterilization and their formation can be cut down to very low levels by sterilization at low pH with no electrolytes present and at high glucose concentrations. These conditions can be achieved by using two bag systems. The exposure of the peritoneal membrane to high concentration of glucose and AGE products may cause deposition of AGE products, capillary changes and fibrosis of the peritoneal membrane even in non-diabetic patients, so to speak as a consequence of "local diabetes mellitus" [53].

The proportion of diabetic patients treated by peritoneal dialysis varies largely between countries. According to the US Renal Data System [54] 13.8% of all patients with diabetes receiving renal replacement therapy are treated by CAPD, whilst 68.8% receive maintenance hemodialysis and 18% undergo transplantation. The proportion of diabetics receiving peritoneal dialysis varies in Denmark, Catalunia, Lombardy, France and Norway between 25.%, 5.5%, 32.6%, 14,9% and 6.5% respectively, clearly illustrating that selection of treatment modalities is influenced at least as much, if not more, by logistics and reimbursement policies than by medical considerations. Large data bases, e.g. the CANUSA Study for peritoneal dialysis and the RKPD Minneapolis HD Data Base, show that comparable survival is achieved in diabetic patients on hemodialysis and peritoneal dialysis as long as therapy dose, as reflected by Kt/V, is matched [41]. This is illustrated in table 40-4. In small regional registries with excellent data acquisition, one year survival adjusted for age and cormorbid factors is comparable between diabetic patients on HD (87%) and PD (86%), compared to 83% in non-diabetic patients. The respective three year survival rates are 65% on HD, 50% on PD for diabetics and 72% for non-diabetics. In Lombardy, 68.6% of diabetic patients are on HD and 29.8% on CAPD, particularly elderly diabetics (25-44 years 24.2%; 45-64 years 33.7% and > 64 years 41.2%; F. Locatelli, Lecco, personal communication).

Table 40- 4: Two year survival on haemodialysis (HD) and CAPD in relation to dialysis dose and age (after Ref. 41).

	HD Kt/V 1.0-1.5	CAPD Kt/V 1.7-2.1	HD Kt/V>1.5	CAPD Kt/V>2.1
> 61 years	56 ± 4	64 ± 8	74 ± 3	74 ± 6
46-60 Years	70 ± 4	79 ± 6	83 ± 3	85 ± 4
> 45 years	87 ± 3	87 ± 5	93 ± 2	91 ± 3

TRANSPLANTATION IN THE DIABETIC PATIENT

There is agreement that medical rehabilitation for the diabetic uremic patient is best after transplantation [55]. Port et al. [56] had shown that the relative survival benefit from transplantation over hemodialysis was significant, but modest, for patients with glomerulonephritis; in contrast it was much more pronounced in diabetics. This has been confirmed by others [9] and recently by Wolfe and Port in a larger data base [57]. Transplantation provides superior survival and rehabilitation not only in the younger type I, but increasingly also the elderly type II diabetic, if severe vascular disease has been excluded [58, 59].

Outcome after transplantation is poorer in diabetic compared to non-diabetic patients (fig. 40-3), but in view of the pronounced survival benefit [56], an effort should be made to transplant diabetic patients, both type I (simultaneous pancreas and kidney graft) and type II (kidney alone). Today the latter are not necessarily very old and very handicapped. Successful pancreas transplants undoubtedly improve the quality of life and recent studies suggest that they may also improve survival over kidney transplantation alone [60]. Whether delayed diabetic complications are favourably influenced has remained uncertain, but there is very suggestive evidence for amelioration of autonomic polyneuropathy. Since combined kidney/pancreas transplantation has become a relatively safe procedure, the numbers have recently increased substantially [55].

SUMMARY

The number of diabetic patients entering renal replacement programs is increasing in all Western countries. Hemodialysis is the preferred modality of treatment, hemofiltration and CAPD being used only in a minority. The proportion of patients undergoing renal or combined renal and pancreatic transplantation is rising encouragingly. Survival in diabetic compared to non-diabetic patients is worse for all renal replacement modalities.

This is mainly due to cardiovascular death. Cardiac death is predicted by a history of vascular disease, echocardiographic abnormalities, smoking and lipid abnormalities. Common clinical problems in the dialysed diabetic include difficulties in metabolic control, sequelae of autonomic polyneuropathy, amputation and vascular access.

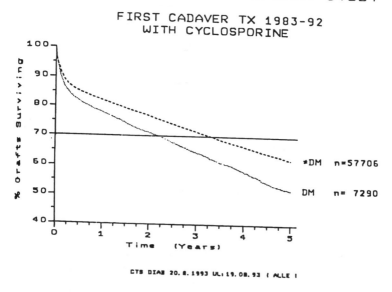

Figure 40-3. Renal graft survival in patients with type 1 diabetes (first graft) – results of the CTS study, courtesy Professor Opelz, Heidelberg

REFERENCES

1.   Ghavamian M, Gutch CG, Kopp KF, Kolff WJ. The sad truth about hemodialysis in diabetic nephropathy. JAMA 1972; 222: 1386-1389.
2.   Koch M, Kutkuhn B, Grabensee B, Ritz E. Apolipoprotein A, fibrinogen, age, and history of stroke are predictors of death in dialysed diabetic patients: a prospective study in 412 subjects. Nephrol Dial Transplant 1997; 12: 2603-2611.
3.   Ritz E, Rychlik I, Locatelli F, Halimi S. End-stage renal failure in type 2 diabetes- a medical catastrophe of worldwide dimensions. Am J Kidney Dis 1999; 34: 795-808.
4.   Pirson Y. The diabetic patient with ESRD: how to select the modality of renal replacement. Nephrol Dial Transplant 1996; 11: 1511-1514.

5.	Ritz E, Orth S. Nephropathy in patients with type 2 diabetes mellitus. N Engl J Med 1999; 341: 1127-1133.
6.	Ritz E. Nephropathy in type 2 diabetes. J Intern Med 1999; 245: 111-126.
7.	Ismail N, Becker B, Strzelczyk P, Ritz E. Renal disease and hypertension in non-insulin-dependent diabetes mellitus. Kidney Int 1999; 55: 1-28.
8.	United States Renal Data System (USRDS): 1999 Annual Data Report. National Institutes of Health, National Institute of Diabetes and Digestive and Kidney Diseases, Division of Kidney, Urologic, and Hematologic Diseases, Bethesda MD. NIH Publication No. 99-3176.
9.	Rodriguéz JA, Clèries M, Vela E and Renal Registry Committee. Diabetic patients on renal replacement therapy: analysis of Catalan Registry Data. Nephrol Dial Transplant 1997; 12: 2501-2509.
10.	Frei U, Schober-Halstenberg HJ and the QuaSi-Niere Task Group for Quality Assurance in Renal Replacement Therapy. Annual Report of the German Renal Registry 1998. QuaSi-Niere Task Group for Quality Assurance in Renal Replacement Therapy. Nephrol Dial Transplant 1999, 14, 1085-1090.
11.	Benhamou PY, Marwah T, Balducci F, Zmirou D, Borgel F, Cordonnier D, Halimi S, Papoz L. Classification of diabetes in patients with end-stage renal disease. Validation of clinical criteria according to fasting plasma C-peptide. Clin Nephrol 1992; 38: 239-244.
12.	Ritz E, Stefanski A. Diabetic nephropathy in type II diabetes. Am J Kidney Dis 1996; 27: 167-194.
13.	Cordonnier DJ, Pinel N, Barro C, Maynard M, Zaoui P, Halimi S, de Ligny BH, Reznic Y, Simon D, Bilous RW. Expansion of cortical interstitium is limited by converting enzyme inhibition in type 2 diabetic patients with glomerulosclerosis. The diabiopsies Group. J Am Soc Nephrol 1999; 10: 1253-1263.
14.	Chantrel F, Enache I, Bouiller M, Kolb I, Kunz K, Petitjean P, Moulin B, Hannedouche T. Abysmal prognosis of patients with type 2 diabetes entering dialysis. Nephrol Dial Transplant 1999; 14: 129-136.
15.	Keller C, Ritz E, Pommer W, Stein G, Frank J, Schwarzbeck A. Behandlungsqualität niereninsuffizienter Diabetiker in Deutschland. Dtsch Med Wochenschr, 2000; 125:240-44.
16.	Koch M, Thomas B, Tschöpe W. Survival and predictors of death in dialysed diabetics. Diabetologia 1993; 36: 1113-1117.
17.	Foley RN, Culleton BF, Parfrey PS, Harnett JD, Kent GM, Murray DC, Barre PE. Cardiac disease in diabetic end-stage renal disease. Diabetologia 1997; 40: 1307-1312.
18.	Foley RN, Parfrey PS. Cardiac disease in the diabetic dialysis patient. Nephrol Dial Transplant 1998; 13: 1112-1113.
19.	Maiorca R, Vonesh E, Cancarini GC, Cantaluppi A, Manili L, Brunori G, Camerini C, Feller P, Strada A. A six year comparison of patient and technique survivals in CAPD and HD. Kidney Int 1988; 34: 518-524.
20.	Herzog CA, Ma JZ, Collins AJ. Poor long-term survival after acute myocardial infarction among patients on long-term hemodialysis. N Engl J Med 1998; 339: 799-805.
21.	Ritz E, Strumpf C, Katz F, Wing AJ, Quellhorst E. Hypertension and cardiovascular risk factors in hemodialyzed diabetic patients. Hypertension 1985; 7 (S2): S118-S124.
22.	Kikkawa A, Arimura T, Haneda M, Nkshio T, Katsunori S, Yagisawa M, Shigeta Y. Current status of type II (non-insulin dependent) diabetic subjects on dialysis therapy in Japan. Diabetologia 1993; 36: 1105-1108.
23.	Tschöpe W, Koch M, Thomas B, Ritz E. Serum lipids predict cardiac death in diabetic patients on maintenance hemodialysis. Nephron 1992; 64: 354-358.

24.   Attman PO, Knight-Gibson C, Travella M, Samuelsson O, Alaupovic P. The compositional abnormalities of lipoproteins in diabetic renal failure. Nephrol Dial Transplant 1998; 13: 2833-2841.

25.   Koch M, Kutkuhn B, Trenkwalder E, Bach D, Grabensee B, Dieplinger H, Kronenberg F. Apolipoprotein B, fibrinogen, HDL cholesterol, and apolipoprotein(a) phenotypes predict coronary artery disease in hemodialysis patients. J Am Soc Nephrol 1997; 8: 1889-1898.

26.   Mc Millan MA, Briggs JD, Junor BS. Outcome of renal replacement therapy in patients with diabetes mellitus. Brit Med J 1990; 301: 540-544.

27.   Wu CC, Wu MS, Wu CH, Yang CW, Huang JY, Hong JJ, Chian CYF, Leu ML, Huang CC. Predialysis glycemic control is an independent predictor of clinical outcome in type II diabetics on continuous ambulatory peritoneal dialysis. Periton Dial Internat 1997; 17: 262-268.

28.   Wu MS, Yu CC, Wang CW, Wu CH, Haung JY, Hong JJ, Fan Chiang CY, Huang CC, Leu ML. Poor predialysis glycemic control is a predictor of mortality in type II diabetic patients on maintenance hemodialysis. Nephrol Dial Transplant 1997; 12: 2105-2110.

29.   Fujisawa T, Ikegami H, Shen GG. Angiotensin I converting enzyme polymorphism is associated with myocardial infarction, but not with retinopathy or nephropathy, in NIDDM. Diabetes Care 1995; 18: 983-985.

30.   De Fronzo RA, Alvestrand A, Smith D, Hendler E, Waren J. Insulin resistance in uremia. J Clin Invest 1981; 67: 563-568.

31.   Hörl WH, Haag-Weber M, Georgopoulos A, Block LH. The physicochemical characterization of a novel polypeptide present in uremic serum that inhibits the biological activity of polymorphnuclear cells. Proc Natl Acad Sci 1990; 87: 6353-6357.

32.   Zuanetti G, Maggioni AP, Keane W, Ritz E. Nephrologists neglect administration of betablockers to dialysed diabetic patients. Nephrol Dial Transplant 1997; 12: 2497-2501.

33.   Koch M, Gradaus F, Schoebel FC, Leschke M, Grabensee B. Relevance of conventional cardiovascular risk factors for the prediction of coronary artery disease in diabetic patients on renal replacement therapy. Nephrol Dial Transplant 1997; 12: 1187-1191.

34.   Manske CL, Thomas W, Wang Y, Wilson RF. Screening diabetic transplant candidates for coronary artery disease: Identification of a low risk subgroup. Kidney Int 1993; 44: 617-621.

35.   Manske Cl, Wang Y, Rector T, Wilson RF, White CW. Coronary revascularisation in insulin-dependent diabetic patients with chronic renal failure. Lancet 1992; 340: 998-1002.

36.   Wanner C, Krane V, Ruf G, März W, Ritz E. Rationale and design of a trial improving outcome of type 2 diabetics on hemodialysis. Die Deutsche Diabetes Dialyse Studie Investigators. Kidney Int Suppl. 1999; 71: 222-226.

37.   Ritz E, Rychlik I. Management of the patient with type 2 diabetes and renal failure. In: Ritz E, Rychlik I: Nephropathy of Type 2 Diabetes. Oxford Clinical Nephrology Series, Oxford University Press 1999.

38.   Wizemann V, Kaufmann J, Kramer W. Effect of erythropoietin on ischemia tolerance in anemic hemodialysis patients with confirmed coronary artery disease. Nephron 1992; 62: 161-165.

39.   Uusitupa M, Siitonen O, Pyorala K, Mustonen F, Voutilainen E, Hersio K, Penttila I. Relationship of blood pressure and left ventricular mass to serum insulin levels in newly diagnosed non-insulin-dependent (type II) diabetic patients and in non-diabetic subjects. Diabetes Res 1987; 4: 19-25.

40.   Ritz E, Ruffmann K, Rambausek M, Mall G, Schmidly M. Dialysis hypotension – is it related to diastolic left ventricular malfunction? Nephrol Dial Transplant 1987; 2: 193-197.

41.   Feriani M, Dell'Aquila R, La Greca G. The treatment of diabetic end-stage renal disease with peritoneal dialysis. Nephrol Dial Transplant 1998; 13(S8): 53-56.

42.   Tzamaloukas AH, Murata GH, Lewis SL, Fox L, Bonner PN. Severity and complications of continuous ambulatory peritoneal dialysis peritonitis in diabetic and nondiabetic patients. Peritoneal Dial Int 1993; 13(S2): 236-238.

43.   Wideroe T, Smeby LC, Berg KJ, Jorstad S, Svartas IM. Intraperitoneal insulin absorption during intermittent and continuous peritoneal dialysis. Kidney Int 1983; 23:22-26.

44.   Daniels ED, Markell MS. Blood glucose control in diabetics. Semin Dial 1993; 6:394.

45.   Lindblad AS, Nolph KD, Novak JW, Friedman EA. A survey of the NIH CAPD Registry population with end-stage renal disease attributed to diabetic nephropathy. J Diabet complications 1988; 2: 227-232.

46.   Twardowski ZJ Nolph KD, McGary TJ, Moore HL, Collin P, Ausman RK, Slimack WS. Insulin binding to plastic bags: A methodologic study. Am J Hosp Pharm 1983; 40: 575-579.

47.   Khanna R, Oreopoulos DG. CAPD in patients with diabetes mellitus. In: Gokal R, ed. Continuous Ambulatory Peritoneal Dialysis. London: Churchill Livingstone. 1986; 12: 291-306.

48.   Nevalainen PI, Lahtela JT, Mustonen J, Pasternak A. Subcutaneous and intraperitoneal insulin therapy in dabetic patients on CAPD. Peritoneal Dial Int 1996; 16(S1): 288-291.

49.   Wanless IR, Bargman JM, Oreopoulos DG, Vas SI. Subcapsular steatonecrosis in response to peritoneal insulin delivery: a clue to the pathogenesis of steatonecroses in obesity. Mod Pathol 1989; 2: 69-74.

50.   Matthijs E, Dolkart R, Lameire N. Potential hazards of glycerol dialysate in diabetic CAPD patients. Peritoneal Dial Bull 1987; 7: 16-19.

51.   Van Biesen W, Faict D, Boer W, Lameire N. Further animal and human ecperience with a 0.6% amino acid/1.4% glycerol peritoneal dialysis solution. Peritoneal Dial Int 1997; 17(S2): 56-62.

52.   Mistry CD, Gokal R, Peers EM and the MIDAS study group. A randomized multicenter clinical trial comparing isoosmolar Icodextrin with hyperosmolar glucose solutions in CAPD. Kidney Int 1994; 45: 1163-1169.

53.   Wieslander AP. Cytotoxicity of peritoneal dialysis fluid-is it related to glucose breakdown products? Nephrol Dial Transplant 1996; 11: 958-959.

54.   US Renal Data System: USRDS 1997 Annual Data Report. The National Institutes of Health, National Institute of Diabetes and Digestive and Kidney Diseases, Behtesda, MD, 1997.

55.   Ringe B, Braun F. Pancreas transplantation: where do we stand in Europe in 1997? Nephrol Dial Transplant 1997; 12: 1100-1104.

56.   Port FK, Wolfe RA, Mauger EA, Berling DP, Jiang K. Comparison of survival probabilities for dialysis patients vs cadaveric renal transplant recipients. JAMA 1993; 270: 1339-1243.

57.   Wolfe RA, Ashby VB, Milford EL, Ojo AO, Ettenger RE, Agodoa LYC, Held PJ, Port FK. Comparison of mortality in all patients on dialysis, patients on dialysis awaiting transplantation, and recipients of a first cadaveric transplant. N Engl J Med 1999; 341: 1725-1730.

58.   Hirschl MM, Derfler K, Heinz G, Sunder-Plassmann G, Waldhäusl W. Longterm follow-up of renal transplantation in type I and type II diabetic patients. Clin Invest 1992; 70: 917-921.

59.   Parving HH, Osterby R, Ritz E. Diabetic nephropathy. In: Brenner BM, Rector FC. The Kidney. 6th Edition, WB Saunders Co., 1999.

60.   Smets YF, Westendorp RG, van der Pijl JW, de Charro FT, Ringers J, de Fijter JW, Lemkes HH. Effect of simultaneous pancreas kidney transplantation on mortality of patients with type-1 diabetes mellitus and end-stage renal failure. Lancet 1999; 353: 1915-1919.

41.   RENAL TRANSPLANTATION FOR DIABETIC NEPHROPATHY

Amy L. Friedman, M.D. , Eli A. Friedman, M.D*.
*Department of Surgery, Yale University College of Medicine, New Haven, Connecticut, AND *Department of Medicine, State University of New York, Health Science Center at Brooklyn*

BACKGROUND

Throughout the industrialized world, as reported in the United States, Japan, and western Europe, diabetes mellitus is the leading cause of end-stage renal disease (ESRD). According to the United States Renal Data System (USRDS) 1999 Report, of 79,102 patients begun on therapy for ESRD during 1997, 33,096 (44.4%) had diabetes, an *incidence* rate of 120 per million population (USRDS, 1999) (figure 41-1). Once begun on treatment, whether by dialysis or a kidney transplant, diabetic patients suffer a higher death rate compared to other causes of ESRD, resulting in their lower *prevalence* among U.S. diabetic ESRD patients (on December 31, 1997) of 33.2% (100,892 of 304,083 patients) [1]. Glomerulonephritis and hypertensive renal disease rank below diabetes in incidence of ESRD patients, substantiating Mauer and Chavers's early recognition in 1985 that "Diabetes is the most important cause of ESRD in the Western world [2]"

More than 16 million people in the United States have diabetes - at least one third of whom are unaware of their malady. According to the National Diabetes Fact Sheet of the Centers for Disease Control [3], during 1999, in the United States, 798,000 people developed   newly diagnosed diabetes while 187,000 people will die from diabetes. Depending on age, race, and gender, diabetes in 1996 ranked from 8th (White men 45 to 65 years) to 4th (Black women 45 years and over) leading cause of death [4]. Health care expenditures for diabetes in the United States amount to a minimum of $98 billion and may be as high as $150 billion annually. The American Diabetes Association projects the full impact of diabetic complications to include in addition to 33,096 new cases of ESRD, 56,000 lower limb amputations, and 24,000 cases of blindness [5].

Extreme morbidity and mortality encountered in the exploratory treatment of people with diabetes and failed kidneys previously discouraged and even today, in some programs, retards their acceptance for renal transplantation due to the mistaken conviction that their rehabilitation is inescapably poor. By the 1990s, however, appreciation of the importance of careful medical regulation of hypertension and

Mogensen C.E. (ed.), THE KIDNEY AND HYPERTENSION IN DIABETES MELLITUS.
Copyright© 2000 by Kluwer Academic Publishers, Boston • Dordrecht • London All rights reserved.

hyperglycemia improved the peri- and post-transplant outcome in diabetic recipients to the extent that renal transplantation is viewed as the preferred therapy for ESRD in diabetes. Furthermore, growing success in patient and allograft survival - at least for the first five years - of combined/sequential kidney-pancreas transplants in type 1 diabetes is transforming this approach from experimental to established therapy [6].

ESRD Incidence: US 1997

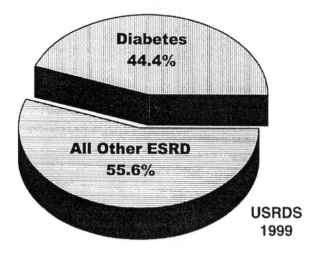

Figure 41-1. Demographic data presented in the 1999 report of the United States Renal Data System (USRDS), shows that the proportion of incident ESRD patients whose diagnoses was listed as diabetes was 44.4% in 1997 [1]. The USRDS does not accurately distinguish between type 1 and type 2 diabetes in their reporting forms. Registries in Europe and Japan also list diabetes as the disease accounting for the greatest number of incident and prevalent ESRD cases.

Diabetic nephropathy was the diagnosis listed for 1607 of 8058 (20.7 per cent) kidney transplants performed in 1989 in the United States, the proportion of kidney recipients with diabetes rose progressively to 24.1% (2896 of 11996) by 1996. In Europe, kidney transplants are less frequently performed in diabetic recipients (about 18% of all transplants).

   The American Diabetes Association (ADA), recently reclassified diabetes [7]; these "new" diagnostic criteria are designed to remedy the problem of undiagnosed diabetes, while transforming a system of diagnosis based on treatment to one based on disease etiology. As outlined by the ADA, there are 4 major categories of diabetes: (1)

type 1 (absolute insulin deficiency); (2) type 2 (insulin resistance with an insulin secretory defect); (3) other specific types; and (4) gestational diabetes mellitus. Key changes from former diagnostic criteria are the fasting glucose (> or = 126 mg/dL) for diagnosis of diabetes plus the suggestion that oral glucose tolerance tests are not essential for routine practice to make the diagnosis of diabetes.

The incidence to prevalence ratio of 1.34 in 1997 in diabetic ESRD patients reflects their disproportionately high mortality during the course of treatment. Because early trials of maintenance hemodialysis in diabetic ESRD patients were disasters, neither prolonging useful life nor gaining rehabilitation [8], individuals with diabetic nephropathy were excluded from ESRD therapy. This excess morbidity and mortality likewise discouraged acceptance of uremic diabetic patients for renal transplantation in the belief that their rehabilitation was unobtainable. A decidedly negative view of the value of proffering renal transplants to diabetic ESRD patients persists into the 1990s in many locations as evidenced by a 1993 report from Groote Schuur Hospital which concludes: "Despite very strict selection criteria, the results of renal transplantation in diabetic patients remains poor. Better treatment strategies are needed to justify acceptance of these patients for transplantation [9]"

Elsewhere in the world, a more favorable assessment of the utility of renal transplantation in the diabetic ESRD patient is the opinion of groups with a large experience. As summarized by surgeons at the University of Minnesota, the center pioneering treatment kidney failure in diabetes: "Kidney transplant results in diabetic recipients have exceeded the expectations of 20 years ago, both at our institution and others. We currently advocate a kidney transplant for all uremic diabetic patients. [10] "

Caution is appropriate when extrapolating results in treating the uremic diabetic from one institution to another. Comparing treatment of diabetic ESRD patients in Norway and the US illustrates this caveat. Firstly, fewer than 10% of Americans with diabetes have insulin-dependent diabetes mellitus (type 1) while as many as 50% of Norwegians with diabetes have type 1. As detailed elsewhere in this text, distinguishing type 1 from the predominant form of diabetes mellitus (type 2) separates two disorders with markedly different inheritance and clinical courses. To illustrate, we surveyed the race and gender of 232 of 1450 (16%) diabetic patients undergoing maintenance hemodialysis at 14 centers in Brooklyn and found the largest patient subset consisted of 87 black woman, who comprised 37.5% of the total study population [11]. Type 2 diabetes was clearly diagnosed in 139 or 59.9% of surveyed diabetic patients on hemodialysis, but diabetes type could not be determined in 24 (10.3%) of patients.

Secondly, what is applicable for younger type 1 patients may be inappropriate for older persons with type 2 diabetes. However, an extensive overlap in signs and symptoms often blurs distinction between diabetes types. Nagai found that of 551 patients diagnosed as having diabetes with onset before the age of 30 years, 337 (61.2%) had type 2 [12]. In Japanese diabetic individuals, diabetic retinopathy and nephropathy are as frequent in those who are young at onset of type 2 as in type 1 diabetes. Underscoring the faulty limits of present diabetes classification systems, Abourizk and Dunn remarked that: "Clinicians treating diabetic patients encounter numerous insulin-taking diabetic subject who clinically are neither Type 1 nor Type 2 [13]." Further to the point, these workers reviewed 348 consecutive diabetic patients of mean age 53 years, evaluated in the northeastern US, and concluded that diabetes type could not be established in 35% of whites, 57% of blacks, and 59% of Hispanics. Even applying the revised Report of the Expert Committee on the Diagnosis and Classification of Diabetes Mellitus [14], recommendations pertaining to kidney transplantation in diabetics *by diabetes type* must be interpreted cautiously. For example, a combined pancreas-kidney transplant generally thought of as applicable only in type 1 diabetes may have a role in therapy of individuals with type 2 diabetes who no longer evince insulin synthesis (C-peptide negative) (vide infra).

TYPE 1 VERSUS TYPE 2 DIABETES

As a generalization, the majority (70 to 95% depending upon race) of those with diabetes in Europe and the US have type 2 diabetes: some population subsets such as 100% full blooded Native American have absolutely no persons afflicted with type 1 despite a high endemicity (exceeding 50% of the population) of type 2 diabetes. In both type 1 and type 2 diabetes, ESRD is the end-point of a well described progression following, in sequence, microalbuminuria, fixed proteinuria and azotemia [15,16,17], associated with the pathologic changes of nodular and diffuse intercapillary glomerular sclerosis and afferent and efferent arteriolonephrosclerosis.

After 20-30 years of type 1diabetes, about 30-40% of patients manifest irreversibly failed kidneys [18]. Over the past forty years, a decreasing proportion of diabetic individuals with type 1 develop ESRD, reflecting the impact of enhanced blood pressure and blood glucose control. While previously, renal failure was thought relatively rare in type 2 [19], longitudinal observation of a defined population reveal an approximately equal risk of nephropathy in both major diabetes types. For example, in Rochester, Minnesota, Humphrey et al. found renal failure equally probable over 30 years in cohorts of 1,832 type 2 and 136 type 1 diabetic patients [20]. A similar study in Heidelberg, Germany reached the same conclusion, noting that after 20 years of diabetes, a serum creatinine level >1.4 mg/dl was present in 59% of type 1 and 63% of type 2 diabetic subjects [21]. From these and other studies, the message is that ESRD is not unusual in type 2 diabetes and probably has an incidence equivalent to that in type 1 diabetes. Whatever the incidence of ESRD in type 2 diabetes, in the US, Europe, and Japan, the large majority of new diabetic ESRD cases occur in persons with type 2 diabetes. Indeed, among 550 diabetic individuals (91% were Black or Hispanic) undergoing maintenance hemodialysis in seven ambulatory dialysis units in Brooklyn in October 1997, 97% had type 2 diabetes. While the ratio of type 2 to type 1 diabetes in the general population is lower in Caucasians than in Blacks, Hispanics, or Native Americans, the much greater prevalence of type 2 compared to type 1 diabetes is present in all ESRD programs reported thus far.

While the subset of ESRD with diabetes has progressively increased absolutely throughout the past forty years (type 2 diabetes is now pandemic [22,23]), the relative proportion (attack rate) of all diabetic individuals who ultimately become uremic is declining due to improved metabolic regulation and effective antihypertensive regimens.

Medical texts of the 1960s and 1970s described the rapid and inexorable deterioration of diabetic individuals once proteinuria was discovered. These earlier observations state that after 20-30 years of type 1 diabetes, about 30-40% of patients manifest irreversibly failed kidneys [24]. By the 1990s, however, proteinuric type 1 and type 2 diabetic individuals commonly experience pre-ESRD intervals of a decade or longer. Uremic symptoms and signs in diabetic individuals are manifested at higher creatinine clearances than in non-diabetic subjects; renal replacement therapy is usually needed within 3-5 years following onset of the nephrotic syndrome. Uremia therapy, is often postponed for years with correction of hypertension, reduction of proteinuria by administering angiotensin converting enzyme inhibitors [25], dietary protein restriction [26], and erythropoietin in those patients who have symptoms largely related to anemia.

UREMIA THERAPY
Planning long-term management for the uremic diabetic patient requires matching life style, availability of desired regimen, and social support systems. Understandably, a small proportion of uremic diabetic patients (usually those with extensive extrarenal complications) opt for passive suicide by declining further dialysis or a kidney transplant [27]. After exclusion of a reversible, profound depression, those individuals wishing to terminate ESRD care - a blind, double lower limb amputee with intractable heart failure, for example - should be guided to a hospice or provided with emotional support at home to minimize agonal discomfort. Variables impacting on the choice and outcome of a kidney transplant are listed in Table 41-1.

Table 41-1

VARIABLES IN COMPARING DIABETIC KIDNEY TRANSPLANT RECIPIENTS

DIABETES TYPE
MEAN AGE
RACE
SOCIOECONOMIC STATUS
CO-MORBID CONDITIONS
SKILL OF SURGEON AND GROUP
IMMUNOSUPPRESSIVE REGIMEN
AVAILABLE SUPPORT SERVICES
(podiatry, ophthalmology, cardiology, nephrology, psychiatry)

Interventional options in therapy must be presented in clearly understood terms in order to enlist the patient as an active member of the renal team. Table 41-2 lists options in ESRD therapy available to diabetic patients including kidney transplantation and peritoneal or hemodialysis, performed at a facility or in the patient's home. The decision to perform self-dialysis at home demands unusually strong patient motivation, appropriate space, and an empathetic partner.

Table 41-2

CHOICES FOR ESRD MANAGEMENT IN DIABETIC NEPHROPATHY

HEMODIALYSIS
    Home hemodialysis
    Facility hemodialysis
PERITONEAL DIALYSIS
    Intermittent (IPD)
    Continuous Ambulatory (CAPD)
    Continuous Cyclic (machine) (CCPD)
KIDNEY TRANSPLANTATION
    Living donor kidney
    Cadaver donor kidney
KIDNEY and PANCREAS TRANSPLANTATION
HEMOFILTRATION (Europe)

As reported by the USRDS in 1999 [1], for patients under treatment in 1997, survival and rehabilitation of those few (0.5%) diabetic persons who elect home hemodialysis is markedly superior to facility hemodialysis. Approximately 72% of diabetic individuals with ESRD in the US in 1997 were treated with facility hemodialysis. Peritoneal dialysis in 1997, was utilized to treat about 9% of diabetic ESRD patients attaining survival equivalent to that of maintenance hemodialysis. Kidney transplantation, the best ESRD option in diabetes, in 1997 in the US was applied to fewer than one in five ESRD patients with diabetes (18%).

KIDNEY TRANSPLANTATION

The combination of diabetes and uremia presents a major challenge in surgical management [28]. With minimal debate, renal transplantation is the treatment of choice for the uremic diabetic patient [29]. Long-term survival of the uremic diabetic patient with a well functioning renal transplant is much better than that achieved in diabetic patients using other forms of renal replacement therapy [30]. Diabetic patients are not - as previously thought - significantly more prone to major complications following transplant surgery than are non-diabetic patients providing that modifications are made prior to, during, and after the transplantation procedure to accommodate to their unique problems [31].

    Comorbidity expressed as extrarenal vasculopathy is an expected component of the total impact of diabetes in individuals under consideration for a kidney transplant. As a prelude to allografting, therefore, careful attention must be devoted to pre-surgical evaluation of the cardiovascular system in the diabetic patient before kidney and/or pancreas whole organ transplantation. Cancellation of contemplated transplant surgery due to detection of severe coronary artery disease is reason to perform coronary artery bypass or angioplasty as a condition permitting reconsideration of kidney transplantation [32].

Khauli et al. believe it wise to "discourage transplantation" in patients who have "the simultaneous presence of >70 per cent arterial stenosis and left ventricular dysfunction [33]." Further to the point, Philipson et al. evaluated 60 diabetic patients prior to a kidney transplant and concluded that "patients with diabetes and end-stage renal disease who are at highest risk for cardiovascular events can be identified, and these patients probably should not undergo renal transplantation [34]." Only seven patients had a negative thallium stress test, four of whom received a kidney transplant, without subsequent "cardiovascular events". Of the 53 diabetic patients with positive or nondiagnostic stress thallium tests, cardiac catheterization identified 26 patients with mild or no coronary disease or left ventricular dysfunction; 16 of these received transplants with no cardiovascular events. By contrast of ten patients with moderate heart disease of whom 8 received transplants, two died of heart disease, while eight of thirteen patients with severe coronary artery disease or left ventricular malfunction died before receiving a transplant, three from cardiovascular disease. An important aspect of this series was the finding that 38% of diabetic ESRD patients being considered for a kidney transplant had coronary artery disease. It is sensible defensive medicine when contemplating a kidney transplant in a diabetic ESRD patient to conduct pretransplant cardiac evaluation including an electrocardiogram, echocardiogram, thallium stress test, and, if needed, coronary artery catheterization and Holter monitoring [35,36]. The transplant should be postponed upon finding arrhythmias on minimal exercise, EKG changes on stress, and/or an ischemic myocardium with occluded coronary vessels.

Peripheral vascular disease, if symptomatic, should be evaluated pre-operatively with noninvasive Doppler flow studies, and in some instances, angiography to help determine where the renal allograft should be placed. Arteries found to be supplying a lower extremity with marginal peripheral flow must not be used to revascularize an organ allograft, because the extremity may be placed in jeopardy [37] Frequently, diabetic recipients have atherosclerotic narrowing of the internal iliac artery forcing use of the external iliac artery, for the arterial anastomosis. Local proximal endarterectomy of the external iliac artery during transplant surgery may be required to relieve severe atherosclerotic narrowing.

Prior assessment of coronary and peripheral vascular systems prior to renal transplantation does not eliminate the substantive risk of extremity amputation and cardiovascular death in diabetic renal allograft recipients followed for three or more years [38,39]. Overall, as depicted in figures 41-2, 41-3, survival in ESRD in diabetes is better with a kidney transplant than with dialytic therapy.

POST-TRANSPLANT MANAGEMENT
Distinguishing between acute allograft rejection, acute tubular necrosis, and cyclosporine drug nephrotoxicity in an oliguric recipient undergoing broad swings between hyper- and hypoglycemia can render post-transplant management a challenge (Table 41-3). Interpretation of renal scans, sonograms, biopsies, and tests of glomerular

and tubular function is largely an art based on experience. Metabolic control of plasma glucose concentration is best effected by frequent - hourly when needed - measurements of glucose and an intravenous infusion of insulin. Postoperative protracted gastric atony from gastroparesis may delay resumption of oral feeding. Administration of a liquid suspension of metoclopramide or cisapride pre-meals usually enhances gastric motility improving gastric emptying. Bethanechol, which may be given in combination with metoclopramide, also improves gastric motility. Constipation, sometimes evolving into obstipation, is a frequent problem following transplantation; To resume spontaneous defecation, early ambulation, stool softening agents, and suspension of cascara are effective. At the other extreme, explosive and continuous liquid diarrhea - a manifestation of autonomic neuropathy, may enervate and dehydrate the post-operative diabetic patient.

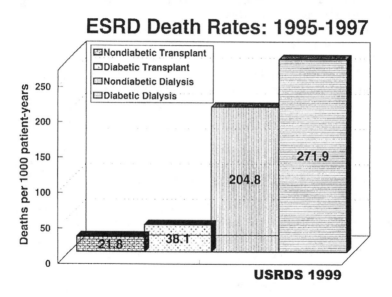

Figure 41-2. Extracted from the 1999 report of the United States Renal Data System (USRDS) [1], the fate of diabetic and nondiabetic ESRD patients treated between 1995 and 1997 is shown by treatment modality. For this analysis, survival of peritoneal and hemodialysis patients was grouped. Note that within both transplant and dialysis subsets, diabetic patients had much greater mortality than did nondiabetic patients.

Loperamide given hourly in doses as high as 4 mg/hr almost always halts "diabetic" diarrhea. Urinary retention, a functional outflow obstruction, is also a manifestation of autonomic neuropathy expressed as diabetic cystopathy. Insistence on frequent voiding, self-application of manual external pressure above the pubic symphysis (Credé Maneuver) and administration of oral bethanechol usually permit resumption of spontaneous voiding. Rarely, repeated self-catheterization is required for an unresponsive atonic bladder.

Interrelated neuropathic, vasculopathic, and psychogenic factors contribute to the common complaint of impotence in diabetic patients on dialysis. Following a successful kidney transplant, a minority of impotent patients report improvement especially after treatment with sildenafil. Resort to a penile prostheses, or pre-coital intrapenile injections of prostaglandins may restore sexual function though data are sparse consisting largely of uncontrolled testimonials

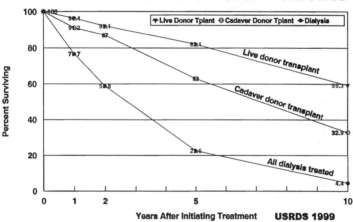

Figure 40-3. Long-term observation of diabetic ESRD patients shown in selected data from the 1999 report of the United States Renal Data System (USRDS) [1], depicts two key points: 1. Few dialysis patients live for a decade. Renal transplant recipients have superior survival though more than one-half die within a decade whether treated with a living donor or cadaver donor kidney. The burden of advanced glycosylated end-product (AGE) toxicity in dialysis patients may explain the difference in outcome between modalities.

Subjective assessment of their own quality of life by diabetic renal transplant recipients compares favorably to that of an age-matched general population in the United States. Nevertheless, rehabilitation of the diabetic patient with ESRD can be blocked by vision loss and debilitating, painful motor and autonomic neuropathy. The renal transplant team depends upon collaboration with an ophthalmologist skilled in laser surgery and a podiatrist experienced in preventative management of diabetic feet. Even with early renal transplantation prior to initiation of a dialysis regimen, many diabetic patients become increasingly disabled due to progressive extrarenal disease processes [40].

An additional threat to renal allograft integrity is imposed by recurrent diabetic glomerulopathy detectable, first detectable as GBM thickening with mesangial expansion after two years [41] and later as characteristic glomerulosclerosis in long-term type 1 diabetes recipients [42]. Loss of renal allografts in diabetic recipients after as short an interval as five years may mirror the original syndrome of diabetic nephropathy with sequential nephrotic syndrome, progressive azotemia and finally, ESRD. Najarian et al. provided encouraging evidence that survival of diabetic kidney transplant recipients may exceed a decade [43]. The Minnesota team reported that of 265 ESRD patients with type 1 diabetes given a renal transplant, 100 were alive with a functioning graft 10 years later, an actual patient and primary graft survival of 40% and 32%, respectively. In HLA-identical recipients of living related kidneys, the actual 10-year functional graft survival was a remarkable 62%. Cardiovascular disease caused 10 of 23 deaths in the second decade after kidney transplantation, persisting as the most frequent risk for death in diabetic renal graft recipients.

Table 41-3

PROGRESSIVE DIABETIC COMPLICATIONS POST RENAL TRANSPLANTATION

1.   Retinopathy, glaucoma, cataracts.
2.   Coronary artery disease. Cardiomyopathy.
3.   Cerebrovascular disease.
4.   Peripheral vascular disease: limb amputation.
5.   Motor neuropathy. Sensory neuropathy.
6.   Autonomic dysfunction: diarrhea, dysfunction, hypotension.
7.   Myopathy.
8.   Depression.

CO-MORBIDITY

Co-morbidity, extrarenal coincident disease, distinguishes diabetic ESRD from nondiabetic ESRD patients (Table 41-4). By means of a scoring system the severity of co-morbid illness in two patients or groups of patients can be expressed quantitatively and compared. We find the co-morbid index to be a useful tool in the pre-transplant assessment of diabetic ESRD patients whether receiving dialytic therapy or a renal allograft as therapy.

PANCREAS TRANSPLANTATIOM

Holding the possibility of actual cure of diabetes, simultaneous pancreas and kidney transplantation is a logical extension of renal transplantation in uremic patients with type 1 diabetes is. A key expectation of pancreatic transplantation is cessation or at least retarding of progression of diabetic micro- and macrovascular extrarenal complications. Combining pancreas and kidney transplants does not raise immediate perioperative mortality; however, perioperative morbidity is increased [44] Pancreas transplantation is "life enriching" for patients with type 1 diabetes who discontinue self-administered insulin injections while experiencing improved well being.

Hedon, reported that grafting of a portion of native pancreas prior to total resection of the organ prevented diabetes in a dog [45]. It was the failure to maintain normal glycemic conditions with the intermittent exogenous delivery of insulin and the development of secondary complications, especially end stage renal disease due to diabetes, that stimulated surgical exploration of kidney transplantation for diabetic nephropathy [46]. Disappointed in the persistent abnormal glucose metabolism despite restoration of renal function after a kidney transplant focused attention on the potential benefit of a pancreas transplant.

Table 41-4.

VARIABLES IN MORBIDITY IN DIABETIC KIDNEY TRANSPLANT RECIPIENTS

THE CO-MORBIDITY INDEX

1)	Persistent angina or myocardial infarction.
2)	Other cardiovascular problems, hypertension, congestive heart failure, cardiomyopathy.
3)	Respiratory disease.
4)	Autonomic neuropathy (gastroparesis, obstipation, diarrhea, cystopathy, orthostatic hypotension.
5)	Neurologic problems, cerebrovascular accident or stroke residual.
6)	Musculoskeletal disorders, including all varieties of renal bone disease.
7)	Infections including AIDS but excluding vascular access-site or peritonitis.
8)	Hepatitis, hepatic insufficiency, enzymatic pancreatic insufficiency.
9)	Hematologic problems other than anemia.
10)	Spinal abnormalities, lower back problems or arthritis.
11)	Vision impairment (minor to severe - decreased acuity to blindness) loss.
12)	Limb amputation (minor to severe - finger to lower extremity).
13)	Mental or emotional illness (neurosis, depression, psychosis).

To obtain a numerical Co-Morbidity Index for an individual patient, rate each variable from 0 to 3 (0 = absent, 1 = mild - of minor import to patient's life, 2 = moderate, 3 = severe). By proportional hazard analysis, the relative significance of each variable can be isolated from the other 12.

In 1966, William Kelly and Richard C. Lillehei at the University of Minnesota performed the first reported vascularized transplant of the body and tail of a cadaveric pancreas in a human causing the recipient to become normoglycemic and insulin independent immediately [47]. This team subsequently performed 13 pancreatic transplants between 1966 and 1973 but only one of these allografts functioned for over one year [48]. Gliedman and associates attained long-term pancreas function by joining the severed duct of the segmental pancreatic allografts to the recipient's ureter rather than the bowel, 2 of 6 recipients evinced sustained function for 2 and 4 years following allografting [49]. Other approaches to diverting secretions of the exocrine pancreas were enteric exocrine drainage [50] and occluding the pancreatic duct by injecting it with the polymer neoprene in vascularized segmental grafts [51]. Presently, the most popular techniques for management of the exocrine pancreas are enteric drainage, bladder drainage and to a lesser extent polymer injection [52].

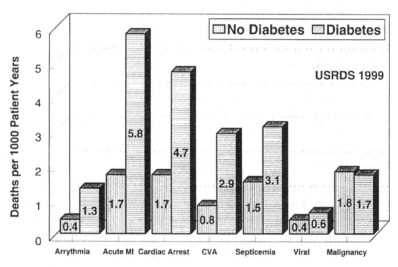

Figure 41-4. Management of renal transplant recipient with diabetes demands the inventory and treatment of progressive comorbid conditions especially coronary artery disease. As shown in selected data from the 1999 report of the United States Renal Data System (USRD) [1], deaths following a kidney transplant (performed in 1991-1993) were greater in diabetic than in non-diabetic patients from myocardial infarction, septicemia, and cerebrovascular disease. Acute MI = myocardial infarction, CVA = cerebrovascular accident, viral = fatal viral infection.

Recent evaluations of large groups of pancreas transplant recipients indicate that enteric drainage increases survival without the dysuria, hematuria and metabolic acidosis associated with bladder drainage [53]. Whole organ rather than segmental pancreatic transplantation is preferred because of the technical ease of the donor and recipient operation and the larger islet dose for the recipient).

The pancreas is a fragile gland susceptible to permanent damage by trauma, hypoperfusion or duct obstruction, responding to such insult with acute pancreatitis, . pseudocyst formation and/or leakage of digestive pancreatic enzymes intra-abdominally or cutaneously (pancreatic fistula), all feared complications of a pancreas transplant. Surgical management centers on minimizing technical adverse consequences of transplantation, obviating rejection and expediting diagnosis of complications as they occur. As for an isolated kidney transplant detection and management of vascular disease of the coronary, cerebrovascular and/or peripheral beds is a major determinant of recipient longevity. Cardiac assessment of both left ventricular function and coronary arterial flow within 6-12 months of a pancreas transplant is mandatory. Heart disease often remains unnoticed as a consequence of autonomic neuropathy. Coronary angiography is highly sensitive and may detect insignificant anatomic lesions while non-invasive nuclear isotope or ultrasound examinations may miss subtle myocardial disease. Determination of the left ventricular ejection fraction and coronary vascular supply are minimal pre-operative necessities. If abnormalities are identified coronary angiography is performed.

Living related donor pancreatic transplants [54] can be performed safely providing an option for a limited group of diabetic patients i.e.: those diabetic patients who must avoid high immunosuppression, patients who are highly sensitized and have a low probability of receiving a cadaver graft, recipients with a donor who is a non-diabetic non-identical twin and uremic patients who want one operation with no waiting time in order to remain or become dialysis free as well as insulin independence [55]. Criteria for living related pancreas donors include being at least 10 years older than the age of onset of diabetes in the sibling recipient, absence of a diabetic immediate family member other than the recipient and a post intravenous glucose first phase insulin level above the 30th percentile of normal. Donors meeting these have remained normoglycemic and metabolically stable [56]. Also under evaluation is the remarkable simultaneous kidney and segmental pancreas transplantation from living related donors [57]. Recipients of living related pancreas transplants require lower doses of immunosuppressive drugs and have superior graft survival and function compared with those from cadaver donors [58]. Pancreas transplantation is "rugged" surgery affording a difficult "cure" for a terrible disease and the only hope for freedom from dependency on exogenous insulin in type 1 diabetes.

OUTCOME OF PANCREAS TRANSPLANTAION

The world's cumulative experience in pancreas grafting is contained in, The International Pancreas Transplant Registry (IPTR) detailing 9,891 transplants (7,437 from the U.S.). Solitary pancreas transplantation (PTA; pancreas transplant alone) represents only 3% of reported cases with the lowest one year patient (93%) survival and allograft (62%) survival. Transplanting a cadaver donor pancreas in a recipient with a functioning renal allograft (PAK; pancreas after kidney) is the most popular strategy for candidates with a living kidney donor even though two separate operations are required. Superior pancreatic graft survival is reported for SPK (simultaneous cadaveric pancreas and kidney) over than PAK recipients; 82 vs. 71%, inter group differences such as 1) duration of pre-transplant maintenance dialysis 2) duration of state of immunosuppression prior to pancreas transplantation and 3) HLA identity or difference of renal and pancreatic donors probably contribute to this perhaps insignificant difference. Pancreatic duct management in the US is almost exclusively limited to bladder or enteric drainage with the latter increasingly popular. Graft survival at 1 year between 1994 and 1997 was equivalent for both drainage techniques; 83% versus 80% for SPK versus PAK transplants. Pancreatic allograft loss from rejection is declining in frequency.

Unfortunately, pancreas transplantation performed in patients with extensive extrarenal disease, has neither arrested nor reversed diabetic retinopathy, diabetic cardiomyopathy, or extensive peripheral vascular disease [59]. Nevertheless, most importantly, a functioning pancreas transplant frees patients with type 1 diabetes from the daily burden of balancing diet, exercise, and insulin dosage [60,61]. From December, 1966 through December, 1990, the International Pancreas Transplant Registry lists a total of 3,082 pancreas transplants of which a detailed analysis was possible in 2,087 [62] . Overall one year recipient and graft functional survival rates were 89% and 62%. Individual programs attained better results as exemplified by the Goteborg team who reported 67 transplants, of which 50 were combined with kidney transplants and 17 were pancreas after kidney transplants, with one year patient and graft survival rates of 95% and 83% [63].

PANCREAS TRANSPLANTATION FOR TYPE 2 DIABETES

Until the past five years, pancreas transplantation in type 2 diabetic recipients was thought contraindicated because of their persistent secretion of insulin. The pathophysiologic problem in type 2 disease is thought to be insulin resistance rather than insulin lack (see chapters 7 and 12). Furthermore, advanced age and obesity, usually present in type 2, diabetes are associated with increased morbidity and mortality from all surgical procedures and specifically following pancreas transplantation [64]. Difficulty in obtaining adequate anatomic visualization, poor healing and peri-operative complications such as deep vein thrombosis raise the rate of technical complications in obese subjects. Exogenous obesity greater than 20% of normal weight, (present in most type 2 diabetic individuals) is reason to deny a pancreas transplant. Also generating apprehension over the wisdom of performing a pancreas transplant in type 2 recipients is the fear that exposure of donor beta cells to an environment of insulin resistance (whatever its pathogenesis) will overstimulate and ultimate exhaust their insulin secreting capacity [65]. Thus, in view of the limited supply of suitable cadaver pancreas glands, limiting their grafting to type 1 diabetic recipients is understandable and consistent with the goal of maximizing duration of graft function.

At variance with the foregoing, after reviewing the outcome of inadvertent pancreas transplantation in type 2 diabetes, Sasaki et al. report a fascinating experience with 13 intentional simultaneous pancreas-kidney transplants in recipients with elevated C-peptide levels - establishing their diabetes as type 2. Graft survival in these type 2 diabetic recipients was an impressive 100% with a mean follow-up of 45.5 months. Our experience with a single patient, also identified as having type 2 diabetes, following inadvertent pancreas transplantation has been similarly encouraging; the recipient lost a primary pancreas graft to venous thrombosis but is insulin independent 6 months after transplantation of a second pancreas. Sasaki et al.'s initial experience justifies further exploration of this approach

COMBINED PANCREAS PLUS KIDNEY TRANSPLANTATION

For many uremic individuals with type 1 diabetes, a combined kidney plus pancreas transplant has evolved as an important option because of its ability to offer superior glycemic control and improved quality of life. As both kidney graft survival and overall mortality are approximately equivalent following kidney alone versus dual organ transplantation alone at many centers, neither the survival of the patient nor the success of the kidney transplant need be jeopardized by the addition of a pancreas graft. Further on the positive side of the ledger, anecdotal reports indicate that recipients of combined pancreas and kidney transplants have greater stabilization of diabetic eye disease than do kidney recipients. On the other hand, a somber review of the surgical risk of 445 consecutive pancreas transplants noted that relaparotomy was required in 32 % of recipients while perioperative mortality was 9% [66]. Based on a "serious surgical complication" rate of 35%, these workers advise that donors over 45 years old not be used while recipients over 45 years old be given a kidney graft alone.

Evidence that a pancreas graft will both prevent recurrent diabetic nephropathy, and may result in improvements in sensory/motor neuropathy justifies (with informed consent) exposure to the greater morbidity of dual organ transplantation. Newer immunosuppressive drug regimens may improve the outlook for pancreas transplantation. For example, matched-pair analysis of pancreas and kidney graft recipients immunosuppressed with tacrolimus plus prednisone had an 88% first year survival compared with 73% immunosuppressed cylclosporine plus prednisone [67] . Switching from cyclosporine to tacrolimus with or without mycopheolate mofetil increased graft survival rates with a low rate of rejection episodes.

Following simultaneous pancreas kidney transplants, but not after a kidney transplant alone, hyperlipidemia reverts to normal affording a hint of perhaps better cardiovascular outcomes as well. In those with normal or only "mild" renal disease, the decision to proffer an isolated pancreas transplant is more complex. In several reports, success rates for solitary pancreas transplants are lower than after combined organ replacement. Suitable candidates for an isolated pancreas graft are those younger than 45 years suffering repeated bouts of disabling hypoglycemia or ketoacidosis unresponsive to other measures. More difficult to judge is whether or when individuals who have advancing diabetic complications with relatively intact renal function (creatinine clearance > 70 mL/min) should be considered for an isolated pancreas transplant.

TRANSPLANTATION OF PANCREAS ISLETS

The main attraction of pancreatic islet over whole organ pancreas transplantation as a diabetes cure is the potential technical simplicity and avoidance of the risks of a major surgical procedure by simple injection of a small volume suspension of islets. To date, however, clinical success, indicated not only by some signs of persistent islet function but by true insulin independence, has been achieved in only a small fraction of diabetic islet recipients. Nevertheless, enthusiasm for this attractive approach to ameliorating type 1 diabetes persists in many active investigators.

Pancreatic islets are durable. Insulin-producing islets can be isolated with a relatively simple and reproducible technique utilizing enzymatic digestion (trypsin) of the whole pancreas in rodent, canine and primate species. Human islets are also culled by mincing and enzyme digestion of normal pancreas glands obtained from cadaver donors [68], or resected for disease [69]. Freshly isolated islets can be safely transported across great distances meaning that the isolation laboratory need not be located at or even in proximity to the transplant center.

Heterotopic sites employed in rodent, dog and primate trials of islet implantation included: the peritoneum [70], thymus [71], testicle [72], spleen [73], kidney capsule [74], and liver [75] but only the last two are clinically practical; the liver is preferred. Underscoring the longevity of pancreatic islets is the use of intrahepatic autotransplanted islets from pancreas glands removed to treat chronic pancreatitis successfully preventing endocrine insufficiency [76]. Technically successful islet transplants may undergo progressive graft loss presumed associated with their ectopic location such as nutritional toxins, intestinal bacteria and endotoxins. Transplanted islets are also subject to recurrence of the same T-cell mediated autoimmune beta-cell destruction that originally caused the host's type 1 diabetes. Recipients of pancreatic segments from identical twins can experience rapidly recurrent diabetes without any evidence of rejection, strongly implicating such an autoimmune mechanism in the graft failure [77]. So called *gentle* immunosuppression may have protected one identical twin recipient of a simultaneous pancreas kidney graft from autoimmune mediated insulitis [78]. Exploratory attempts to use porcine islet xenotransplants provoked the worry that a porcine retrovirus may infect the human host resulting in a halt (at present in late 1999) of further trials [79,80]. Analysis of the infectious risks to both individual patients and the whole human species is underway [81,82]. Strictly controlled, islet xenotransplantation may very well become a cost effective therapy for diabetes in the new millennium. Immunoisolation barriers and other imaginative approaches such as islet immunomodulation prior to transplantation through tissue culture, antibody application and even ultraviolet irradiation [83].

PATHOGENESISE OF DIABETIC MICROVASCULOPATHY

Kidneys in diabetic individuals are under stress induced by hemodynamic and metabolic perturbations. Debate is intense over the relative importance of intraglomerular hypertension [84] versus hyperglycemia as key causes of glomerulosclerosis. Lacking a reliable indicator of renal morphologic damage, however, precise timing of the transition from diabetes as a purely metabolic disease to that of a multisystem vasculopathy is often a clinical guess. The relative importance of capillary hypertension, hyperglycemia, hyperlipidemia, glycation, advanced glycated end-product formation, sorbitol synthesis, nitric oxide formation and genetic predetermination to the pathogenesis of intercapillary glomerulosclerosis is unknown.

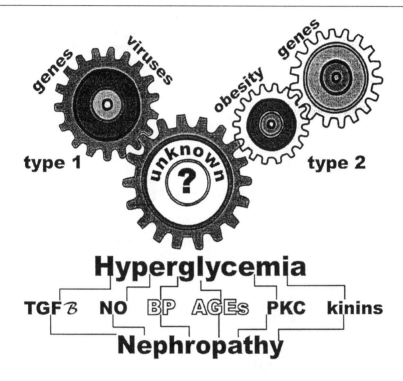

Figure 41-5. Both type 1 and type 2 diabetic persons are at risk of diabetic nephropathy though within racial, gender, and family subsets, genetic variability governs expression of susceptibility. The link between hyperglycemia and nephropathy is imprecisely defined though hypertension and advanced glycosylated end-products (AGEs) are at the least, contributing factors. Other suspected agents of injury include TGFß (transforming growth factor beta), NO (nitric oxide), and PKC (protein kinase C).

No single mechanism explains a large body of seemingly incompatible experimental data (figure 41-6). The *hyperglycemia school* holds that a high ambient glucose concentration is the main risk factor for glomerular damage. Support for this thesis is drawn from several observations: 1. Recurrent intercapillary glomerulosclerosis and renal failure can develop in kidneys obtained from nondiabetic donors that are transplanted into diabetic recipients [85] 2. Kidney graft recipients who become diabetic only after administration of corticosteroid drugs (steroid diabetics) may develop typical diabetic glomerulopathy - nodular and diffuse intercapillary glomerulosclerosis. 3. In isolated case reports, early diabetic glomerulopathy may be reversed by establishment of a euglycemic environment, as shown by disappearance of glomerulosclerosis in two cadaveric donor kidneys obtained from a diabetic donor after transplantation into nondiabetic recipients [86]. Further to the point, if nephromegaly is accepted as an early morphologic change in diabetic nephropathy, then the reduction in renal size induced by sustained euglycemia in type 1 diabetes is evidence that correction of euglycemia reverses morphologic injury [87]. 4. Kidneys transplanted into recipients who have become diabetic only after transplantation (steroid diabetics) may subsequently show characteristic nodular intercapillary glomerulosclerosis. 5. Lastly and surprisingly, renal biopsies obtained after a decade of euglycemia afforded by a pancreas transplant show disappearance of previously documented nodular and diffuse intercapillary glomerulosclerosis [88].

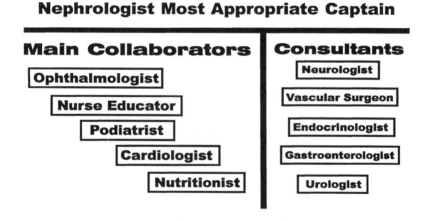

Diabetic Nephropathy Team
Nephrologist Most Appropriate Captain

Main Collaborators	Consultants
Ophthalmologist	Neurologist
Nurse Educator	Vascular Surgeon
Podiatrist	Endocrinologist
Cardiologist	Gastroenterologist
Nutritionist	Urologist

Figure 41-6. Defining a Life Plan for each ESRD patient reduces stress imparted by indecision and confusion. Key collaborators are listed on the left while frequent consultants are listed on the right. Not included though perhaps equally important is "The Patient" who should be an active participant in all decision making. A team captain B most appropriately, a nephrologist B coordinates care avoiding duplicate testing, wasted time, and patient frustration.

ADVANCED GLYCOSYLATION END-PRODUCTS (AGEs)

As a constantly occurring process, reducing sugars such as glucose react nonenzymatically and reversibly with free amino groups in proteins to form small amounts of stable Amadori products through Schiff base adducts. With progressive aging, spontaneous further irreversible modification of proteins by glucose results in the formation of a series of compounds termed advanced glycosylated end-products (AGEs), a heterogeneous family of biologically and chemically reactive compounds with crosslinking properties. In diabetes, this continuous process of protein modification is magnified by high ambient glucose concentrations [89]

Hyperglycemia is the prime determinant of protein binding by Amadori products [90]. After dehydration and rearrangements Amadori products become highly reactive carbonyl compounds including 3-deoxyglucosane (3-deoxy-D-erythro-hexos-2-ulose, 3-DG) [91] which in turn reacts with free amino groups, leading to crosslinking and so called "browning" of proteins as AGEs accumulate in the Maillard reaction. Determining which AGE compounds are the active mediators of protein injury has produced inferential evidence indicting N^ε-(carboxymethyl)-L-lysine (CML) [92], pyrraline, pentosidine [93], and crosslinks [94]. Niwa and coworkers infer that several imidazolones, the reaction products of the guanidino group of arginine with 3-DG, are common epitopes of AGE-modified proteins produced in vitro and are significantly increased in erythrocytes of diabetic patients. Employing immunologic histopathologic techniques, imidazolone has been demonstrated in nodular lesions and expanded mesangial matrix of glomeruli and renal arteries in diabetic nephropathy [95]. CML, an oxidative product of glycated proteins, accumulates in arteries, atherosclerotic plaques, and in foam cells and serum proteins in diabetic patients suggesting that it may be an endogenous marker of oxidative tissue damage and glomerulopathy in diabetic individuals [96].

Binding to specific receptors on endothelial cells [97], AGEs increase vascular permeability, procoagulant activity, adhesion molecule expression, and monocyte influx, actions that may contribute to vascular injury [98]. Normally excreted by the kidney, the plasma concentration of AGEs is inversely proportional to the glomerular filtration rate. As diabetic patients develop renal renal insufficiency, there is a progressive and marked increase in plasma and tissue levels of AGEs. Compounding the complexity of AGE action is the demonstration by Vlassara's group that renal excretion of AGEs in digested foods is suppressed in individuals with diabetic nephropathy, a perturbation that may contribute to progressive elevation of plasma AGE levels as residual renal function declines [99].

Following administration of AGEs to nondiabetic rabbits and rats, vascular dysfunction resembling that seen in diabetes is observed [100]. Furthermore, treatment of nondiabetic rats for four weeks with AGE-modified albumin causes glomerular hypertrophy and increased extracellular matrix production in association with activation of the genes for collagen, laminin, and transforming growth factor-ß [101].

Treatment with AGEs alone in concentrations that achieve plasma concentrations equivalent to those seen in diabetic animals [102]. AGE-treated rats had a 50 percent expansion in glomerular volume, basement membrane widening, and increased mesangial matrix, indicating significant glomerulosclerosis compared to untreated controls.

AGEs in the rat impair a variety of important nitric oxide-mediated processes including neurotransmission, wound healing [103], blood flow in small vessels, and decreased cell proliferation [104]. It follows that, the toxicity of AGEs may be mediated in part by their interference with the actions of nitric oxide [105]. Brownlee reviewed the importance of glycosylation of proteins to the progression of diabetic microangiopathy through the mechanism of formation of advanced glycosylation end-products (AGEs) [106].

Renal failure is associated with both a high serum level of AGEs and accelerated vasculopathy in diabetes. Vlassara et al., injected AGEs to nondiabetic rats and rabbits and showed that physiologic and morphologic changes typical of diabetes resulted [107]. Diabetic uremic patients accumulate advanced glycosylated end-products in "toxic" amounts that are not decreased to normal by hemodialysis or peritoneal dialysis, but fall sharply, to within the normal range, within days of restoration of renal function by renal transplantation [108]. *It is this persistent high level of AGEs in dialysis patients which we postulate is responsible to the greater mortality in diabetics of dialytic therapy as compared with a functioning renal transplant* (figures 41-2,41-3).

AMINOGUANIDINE

Aminoguanidine (empirical formula of CH6N4) is a nucleophilic hydrazine derivative. It has an.HCl, a molecular weight of 110.5 and a chemical structure as depicted:

$$H_2N - C - NHNH_2 = NH$$

Given to Aminoguanidine streptozotocin-induced diabetic rats aminoguanidine pharmacologically inhibits formation of AGEs. In a 9 month trial from the onset of experimental diabetes, aminoguanidine prevented the widening of the glomerular basement membrane that is typical of diabetes [109]. Induced diabetic retinopathy is also prevented in rats by treatment with aminoguanidine which blocks retinal capillary closure, the principal pathophysiologic abnormality underlying diabetic retinopathy [110]. Similarly, experimental diabetic neuropathy in the rat also is minimized by treatment with aminoguanidine as judged by motor nerve conduction velocity and the accumulation of AGEs in nerves [111]. Streptozotocin-induced diabetic rats made azotemic by surgical reduction of renal mass, aminoguanidine treated rats have significantly ($p < 0.04$) superior survival over that of untreated azotemic diabetic rats [112].

The rationale for preventing AGE formation as a means of impeding development of diabetic complications has been reviewed [113,114]. An especially appealing aspect of this approach to preventing diabetic complications is the elimination of the necessity for the patient to attain euglycemia [115]. Aminoguanidine treatment significantly prevents NO activation and limits tissue accumulation of AGEs. Corbett et al. speculate that aminoguanidine inhibits interleukin-1 beta-induced nitrite formation (an oxidation product of NO) [116].

In a derivative study [117], aminoguanidine but not methylguanidine, inhibited AGE formation from L-lysine and G6P while both guanidine compounds were equally effective in normalizing albumin permeation in induced-diabetic rats. A role for a relative or absolute increase in NO production in the pathogenesis of early diabetic vascular dysfunction was also inferred as was the possibility that inhibition of diabetic vascular functional changes by aminoguanidine may reflect inhibition of NO synthase activity rather than, or in addition to, prevention of AGE formation. Aminoguanidine is also a glucose competitor for the same protein-to-protein bond [118] that becomes the link for the formation and accumulation of irreversible and highly reactive advanced glycation end-products (AGE) over long-lived fundamental molecules such as the constituents of arterial wall collagen, GBM, nerve myelin, DNA and others. How aminoguanidine prevents renal, eye, nerve, and other microvascular complications in animal models of diabetes is under active investigation by Brownlee and associates [119], and others in diverse specialties [120].

Yang et al. believe that aminoguanidine acts mainly by preventing formation of reactive AGEs and their subsequent crosslinking with albumin, thereby leading to a reduction in AGE levels while blocking synthesis of nitric oxide [121]. Initial clinical trials of aminoguanidine in type 1 and type 2 diabetes as well as in diabetic hemodialysis patients have been inconclusive due to hepatotoxicity (type 1 diabetes) and problems with experimental design. Derivative trials are in the planning stage.

LIFE QUALITY

Diabetic renal transplant recipients enthusiastically rate their quality of life as equivalent to that of the general population in the US. Rehabilitation of the diabetic transplant recipient often hinges on a team approach to management which minimizes the time devoted to multiple visits to different specialists. Typically, the diabetic transplant recipient is expected to make repeated visits to ophthalmologist, podiatrist, endocrinologist, nephrologist and internist (figure 41-6). Success of the renal transplant team depends upon collaboration with an ophthalmologist skilled in laser surgery and a podiatrist experienced in preventative management of diabetic feet. Progressive vasculopathy, even in those given a renal transplant before initiation of a dialysis regimen, does not prevent worsening many diabetic patients become increasingly disabled due to progressive extrarenal disease processes [122].

RECURRENT NEPHROPATHY

Recurrent diabetic glomerulopathy, along with allograft rejection, cyclosporine toxicity and single kidney hyperfiltration pose threats to renal allograft integrity. First detectable as GBM thickening with mesangial expansion after two years [123] and later as characteristic glomerulosclerosis in recipients with Type 1 [124], after five or more years [125], recurrent diabetic nephropathy may present as a nephrotic syndrome followed by progressive azotemia and finally and sadly as recurrent ESRD. Approximately half of those given a living related kidney survive their first post-transplant decade. After kidney transplantation, survival of diabetic recipients may be longer than a decade [126]. Of 265 ESRD patients with Type 1 at the University of Minnesota, who were given a renal transplant between December 1966 and April 1978, 100 were alive with a functioning graft 10 years later, an actual patient and primary graft survival of 40% and 32%, respectively. HLA-identical recipients of living related kidneys attained a remarkable actual 10-year functional graft survival of 62%. 23 recipients died in the second decade after kidney transplantation; death from cardiovascular disease occurred in 10, continuing the pattern observed during the first decade.

CONCLUSION

Diabetes is the disorder most often linked with development of end-stage renal disease (ESRD) in the USA, Europe, South America, Japan, India, and Africa. Kidney disease is as likely to develop in long-duration Type 2 as in Type 1 diabetes mellitus. Nephropathy in diabetes follows a predictable course starting with microalbuminuria through proteinuria, azotemia and culminating in ESRD. When compared with other causes of ESRD, the diabetic patient sustains greater mortality and morbidity due to concomitant (co-morbid) systemic disorders especially coronary artery and cerebrovascular disease. A functioning kidney transplant provides the uremic diabetic patient better survival with superior rehabilitation than does either peritoneal or maintenance hemodialysis. For the minority (<8%) of diabetic ESRD patients who have Type 1 diabetes, performance of a combined pancreas and kidney transplant may cure diabetes and permit full rehabilitation. No matter which ESRD therapy has been elected, optimal rehabilitation in diabetic ESRD patients requires that effort be devoted to recognition and management of co-morbid conditions.

Survival in treating ESRD in diabetes by dialytic therapy and renal transplantation is continuously improving. This inexorable progress in therapy reflects multiple small advances in understanding of the pathogenesis of extrarenal micro- and macrovasculopathy in an inexorable disease, coupled with safer immunosuppression. perturbed biochemical reactions underlying the pathogenesis of diabetic vasculopathy - especially the adverse impact of accumulated advanced glycosylated end-products (AGEs) - raises the possibility of blocking end-organ damage without necessarily correcting hyperglycemia. A functioning kidney transplant provides the uremic diabetic patient a greater probability for survival with better rehabilitation than does either CAPD or maintenance hemodialysis (figure 41-7). Reflecting multiple incremental improvements in overall care, the two-year survival during maintenance hemodialysis or after a cadaveric kidney transplant is continuously increasing (figure 41-8).

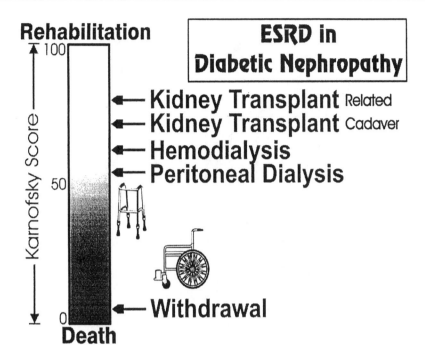

Figure 41-7. Rehabilitation of the diabetic ESRD patient can be ranked using the Karnofsky scoring system from 0 to 100 where 100 equals perfect health and 0 equals death. A score below 70 indicates the need for substantive assistance in everyday activities while a score below 60 defines invalidism. Arrows reflect the author=s bias as to the usual outcome for kidney transplant recipients, versus hemodialysis versus peritoneal dialysis treated diabetic ESRD patients. The walker and wheelchair symbols respectively connote moderate and severe disability.

For the minority (<10%) of diabetic ESRD patients who have type 1 diabetes, serious consideration should be devoted to performance of a combined pancreas and kidney transplant to effect a cure of the diabetes so long as the pancreas functions [127]

No matter which ESRD therapy has been elected, optimal rehabilitation in diabetic ESRD patients requires that effort be devoted to recognition and management of co-morbid conditions. Uremia therapy, whether CAPD, hemodialysis or a kidney transplant should be individualized to the patient's specific medical and family circumstances.

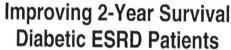

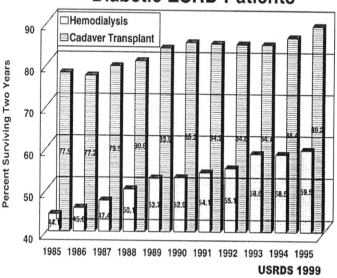

Figure 41-8. Survival data from the 1999 report of the United States Renal Data System (USRDS) [1] shows that diabetic ESRD patients treated by dialysis or kidney transplantation have an increasingly greater chance of living for at least two years.

REFERENCES

1.   United States Renal Data System, USRDS 1999Annual Data Report, The National Institutes of Health, National Institute of Diabetes and Digestive and Kidney Diseases. Bethesda, MD, August 1999.
2.   Mauer SM, Chavers BM. A comparison of kidney disease in type I and type II diabetes. Adv Exp Med Biol 1985; 189:299-303.
3.   National Diabetes Fact Sheet, 1998. Centers for Disease Control and Prevention. National Diabetes Fact Sheet: National estimates and general information on diabetes in the United States. Revised edition. Atlanta, GA: U.S. Department of Health and Human Services, Centers for Disease Control and Prevention, 1998.
4.   National Center for Health Statistics. Health, United States, 1998. Hyattsville, Maryland: Public Health Service. 1999.
5.   American Diabetes Association: clinical practice recommendations 1999. Diabetes Care 1999;22 Suppl 1:S1-114.

6. Robertson RP, Sutherland DE, Lanz KJ. Normoglycemia and preserved insulin secretory reserve in diabetic patients 10-18 years after pancreas transplantation. Diabetes 1999;48:1737-1740.

7. American Diabetes Association: clinical practice recommendations 1999. Diabetes Care 1999;22 Suppl 1:S1-114.

8. Ghavamian, M., Gutch, C. F., Kopp, K. F., and Kolff, W. J. 1972. The sad truth about hemodialysis in diabetic nephropathy. JAMA, 222:1386-1389.

9. Lemmer ER, Swanepoel CR, Kahn D, van-Zyl-Smit R. Transplantation for diabetic nephropathy at Groote Schuur Hospital. S Afr med J 1993;83:88-90.

10. Basadonna G, Matas AJ, Gillingham K, Sutherland DE, Payne WD, Dunn Dl, Gores PF, Gruessner RW, Arrazola I, Najarian JS. Kidney transplantation in patients with type I diabetes: 26-year experience at the University of Minnesota. Clinical Transplants 1992, 1993. Paul I. Terasaki, J.M. Cecka Eds, UCLA Tissue Typing Laboratory, Los Angeles, California, pp227-235.

11. Lowder GM, Perri NA, Friedman EA. 1988. Demographics, diabetes type, and degree of rehabilitation in diabetic patients on maintenance hemodialysis in Brooklyn. J Diabetic Complications 2:218-226.

12. Nagai N. 1982. Clinical statistics of 551 patients with diabetes mellitus found before 30 years of age. J. Tokyo Wom. Med. Coll. 52:904-915.

13. Abourizk NN, Dunn JC. Types of diabetes according to National Diabetes. Data Group Classification. Limited applicability and need to revisit. 1990 Diabetes Care 13:1120-1123.

14. The Expert Committee on the Diagnosis and Classification of Diabetes Mellitus. Report of the Expert Committee on the Diagnosis and Classification of Diabetes Mellitus. Diabetes Care 1997;20:1183-1197.

15. Mogensen CE. Management of early nephropathy in diabetic patients. Annu Rev Med 1995;46:79-93.

16. Christensen CK, Christiansen JS, Schmitz A, Christensen T, Hermansen K, Mogensen CE. 1987. Effect of continuous subcutaneous insulin infusion on kidney function and size in Type 1 patients. A 2 year controlled study. J Diab Compl, 1: 91-95.

17. Mogensen CE. 1992. Angiotensin converting enzyme inhibitors and diabetic nephropathy. BMJ, 304:327-328.

18. Balodimus MC. 1971. Diabetic nephropathy. In :"Joslin's Diabetes" (Eds A Marble, P White, RF Bradley, LP Krall), Lea and Febiger, Philadelphia, pp 526-561.

19. Grenfell A, Watkins PJ. 1986. Clinical diabetic nephropathy: natural history and complications. Clin Endocrin Metab 15:783-805.

20. Humphrey LL, Ballard DJ, Frohnert PP, Chu CP, O'Fallon WM, Palumbo PJ. 1989. Chronic renal Failure in non-insulin-dependent diabetes mellitus. Ann Intern Med, 10:788-796.

21. Hasslacher CH, Ritz E, Wahl P, Michael C. 1989. Similar risks of nephropathy in patients with type I or type II diabetes mellitus. Nephrol Dial Transplant, 4: 859-863.

22. Ritz E, Nowack D, Fliser D, Koch M, Tschope W. 1991. Type II diabetes mellitus: Is the renal risk adequately appreciated? Nephrol Dial Transplant, 6: 679-682.

23. Rosenbloom AL, Joe JR, Young RS, Winter WE. 1999. Emerging epidemic of type 2 diabetes in youth. Diabetes Care 1999;22:345-354.

24. Balodimus MC. 1971. Diabetic nephropathy. In :"Joslin's Diabetes" (Eds A Marble, P White, RF Bradley, LP Krall), Lea and Febiger, Philadelphia, pp 526-561.

25. De Jong PE, Navis G, de Zeeuw Renoprotective therapy: titration against urinary protein excretion. 1999 Lancet;354:352-353.

26. Locatelli F, Del Vecchio L How long can dialysis be postponed by low protein diet and ACE inhibitors? 1999 Nephrol Dial Transplant 14:1360-1364.

27. Neu S, Kjellstrand CM. Stopping long-term dialysis. An empirical study of withdrawal of life-supporting treatment. N Engl J Med 1986;314:14-20.

28. Khauli RB, Steinmuller DR, Novick AC, et al. 1986. A Critical Look at Survival of Diabetics with End-Stage Renal Disease: Transplantation Versus Dialysis Therapy. Transplantation 41: 598-602.

29. Sutherland DER, Morrow CE, Fryd DS, Ferguson R, Simmons RL, Najarian JS. 1982. Improved patient and primary renal allograft survival in uremic diabetic recipients. Transplantation 34:319-325.

30. Reltig and Levinsky ed. 1991. Institute for Medicine (U.S.) Kidney Failure and the Federal Government Access to Kidney Transplantation. Nat. Academy of Sciences p. 167-186.

31. Paterson AD, Dornan TL, Peacock I, Burden RP, Morgan AG, Tattersall RBl. 1987. Cause of death in diabetic patients with impaired renal function. An audit of a hospital diabetic clinic population. Lancet 1: 313-316.

32. Braun WE, Phillips D, Vidt DG. 1983. The Course of Coronary Artery Disease in Diabetics with and without Renal Allografts. Transplant Proc 15: 1114-1119.

33. Khauli RB, Steinmuller DR, Novick AC, et al. 1986. A Critical Look at Survival of Diabetics with End-Stage Renal Disease: Transplantation Versus Dialysis Therapy. Transplantation 41: 598-602.

34. Philipson JD, Carpenter BJ, Itzkoff J, Hakala TR, Rosenthal JT, Taylor RJ, Puschett JB.1986. Evaluation of cardiovascular risk for renal transplantation in diabetic patients. Am J Med 81:630-634.

35. Corry RJ, Nghiem DD, Schanbacher B, et al. 1987. Critical Analysis of Mortality and Graft Loss Following Simultaneous Renal - Pancreatic Duodenal Transplantation. Transplant Proc 19: 2305-2306.

36. Gill JB, Ruddy TD, Newell JB, et al. 1987. Prognostic Importance of Thallium Uptake by the Lungs During Exercise in Coronary Artery Disease. N Engl J Med 317: 1485-1489.

37. Fanning WJ, Henry ML, Sommer BG, et al. 1986. Lower Extremity and Renal Ischemia Following Renal Transplantation. Vascular Surg 23: 231-234.

38. Gonzalez-Carrillo M, Moloney A, Bewick M, et al. 1982. Renal Transplantation in Diabetic Nephropathy. Br Med J 285: 1713-1716.

39. Abendroth D, Landgraf R, Illner WD, Land W. 1990. Beneficial Effects of Pancreatic Transplantation in Insulin -Dependent Diabetes Mellitus Patients. Transplant Proc 22: 696-697.

40. Sutherland DER. 1988. Who should get a Pancreas Transplant? Diabetes Care 11: 681-685.

41. Osterby R, Nyberg G, Hedman L, Karlberg I, Persson H, Svalander C. 1991. Kidney transplantation in type 1 (insulin-dependent) diabetic patients. Diabetelogia, 9:668-674.

42. Mauer SM, Goetz FC, McHugh LE, et al. 1989. Long-term Study of Normal Kidneys Transplanted into Patients with Type I Diabetes. Diabetes 38: 516-523.

43. Najarian JS, Kaufman DB, Fryd DS, McHugh L, Mauer SM, Ramsay RC, Kennedy WR, Navarro X, Goetz FC, Sutherland DE. 1989. Long-term survival following kidney transplantation in 100 type 1 diabetic patients. Transplantation, 1:106-113.

44. United States Renal Data System, USRDS 1992 Annual Data Report, The National Institutes of Health, National Institute of Diabetes and Digestive and Kidney Diseases. Bethesda, MD, August 1992.

45. Hedon E (1893) Sur la consommation du sucre ches le chien apres l'extirpation du pancreas. Arch Physiol Norm Pathol 5: 154-163.

46. Najarian JS, Sutherland DER, Simmons RL, Howard RJ, Kjellstrand CM, Ramsay RC, Goetz FC, Fryd DS, Sommer BG (1979) Ten year experience with renal transplantation in juvenile onset diabetes. Ann Surg 190:487-500.

47. Kelly WD, Lillehei RC, Merkel FK, et al. 1967. Allotransplantation of the Pancreas and Duodenum along with the Kidney in Diabetic Nephropathy. Surgery 61: 827-837.

48. Lillehei RC, Ruiz JO, Acquino C, Goetz FC (1976) Transplantation of the Pancreas. Acta Endocrinol 83 (Suppl 205): 303-318.

49. Gliedman ML, Gold M, Whittaker J, Rifkin H, Soberman R, Freed S, Tellis V, Veith FJ (1973) Clinical segmental pancreatic transplantation with ureter-pancreatic duct anastomosis for exocrine drainage. Surgery 74: 171-180.

50. Groth CG, Collste H, Lundgren G, Wilczek H et al: (1982) Successful outcome of segmental human pancreatic transplantation with enteric exocrine diversion after modifications in technique. Lancet 2: 522-24.

51. Dubernard JM, Traeqer J, Neyra P, Touraine JL, Tranchant D, Blanc-Brunat N: (1978) A new preparation of segmental pancreatic grafts for transplantation: Trials in dogs and in man. Surgery 84: 633-640.

52. DiCarlo V, Castoldi R, Cristallo M, Ferrari G, Socci C, Baldi A, Molteni B, Secchi A, Pozza G, (1998) Techniques of Pancreas Transplantation through the World: An IPITA Center Study. Transplant Proc 30: 231-241.

53. Sugitani A, Gritsch HA, Shapiro R, Bonham, CA, Egidi CA, Corry RJ (1998) Surgical Complications in 123 Consecutive Pancreas Transplant Recipients: Comparison of Bladder and Enteric Drainage Transplant Proc 30: 293 - 294.

54. Sutherland DER, Goetz FC, Najarian JS, (1980) Living related donor segmental pancreatectomy for transplantation. Transplant Proc 12 (Suppl 2) 19 - 25.

55. Humar A, Gruessner RW, Sutherland DE, (1997) Living related donor pancreas and pancreas-kidney transplantation. Br Med Bull 53: 879 - 91.

56. Seaquist ER, Robertson RP, (1992) Effects of hemipancreatectomy on pancreatic alpha and beta cell function in healthy human donors. J. Clin Invest 89: 1761 - 1766.

57. Gruessner AC and Sutherland DER. 1998. Pancreas transplants for United States (US) and non-US cases as reported to the international pancreas transplant registry (IPTR) and to the United Network for Organ Sharing (UNOS). In:"Clinical transplants 1997". (Ed JM Cecka and PI Terasaki), UCLA Tissue Typing Laboratory, Los Angeles, pp 45-58.

58. Sutherland DER, Gruessner R, Dunn D, Moudry-Munns K, Gruessner A, Najarian JS, (1994) Pancreas Transplantation from living-related donors. Transplant Proc 26: 443-445.

59. Ramsay RC, Goetz FC, Sutherland DE, Mauer SM, Robison LL, Cantrill HL, Knobloch WH, Najarian JS. 1988. Progression of Diabetic Retinopathy After Pancreas Transplantation for Insulin - Dependent Diabetes Mellitus. N Engl J Med 318: 208-214.

60. Katz H, Homan M, Velosa J, et al. 1991. Effects of Pancreas Transplantation on Postprandial Glucose Metabolism. N Engl J Med. 325: 1278-1283.

61. Piehlmeier W, Bullinger M, Nusser J, Konig A, Illner WD, Abendroth D, Land W, Landgraf R et al. 1992. Quality of Life in Diabetic Patients Prior to or After Pancreas Transplantation in Relation to Organ Function. Transplant Proc 24: 871-873.

62. Sutherland DE. 1991. Report from the International Pancreas Transplant Registry. Diabetologia, 34 (Suppl 1):S28-39.

63. Olausson M, Nyberg G, Norden G, Frisk B, Hedman L. 1991. Outcome of pancreas transplantations in Goteberg, Sweden 1985-1990. Diabetologia, 34(Suppl 1):S1-3.

64.   Odorico JS, Becker YT, Van der Werf W, Collins B, D'Alessandro AM, Knechtle SJ, Pirsch JD and Sollinger HW. Advances in pancreas transplantation: the University of Wisconsin experience. In Clinical Transplants 1997, Cecka and Terasaki, Eds. UCLA tissue typing laboratory, Los Angeles, California.

65.   Sasaki TM, Gray RS, Ratner RE, Currier C, Aquino A, Barhyte DY, Light JA. 1998. Successful long-term kidney-pancreas transplants in diabetic patients with high C-peptide levels. Transplantation 65:1510-1512.

66.   Gruessner RW, Sutherland DE, Troppmann C, Benedetti E, Hakim N, Dunn DL, Gruessner AC. The surgical risk of pancreas transplantation in the cyclosporine era: an overview. J Am Coll Surg 1997;185:128-144.

67.   Gruessner RW.   Tacrolimus in pancreas transplantation: a multicenter analysis. Tacrolimus Pancreas Transplant Study Group. Clin Transplant 1997;11:299-312.

68.   Marshak S, Leibowitz G, Bertuzzi F, Socci C, Kaiser N, Gross DJ, Cerasi E, Melloul D. 1999. Impaired beta-cell functions induced by chronic exposure of cultured human pancreatic islets to high glucose. Diabetes, 48(6):1230-1236.

69.   Rabkin JM, Leone JP, Sutherland DE, Ahman A, Reed M, Papalois BE, Wahoff DC. 1997. Transcontinental shipping of pancreatic islets for autotransplantation after total pancreatectomy. Pancreas, 15(4):415-9.

70.   Sutherland DE. 1994 Intraperitoneal transplantation of microencapsulated canine islet allografts with short-term, low-dose cyclosporine for treatment of pancreatectomy-induced diabetes in dogs. Transplantation Proceedings.. 26(2):804.

71.   Tuch BE, Wright DC, Martin TE, Keogh GW, Deol HS, Simpson AM, Roach W, Pinto AN. 1999. Fetal pig endocrine cells develop when allografted into the thymus gland. Transplantation Proc, 31(1-2):670-674.

72.   Ar'Rajab A, Dawidson IJ, Harris RB, Sentementes JT Immune privilege of the testis for islet xenotransplantation (rat to mouse). Transplant Proc 1994 Dec;26(6):3446 .

73.   Gray DW. 1990Islet isolation and transplantation techniques in the primate.. Surgery, Gynecology and Obstetrics, 170(3):225-232.

74.   Leow CK. Shimizu S. Gray DW. Morris PJ. 1994Successful pancreatic islet autotransplantation to the renal subcapsule in the cynomolgus onkey.. Transplantation. 57(1):161-4.

75.   Stevens RB. Lokeh A. Ansite JD. Field MJ. Gores PF. Sutherland DE. 1994.Role of nitric oxide in the pathogenesis of early pancreatic islet dysfunction during rat and human intraportal islet transplantation.. Transplantation Proceedings. 26(2):692.

76.   Robertson GS, Dennison AR, Johnson PR et al. 1998. A review of pancreatic islet autotransplantation. Hepatogastroenterology 45:226-235.

77.   Sibley R, Sutherland DER, Goetz F, Michael AF. 1985. Recurrent diabetes mellitus in the pancreas iso- and allograft. A light and electron microscopic and immunohistochemical analysis of four cases. Lab Invest 53:132-144.

78.   Benedetti E, Dunn T, Massad MG, Raofi V, Bartholomew A, Gruessner RW, Brecklin C. 1999.Successful living related simultaneous pancreas-kidney transplant between identical twins. Transplantation 67(6):915-8.

79.   Butler D. FDA warns on primate xenotransplants. Nature 1999;398:549.

80.   Bach FH and Fineberg HV. 1998. Call for moratorium on xenotransplants. Nature 391:326. Bakris GL, Barnhill BW, Sadler R: Treatment of arterial hypertension in diabetic humans: Importance of therapeutic selection. Kidney Int 41:912-919, 1992.

81.   Weiss RA. Xenografts and retroviruses. Science 1999;285:1221-1223.

82. Paradis K, Langford G, Long Z, Heneine W, Sandstrom P, Switzer WM, Chapman LE, Lockey C, Onions D, The XEN 111 Study Group, and Otto E. Search for Cross-Species Transmission of Porcine Endogenous Retrovirus in Patients Treated with Living Pig Tissue. Science 1999; 285: 1236-1241.

83. Lau H, Reemtsma K, Hardy MA. 1984. Prolongation of rat islet allograft survival by direct ultraviolet irradiation of the graft. Science 223:607-609.

84. Lewis EJ, Hunsicker LG, Bain RP, Rhode RD. The effect of angiotensin-converting-enzyme inhibition on diabetic nephropathy. N ENGL J Med 1993;329:1456-1462.

85. Maryniak RK, Mendoza N, Clyne D, Balakrishnan K, Weiss MA. 1985. Recurrence of diabetic nodular glomerulosclerosis in a renal transplant. Transplantation 39:35-38.

86. Abouna G, Adnani MS, Kumar MS, Samhan SA. 1986. Fate of transplanted kidneys with diabetic nephropathy. Lancet, 1: 622-624.

87. Tuttle KR, Bruton L, Perusek MC, Lancaster JL, Kopp DT, DeFronzo R. 1991. Effect of strict glycemic control on renal hemodynamic response to amino acids and renal enlargement in insulin-dependent in insulin-dependent diabetes mellitus. N Engl J Med, 324: 1626-1632.

88. Fioretto P, Steffes MW, Sutherland DE, Goetz FC, Mauer M. 1999. Reversal of lesions of diabetic nephropathy after pancreas transplantation. N Engl J Med 1998;339:69-75.

89. Brownlee, M. Glycation and diabetic complications. Diabetes 1994; 43:837-841.

90. Vlassara, H. Protein glycation in the kidney: Role in diabetes and aging. Kidney Int 1996; 49:1795-1804.

91. Kato H, Hayase F, Shin DB, Oimomi M, Baba S 3-Deoxyglucosone, an intermediate product of the Maillard reaction. 1989;Prog Clin Biol Res 304:69-84.

92. Reddy S, Bichler J, Wells-Knecht KJ, Thorpe SR, Baynes JWReddy S, Bichler J, Wells-Knecht KJ, Thorpe SR, Baynes JW N^{ε}-(carboxymethyl)lysine is a dominant advanced glycation end product (AGE) antigen in tissue proteins. Biochemistry 1995;34:10872-10878.

93. Friedlander MA, Witko-Sarsat V, Nguyen AT, Wu YC, Labrunte M, Verger C, Jungers P, Descamps-Latscha B The advanced glycation endproduct pentosidine and monocyte activation in uremia. Clin Nephrol 1996;45:379-382.

94. Sell, DR, Monnier, VM,. Structure elucidation of a senescence cross-link from human extracellular matrix. J Biol Chem 1989;264:21597-21602.

95. Niwa, T, Kaatsuzaki, T, Miyazaki S, et al. Immunohistochemical detection of imidazolone, a novel advanced glycation end product, in kidneys and aortas of diabetic patients. J Clin Invest 1997;99:1272-1280.

96. Schleicher, ED, WagnerE, Nerlich, AG. Increased accumulation of the glycoxidation product N(epsilon)-(carboxymethyl)lysiine in human tissues in diabetes and aging. J Clin Invest 1997;99:3:457-468.

97. Schmidt, AM, Hori, O, Chen, JX, et al. Advanced glycation endproducts interacting with their endothelial receptor induce expression of vascular cell adhesion molecule-1 (VCAM-1) in cultured human endothelial cells and in mice. J Clin Invest 1995; 96:1395-1403.

98. Renard C, Chappey O, Wautier MP, Nagashima M, Lundh E, Morser J, Zhao L, Schmidt AM, Scherrmann JM, Wautier JL. Recombinant advanced glycation end product receptor pharmacokinetics in normal and diabetic rats. Mol Pharmacol 1997;52:54-62.

99. Koschinsky T, He CJ, Mitsuhashi T, Cucala R, Liu C, Buenting C, Heitmann K, Vlassara H. Orally absorbed reactive glycation products (glycotoxins): an environmental risk factor in diabetic nephropathy. Proc Natl Avcad Sci USA 1997;94:6474-6479.

100. Vlassara H, Fuh H, Makita Z, Krungkrai S, Cerami A, Bucala R. Exogenous advanced glycosylation end products induce complex vascular dysfunction in normal animals: A model for diabetic and aging complications. Proc Natl Acad Sci U S A 1992; 89:12043-12047.

101. Yang CW, Vlassara H, Peten EP, He CJ, Striker GE, Striker LJ Advanced glycation end products up-regulate gene expression found in diabetic glomerular disease. Proc Natl Acad Sci U S A 1994; 91:9436-9440.

102. Vlassara, H. Serum advanced glycosylation end products: A new class of uremic toxins? Blood Purif 1994; 12:54-59.

103. Knowx, LK, Stewart, AG, Hayward, PG, Morrison, WA. Nitric oxide synthase inhibitors improve skin flap survival in the rat. Microsurgery 1994; 15:708-711.

104. Tilton, RG, Chang, K, Corbett, JA, Misko TP, Currie MG, Cora NS, Kaplan HJ, Williamson JR Endotoxin–induced uveitis in the rat is attenuated by inhibition of nitric oxide production. Invest Ophthalmol Vis Sci 1994; 35:3278-3288.

105. Hogan, M, Cerami, A, Bucala, R. Advanced glycosylation end products block the antiproliferative effect of nitric oxide. Role in the vascular and renal complications of diabetes mellitus. J Clin Invest 1992; 90:1110-1105.

106. Brownlee M. Glycosylation of proteins and microangiopathy. Hosp Pract (Off Ed) 27 (Suppl 1):46-50, 1992.

107. Vlassara H, Fuh H, Makita Z, Krungkrai S, Cerami A, Cucala R. Exogenous advanced glycosylation end products induce complex vascular dysfunction in normal animals: a model for diabetic and aging complications. Proc Natl Acad Sci USA. 89:12043-12047, 1992.

108. Makita Z, Radoff S, Rayfield EJ, Yang Z, Skolnik E, Delaney V, Friedman EA, Cerami A, Vlassara H. 1991. Advanced glycosylation end products in patients with diabetic nephropathy. New Engl J Med 325:836-842.

109. Ellis EN, Good BH. Prevention of glomerular basement membrane thickening by aminoguanidine in experimental diabetes mellitus. Metabolism 40:1016-1019, 1991.

110. Hammes HP, Martin S, Federlin K, Geisen K, Brownlee M. Aminoguanidine treatment inhibits the development of experimental diabetic retinopathy. Proc Natl Acad Sci USA. 88:11555-11558, 1991.

111. Yagihashi S, Kamijo M, Baba M, Yagihashi M, Nagai K. Effect of aminoguanidine on functional and structural abnormalities in peripheral nerve of STZ-induced diabetic rats. Diabetes 41:47-52, 1992.

112. Friedman EA, Distant DA, Fleishhacker JF, Boyd TA, Cartwright K. Aminoguanidine prolongs survival in azotemic induced diabetic rats. Amer J Kidney Dis 1997;30:253-259.

113. Brownlee M. 1989. Pharmacological modulation of the advanced glycosylation reaction. Prog Clin Biol Res, 304:235-248.11

114. Nicholls K, Mandel TE. 1989. Advanced glycosylation end-products in experimental murine diabetic nephropathy: effect of islet isografting and of aminoguanidine. Lab Invest, 60:486-491.

115. Lyons TJ, Dailie KE, Dyer DG, Dunn JA, Baynes JW. 1991. Decrease in skin collagen glycation with improved glycemic control in patients with insulin-dependent diabetes mellitus. J Clin Invest, 87:1910-1915.

116. Corbett JA, Tilton RG, Chang K, Hasan KS, Ido Y, Wang JL, Sweetland MA, Lancaster Jr., Williamson JR, McDaniel ML. Aminoguanidine, a novel inhibitor of nitric oxide formation, prevents diabetic vascular dysfunction. Diabetes 1992;4:552-556.

117. Tilton RG, Chang K, Hasan KS, Smith SR, Petrash JM, Misko TP, Moore WM, Currie MG, Corbett JA, McDaniel ML et al. Prevention of diabetic vascular dysfunction by guanidines. Inhibition of nitric oxide synthase versus advanced glycation end-product formation. Diabetes 42:221-232, 1993.

118. Sensi M, Pricci F, Andreani D, DiMario U. Advanced nonenzymatic glycation endproducts (AGE): their relevance to aging and the pathogenesis of late diabetic complications. Diabetes Res 1991; 16:1-9.

119. Edelstein D, Brownlee M. 1992. Mechanistic studies of advanced glycosylation end product inhibition by aminoguanidine. Diabetes, 41:26-29.

120. Eika B, Levin RM, Longhurst PA. Collagen and bladder function in streptozotocin-diabetic rats: effects of insulin and aminoguanidine. J Urol 1992;148:167-172.

121. Yang, CW, Yu, CC, Ko, YC, Huang, CC. 1998. Aminoguanidine reduces glomerular inducible nitric oxide synthase (iNOS) and transforming growth factor-beta 1 (TGF-beta 1) mRNA expression and diminishes glomerulosclerosis in NZB/W F1 mice. Clin Exp Immunol 1998; 113:258.

122. Milde FK, Hart LK, Zehr PS. Pancreatic transplantation. Impact on the quality of life of diabetic renal transplant recipients. Diabetes Care 1995;18:93-95.

123. Østerby R, Nyberg G, Hedman L, Karlberg I, Persson H, Svalander C. 1991. Kidney transplantation in type 1 (insulin-dependent) diabetic patients. Diabetelogia, 9:668-674.

124. Bohman SO, Wilczek H, Jaremko G, et al. 1984. Recurrence of Diabetic Nephropathy in Human Renal Allografts: Preliminary Report of a Biopsy Study. Transplant Proc 16: 649-653.

125. Mauer SM, Goetz FC, McHugh LE, et al. 1989. Long-term Study of Normal Kidneys Transplanted into Patients with Type I Diabetes. Diabetes 38: 516-523.

126. Najarian JS, Kaufman DB, Fryd DS, McHugh L, Mauer SM, Ramsay RC, Kennedy WR, Navarro X, Goetz FC, Sutherland DE. 1989. Long-term survival following kidney transplantation in 100 type 1 diabetic patients. Transplantation, 1:106-113.

127. Remuzzi G, Ruggenenti P, Mauer SM. Pancreas and kidney/pancreas transplants: experimental medicine or real improvement? Lancet 1994;343:27-31.

42. COMBINATION THERAPY FOR HYPERTENSION AND RENAL DISEASE IN DIABETES

Unini O. Odama,M.D and George L. Bakris, MD, F.A.C.P
The Rush Hypertension Center, Department of Preventive Medicine, Rush-Presbyterian-St. Luke's Medical Center, 1700 W. Van Buren Street, Suite #470, Chicago, IL 60612.

INTRODUCTION

The incidence of diabetic nephropathy is increasing, with cardiovascular disease still accounting for more than half of the morbidity and mortality seen in diabetes. Maintaining blood pressure levels to less than 130/85 mmHg is an important measure in patients with diabetes and hypertension in order to prevent a rise in the incidence of cardiac death and diabetic nephropathy.

More than 65% of individuals with diabetes, micro or macroalbuminuria and hypertension require at least two antihypertensive medications to attain the currently recommended arterial pressure goal i.e., less than 130/85 mmHg [1-3]. This observation is supported by data from clinical trials that randomized to two different levels of blood pressure. These trials show that those with renal insufficiency and/or diabetes required a minimum of three different antihypertensive medications, in moderate to high doses to achieve the lower blood pressure goal, figure 42-1. Moreover, in these trials as well as other studies, it was common to add a medication whose antihypertensive action provides complementary, additive or synergistic antihypertensive effects through different mechanisms [3-5].

To further improve compliance and reduce drug side effect profiles, fixed-dose combinations of antihypertensive drugs with complementary modes of action have been recently developed [5]. These medications combine a lower dose of two different antihypertensive drugs that, in a fixed dose combination, reduce arterial pressure to a greater extent compared to either alone. The history of various fixed-dose antihypertensive drug combinations is shown in Table 42-1.

The evolution of fixed-dose combination antihypertensive therapy is beyond the scope of this chapter. The reader, however, is referred to a recent review on the topic [5]. This chapter will focus on the available evidence from both animal models of hypertension and renal disease as well as clinical studies that examine the efficacy of

Mogensen C.E. (ed.), THE KIDNEY AND HYPERTENSION IN DIABETES MELLITUS.
Copyright© 2000 by Kluwer Academic Publishers, Boston ● Dordrecht ● London. All rights reserved.

different classes of antihypertensive medications, either alone or combined, to either halt or prevent development of renal disease. The discussion will primarily, but not exclusively, focus on combination therapy with angiotensin converting enzyme (ACE) inhibitors and calcium channel blockers (CCBs) as well as ACE inhibitors and angiotensin II receptor blockers (ARBs).

Table 42-1. Historical Evolution of Fixed Dose Combination

1960's
Ser-Ap-Es (reserpine-hydralazine-hydrochlorothiazide)
Methyldopa/thiazide diuretic
1970's
Thiazide/ Various [K+] Sparing Diuretic
Thiazide/Spironolactone
 Beta blocker/thiazide diuretic
Clonidine/thiazide diuretic
1980's
ACE inhibitor/thiazide diuretic
1990's
(Low dose) β Blocker /thiazide diuretic
Calcium Channel Blocker/ACE inhibitor
β Blocker/Dihydropyridine Calcium Channel Blocker
Angiotensin II Receptor Blocker/Diuretic

RENAL MORPHOLOGY AND HEMODYNAMICS
Brief overviews of the renal hemodynamic and morphologic changes that occur in the diabetic kidney are presented. This is done in an effort to improve the understanding of how and why, at a comparable blood pressure level, combinations of various antihypertensive medications slow progression of diabetic nephropathy to a greater extent than either of the individual components.

Early changes observed in the diabetic kidney include an increase in efferent arteriolar tone and a loss of autoregulation [6-7]. These changes lead to an increase in intraglomerular capillary pressure, which results in cell stretch and activation of various autocrine and paracrine factors associated with tissue injury [7-8]. In addition, glomerular membrane permeability is increased and microalbuminuria ensues, a surrogate marker for the presence and progression of diabetic nephropathy [9-12]. The earliest morphologic change is mesangial matrix expansion and in some cases interstitial inflammation, the latter portends a poor renal prognosis [12,13].

The role of the renin angiotensin system (RAS) in diabetic nephropathy cannot be overemphasized. Blocking the RAS slows down the progression of established diabetic nephropathy in type I diabetes mellitus and inhibiting angiotensin II formation retards or impedes the progression from microalbuminuria to established diabetic nephropathy in people with type I diabetes mellitus. The situation could be the same for type 2 diabetes mellitus [12,14].

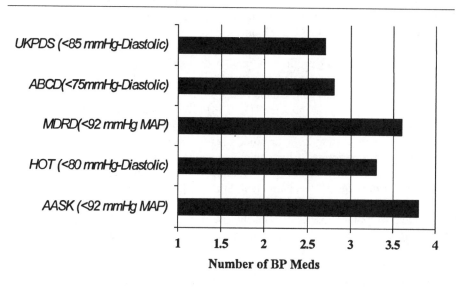

Figure 42-1- A summary of all randomized trials to level of blood pressure control and the average number of antihypertensive medications per person in each trial. Note the average number is *three* different medications in moderate to high doses.

INDIVIDUAL ANTIHYPERTENSIVE AGENTS

Experimental evidence demonstrates that reductions in intraglomerular capillary pressure, through either profound reductions in arterial pressure or dilation of the efferent arteriole, slow progression of diabetic renal disease [7,12,14]. Drugs that reduce efferent arteriolar tone and intraglomerular pressure include the ACE inhibitors, ARB and potassium channel openers [7,12,14-15]. In long-term clinical trials, however, only the ACE inhibitors have, thus far, demonstrated a consistent and persistent reduction in both proteinuria as well as an attenuated progression in nephropathy associated in association with type I diabetes and possibly from type 2 diabetes [16-25]. Moreover, while blood pressure reduction itself slows progression of both diabetic and non-diabetic renal disease, the ACE inhibitors appear to preserve renal function to even greater extent than other agents do when the achieved blood pressure approximates 140/90 mmHg [16,18,23-26].

The benefit of ACE inhibitors on diabetic glomerulosclerosis is thought to result from attenuation of angiotensin II effects on blood pressure, glomerular hemodynamics and hypertrophy and tissue fibrosis [12,14-15]. Inhibition of angiotensin II occurs with ACE inhibitors and ARBs. Clinical trials have demonstrated that ARBs are a safe and effective treatment for hypertension in people with renal impairment and produce renal hemodynamic effects akin to those seen with ACE inhibitors (15,27-28). Moreover, ARBs do not directly interfere with any enzymatic process in the renin angiotensin system (RAS). In contrast to ACE inhibitors, ARB have no direct effect on angiotensin II production or bradykinin metabolism. This more targeted mechanism, may account for the excellent tolerability profiles observed with ARB [29-32].

Antihypertensive agents that do not reduce intraglomerular pressure will not slow progression of nephropathy unless blood pressure is lowered well below that of agents that lower intraglomerular pressure [7,12,14]. To further bolster this argument, dihydropyridine CCBs are well known not to protect against morphologic progression of renal disease. Studies using 24 hour blood pressure monitoring in a rat model of renal insufficiency were performed where animals were randomized to four different CCBs, two long acting dihydropyridines, amlodipine or felodipine, as well as the nondihydropyridine agents, verapamil and diltiazem [33]. In this and four other studies, given similar levels of blood pressure reduction, verapamil and diltiazem prevented development of glomerulosclerosis and the rise in proteinuria [33-37]. Conversely, the long acting CCBs, amlodipine and felodipine did not protect against development of renal injury or proteinuria at comparable blood pressure levels, figure 42-2. A lack of morphologic protection by dihydropyridine CCBs and increase in proteinuria has also been noted in a salt-sensitive, DOCA-salt, rat model as well as the SHR model [38]. It should also be noted that in addition to dihydropyridine CCBs, prevention of mesangial expansion or glomerulosclerosis has also never been shown for alpha-blockers in either clinical studies or animal models of diabetes [12,38-40]. This has also been confirmed by the recent action of the data safety monitoring board of the ALLHAT trial, where they stopped the alpha-blocker arm due to a 25% higher cardiovascular event rate in those who developed heart failure.

This lack of effect on albuminuria by dihydropyridine CCBs is also seen clinically [9,10,41]. Results from a recent clinical trial of patients with type 2 diabetes and microalbuminuria randomized to either lisinopril or nifedipine-retard were found to have a significantly greater reduction in albumin excretion when compared to the CCB [25]. Moreover, this occurred in spite of similar reductions in blood pressure. In a separate study, an increase in protein excretion of as much as 50 % has also been shown in Type 2 diabetic African-Americans with albuminuria randomized to isradipine [24].

The reason for this absence of effect on albuminuria by dihydropyridine CCBs relates to a lack of effect on glomerular membrane permeability, in spite of blood pressure reduction to levels around 140/90 mmHg [9,10,12,33]. Results from a recently completed two year randomized, prospective trial in 28 type 2 diabetic patients with nephropathy, demonstrates no alteration of glomerular membrane permeability or albuminuria with once-daily nifedipine whereas there was a clear reduction in membrane permeability and albuminuria with once-daily diltiazem [9].

There are five long-term (> 3 year follow-up) clinical studies that examine the effects of long-acting dihydropyridine CCBs on both changes in albuminuria as well as progression of renal disease [42-47]. Two of the longest-term studies with dihydropyridine CCBs followed patients with both incipient and established diabetic nephropathy for a period of four or more years. Both these studies noted that the initial reductions in albuminuria seen with a dihydropyridine CCB did not persist beyond the first year [43,47]. Moreover, in one of these studies, the rate of decline in renal function in the group randomized to nifedipine was significantly faster than the group randomized to the ACE inhibitor [43]. In a separate study, Zucchelli et.al. followed patients with chronic renal disease, randomized to either nifedipine or an ACE inhibitor, for three years [44].

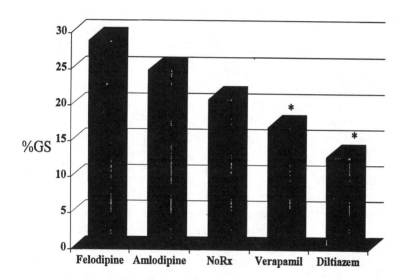

Figure 42-2. The effects of four different calcium channel blockers on glomerulosclerosis at a systolic blood pressure of 140 mmHg in a rat remnant kidney model. Note these data are derived from a slope analysis of blood pressure versus glomerulosclerosis Data are taken from reference 33. * P< 0.05 compared to felodipine, amlodipine ^ P< 0.05 compared to no therapy.

At study end, no significant differences in proteinuria or the slopes of glomerular filtration rate (GFR) declines were noted. However, in the third year, people randomized to nifedipine were more than five times more likely to start dialysis. A third study of patients with early diabetic nephropathy, randomized to either an ACE inhibitor or amlodipine and followed for three years, noted no difference between groups in reduction of microalbuminuria [45]. Interestingly, however, this is the only study, to date, that demonstrates an acute reduction in GFR with amlodipine. Thus, the results of this small study may be the result of a reduction in GFR. A sub-analysis of a recent international trial among patients with non-diabetic renal disease also demonstrated that the placebo group, those who received nifedipine retard to control blood pressure, had a significantly faster rate of decline in GFR as well as a much shorter time to dialysis [46]. Lastly, a four-year randomized double-blinded trial in people with mild renal insufficiency and Type I diabetes showed no substantive reduction from baseline albuminuria and no worsening of left ventricular hypertrophy with a dihydropyridine CCB as compared to an ACE inhibitor [47]. This was spite of reasonable blood pressure control.

In contrast to the dihydropyridine CCBs, three different meta-analyses note that nondihydropyridine CCBs reduce albuminuria and slow the decline in GFR among people with established diabetic nephropathy [48-50]. This observation is further supported by two recent long-term ($\geq$ 5 years) studies in people with established nephropathy from type 2 diabetes. These studies demonstrated that long acting verapamil or diltiazem slowed progression of established diabetic renal disease to a degree similar to an ACE inhibitor [21,51].

Many factors may contribute to the disparate effects of the different subclasses of CCBs on both surrogate end-points as well as progression of renal disease. These differences are reviewed, in detail, elsewhere [52]. It is clear, however, that arterial pressure reduction is the ultimate goal that uniformly leads to preservation of renal function. Moreover, once arterial pressure reaches levels of less than 120 mmHg systolic or dihydropyridine CCBs are combined with an ACE inhibitor, significant differences in renal protection between the subclasses of CCBs are no longer present [2,33,53]. Thus, since the majority of patients with diabetic nephropathy require two or more medications to reduce arterial pressure, a combination of antihypertensive agents, individually shown to reduce arterial pressure and albuminuria as well as preserve renal morphology and function, is preferred, figure 42-3. Since preliminary evidence supports the notion that both ACE inhibitors and nondihydropyridine CCBs slow progression of diabetic renal disease to a greater extent than conventional blood pressure lowering agents, it is predicted that a combination of these two classes of agents will provide better renal protection than either alone. Unfortunately, few animal or human studies have examined this hypothesis.

ARBs are agents with a benefit profile similar to ACE inhibitors yet with a side effect profile similar to placebo. The effects of ARBs on blood pressure and renal function were compared with those of the CCB, amlodipine. A small pilot study of hypertensive patients with type 2 diabetes and microalbuminuria demonstrated that those randomized to the ARB had significantly less urine protein excretion and stable creatinine clearance values compared to amlodipine [54]. This effect was observed in spite of similar blood pressure reduction with the two agents. These results were further corroborated by pilot data from a clinical trial that demonstrated the same results in people with type 2 diabetes [55].

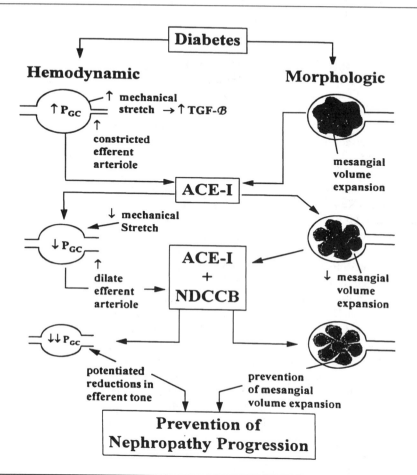

Figure 42-3-A representation of the renal hemodynamic and morphologic effects of ACE inhibitors (ACE-I) and nondihydropyridine calcium channel blockers (NDCCB), PGC-Intraglomerular capillary pressure

****Adapted from Kilaru PK and Bakris GL. Calcium channel blockade and/or ACE inhibition in diabetic hypertensive nephropathy. IN Combination Drug Therapy for Hypertension . Opie LH and Messerli F, (eds). Lippincott-Raven Publ., Philadelphia, 1997, pp.123-138.*

These results suggest that, ARBs are at least equivalent to the CCB, amlodipine, with respect to antihypertensive efficacy and that they provide better renoprotective benefits than amlodipine. The data from two ongoing clinical trials in people with nephropathy associated with Type 2 diabetes will answer the question of long-term renoprotective benefits of ARBs when completed in 2002.

COMBINATION ANTIHYPERTENSIVE THERAPY

Few animal studies have evaluated the effects of an ACE inhibitor/CCB combination on various aspects of renal disease [34,38,53,56]. Unfortunately, only two of these studies actually controlled for blood pressure differences, so that a meaningful comparison could be made between the combination and its individual components [36,53]. One of these studies showed that combination therapy with a fixed-dose of an ACE inhibitor, benezapril, and dihydropyridine CCB, amlodipine, prevented progression to glomerulosclerosis observed with amlodipine alone. This combination also blunted the rise in albuminuria in contrast to amlodipine alone, which had no effect on this variable. These findings were also observed in a recent clinical study that examined changes in proteinuria and GFR with this combination [57]. Lastly, a series of case reports demonstrate a reduction in proteinuria after cessation of once daily nifedipine among patients with diabetic nephropathy who were also receiving other antihypertensive therapy [58]. Interestingly, while proteinuria dropped in these patients, mean arterial pressure increased by an average of 7 mmHg.

In contrast to dihydropyridine CCB/ACE inhibitor combinations, animal studies that combine a nondihydropyridine CCB with an ACE inhibitor have demonstrated a potentiation of ACE inhibitor associated reductions in proteinuria [34,38,39]. Two of these studies also showed relatively greater preservation of renal morphology [34,38]. Moreover, in one animal study, the fixed-dose combination of verapamil with trandolapril showed protection of glomerular morphology, in the absence of blood pressure reduction [38]. The additive antiproteinuric effects of the fixed-dose combination, verapamil plus trandolapril, has also been observed in a recent randomized, multicenter, clinical trial of patients with nephropathy secondary to type 2 diabetes with comparable blood pressure control [59]. Thus, while ACE inhibitors appear to protect the kidney from the neutral effects of dihydropyridine CCBs, they potentiate the positive effects of nondihydropyridine CCBs.

Aside from the additive antiproteinuric effects of fixed-dose nondihydropyridine CCB/ACE inhibitor combinations, clinical studies have also shown that fixed-dose combinations have a side effect profile generally less than that the individual components used separately [60]. Schneider, et al has shown that in patients with type 2 diabetes and hypertension, this combination did not aggravate insulin resistance nor elevate lipid levels unlike patients who were treated with beta-blockers and chlorthalidone [61]. Additionally, a four-year follow-up study of patients with nephropathy secondary to type 2 diabetes demonstrated that the combination of verapamil plus lisinopril resulted in a slower decline in GFR, a lower amount of albuminuria and the lowest side effect profile [62]. No other long-term clinical studies have formally evaluated either fixed-dose or reduced dose combination therapy on progression of diabetic renal disease.

Lastly, the most common cause of death in people with type 2 diabetes and nephropathy results from cardiovascular causes [63]. In anesthetized dogs, the verapamil-trandolapril combination prevented hypoxemia-induced vasoconstriction of the coronary arteries [64]. It is important to note that in all clinical trials where a CCB, regardless of subclass was used with an ACE inhibitor to achieve blood pressure control there was a reduction in mortality. This includes the diabetes subgroup of the HOT and Syst-Eur trials [65-66]. Keep in mind, however, that unlike non-dihydropyridine CCBs that restrict elevations in heart rate to exercise, there is no evidence of cardiovascular risk reduction with a dihydropyridine among individuals with diabetes. However, with the addition of an ACE inhibitor or beta-blocker to inhibit the renin-angiotensin and/or sympathetic nervous system reduction in cardiovascular events occurs without further substantive reduction in blood pressure. This may relate to the fact that dihydropyridine CCBs; regardless of duration of action increase sympathetic neural tone [67].

Decreased angiotensin II formation or action is beneficial in diabetic nephropathy in that it reduces both systemic and glomerular hypertension, proteinuria, the tendency to form abnormal amounts of glomerular and interstitial matrix protein and decreases in aldosterone formation. Thus, a therapeutic goal in diabetic nephropathy might be to inhibit angiotensin II effects as completely as possible. ACE inhibitor therapy reduces the impact but do not totally eliminate angiotensin II effects [68-69].

With the advent of ARBs, it seems logical to combine ACE inhibitors and ARBs to eliminate the effects of angiotensin II and still take advantage of the positive effects of bradykinin stimulation of ACE inhibitors and further aldosterone reduction by both agents. The data, however, with such combinations is mixed. Hebert et al did not observe additive acute effects of the combination of an ACE and ARB on glomerular filtration rate preservation or proteinuria in their small, short-term study [70]. Conversely, A recent study examined the effects on blood pressure and plasma renin of a single dose of enalapril 10mg, enalapril 10mg combined with losartan 50mg, or enalapril 20mg in salt depleted normal subjects to assess whether combination therapy with an ACE inhibitor/ARB is more effective than higher doses of ACE inhibitors alone [71]. The study demonstrated that combination therapy decreased blood pressure to a greater extent than the single agent and increased plasma renin more than either dose of enalapril given alone. Additionally, Ruilope et.al randomized 108 people with renal insufficiency to either an ARB alone, in two different doses, or these same doses in combination with a low dose ACE inhibitor. They demonstrated that the blood pressure lowering effects of the combination were significantly better with no significant adverse effects on measures of renal function including serum creatinine and potassium [72]. Thus, long-term combination therapy might result in less glomerular and interstitial fibrosis than ACE inhibitors alone because of the greater attenuation of angiotensin II effects in combination [73].

CONCLUSIONS

It is critically important that arterial pressure levels of <130/85 mmHg be achieved in diabetic patients to not only preserve renal function but to also reduce cardiovascular mortality. Since more than two-thirds of patients with diabetic nephropathy require a minimum of two medications to control their blood pressure to the newly recommended goal, combination therapy is highly recommended. Given the difficulties with medication compliance in this patient group along with the socioeconomic cost of diabetic nephropathy and its impact on the quality of life, the advantages of fixed dose combinations are obvious [74]. Of the many possible combinations, an ACEI/ARB combination or a non-dihydropyridine CCB/ACE inhibitor combination may be preferred not only because of a low side effect profile but also because each agent has been individually shown to reduce cardiovascular mortality following myocardial infarctions [75]. This has not been shown for dihydropyridine CCBs [76]. However, a dihydropyridine CCB combined with an ACE inhibitor has been shown to reduce cardiovascular events in those with hypertension and diabetes as in the Hypertension Optimal Treatment Trial (HOT), and the Syst-Eur trial.

In light of these few studies, however, there are insufficient data to assess whether fixed-dose antihypertensive therapy offers a distinct advantage to reduce renal and cardiovascular mortality over use of the individual components together. However, it is clear from data on patient adherence to medication regimens that there would be fewer missed doses of medication. Moreover, the evidence suggests that an ACEI/ARB combination therapy or low dose combinations of a nondihydropyridine CCB with an ACE inhibitor yields additive effects on glomerular membrane permeability as evidenced by reductions in proteinuria independent of blood pressure reduction. This may, in longer-term studies, result in slowed progression of diabetic nephropathy to a greater extent than an ACE inhibitor alone. This hypothesis is further supported by a recent meta-analysis of experimental and clinical studies that examined changes in glomerular permeability in the context of renal disease progression as well as a review of clinical trial data for cardiovascular and renal events [77,78]. Additionally, the most recent recommendations of the National Kidney Foundation recommend a fixed-dose combination of an ACE inhibitor with a diuretic in all patients with diabetes and hypertension whose blood pressure is > 15/10 mmHg above goal blood pressure, i.e. the new lower goal of 130/80 mmHg [79].

REFERENCES

1.   National High Blood Pressure Education Program Working Group on Hypertension and Renal Disease. 1995 Update of the working group reports on chronic renal failure and renovascular hypertension. Arch Intern Med. 1996;156 :1938-1947.
2.   Sheinfeld GR and Bakris GL. Benefits of combination angiotensin-converting enzyme inhibitor and calcium antagonist therapy for diabetic patients. Am J Hypertension 1999;12:80S-85S.

3. The Sixth Report of the Joint National Committee on Prevention, Detection, Evaluation, and Treatment of High Blood Pressure (JNC VI). Arch Intern Med, 1997;157:2413-2446

4. Waeber B, Brunner HR. Main objectives and new aspects of combination treatment of hypertension. J Hypertens 1995; 13 (Suppl):S15-S19.

5. Epstein M and Bakris GL. Newer approaches to antihypertensive therapy using fixed dose combination therapy: Future perspectives. Arch Intern Med. 1996;156:1969-1978.

6. Griffin KA, Picken MM and Bidani AK. Deleterious effects of calcium channel blockade on pressure transmission and glomerular injury in rat remnant kidneys. J Clin. Invest 1995; 96: 793-800.

7. Makrilakis K and Bakris GL. New therapeutic approaches to achieve the desired blood pressure goal. Cardiovasc Rev. & Reports 1997;18:10-16.

8. Bakris GL, Walsh MF, Sowers JR. Endothelium,mesangium interactions:Role of insulin-like growth factors . IN: Endocrinology of the Vasculature (Sowers JR, ed). Humana Press Inc. New Jersey, 1996, pp.341-356.

9. Smith AC, Toto R, Bakris GL Differential effects of calcium channel blockers on size selectivity of proteinuria in diabetic glomerulopathy. Kidney Int. 1998;54:889-896

10. Bakris GL. Microalbuminuria: Prognostic Implications. Curr Opin in Nephrol and Hypertens 1996;5(3):219-233.

11. Drumond MC , Kristal B , Myers BD , Deen WM Structural basis for reduced glomerular filtration capacity in nephrotic humans. J Clin Invest 1994 ;94(3):1187-1195

12. Bakris GL, Mehler P, and Schrier R. Hypertension and Diabetes. IN Schrier RW and Gottschalk CW (eds.) Diseases of the Kidney 6th ed., Little Brown and Company, 1996, Chapter 54, pp.1281-1328

13. Steffes MW, Osterby R, Chavers B, and Mauer SM. Mesangial expansion as a central mechanism for loss of kidney function in diabetic patients. Diabetes 1989;38:1077-1081.

14. Anderson S, Rennke HG, Brenner BM. Nifedipine versus fosinopril in uninephrectomized diabetic rats. Kidney Int 1992;41:891-897.

15. Tarif N and Bakris GL. Angiotensin II receptor blockade and progression of renal disease in nondiabetic patients. Kidney Int 1997; 52(Suppl. 63): S-67-S-70

16. Ravid M, Lang R, Rachmani R, Lishner M. Long-term renoprotective effect of angiotensin-converting enzyme inhibition in non-insulin-dependent diabetes mellitus. Arch Intern Med 1996;156:286-289

17. Parving H, Hommel E, Nielsen M, Giese J: Effect of captopril on blood pressure and kidney function in normotensive insulin dependent diabetics with nephropathy. Br Med J 1989;299:533-536.

18. Bakris GL, Slataper R, Vicknair N, Sadler R: ACE inhibitor mediated reductions in renal size and microalbuminuria in normotensive, diabetic subjects. J Diab Compl 1994;8:2-6.

19. Viberti G; Mogensen CE; Groop LC; Pauls JF. Effect of captopril on progression to clinical proteinuria in patients with insulin-dependent diabetes mellitus and microalbuminuria. European Microalbuminuria Captopril Study Group JAMA 1994;271(4):275-9.,

20. Sakamoto N: Effects of long-term enalapril treatment on persistent microalbuminuria in well- controlled hypertensive and normotensive NIDDM patients. Diabetes Care 1994;17:420-424

21. Bakris GL, Copley JB, Vicknair N, Sadler R, Leurgans S. Calcium channel blockers versus other antihypertensive therapies on progression of NIDDM associated nephropathy: Results of a six year study. Kidney Int. 1996;50:1641-1650.

22.   Lebovitz HE, Wiegmann TB, Cnaan A: Renal protective effects of enalapril in hypertensive NIDDM: role of baseline albuminuria. Kidney Int Suppl 1994;45:S150-S155.

23.   Lewis EJ, Hunsicker LG, Bain RP, Rohde RD for the Collaborative Study Group. The effect of angiotensin converting enzyme inhibition on diabetic nephropathy. N Engl J Med 1993;329:1456-1462.

24.   Guasch A, Parham M, Zayas CF, Campbell O, Nzerue C, Macon E. Contrasting effects of calcium channel blockade versus converting enzyme inhibition on proteinuria in African Americans with non-insulin dependent diabetes mellitus and nephropathy. J Am Soc Nephrol 1997;8: 793-798.

25.   Agardh CD, Garcia-Puig J, Charbonnel B, Angelkort B, Barnett AH. Greater reduction of urinary albumin excretion in hypertensive Type II diabetic patients with incipient nephropathy by lisinopril than by nifedipine. J Human Hypertens 1996;10:185-192.

26.   Maschio G, Alberti D, Janin G, Locatelli F, Mann JEF, Motolese M, Ponticelli C, Ritz E, Zucchelli P, and the Angiotensin-Converting-Enzyme Inhibition in Progressive Renal Insufficiency Study Group. Effect of the angiotensin-converting-enzyme inhibitor benazepril on the progression of chronic renal insufficiency. N Engl J Med 1996;334:939-945

27.   Venkart C, Ram S, Fierro G. The Benefits of Angiotensin II Receptor Blockers in patients with renal insufficiency of failure. Am J Ther.1998;5(2): 101-105

28.   Pitt B, Segal R, Martinez FA, Meurers G, Cowley AJ, Thomas I, Deedwania PC, Ney DE, Snavely DB, Chang PI Randomised trial of losartan versus captopril in patients over 65 with heart failure. Lancet 1997;349:747-752

29.   Bauer JH, Reams GP: the angiotensin II type I receptor antagonists: a new class of antihypertensive drugs. Arch Intern Med 1995;155: 1361-1368.

30.   Kang PM, Landau AJ, Eberhardt RT, Frishman WH: Angiotensin II receptor antagonists: a new approach to blockade of the renin-angiotensin system. Am Heart J 1994;127:1388-1401

31.   Goldberg AI, Dunlay MC, Sweet CS: safety and tolerability of Losartan potassium, an angiotensin II receptor antagonist, compared with hydrocholothiazide, atenolol, felodipine ER, and angiotensin –converting enzyme inhibitors for the treatment of systemic hypertension. Am J Cardiol 1995;75:793-795.

32.   Dahlof B, Keller SE, Makris L, et al: Efficacy and tolerability of Losartan potassium and atenolol in patients with mild to moderate essential hypertension. Am J Hypertens 1995:8:578-583

33.   Griffin KA, Picken MM, Bakris GL, Bidani AK Class differences in the effects of calcium channel blockers in the rat remnant kidney model. Kidney Int 1999; 55(5):1849-1860.

34.   Gaber L, Walton C, Brown S, Bakris, GL: Effects of different antihypertensive treatments on morphologic progression of diabetic nephropathy in uninephrectomized dogs. Kidney Int 1994;46:161-169

35.   Jyothirmayi GN, Reddi AS: Effect of diltiazem on glomerular heparan sulfate and albuminuria in diabetic rats. Hypertension 1993; 21:765-802.

36.   Munter K, Hergenroder S, Jochims K, Kirchengast M. Individual and combined effects of verapamil or trandolapril on glomerular morphology and function in the stroke prone rat. J Am Soc Nephrol 1996;7:681-686

37. Brown SA, Walton CL, Crawford P & Bakris GL. Long-term effects of different anti-hypertensive regimens on renal hemodynamics and proteinuria. Kidney Int 1993, 43:1210-1218.

38. Dworkin LD, Tolbert E, Recht PA, Hersch JC, Feiner H, Levin RI. Effects of amlodipine on glomerular filtration, growth and injury in experimental hypertension. Hypertension 1996; 27:245-250

39. Jyothirmayi GN, Alluru I, Reddi AS. Doxazosin prevents proteinuria and glomerular loss of heparan sulfate in diabetic rats. Hypertension 1996;27:1108-1114

40. Rachmani R, Levi Z, Slavachevsky I, Half-Onn E, Ravid M Effect of an alpha-adrenergic blocker, and ACE inhibitor and hydrochlorothiazide on blood pressure and on renal function in type 2 diabetic patients with hypertension and albuminuria. A randomized cross-over study. Nephron 1998;80(2):175-182

41. Abbott K, Smith AC, Bakris GL. Effects of dihydropyridine calcium antagonists on albuminuria in diabetic subjects. J. Clin Pharmacol. 1996;36:274-279.

42. Gilbert RE, Jerum G, Allen T, Hammond J, Cooper ME on behalf on Diabetic Nephropathy Study Group. Effect of different antihypertensive agents on normotensive microalbuminuria patients with IDDM and NIDDM. J Am Soc Nephrol 1994;5:377 (abstract).

43. Campbell D on behalf of the Melbourne Nephropathy Study Group. ACE inhibitors versus calcium channel blockade. Fifth International Symposium on Hypertension associated with Diabetes Mellitus. International Society of Nephrology 1997, pp.32.

44. Zucchelli P, Zuccala A, Borghi M, et. al., Long term comparison between captopril and nifedipine in the progression of renal insufficiency Kidney Int 1992 42:452-458.

45. Velussi M, Brocco E, Frigato F, Zolli M, Muollo B, Maioli M, Carraro A, Tonolo G, Fresu P, Cernigoi A, Fioretto P, Nosadini R. Effects of cilazapril and amlodipine on kidney function in hypertensive NIDDM patients. Diabetes 1996;45:216-222

46. Locatelli F, Carbarns IR, Maschio G, Mann JF, Ponticelli C, Ritz E, Alberti D, Motolese M, Janin G, Zucchelli P Long-term progression of chronic renal insufficiency in the AIPRI Extension Study. The Angiotensin-Converting-Enzyme Inhibition in Progressive Renal Insufficiency Study Group. Kidney Int Suppl, 1997;63:S63-S66

47. Tarnow L, Sato A, Ali S, Rossing P, Nielsen FS, Parving HH Effects of nisoldipine and lisinopril on left ventricular mass and function in diabetic nephropathy. Diabetes Care 1999;22(3):491-494

48. Gansevoort RT, Sluiter WJ, Hemmelder MH, de Zeeuw D, de Jong PE. Antiproteinuric effect of blood pressure lowering agents: a meta-analysis of comparative trials. Nephrol Dial Transplant 1995;10:1963-1974

49. Maki DD, Ma JZ, Louis TA, Kasiske BL: Effect of antihypertensive agents on the kidney. Arch Intern Med 1995 ;155:1073-1082.

50. Kloke HJ, Branten AJ, Huysmans FT, Wetzels JF Antihypertensive treatment of patients with proteinuric renal diseases: risks or benefits of calcium channel blockers? Kidney Int 1998;53(6):1559-1573

51. Bakris GL, Mangrum A, Copley JB, Vicknair N, Sadler R. Calcium channel or beta blockade on progression of diabetic renal disease in African-Americans. Hypertension 1997;29:744-750

52. Tarif N and Bakris GL Preservation of renal function: the spectrum of effects by calcium channel blockers. Nephrol Dial Transpl, 1997;12:2244-2250.

53.   Bakris GL, Griffin KA, Picken MM, and Bidani AK. Combined effects of an angiotensin converting enzyme inhibitor and a calcium antagonist on renal injury. J Hypertension 1997;15:1181-1185

54.   Holdaas H, Hartman A, Berg KJ, Lund K, Fauchald P, Renal effects of losartan and amlodipine in hypertensive patients with non- diabetic nephropathy; Nephrol Dial Transplant. 1998;13(12):3096-3102.

55.   Pohl M, Cooper M, Ulrey J, et al: Safety and efficacy of Irbesartan in hypertensive patients with type II diabetes and proteinuria (abs). Am J Hypertens 1997;10 (4, part 2):105A

56.   Wenzel RO, Helmchen U, Schoeppe W, Schwietzer G. Combination treatment of enalapril with nitrendipine in rats with renovascular hypertension. Hypertension 1994;23: 114-122.

57.   Fogari R, Zoppi A, Mugellini A, Lusardi P, Destro M, Corradi L. Effect of benazepril plus amlodipine vs. benazepril alone on urinary albumin excretion in hypertensive patients with type II diabetes and microalbuminuria. Clin Drug Invest 1996:11:50-55.

58.   Hess B. Reduced proteinuria after cessation of long acting osmotic release nifedipine GITS in diabetic nephropathy. Nephrol Dial Transplant. 1997;12:1772 (letter).

59.   Bakris GL, Weir MR, DeQuattro V, McMahon FG. Effects of an ACE inhibitor/calcium antagonist combination on proteinuria in diabetic nephropathy. Kidney Int.1998; 54:1283-1289

60.   Holzgreve H.   Safety profile of the combination of verapamil and trandolapril. J Hypertens. 1997;15(suppl 2): S51-S53.

61.   Schneider M, Lerch M, Papiri M, Buechel P, Boehlen L, Shaw S, Risen W, Weidmann P. Metabolic neutrality of combined verapamil-trandolapril treatment in contrast to beta-blocker-low-dose chlorthalidone treatment in hypertensive type II diabetes. J Hypertens. 1996;14:669-677.

62.   Lash JP and Bakris GL. Effects of ACE inhibitors and calcium antagonists alone or combined on progression of diabetic nephropathy. Nephrol. Dial and Transpl.1995;10 (Suppl.9):56-62

63.   Nelson RG, Knowler WC, Pettitt DJ, Bennett PH. Kidney diseases in diabetes. In Diabetes In America National Institutes of Health Pub. No.95-1468, 2nd edition, 1995, pp. 349-400

64.   Lee JJ, Boulanger CM, Kirchengast M, Vanhoutte PM.   Trandolapril plus verapamil inhibits the coronary vasospasm induced by hypoxia following ischemia-reperfusion injury in dogs. Gen Pharm. 1996;27(6):1057-1059.

65.   Hansson L, Zanchetti A, Carruthers SG, Dahlof B, Elmfeldt D, Julius S, Menard J, Rahn RK, Wedel H, Westerling S. Effects of intensive blood-pressure lowering and low dose aspirin in patients with hypertenstion: principal results of the Hypertension Optimal Treatment (HOT) randomised trial. HOT Study Group Lancet, 1998; 351: 1755-1762.

66.   Staessen JA, Thijs L, Gasowski J, Cells H, Fagard RH. Treatment of isolated systolic hypertension in the elderly: further evidence from the systolic hypertension in Europe (Syst-Eur) trial. Am J Cardiol 1998; 82(9B):20R-22R.

67.   Ligtenberg G, Blankenstijn PJ, Oey PL, Klein IH, Dijkhorst-Oei LT, Boomsma F, Wieneke GH, van Huffelen AC, Koomans HA. Reduction of sympathetic hyperactivity by enalapril in patients with chronic renal failure. N Engl J Med 1999; 340: 1321-1328.

68.   Nussberger J, Brunner DB, Waeber B, Brunner HR: True versus immunoreactive angiotensin II in human plasma. Hypertension 1985;7(suppl D):11-17

69.   Nussberger J, Brunner DB, Waeber B, Brunner HR: Specific measurement of angiotensin metabolites and in vitro generated angiotensin II in plasma. Hypertension 1986;6:476-482.

70. Herbert LA, Falkenhain ME, Nahman Jr NS, Cosio FG, O' Dorisio TM. Combination ACE inhibitor and angiotensin II receptor antagonist therapy in diabetic nephropathy. Am J Nephrol. 1999; 19(1):1-6

71. Azizi M, Guyene TT, Chatellier G, Wargon M, Menard J: Additive effects of losartan and enalapril on blood pressure and plasma active renin. Hypertension 1997;29:634-640.

72. Ruilope LM, Aldigier JC, Ponticelli C, Oddou-Stock P, Botten F, Mann JF for the European Group for the Investigation of valsartan in chronic renal disease. Safety of the combination of valsartan and benazepril in patients with chronic renal disease. J Hypertens, 2000;18(1):89-95.

73. Azizi M, Guyene TT, Chatellier G, Menard J; Pharmacological demonstration of the additive effects of angiotensin-converting enzyme inhibition and angiotensin II antagonism in sodium depleted healthy subjects. Clin Exp Hypertens. 1997;19:937-951.

74. Simeon G, Bakris G. Socioeconomic impact of diabetic nephropathy: can we improve the outcome? J Hypertens 1997;15 (Suppl 2):S77-S82.

75. Yusuf S, Lessem J, Jha P, Lonn E. Primary and secondary prevention of myocardial infarction and strokes: an update of randomly allocated, controlled trials. J Hypertens 1993; 11 (Suppl 4):S61-S73.

76. Furberg CD, Psaty BM and Meyer JV. Dose-related increase in mortality in patients with coronary heart disease. Circulation 1995;92:1326-1331.

77. Perna A and Remuzzi G. Abnormal permeability to proteins and glomerular lesions: a meta-analysis of experimental and human studies. Am J Kidney Dis 1996;27:34-41.

78. Keane WF, Eknoyan G. Proteinuria, albuminuria, risk, assessment, detection, elimination (PARADE): a position paper of the National Kidney Foundation. Am J Kidney Dis 1999;33 :1004-1010

79. The National Kidney Foundation Hypertension and Diabetes Councils-A position paper on the treatment of hypertension in diabetes to preserve renal function. Am J Kidney Dis, In Press

43. MICROALBUMINURIA IN ESSENTIAL HYPERTENSION.
SIGNIFICANCE FOR THE CARDIOVASCULAR AND RENAL SYSTEMS

Vito M. Campese*, Roberto Bigazzi, and Stefano Bianchi
* Division of Nephrology, University of Southern California, Los Angeles, USA.
and Unita' Operativa di Nefrologia, Spedali Riuniti, Livorno, Italy

INTRODUCTION
It is now well recognized that microalbuminuria in patients with insulin-dependent (IDDM) and non-insulin-dependent diabetes mellitus (NIDDM) is a marker of generalized microvascular and glomerular damage, and, as such, it predicts overt proteinuria and progressive renal failure [1] as well as cardiovascular morbidity and mortality [2,3,4].

In recent years, evidence has been accumulating that microalbuminuria may also predict cardiovascular and renal events in patients with essential hypertension. Given the very high prevalence of essential hypertension in most industrialized countries, the recognition of prognostic tools for cardiovascular diseases assumes extreme clinical importance. Evidence indicates that measurements of urinary albumin excretion (UAE) may be a useful tool to predict cardiovascular disease in patients with essential hypertension.

MICROALBUMINURIA IN ESSENTIAL HYPERTENSION: INCIDENCE AND RELATIONSHIP WITH LEVELS OF BLOOD PRESSURE
The prevalence of microalbuminuria in patients with essential hypertension varies enormously among different studies with rates ranging between 5 and 37 percent. [5,6,7,8] In a study of 11 343 non-diabetic hypertensive patients with a mean age of 57 years, microalbuminuria was present in 32% of men and 28% of women ($P < 0.05$) and increased with age, severity and duration of hypertension [9]. Most studies have demonstrated a significant relationship between severity of blood pressure elevation and UAE [10,11,12,13], whereas other studies have failed to find such a relationship [7,14]. The correlation between UAE and levels of blood pressure improves when average 24 hr blood pressure levels are obtained by continuous ambulatory recordings [15,16]. Also, UAE seems to correlate with abnormal patterns of ambulatory blood pressure recordings. We observed that patients with essential hypertension and microalbuminuria

manifest a blunted nocturnal dipping of blood pressure. Hypertensive patients with no nocturnal dipping of blood pressure (non-dippers) displayed greater UAE than "dippers" (fig. 43-1) [17].

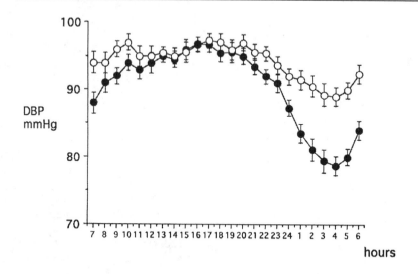

Figure 43-1   Mean hourly diastolic blood pressure (DBP) values in patients with essential hypertension with   (open circle) and without (closed circles) microalbuminuria. [Adapted from Ref. 18].

MICROALBUMINURIA AND SERUM LIPIDS

Microalbuminuria and hyperlipidemia frequently coexist in patients with essential hypertension. We have observed that serum levels of lipoprotein (a), low-density lipoprotein (LDL) cholesterol, and triglycerides are higher whereas levels of HDL-cholesterol are lower in hypertensive patients with microalbuminuria compared with patients without microalbuminuria (Figure 43-2). Using multiple regression analyses we observed that lipoprotein (a) and nocturnal blood pressure values were the variables that best correlated with UAE. [18] Haffner et al [19] also observed higher serum levels of triglycerides and lower HDL cholesterol in non diabetic subjects with microalbuminuria compared with subjects without microalbuminuria. Others observed a significant correlation between UAE and levels of triglycerides and apolipoprotein B [20-21].

The reasons for the frequent association between microalbuminuria and serum lipid abnormalities are not clear. One possible explanation is that the urinary loss of protein causes the rise in serum levels of lipoproteins. This hypothesis is supported by the evidence that urinary losses of large amounts of proteins may lead to increased serum levels of total and LDL cholesterol [22,23] as well as of lipoprotein(a) [24,25]. Moreover, some studies have suggested that urinary loss of small amounts of albumin in diabetic patients may cause substantial alterations of serum lipoproteins [26,27].

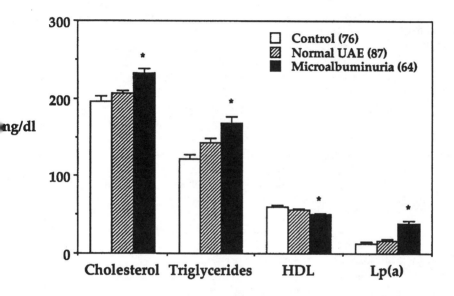

Figure 43-2. Serum levels of lipoproteins in 76 normotensive healthy subjects, 87 patients with essential hypertension and normal urinary albumin excretion (UAE) and 64 hypertensive patients with microalbuminuria. Values in patients with microalbuminuria were significantly (p<0.001 by ANOVA) greater than in hypertensive patients with normal UAE and normotensive healthy subjects.

An alternative hypothesis to explain the frequent association between microalbuminuria and hyperlipidemia is that hyperlipidemia causes renal damage resulting in increased UAE. This hypothesis is supported by experimental evidence that lipid abnormalities may contribute to the progression of renal disease [28] both in experimental nephropathy in animals [29] as well as in patients with diabetic [30] or with nondiabetic nephropathy [31], by a mechanism analogous to atherogenesis. Patients with familial type III hyperlipoproteinemia may manifest generalized atherosclerosis and glomerulosclerosis with massive foam cells accumulation within the glomeruli [32]. Alternatively, some patients with type III hyperlipoproteinemia may manifest a lipoprotein glomerulopathy characterized by intraglomerular lipoprotein thrombi in the absence of generalized atherosclerosis [33]. Recent studies have suggested that this form of lipoprotein glomerulopathy may be linked to some variants in apoE molecule

[34,35]. The mechanism(s) responsible for the deleterious effects of lipids on glomerular injury are not well established. The resemblance between glomerular mesangial cells and vascular smooth muscle cells and the important role played by the latter cells in the process of atherosclerosis suggests that accumulation of lipids in the mesangial cells may cause or accelerate glomerulosclerosis. The accumulation of lipids in mesangial cells or glomerular macrophages, along with collagen, laminin and fibronectin, also supports some similarities between the process of atherosclerosis and glomerulosclerosis. Klahr et al [36] have suggested that mesangial cells exposed to increased amounts of lipoproteins may incorporate lipids which, in turn, may stimulate their proliferation and excessive glomerular basement membrane deposition leading to progressive glomerulosclerosis. The experimental evidence suggests that it is the elevated concentration of apoB-containing lipoproteins that contributes to further progression of renal injury [37]. LDL, VLDL and IDL promote the proliferation of human mesangial cells in vitro [38]. The chemokine monocyte chemoattractant protein-1 (MCP-1), has been suggested to play a pivotal role in mediating lipid-induced nephrotoxicity, and lovastatin reduces gene expression of this protein [38]. A high cholesterol diet caused a marked upregulation of macrophage-colony stimulating factor (M-CSF), vascular adhesion molecules-1 (VCAM) and intracellular adhesion molecule-1 (ICAH-1) in glomerular mesangial cells from ExHC rats [40]. These studies suggest that hypercholesterolemia can induce a proinflammatory response within the glomeruli, which involves the recruitment of macrophages via activation of chemotactic and adhesion molecules, resulting in renal injury.

Pharmacological agents that lower serum lipids ameliorate renal injury in several experimental models of renal disease [41]. In subtotally nephrectomized rats, the beneficial effect of atorvastatin on proteinuria was associated with reduced renal TGF-1 expression and less macrophage infiltration in both glomeruli and the tubulointerstitium [41]. Statins appear to influence important intracellular pathways that are involved in the inflammatory and fibrogenic responsible for progressive renal injury [42]. Statins seem to reduce mesangial cell expression and production of chemokines such as MCP-1 and macrophage-colony stimulating factor (M-CSF), as well as vascular adhesion molecules-1 (VCAM) and intracellular adhesion molecule-1 (ICAM-1). Moreover, lovastatin inhibited the activation of transcription nuclear factor-kB (NKF-kB), which plays a major role in the gene expression involved in mesangial cell inflammatory response.

MICROALBUMINURIA, INSULIN RESISTANCE AND HYPERINSULINEMIA IN ESSENTIAL HYPERTENSION

Several investigators have described the presence of insulin resistance and hyperinsulinemia in a substantial number of patients with essential hypertension [44,45], and suggested hyperinsulinemia as a risk factor for atherosclerotic cardiovascular diseases [46].

The mechanisms by which insulin resistance, hyperinsulinemia, or both may increase the risk of cardiovascular disease are not well established. The plasma insulin response to an oral glucose load was enhanced in hypertensive patients compared with control subjects [47]. A significant direct correlation was present between insulin area-under-the-curve and urinary albumin excretion rate. Using the euglycemic clamp technique, we also observed a 35% reduction of the peripheral glucose uptake stimulated by insulin in patients with essential hypertension and microalbuminuria [48]. This appeared to be secondary to a reduction of glycogen synthesis in skeletal muscle cells. Nosadini et al showed a significant correlation between UAE and insulin resistance in patients with essential hypertension [49]. An association between insulin resistance and microalbuminuria has also been described by Falkner et al [50] in young African-Americans. In all, the data supports microalbuminuria as a consistent correlate of iperinsulinemia and insulin resistance in normotensive and hypertensive individuals.

The significance of the association between hyperinsulinemia, insulin resistance and microalbuminuria in essential hypertension is uncertain. Because microalbuminuria and insulin resistance [51,52] occur in nondiabetic normotensive subjects with genetic predisposition for hypertension, microalbuminuria and enhanced plasma insulin response to glucose could be both genetically determined and cosegregate with the hypertensive status. Alternatively, insulin resistance and hyperinsulinemia, or both, could be causally related to microalbuminuria. Finally, enhanced plasma insulin response to glucose, insulin resistance and microalbuminuria could be a consequence of hypertension.

Insulin could increase UAE directly or indirectly through a variety of mechanisms. Insulin could contribute to arteriosclerosis, renal damage and microalbuminuria through its effects on blood pressure, lipid metabolism, or through its throphic actions on vascular smooth muscle cells. Insulin infusion into femoral arteries of animals induced intimal and medial proliferation and accumulation of cholesterol and fatty acids [53]. In vitro, insulin can stimulate the proliferation of smooth muscle cells and collagen deposition by growth-promoting factors [54]. Insulin can increase cholesterol and triglycerides synthesis and enhance LDL-receptor activity in arterial smooth muscle cells, fibroblasts and mononuclear cells [55,56].

An alternative hypothesis is that insulin may alter glomerular hemodynamics and/or glomerular permeability directly or in association with other factors such as catecholamines, angiotensin II, glucagone or sodium retention. Insulin may contribute to the salt-sensitivity of blood pressure by causing sodium retention [57] or via activation of the sympathetic nervous system [58]. Salt-sensitive individuals manifest an abnormal renal hemodynamic response to high salt intake characterized by increased filtration fraction and intraglomerular pressure, and greater UAE than salt resistant patients [59]. Insulin could increase UAE by altering glomerular membrane permeability [60], or endothelial function [61,62]. Finally, both insulin resistance and microalbuminuria could be the result of alterations of the microcirculation caused by long standing hypertension. This explanation seems less likely, because hyperinsulinemia, insulin resistance and microalbuminuria may precede the appearance of high blood pressure and are not found in all patients with established hypertension.

MICROALBUMINURIA AND CARDIOVASCULAR DISEASE

The increasing interest in the significance of microalbuminuria in essential hypertension derives, in large part, from the recognition that an increase in UAE is associated with an increased incidence of cardiovascular morbid events, such as left ventricular hypertrophy, [63,64] thickness of the carotid artery (fig. 43-3), [18, 65] myocardial ischemia, [66,67], coronary heart disease, [68] peripheral vascular disease, [69] stroke, and hypertensive retinopathy. [70].

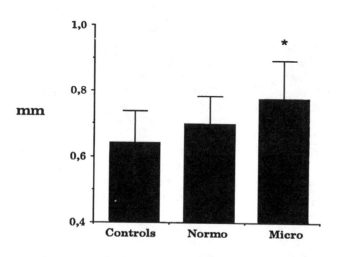

Figure 43-3 Thickness of the media-intima carotid artery in hypertensive patients with normal urinary albumin excretion (normo), patients with microalbuminuria (micro) and normotensive healthy subjects (control). the difference between patients with microalbuminuria and patients with normal urinary albumin excretion was significant (P<0.01). [From Ref. 18 with permission].

In a study of 11 343 non-diabetic hypertensive patients, among patients with microalbuminuria, 31% had coronary artery disease, 24% had left ventricular hypertrophy, 6% had had a stroke, and 7% had peripheral vascular disease. In patients without MAU, these rates were 22%, 14%, 4%, and 5% respectively [P < 0.001]. Further, in patients with coronary artery disease, left ventricular hypertrophy, stroke, and peripheral vascular disease, MAU was significantly greater than in patients who did not have these complications (P < 0.001) [9].

We performed a retrospective cohort analysis of 141 hypertensive individuals followed-up for approximately 7 years. Fifty-four patients had microalbuminuria and 87 had normal UAE. At baseline, the two groups had similar age, weight and blood pressure, but serum cholesterol, triglycerides, and uric acid were higher and HDL cholesterol lower in patients with microalbuminuria than those with normal UAE. During follow-up, 12 cardiovascular events occurred in the 54 patients with microalbuminuria and only 2 events in the 87 patients with normal UAE. Multiple regression analysis showed that UAE, cholesterol and diastolic blood pressure were independent predictors for the cardiovascular outcome [71].

In conclusion, the presence of microalbuminuria in patients with essential hypertension carries an increased risk of cardiovascular events. Although the mechanisms underscoring this association are not clear, it is plausible that the increased incidence of cardiovascular events in these patients may be due, at least in part, to the presence of lipid abnormalities.

MICROALBUMINURIA AND NEPHROANGIOSCLEROSIS

Data from the United States Renal Data System (USRDS) show that over the past decade, the incidence of renal failure as a consequence of essential hypertension has steadily increased.

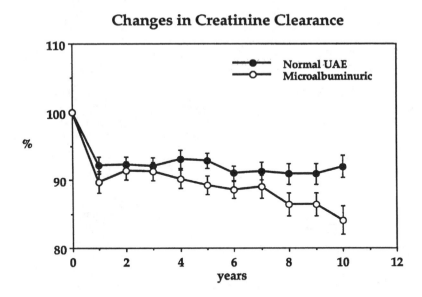

Changes in Creatinine Clearance

Figure 43-4 The line graphs show the changes in rate of clearance of creatinine over time for hypertensive patients with microalbuminuria (open circles) and patients with normal urinary excretion of albumin (closed circles) [From Ref. 71 with permission].

This phenomenon is particularly striking when one considers that definite progress has been made in the treatment of established hypertension and in the prevention of other cardiovascular complications. Can we predict the patients at risk for developing renal failure due to hypertension, and more specifically is microalbuminuria such a predictor?

Schmieder et al followed-up for 6 years a group of hypertensive subjects with normal renal function and observed no correlation between baseline urinary protein excretion and worsening of renal function [72]. Ruilope et al studied hypertensive subjects with and without microalbuminuria maintained on antihypertensive therapy consisting of diuretics and beta-blockers alone or in combination for 5 years. They observed that patients who at baseline evaluation manifested microalbuminuria, showed a greater reduction of renal function then patients without microalbuminuria [72].

In a retrospective analysis of 141 hypertensive individuals followed for approximately 7 years, we observed a greater decrease of creatinine clearance among hypertensive patients with microalbuminuria than among those with normal UAE (-12.12.77 vs. -7.10.88 ml/min; $P<0.05$) [71].

REFERENCES

1.   Mogensen CE. Microalbuminuria predicts clinical proteinuria and early mortality in maturity-onset diabetes. N Engl J Med 1984; 310: 356-360.
2.   Messent JW, Elliot TG, Hill RG, Jarret RJ, Keen H, Viberti GC. Prognostic significance of microalbuminuria in insulin-dependent diabetes mellitus: a twenty-three-year follow-up study. Kidney Int 1992; 41: 836-839.
3.   Mau Pedersen M, Christensen CK, Mogensen CE. Long-term (18 years) prognosis for normo-and microalbuminuric type 1 (insulin-dependent) diabetic patients. Diabetologia 1992; 35: A60.
4.   Schmitz A, Vaeth M. Microalbuminuria: a major risk factor in non-insulin-dependent diabetes. A ten-year follow-up study of 503 patients. Diabet Med 1988; 5: 126-134.
5.   Gerber LM, Shmukler C, Alderman MH. Differences in urinary albumin excretion rate between normotensive and hypertensive white and non white subjects. Arch Intern Med 1992;152: 373-377.
6.   Bigazzi R, Bianchi S, Campese VM, Baldari G. Prevalence of microalbuminuria in a large population of patients with mild to moderate essential hypertension. Nephron 1992; 61: 94-97.
7.   Redon J, Liao Y, Lozano JV, Miralles A, Baldo E. Factors related to the presence of microalbuminuria in essential hypertension. Am J Hypertens 1994; 7(9 Pt1): 801-807.
8.   Jensen JS, Feldt-Rasmussen B, Borch-Johnson K, Clausen P, Appleyard M, Jensen G. Microalbuminuria and its relation to cardiovascular disease and risk factors. A population-based study of 1254 hypertensive individuals. J Human Hypertens 1997;11:727-732.
9.   Agrawal B, Berger A, Wolf K, Luft FC. Microalbuminuria screening by reagent strip predicts cardiovascular risk in hypertension. J Hypertens 1996 Feb;14(2):223-8
10.   Pedersen EB, Mogensen CE. Effect of antihypertensive treatment on urinary albumin excretion, glomerular filtration rate, and renal plasma flow in patients with essential hypertension. Scand J Clin Lab Invest 1976; 36: 231-237.

11. Parving HH, Jensen HE, Mogensen CE, Evrin PE. Increased urinary albumin excretion rate in benign essential hypertension. Lancet 1974; i: 1190-1192

12. James A, Fotherby MB, Potter JF. Screening tests for microalbuminuria in non-diabetic elderly subjects and their relation to blood pressure. Clin Sci 1995;88:185-190.

13. West JNW, Gosling P, Dimmitt SB, Littler WA. Non-diabetic microalbuminuria in clinical practice and its relationship to posture, exercise and blood pressure. Cli Sci 1991;81: 373-377.

14. Opsahl JA, Abraham PA, Halstenson CE, Keane WF. Correlation of office and ambulatory blood pressure measurements with urinary albumin and N-acetyl-beta-D-glucosaminidase excretions in essential hypertension. Am J Hypertens 1988;1: S117-S120.

15. Giaconi S, Levanti C, Fommei E, Innocenti F, Seghieri G, Palla L, Palombo C, Ghione S. Microalbuminuria and casual and ambulatory blood pressure monitoring in normotensives and in patients with borderline and mild essential hypertension. Am J Hypertens 1989; 2: 259-261.

16. Cerasola G, Cottone S, Mule G, Nardi E, Mangano MT, Andronico G, Contorno A, Li Vecchi M, Gaglione P, Renda F, Piazza G, Volpe V, Lisi A, Ferrara L, Panepinto N, Riccobene R. Microalbuminuria, renal dysfunction and cardiovascular complication in essential hypertension. J Hypertens 1996;14: 915-920

17. Bianchi S, Bigazzi R, Baldari G, Sgherri GP, Campese VM. Diurnal variation of blood pressure and microalbuminuria in essential hypertension. Am J Hypertens 1994; 7: 23-29.

18. Bigazzi R, Bianchi S, Nenci R, Baldari D, Baldari G, Campese VM. Increased thickness of the carotid artery in patients with essential hypertension and microalbuminuria. J Hum Hypertens 1995;9: 827-833.

19. Haffner SM, Stern MP, Gruber KK, Hazuda HP, Mitchell BD, Patterson JK. Microalbuminuria. A marker for increased cardiovascular risk factors in nondiabetic subjects? Arteriosclerosis 1990; 10: 727-31.

20. Nosadini R, Cipollina MR, Solini A, Sambataro M, Morocutti A, Doria A, Fioretto P, Brocco E, Muollo B, Frigato F. Close relationship between microalbuminuria and insulin resistance in essential hypertension and non-insulin dependent diabetes mellitus. J Am Soc Nephrol 1992; 3:S56-S63.

21. Mimran A, Ribstein J, DuCailar G. Is microalbuminuria a marker of early intrarenal vascular dysfunction in essential hypertension? Hypertension 1994; 23(part2): 1018-1021.

22. Kaysen GA. Hyperlipidemia of the nephrotic syndrome. Kidney Int 1991;3 (suppl 31): S8-S15.

23. Keane WF, Peter JV St, Kasiske BL. Is the aggressive management of hyperlipidemia in nephrotic syndrome mandatory?. Kidney Int 1992;42 (suppl 38): S134-S141.

24. Newmark SR, Anderson CF, Donadio JV, Ellefson RD. Lipoprotein profiles in adult nephrotics. Mayo Clin Proc 1975; 50: 359-366.

25. Thomas ME, Freestone AL, Persaud JW, Varghese Z, Moorhead JF. Raised lipoprotein(a) [Lp(a)] levels in proteinuric patients. J Am Soc Nephrol 1990; 1: 344A.

26. Jenkins AJ, Steel JS, Janus ED, Best JD. Increased plasma apoprotein(a) levels in IDDM patients with microalbuminuria. Diabetes 1991; 40: 787-790.

27. Kapelrud H, Bangstad HJ, Dahl-Jorgensen K, Berg K, Hanssen KF. Serum Lp(a) lipoprotein concentrations in insulin dependent diabetic patients with microalbuminuria. Brit Med J 1991; 303: 675-678.

28. Keane WF. Lipids and the kidney. Kidney Int 1994; 46: 910-920.

29. Keane WF, Kasiske BL, O'Donnel MP, Kim Y. Hypertension, hyperlipidemia and renal damage. Am J Kidney Dis 1993; 21 (suppl 2): 43-50.

30.   Mulec H, Johnson SA, Bjorck S. Relationship between serum cholesterol and diabetic nephropathy. Lancet 1990; i:1537-1538.

31.   Tolins JP, Stone BG, Raij L. Interactions of hypercholesterolemia and hypertension in initiation of glomerular injury. Kidney Int 1992; 41:1254-1261.

32.   Amatruda JM, Margolis S, Hutchins GM: Type III hyperlipoproteinemia with mesangial foam cells in renal glomeruli. Arch Pathol 1974;98:51-54.

33.   Saito T, Sato H, Kudo K, Oikawa S, Shibata T, Hara Y, Yoshinaga K, Sakaguchi H. Lipoprotein glomerulopathy: Glomerular lipoprotein thrombui in a patient with hyperlipoportinemia. Am J Kidney Dis 1989;13:148-153.

34.   Oikawa S, Suzuki N, Sakuma E, Saito T, Namai K, Kotake H, Fujii Y, Toyota T. Abnormal lipoprotein and apolipoprotein pattern in lipoprotein glomerulopathy. Am J Kidney Dis 1991;18:553-558.

35.   Saito T, Oikawa S, Sato H, Sato T, Ito S, Sasaki J. Lipoprotein glomerulopathy: significance of lipoprotein and ultrastructural features. Kidney Int 1999;55:(Suppl 71):S-37-S41.

36.   Klahr S, Schreiner G, Ichikawa I.   The progression of renal disease. New Engl J Med 1988; 318: 1657-1666.

37.   Attman PO, Alaupovic P, Samuelsson O. Lipoprotein abnormalities as a risk factor for progressive nondiabetic renal disease. Kidney Int 1999;56(Suppl 71):S-14-S17.

38.   Nishida Y, Oda H, Yorioka N. Effect of lipoproteins on mesangial cell proliferation. Kidney Int 1999;56(Suppl 71):S-51-S-53.

39 .   Park YS, Guijarro C, Kim Y, Massy ZA, Kasiske BL, Keane WF, O'Donnell MP. Lovastatin reduces glomerular pacrophage influx and expression of monocyte chemoattractant protein-1 mRNA in nephrotic rats. Am J Kidney Dis 1998;31:190-194.

40.   Hattori M, Nikolic-Paterson DJ, Miyazaki K, Isbel NM, Lan HY, Atkins RC, Kawaguchi H, Ito K. Mechanisms of glomerular macrophage infiltration in lipid-induced renal injury. Kidney Int 1999;55(Suppl 71)S-47-S50.

41.   Keane WF, Mulcahy WS, Kasiske BL, Kim Y, O'Donnell MP. Hyperlipidemia and progressive renal disease. Kidney Int 1991; 39 (Suppl 31): S41-S48.

42.   Jandeleit-Dahm K, Cao Z, Cox AJ, Kelly DJ, Gilbert RE, Cooper ME. Role of hyperlipidemia in progressive renal disease: focus on diabetic nephropathy. Kidney Int 1999;56(Suppl 71):S-31-S-36.

43 .   Oda H, Keane WF. Recent advances in statins and the kidney. Kidney Int 1999;56(Suppl 71):S-2-S-5.

44.   Ferrannini E, Buzzigoli G, Bonadonna R, Giorico MA, Oleggini M, Graziadei L, Pedrinelli R, Brandi L, Bevilacqua S. Insulin resistence in essential hypertension. N Eng J Med 1987; 317: 350-357.

45.   Swislocki AL, Hoffman BB, Reaven GM. Insulin resistance, glucose intolerance and hyperinsulinemia in patients with hypertension. Am J Hypertens 1989; 2: 419-423

46.   Fuller JH, Shipley MJ, Rose G, Jarret RJ, Keen H. Coronary heart disease risk and impaired glucose tolerance: The Whitehall Study. Lancet 1980; i: 1373-1376.

47.   Bianchi S, Bigazzi R, Valtriani C, Chiapponi I, Sgherri G, Baldari G, Natali A, Ferrannini E Campese VM. Elevated serum insulin levels in patients with essential hypertension and microalbuminuria. Hypertension 1994;23: 681-687.

48.   Bianchi S, Bigazzi R, Quinones Galvan A, Muscelli E, Baldari G, Pecori N, Ciociaro D, Ferranini E, Natali A. Insulin resistance in microalbuminuric hypertension: sites and mechanism. Hypertension 1995; 26: 789-795.

49. Doria A, Fioretto P, Avogaro A, Carraro A, Morocutti A, Trevisan R, Frigato F, Crepaldi G, Viberti GC, Nosadini R. Insulin resistance is associated with high sodium-lithium countertransport in essential hypertension. Am J Physiol 1991;261: 684-691.

50. Falkner B, Kushner H, Levison S, Canessa M. Albuminuria in association with insulin and sodium-lithium countertransport in young african americans with borderline hypertension. Hypertension 1995;25: 1315-1321.

51. Ferrari P, Weidmann P, Shaw S, Giachino D, Riesen W, Alleman Y, Heynen G. Altered insulin sensitivity, hyperinsulinemia, and dyslipidemia in individuals with a hypertensive parent. Am J Med 1991;91:589-596.

52. Grunfeld B, Balzareti M, Romo M, Gimenez M, Gutman R. Hyperinsulinemia in normotensive offspring of hypertensive parents. Hypertension 1994; 231 (Suppl 1): I12-I15.

53. Cruz AB, Amatuzio DS, Grande F, Hay LJ. Effect of intraarterial insulin on tissue cholesterol and fatty acids in alloxan diabetic dogs. Circ Res 1961; 9: 39-43

54. Capron L, Jarnet J, Kazandjian S, Housset E. Growth promoting effects of diabetes and insulin on arteries. Diabetes 1988; 35: 973-978.

55. Oppenheumer MJ Sundquist K, Bierman EL. Down-regulation of high-density lipoprotein receptor in human fibroblats by insulin and IGF-I. Diabetes 1989; 38: 117-122.

56. Krone W, Greten H. Evidence for post-transcriptional regulation by insulin of 3 Hydroxy-3-methylglutaryl coenzyme A reductase and sterol synthesis in human mononuclear leucocytes. Diabetologia1984; 26:366-369.

57. DeFronzo RA, Cooke CR, Andres R, Faloona GR, David PJ. The effect of insulin on renal handling of sodium, potassium, calcium, and phosphate in man. J Clin Invest 1975; 55: 845-855.

58. Christensen NJ, Gundersen HJG, Hegedus L, Jacobsen F, Mogensen CE, Osterby R, Vittinghus E. Acute effects of insulin on plasma noradrenaline and the cardiovascular system. Metabolism 1980; 29: 1138-1145.

59. Bigazzi R, Bianchi S, Baldari D, Sgherri G, Baldari G, Campese VM. Microalbuminuria in salt-sensitive patients: a marker for renal and cardiovascular risk factors. Hypertension 1994; 23: 195-199.

60. Hilsted J, Christensen NJ. Dual effect of insulin on plasma volume and transcapillary albumin transport. Diabetologia 1992; 35: 99-103.

61. Elliot TG, Cockcroft JR, Groop PH, Viberti GC, Ritter JM. Inhibition of nitric oxide synthesis in forearm vasculature of insulin-dependent diabetic patients: blunted vasocontriction in patients with microalbuminuria. Clin Sci 1993; 83: 687-693.

62. Stehouwer CDA, Nauta JJP, Zeldenrust GC, Hackeng WHL, Donker AJM, den Ottolander GJH. Urinary albumin excretion, cardiovascular disease, and endothelial dysfunction in non-insulin dependent diabetes mellitus. Lancet 1992; 340: 319-323.

63. Redon J, Gomez-Sanchez MA, Baldo E, Casal MC, Fernandez ML, Miralles A, Gomez-Pajuelo C, Rodicio JL, Ruilope LM. Microalbuminuria is correlated with left ventricular hypertrophy in male hypertensive patients. J Hypertens 1991; 9 (Suppl.6): S148-S149.

64. Pedrinelli R, Bello VD, Catapano G, Talarico L, Materazzi F, Santoro G, Giusti C, Mosca F, Melillo E, Ferrari M. Microalbuminuria is a marker of left ventricular hypertrophy but not hyperinsulinemia in non diabetic atherosclerotic patients. Arteriosclerosis and Thrombosis 1993; 13: 900-906.

65. Mykkanen L, Zaccaro DJ, O'Leary D, Howard G, Robbins DC, Haffner SM. Microalbuminuria and carotid arery intima-media thickness in nondiabetic and NIDDM subjects. Stroke 1997;28:1710-1716.

66. Agewall S, Persson B, Samuelsson O, Ljungman S, Herlitz H, Fageberg B. Microalbuminuria in treated hypertensive men at high risk of coronary disease. The Risk Factor Intervention Study Group. J Hypertens 1993;11: 461-469.

67. Horton RC, Gosling P, Reeves CN, Payne M, Nagle RE. Microalbumin excretion in patients with positive exercise electrocardiogram tests. Eur Heart J 1994; 15: 1353-1355.

68. Kuusisto J, Mykkanen L, Pyorealea K, Laakso M. Hyperinsulinemic microalbuminuria. A new risk indicator for coronary heart disease. Circulation 1995; 9: 831-837.

69. Yudkin JS, Forrest RD, Jackson CA. Microalbuminuria as predictor of vascular disease in non-diabetic subjects. Islington Diabetes Survey. Lancet 1988; ii: 530-533.

70. Cerasola G, Cottone S, D'Ignoto G, Grasso L, Mangano MT, Carapelle E, Nardi E, Andronico G, Fulantelli MA, Marcellino T, Seddio G. Micro-albuminuria as a predictor of cardiovascular damage in essential hypertension. J Hypertens 1989; 7(suppl 6) : S332-S333.

71. Bigazzi R, Bianchi S, Baldari G, Campese VM. Microalbuminuria predicts cardiovascular and renal insufficiency in patients with hypertension. J Hypertens 1998; 16: 1325-1333.

72. Schmieder RE, Veelken R, Gatzka CD, Ruddel H, Schachinger H. Predictors for hypertensive nephropathy: results of a 6-year follow-up study in essential hypertension. J Hypertens 1994; 13: 357-365.

73. Ruilope LM, Campo C, Rodriguez-Artalejo F, Lahera V, Garcia Robles R, Rodicio JL. Blood pressure and renal function: therapeutic implications. J Hypertens 1996; 14: 1259-1263.

44. A COMPARISON OF PROGRESSION IN DIABETIC AND NON-DIABETIC RENAL DISEASE: SIMILARITY OF PROGRESSION PROMOTERS

Gerjan Navis[1,2], Paul De Jong[1], Dick De Zeeuw[1].
Department of Internal Medicine, Division of Nephrology[1] and Department of Clinical Pharmacology[2], State University, Groningen, The Netherlands.

The prevention of progressive renal function loss remains the major challenge for nephrologists today. Traditionally the progressive nature of renal function loss was attributed to the underlying disease, with a major role for hypertension [1]. The hypothesis, however, that common mechanisms account for the progressive renal function loss in many different renal conditions regardless the nature of initial renal damage [2]was fueled by several observations. These include the linear renal function deterioration that occurs in many patients regardless their initial renal disease [3] as well as the similarity in histopathological abnormalities in end-stage kidneys with different underlying diseases. Systemic [4] and glomerular [5] hypertension, proteinuria [6] and lipid abnormalities [7] are assumed to be common mediators in the pathogenesis of focal segmental glomerulosclerosis, the alleged final common pathway of progressive renal disease [8]. Here we will briefly review current knowledge on the determinants of progressive renal function loss in human diabetic and non-diabetic renal disease and on the response to intervention treatment. As to diabetic patients we will, for the sake of brevity, mainly focus on patients with type I (insulin-dependent) diabetes. We will specifically address the question whether current clinical evidence supports the hypothesis that common mechanisms underlie progressive renal function loss in diabetic and non-diabetic renal disease; this will help to devise future prevention strategies.

NATURAL HISTORY

The assessment of progression rate
As progression to end stage renal failure usually takes many years, it is not surprising that few studies provide data in terms of hard end points such as end stage renal failure

Mogensen C.E. (ed.), THE KIDNEY AND HYPERTENSION IN DIABETES MELLITUS.
Copyright© 2000 by Kluwer Academic Publishers, Boston ● Dordrecht ● London. All rights reserved.

or death. In view of the constant rate of renal function loss in many patients, the rate of decline of GFR is usually considered a useful surrogate end point [9], provided it is measured with accuracy, taking into account the methods of measurement, and the frequency and duration of follow-up in relation to the rate of decline [10,11].

The use of progression rate as a surrogate end point, however, entails several pitfalls. The unreliability of creatinine-derived indices has recently extensively been reviewed [12]. When progression rate is used as a surrogate end point, moreover, it should be kept in mind that the assumption of linear deterioration of renal function may not always be true. Whereas in patients with nephropathy due to IDDM, linear progression appears to be the rule [13], among patients with non-diabetic renal disease [6,14] or with NIDDM [15], considerable subpopulations (up to one-fifth or a quarter of the patients) may have stable renal function, or non-linear progression. Such a heterogeneity in patient populations might partly explain the difficulties in reproducing clear-cut renoprotective effects obtained by specific treatment modalities in experimental animals, in particular for nondiabetic renal disease [10,16].

The initiation of renal damage
In diabetic nephropathy the natural history is relatively well-characterized, as, contrary to non-diabetic renal disease, most patients come to medical attention years before renal abnormalities develop. It is still not understood why some 30 to 40 per cent of diabetic patients develop nephropathy whereas others don't; familial clustering, however, suggests genetically determined susceptibility [17]. In patients in whom nephropathy occurs, a typical, biphasic clinical course of renal function has been demonstrated, with elevated glomerular filtration rate in the early stages, followed by microalbuminuria [9]. The elevated GFR presumably reflects glomerular hypertension, due to afferent arteriolar dysfunction with increased transmission of systemic blood pressure to glomerular capillaries. Glomerular hypertension, leading to glomerular capillary damage and protein leakage is thought to play an important role in the initiation and perpetuation of renal damage in these patients [18,19]. These functional abnormalities are accompanied by renal and glomerular enlargement [20,21]. The transition from normoalbuminuria to microalbuminuria is associated with a slight increase in systemic blood pressure [22]. When microalbuminuria progresses to overt proteinuria, usually in association with a further rise in arterial blood pressure, glomerular filtration rate decreases, and gradual progression to end-stage renal failure occurs, albeit with large interindividual differences in progression rate [9,13].

In non-diabetic renal disease the factors that initiate renal damage are of a heterogeneous nature, and can include primarily glomerular or vascular, or tubulo-interstitial damage. Little is known about possible factors preceding the development of non-diabetic renal disease, as by the time patients come to medical attention overt renal damage is usually present. Patients with hypertension may form an exception to this rule. Remarkably, microalbuminuria [23] as well as glomerular hyperfiltration [24], the two hallmarks of incipient diabetic nephropathy, can be found in subsets of patients with essential hypertension. Moreover, a recent cross-sectional analysis in the general population revealed an association between albuminuria and creatinine clearances with a striking similarity to the biphasic pattern in diabetes, with an association between hyperfiltration and the presence of microalbuminuria or a high-normal albumin excretion, with hypofiltration becoming more prevalent among those with macroalbuminuria [25]. For the non-diabetic population however, prospective studies on the prognostic value of albuminuria and glomerular hyperfiltration for long term renal function are still lacking. Nevertheless these data suggest that similar pathways of early renal damage may be involved in diabetic renal disease and some non-diabetic populations. For primary glomerular or tubulo-interstitial disorders, such functional data are lacking altogether. One morphological study revealed an interesting parallel to the morphological sequence of events in diabetic nephropathy, by demonstrating that, in minimal change nephropathy, the presence of glomerular enlargement is a risk factor for the development of focal glomerlosclerosis [26].

If long-term renal function loss is determined by common perpetuating factors one would expect progression of renal function loss to be more or less similar in different renal disorders. Whether or not the underlying disease determines progression rate, however, remains controversial. Some studies found no effect of underlying disease on progression rate [3, 27] but in many other studies progression was related to the diagnostic category. In those studies, glomerulonephritis and diabetic nephropathy invariably had a faster progression rate than chronic pyelonephritis, analgesic nephropathy or hypertensive nephrosclerosis [6,28-33]. In most studies, polycystic kidney disease is associated with a faster progression rate as well [14-30,33-35] although this is not a uniform finding [6][28]. Current evidence, therefore, seems to indicate that the nature of the underlying disease is not indifferent to the long-term course of renal function. Of note, in conditions where the primary cause of damage can be reliably eliminated (such as obstructive uropathy, analgesic abuse, or primary hypertension) the course of renal function is more favorable than in conditions where the initiating factors cannot (or not reliably) be annihilated (such as diabetic nephropathy, glomerulonephritis, or polycystic kidney disease). This suggests that either primary causes still exert effect, or that they trigger the alleged common perpetuating factors to a greater extent than other conditions.

Common progression promoters
In diabetic as well as non-diabetic populations [3] considerable interindividual variability is apparent in the rate of renal function loss for any given disease. Many studies investigated the determinants of this variability (see also Table 44-1), thus attempting to assess the clinical relevance of common progression promoters identified in experimental renal disease, such as systemic and glomerular hypertension, proteinuria and lipid abnormalities. In the interpretation of these studies, however, the close interaction of these factors as to their effects on long-term renal function [2] should be kept in mind. As a consequence, their respective contributions are often hard to dissect.

In both diabetic and non-diabetic renal disease [6,30,34-36] the severity of proteinuria is a predictive factor for progression rate. Interestingly, Wight [34] showed that differences in progression rate between most renal conditions were no longer apparent after correction for proteinuria (with the sole exception of polycystic kidney disease).

Table 44-1. Clinical characteristics of progressive renal function loss in diabetic and non-diabetic renal disease

	diabetic nephropathy	*non-diabetic nephropathy*
Natural history		
renal function loss	invariably progressive	progressive in many patients
Predictors of progression	diabetes control proteinuria blood pressure cholesterol DD genotype ACE gene	underlying disease proteinuria blood pressure cholesterol DD genotype ACE gene
Prevention of progressive renal function loss		
protein restriction	Effective	Effective
Antihypertensive therapy	effective	effective; benefit proportional to severity of proteinuria.
Predictors renoprotection	initial antiproteinuric effect initial renal hemodynamic effect	initial antiproteinuric effect initial renal hemodynamic effect
Response to specific renoprotective drugs		
ACE inhibitors	reduce proteinuria reduce progression rate independent from blood pressure effect??	reduce proteinuria reduce progression rate independent from blood pressure effect??
non-ACE inhibitor antihypertensives	reduce proteinuria in a strongly pressure-dependent fashion	slight, pressure-dependent effect on proteinuria

Moreover, the association between proteinuria and progression not only occurs in conditions where proteinuria might reflect activity of the primary glomerular disorder, such as diabetic nephropathy and glomerulonephritis, but also in chronic pyelonephritis [6], renovascular disease [37], and Wegeners granulomatosis [38].

Taken together, this evidence strongly suggests that, once a certain renal disorder is present, the severity of proteinuria rather than the underlying disorder per se predicts renal outcome. The case of polycystic kidney disease [39,40] however, illustrates that disease-specific mechanisms may predominate over common mechanisms in some conditions.

As to hypertension, in IDDM the development of hypertension is closely associated with transition from normoalbuminuria to microalbuminuria [22] and subsequently with further progression to overt proteinuria and progressive renal function loss [41-43]. In non-diabetic renal disease as well, high blood pressure is usually associated with a poor renal outcome [27,30,34-35], and moreover, the antihypertensive response to treatment is associated with reduction of the rate of renal function loss, as discussed below [4]. Moreover, blood pressure was a strong predictor for end stage renal failure in the large MRFIT cohort [44]. Yet, somewhat surprisingly, several studies in renal patients failed to demonstrate that blood pressure was an independent determinant of progression rate [6,29,30]. In these studies, however, proteinuria and blood pressure were closely related and a predominant effect of proteinuria might obscure the role of a co-linear factor such as blood pressure.

Lipid profile appears to be relevant to progression rate as well: in both diabetic [45-47] and non-diabetic renal disease [48-50] serum cholesterol was found to be associated with a faster progression rate in several studies. Further evidence for a role of hyperlipidemia in progressive renal damage in man is provided by a morphological study in black patients with hypertensive nephropathy, where cholesterol was an independent determinant of the severity of focal segmental glomerulosclerosis [51]. Yet it should be noted that it is still unsure whether the reported associations between lipids and progression rate reflect an effect of hyperlipidemia per se, or the poor prognosis of proteinuria as such, as patients with the more severe hyperlipidemia also tend to be the ones with the more severe hyperlipidemia. [50]

The rapid developments in molecular genetic techniques may in the coming years allow the identification of multiple genetic factors involved in the interindividual differences in rate of renal function loss in diabetic as well as non-diabetic renal disease. So far, most data are available on the insertion/deletion (I/D) polymorphism for the ACE-gene. As reviewed recently [52], the D-allele appears to be a determinant of the rate of renal function loss in patients with *diverse* nondiabetic renal disorders [53] as well as diabetic nephropathy [54] with an increased rate of renal function loss in patients homozygous for the D-allele. The mechanism of the increased renal risk in DD homozygotes is still unknown. As the increased renal risk is apparent in almost any renal condition studied, it appears to be related to the final common pathway of renal damage rather than to the specific causes of initiation of renal damage. It should be noted, however, that it is still unsure whether the ACE genotype is a mere marker of increased renal risk or whether it may play a causal role. Higher serum [55] and kidney

ACE-levels [56] are present in DD-homozygotes, suggesting that increased availability of angiotensin may occur under specific circumstances. Some studies however yielded results that seem discrepant [57]. Differences in genetic background with gene-gene interaction, as well as environmental factors may be involved in the discrepancies between studies. Gene-gene interaction between ACE (I/D) polymorphism with the MT polymorphism for the angiotensinogen gene has been reported for non-diabetic renal disease (i.e IgA nephropathy)[57] as well as diabetic nephropathy [58] although this issue awaits further clarification. Response to renoprotective therapy may be affected by ACE genotype as well. A blunted response to ACE inhibition was reported to be associated with the D-allele in diabetic nephropathy [59,60] as well as non-diabetic proteinuric patients [61] in European studies. Studies from Japan, however, yielded conflicting results [62]. Again, differences in genetic background may be involved. Moreover, gene-environment interaction between ACE genotype and sodium intake may explain some of the discrepancies: as a difference in therapy response to ACE inhibition between the genotypes was only apparent among subjects ingesting excess sodium [61]. Moreover, also differences in angI response between the genotypes were only apparent during high sodium intake [63]. In diabetes similar data are not available yet.

RESPONSE TO RENOPROTECTIVE TREATMENT

As a matter of clinical common sense, renoprotective treatment should, first, aim at eliminating primary damaging factors. This may halt progression in some patients with specific disorders, such as obstructive uropathy [6] and analgesic nephropathy [64]. In diabetes, strict metabolic control can reverse early hyperfiltration, and retard the progression of renal function loss [65]. Progressive renal function loss in the large proportion of patients in whom the initial cause of renal damage is no longer present [3] however, prompted the development of additional treatment strategies aimed at intervention with factors thought to be involved in the alleged final common pathway for progressive renal function loss; i.e, systemic and glomerular pressure, proteinuria and lipid abnormalities.

Research has mainly focussed on two intervention strategies: antihypertensive treatment and reduction of protein intake. Reduction of blood pressure is considered the cornerstone of therapy for renal patients: it effectively slows renal function loss in diabetic [66] and in non-diabetic renal disease [4,27,50] (Table 44-1). Restriction of dietary protein intake has elicited extensive discussion over the last decades as to its efficacy and feasibility, but recent analyses have shown that a low protein intake indeed is associated with a reduction in the rate of renal function loss in both diabetic and non-diabetic renal patients [67,68].

Short-term responses to renoprotective therapy are of interest to see whether they are prognostic for long-term protection. If so, this may not only help to titrate therapy but also to unravel the mechanisms of renoprotection. Indeed, such predictive responses have been identified. The magnitude of the early renal hemodynamic response (i.e a slight drop in GFR that may reflect a fall in glomerular hydostatic pressure) to renoprotective intervention be it antihypertensive treatment [69] or a low protein diet appears to predict the long term course of renal function [70]. Likewise, as reviewed recently [71], the efficacy of the initial antiproteinuric effect consistently predicts the course of long term renal function in both diabetic [72] and non-diabetic nephropathy [73,74]. With the notable exception of the MDRD study [75], the reduction in blood pressure did not predict the subsequent course of renal function. This supports the hypothesis that specific renal effects, such as a reduction in proteinuria, are causally involved in long-term renoprotection [8].

The question whether ACE-inhibitors, by virtue of specific renal effects, offer better renoprotection than other antihypertensives has been subject of many studies. These were motivated by findings in experimental animals that ACE-inhibition protects against progressive renal damage not only by reducing systemic blood pressure, but also by a fall in glomerular capillary pressure [18] and in proteinuria. In man, renoprotective properties of ACE inhibitors beyond reduction of blood pressure are for instance suggested by studies in normotensive diabetic patients where treatment with ACE inhibition was able to reverse microalbuminuria [76] and to prevent progression to overt proteinuria [77], in the absence of a blood pressure effect. In overt diabetic nephropathy as well as non-diabetic renal disease ACE inhibitors can reduce proteinuria [78-80], progression rate [81] and the risk to reach end stage renal failure or death [50,82,83]. Moreover, ACEi provided more effective long-term renoprotection than control antihypertensives in several studies in diabetic and non-diabetic patients [84,85]. Blood pressure effects, however, may explain the differences in long term renoprotection, as in these studies ACE inhibition generally induced more effective blood pressure reduction than the control regimens [85]. Some studies in non-diabetic patients, however, failed to demonstrate an advantage of ACE inhibitors over control antihypertensives [85,86]. Patient selection may be involved in the discrepancies between different comparative trials, as the advantage of ACE inhibitors over other antihypertensives appeared to be most readily apparent in patients with a rapid progression rate associated with proteinuria, that is, in patients with diabetic nephropathy and in non-diabetic patients with overt proteinuria [87]. In fact, the advantage of the ACE-inhibitor appears to be proportional to the severity of pre-treatment proteinuria [73,88]. Taken together with the predictive value of the antiproteinuric response for long term renoprotection, this suggests that the antiproteinuric effect may be pivotal in providing renoprotection.

The antiproteinuric efficacy of ACE inhibitors versus other antihypertensives in diabetic and non-diabetic renal patients has been subject of several reviews [89-91]. From these analyses some interesting inferences emerge. First, the meta-analyses confirmed the notion that the antiproteinuric effect of ACE inhibitors cannot solely be accounted for by their effect on blood pressure. Second, it was shown that non-ACE inhibitor antihypertensives, with the exception of nifedipine, also lower proteinuria (albeit to a lesser extent than ACE-inhibitors) provided a pronounced fall in blood pressure is achieved. Finally, it was shown that this blood pressure-related fall in proteinuria with non-ACE inhibitor therapy was more pronounced in diabetic patients than in non-diabetic patients. This is consistent with the hypothesis that in diabetic nephropathy, due to afferent arteriolar dysfunction, increased transmission of systemic blood pressure to the glomerular capillary bed plays an important role in abnormal glomerular hemodynamics and protein leakage.

Interestingly, in large scale trials in non-diabetic patients the long- term benefit of lower blood pressure (whether or not achieved with ACE inhibitors) on renal function was more pronounced in proteinuric patients [75,82,92]. Thus, like diabetic patients (in whom proteinuria is the hallmark of renal involvement), proteinuric patients with non-diabetic renal disease display greater renal sensitivity to the effect of elevated systemic blood pressure than their non-proteinuric counterparts. Whether this similarity simply reflects the long-term benefits of reduction of proteinuria secondary to the lower blood pressure, or whether proteinuria is a marker (or even a mediator) of the susceptibility of the glomerular vascular bed to hypertensive damage is as yet unknown.

CONCLUSIONS AND IMPLICATIONS FOR RENOPROTECTIVE TREATMENT

From the studies summarized here it appears that promoters for progression in patients with diabetic and non-diabetic nephropathy are remarkably similar. Moreover, predictors for efficacy of long-term renoprotective therapy are similar as well. This supports the hypothesis that common mechanisms underlie progressive renal function loss in diabetic and many non-diabetic renal patients, with the possible exception of specific diagnostic categories, such as polycystic kidneys [40] where disease-specific mechanisms may be the main determinants of progression. The similarities with diabetes are most readily apparent for non-diabetic patients with overt proteinuria, supporting the assumption that proteinuria is pivotal in the alleged common mechanisms [8].

Several implications for renoprotective treatment can be derived from the studies reviewed here. First, these data suggest that to provide renoprotection in proteinuric patients (with or without diabetes) target blood pressure should be lower than in non-proteinuric patients. For diabetic patients the need for a low target blood pressure has already gained acceptance [93]. For non-diabetic proteinuric patients, data from the MDRD study demonstrated that the lowest mean arterial pressure attained ($\leq$92 mmHg, corresponding to 125/75 mmHg) provided improved renoprotection, without signs of a J-shape pattern [94]. From a renal perspective, therefore, target mean arterial blood pressure in proteinuric patients may have to be even lower than 90 mmHg. For such an aggressive approach to be feasible, short-term titration criteria predictive for long-term renoprotection are virtually indispensable.

Second, the predictive value of the antiproteinuric response to antihypertensive treatment for long-term renoprotection implicates that proteinuria is presumably a useful parameter to monitor and titrate blood pressure to a long-term renoprotective level. This may even implicate that, in proteinuric patients, reduction of proteinuria is a major, and perhaps the main target of renoprotective therapy. In fact, for diabetic patients, such an approach has been advocated in the recent recommendations to start ACE-inhibitor therapy in normotensive patients with microalbuminuria, with the purpose of preventing progression to overt nephropathy [77]. Based on current evidence, therefore, it would be of interest to evaluate the long-term renoprotective potential of treatment strategies that target at elimination of proteinuria for non-diabetic patients as well [95].

REFERENCES

1. Ellis A. Natural history of Bright's disease; clinical, histological and experimental observations. The vicious circle in Bright's disease. Lancet 1942; i: 72-76.
2. Klahr S, Schreiner G, Ichikawa I. The progression of renal disease. N Engl J Med 1988; 318:1657-1666
3. Mitch WE, Buffington G, Lemaan J, Walser M. Progression of renal failure: a simple method of estimation. Lancet 1976; ii: 1326-1331.
4. Alvestrand A, Gutierrez A, Bucht H, Bergström J. Reduction of blood pressure retards the progression of chronic renal failure in man. Nephrol Dial Transplant 1988; 3: 624-631.
5. Brenner BM, Meyer TW, Hostetter TW. Dietary protein and the progressive nature of kidney disease: role of hemodynamically mediated glomerular injury in the pathogenesis of progressive glomerular sclerosis of aging, renal ablation and intrinsic renal disease N Engl J Med 1982; 307: 652-659.
6. Williams PS, Fass G, Bone JM. Renal pathology and proteinuria determine progression in untreated mild/moderate chronic renal failure. Quart J Med 1988; 67: 343-354.
7. Keane WF, Kasiske B, O'Donnell MP, Kin Y. The role of altered lipid metabolism in the progression of renal disease. Am J Kidney Dis 1991; 17: S38-S42.
8. Remuzzi G, Bertani T. Is glomerulosclerosis a consequence of altered glomerular permeability to macromolecules? [editorial]. Kidney Int 1990; 38: 384-394.
9. Mogensen CE. Natural history and potential prevention of diabetic nephropathy in insulin-dependent and non-insulin-dependent diabetic patients. In: Prevention of progressive chronic renal failure. El Nahas A, Mallick NP, Anderson S, (eds). Oxford 1993; pp 278-279.
10. Levey AS. Measurement of renal function in chronic renal disease. Kidney Int 1990; 38: 167-184.
11. Apperloo AJ, de Zeeuw D, de Jong PE. Precision of GFR determinations for long term slope calculations is improved by simultaneous infusion of ^{125}I-iothalamate and ^{131}I-Hippuran. JASN 1996; 7: 567-572.
12. Walser M, Drew HH, LaFrance LD. Creatinine measurements often yield false estimates in chronic renal failure. Kidney Int 1988; 34: 412-418.
13. Jones RH, Mackay JD, Hayakawa H, Parsons V, Watkins PJ. Progression of diabetic nephropathy. Lancet 1979; i: 1105-1106.
14. Bergström J, Alvestrand A, Bucht H, Gutierrez A, Stenvinkel P. Is renal failure always progressive? Contrib Nephrol 1989; 75: 60-67.
15. Gall M-A, Nielsen FS, Smidt UM, Parving H-H. The course of kidney function in type 2 (non-insulin-dependent) diabetic patients with diabetic nephropathy. Diabetologia 1993; 36; 1071-1078.
16. Williams PS, Mallick NP. The natural history of chronic renal failure. In: Prevention of progressive chronic renal failure. El Nahas AM, Mallick NP, Anderson S (eds). Oxford 1993, p210-259.
17. Tarnow L. Genetic pattern in diabetic nephropathy. Nephrol Dial Transplant 1996; 11: 410-412.

18. Zatz R, Meyer TW, Rennke HG, Brenner BM. Predominance of hemodynamic rather than metabolic factors in the pathogenesis of diabetic glomerulopathy. Proc Natl Acad Sci 1985; 82; 5963-5967.

19. Parving H-H, Kastrup H, Smidt UM, Andersen AR, Feldt-Rasmussen B, Sandahl Christiansen J. Impaired autoregulation of glomerular filtration rate in type I (insulin-dependent) diabetic patients with nephropathy. Diabetologia 1984; 27: 547-552.

20. Hirose K, Tsuchida H, østerby R, Gundersen HJG. A strong correlation between glomerular filtration rate and filtration surface in diabetic kidney hyperfunction. Lab Invest 1980: 43: 434-437.

21. Feldt-Rasmussen B, Hegedüs L, Mathiesen ER, Deckert T. Kidney volume in type I (insulin-dependent) diabetic patients with normal or increased urinary albumin excretion: effect of long-term improved metabolic control. Scand J Lab Invest 1991: 51: 31-36.

22. Poulsen PL, Hansen KW, Mogensen CE. Ambulatory blood pressure in the transition from normo- to microalbuminuria: a longitudinal study in IDDM. Diabetes 1994; 43: 1248-53.

23. Parving HH, Jensen HE, Mogensen CE. Increased urinary albumin excretion in benign essential hypertension. Lancet 1974; 231-237.

24. du Cailar G, Ribstein J, Mimran A. Glomerular hyperfiltration and left ventricular mass in mild never-treated essential hypertension. J Hypertens 1990; 9: supp 6:S158-S159.

25. Pinto-Sietsma SJ, Janssen WMT, Hillege HL, Navis GJ, de Zeeuw D, de Jong PE. Urinary albumin excretion is associated with renal functional abnormalities in a non-diabetic population. JASN 2000 (in press).

26. Fogo A, Hawkins EP, Berry PL, Glick AD, Chiang ML, MacDonnelll RC, Ichikawa I. Glomerular hypertrophy in minimal change predicts subsequent progression to focal glomerular sclerosis. Kidney Int 1990: 38: 115-123.

27. Brazy PC, Fitzwilliam JF. Progressive renal disease: role of race and antihypertensive medications. Kidney Int 1990; 37: 1113-1119.

28. Ahlem J. Incidence of human chronic renal insuffiency. A study of the incidence and pattern of renal insufficiency in adults during 1966-71 in Gothenburg. Acta Med Scand 1975; supp 582: 1-50.

29. Stenvinkel P, Alvestrand A, Bergström J. Factors influencing progression in patients with chronic renal failure. J Int Med 1989; 226: 183-88.

30. Locatelli F, Marcelli D, Comelli M, Alberti D, Graziani G, Buccianti G, Redaelli B. Giangrande A et al. Proteinuria and blood pressure as causal components of progression to end-stage renal failure. Nephrol Dial Transplant 1996; 11: 461-467.

31. Rutherford WE, Blondin J, Miller JP, Greenwalt AS, Vavra JD. Chronic progressive renal disease: rate of change of serum creatinine concentration. Kidney Int 1977; 11; 62-70.

32. Hannedouche T, Chaveau P, Fehrat A, Albouze G, Jungers. Effect of moderate protein restriction on the rate of progression of renal failure. Kidney Int 1989; 36 (supp 27): S91-95.

33. Rosman JB, Langer K, Brandl M, Piers-Becht TPM, van der Hem GK, ter Wee PM, Donker AJM. Protein-restricted diets in chronic renal failure: a four-year follow-up shows limited indications. Kidney Int 1989; 36 (supp 27): S96-102.

34. Wight JP, Salzano S, Brown CB, El Nahas AM. Natural history of chronic renal failure: a reappraisal. Nephrol Dial Transplant 1992; 7: 379-383.

35. Oldrizzi L, Rugiu C, Valvo E, Lupo A, Loschiavo C, Gammaro L, Tessitore N, Fabris A, Panzetta G, Maschio G. Progression of renal failure in patients with renal disease of diverse etiology on protein-restricted diet. Kidney Int 1985; 27: 553-557.

36. Mallick NP, Short CD, Hunt LP. How far since Ellis? Nephron 1987; 46: 113-124.

37. Halimi J-M, Ribstein J, Du Cailar G, Ennouchi J-M,Mimran A. Albuminuria predicts renal functional outcome after intervention in atheromatous renovascular disease. J Hypertens 1995: 13: 1335-1342.

38. Franssen CFM, Stegeman CA, W Oost-Kort, Tiebosch ATM, de Jong PE, Kallenberg CGM, Cohen Tervaert JW. Determinants of renal outcome in anti-myeloperoxidase-associated crescentic glomerulonephritis. J Am Soc Nephrol 1998: 9:1915-1923.

39. Woo DJ. Apoptosis and loss of renal tissue in polycystic kidney diseases. N Engl J Med 1995; 333: 18-25.

40. Grantham JJ. Polycystic kidney disease: there goes the neighbourhood. N Engl J Med 1995; 333: 56-57.

41. Hasslacher C, Ritz E, Terpstra J, Gallasch G, Kunowski G, Rall C. Natural history of nephropathy in type I diabetes. Hypertension 1985; 7 [supp II]: II74-II78.

42. Mogensen CE, Christensen CK. Blood pressure changes and renal function in incipient and overt diabetic nephropathy. Hypertension 1985; 7 [supp II]: II64-II73.

43. Rossing P, Hommel E, Smidt U, Parving H-H. Impact of blood pressure and albuminuria on the progression of diabetic nephropathy in IDDM patients. Diabetes 1993; 42: 715-719.

44. Klag MJ, Whelton PK, Randall BL, Neaton JD, Brancati FL, Ford CE, Shulman NB, Stamler J. Blood pressure and end stage renal disease in men. N Engl J Med 1996; 334: 13-18.

45. Mulec H, Johnson S-A, Björck S. Relation between serum cholesterol and diabetic nephropathy. Lancet 1990; 335: 1536-1538.

46. Krolewski AS, Warram JH, Christlieb AR. Hypercholesterolemia. A determinant of renal function loss and deaths in IDDM patients with nephropathy. Kidney Int 1994: 45: supp 45: S125-131

47. Breyer JA, Bain RP, Evans JK, Nahman NS Jr, Lewis EJ, Cooper, McGill J, Berl T. The colloborative study group. Predictors of progression of renal insufficiency in patients with insulin-dependent diabetes and overt diabetic nephropathy. Kidney Int 1996: 50: 1651-1658.

48. Apperloo AJ, de Zeeuw D, de Jong PE. Short-term antiproteinuric response to antihypertensive therapy predicts long-term GFR decline in patients with non-diabetic renal disease. Kidney Int 1994; 45 (supp 45): S174-178.

49. Samuelsson O, Aurell M, Knight-Gibson C, Alaupovic P, Attman P-O. Apolipoprotein-B containing lipoproteins and the progression of renal insuffiency. Nephron 1993: 63: 279-285.

50. Maschio G, Alberti D, Janin G, Locatelli F, Mann JFE, Motolese M, Ponticelli C, Ritz E, Zuchelli P et al. Effect of the angiotensin converting enzyme inhibitor benazepril on the progression of chronic renal insufficiency. N Engl J Med 1996; 334; 939-945.

51. Fogo A, Breyer JA, Smith MC, Cleveland WH, Agodoa L, Kirk KA, Glassock R. The AASK pilot Study Investigators: Accuracy of diagnosis of hypertensive neprhosclerosis in African Americans: A report form the African American Study of Kidney Disease (AASK) Trial. Kidney Int 1997: 244-252.

52. Navis GJ, van der Kleij FGH, de Zeeuw D, de Jong PE. Angiotensin converting enzyme gene I/D polymorphism and renal disease. J Mol Med 1999, 77:781-789.

53. van Essen GG, Rensma PL, de Zeeuw D, de Jong PE. Association between angiotensin-converting enzyme gene polymorphism and failure of renoprotective therapy. Lancet 1996; 347: 94-95.

54.   Parving H-H, Jacobsen P, Tarnow L, Rossing PP, Lecrof L, Poirier O, Cambien F. Effect of deletion polymorphism of the angiotensin converting enzyme gene on progression of diabetic nephropathy during inhibition of angiotensin converting enzyme: observational follow-up study. BMJ 313: 591-594.

55.   Rigat B, Hubert C, Alhenc-Gelas F, Cambien F, Corvol P, Soubrier F. An insertion/deletion polymorphism in the angiotensin converting enzyme accounts for half of the variance of serum enzyme levels. J Clin Invest 1990: 86: 1343-1346.

56.   Mizuiri S, Yoshikawa H, Tanegashima M, Miyagi M, Kobayshi M, Sakai K, Hayashi I, Aikawa A, Ohara T, Hasegawa A. Renal ACE immunohistochemical localization in NIDDM patients with nephropathy. Am J Kidney Dis 1998; 31: 301-307.

57.   Pei Y, Scholey J, Thai K, Suzuki M, Cattran D. Association of angiotensinogen gene T235 variant with progression of immunoglobulin A nephropathy in caucasian patients. J Clin Invest 1997: 100: 814-820.

58.   Marre M, Jeunemaitre X, Gallois Y, Rodier M, Chatellier G, Sert C. Contribution of genetic polymorphisms in the renin-angiotensin system to the development of renal complications in insulin-dependent diabetes. J Clin Invest 1997: 99: 1585-1595.

59.   Jacobsen P, Rossing K, Rossing P, Tarnow L, Mallet C, Poirier O, Cambien F, Parving H-H. Angiotensin-converting enzyme (ACE) gene polymorphism and ACE inhibition in diabetic nephropathy. Kidney Int 1998: 53: 1002-1006.

60.   Penno G, Chaturvedi N, Talmud PJ, Coroneo P, Manto A, Nannipieri M, Luong I, Fuller JH and the Euclid Study Group. Effect of angiotensin converting enzyme (ACE) gene polymorphism on progression of renal disease and the influence of ACE inhibition in IDDM patients. Diabetes 1998: 47: 1507-1511

61.   van der Kleij FGH, Schmidt A, Navis GJ, Haas M, Yilmaz N, de Jong PE, Mayer G, de Zeeuw D. ACE I/D polymorphism and short term response to ACE inhibition; role of sodium status. Kidney Int 1997, 52, supp 63: S23-26

62.   Yoshida H, Mitarai T, Kawamura T, Kitajima T, Miyazaki Y, Nagasawa R, Kawaguchi Y, Kubo H, Ichikawa I, Sakai O. Role of the deletion polymorphism of the angiotensin converting enzyme gene in the progression and therapeutic responsiveness of IgA nephropathy. J Clin Invest 1995; 96:2162-2169.

63.   van der Kleij FGH, de Jong PE, Henning RH, de Zeeuw D, Navis GJ. High sodium intake reveals phenotype differences in ACE I/D polymorphism. J Am Soc Nephrol 1998: 9: 349A

64.   Hauser AC, Derfler K, Balcke P. Progression of renal insufficiency in analgesic nephropathy: impact of drug abuse. J Clin Epidemiol 1991; 44: 53-56.

65.   Diabetes Control and Complications Trial Research Group. The effect of intensive treatment of diabetes on the development and progression of long-term complications in insulin-dependent diabetes mellitus. N Engl J Med 1993; 329: 977-986.

66.   Parving H-H, Andersen AR, Smidt UM, Svendsen PA. Early aggressive antihypertensive treatment reduces rate of decline in kidney function in diabetic nephropathy. Lancet 1983; 1175-1179.

67.   Pedrini MT, Levey AS, Lau J, Chalmers TC, Wang PH. The effect of dietary protein restriction on the progression of diabetic and non-diabetic renal disease: a meta-analysis. Ann Int Med 1996:124:627-632.

68.   Levey AS, Adler S, Caggiula AW, England BK, Greene T, Hunsicker LG. Effects of dietary protein restriction on the progression of advanced renal disease in the Modification of Diet in Renal Disease (MDRD) Study. Am J Kidney Dis 1996; 27: 652-663.

69. Apperloo AJ, de Zeeuw D, de Jong PE. A short-term antihypertensive treatment induced fall in glomerular filtration rate predicts long term stability of renal function. Kidney Int 1997; 51: 793-797

70. El Nahas AM, Masters-Thomas A, Brady SA, Farrington K, Wilkinson V, Hilson AJW, Varghese Z, Moorhead JFI. Selective effect of low protein diets in chronic renal diseases BMJ 1984; 289:1337-1341.

71. Wapstra FH, Navis GJ, de Jong PE, de Zeeuw. Short term and long term antiproteinuric response to inhibition of renin angiotensin axis in patients with non diabetic renal disease: prediction of GFR decline. Exp Nephrol 1996; 4: supp 1, 47-52.

72. Rossing P, Hommel E, Smidt UM, Parving H-H. Reduction in albuminuria predicts diminished progression in diabetic nephropathy. Kidney Int 1994; 45 (supp 45): S145-149.

73. The GISEN Group: Randomised placebo-controlled trial of effect of ramipril on decline in glomerular filtration rate and risk of terminal renal failure in proteinuric, non-diabetic nephropathy. Lancet 1997; 349:1857-1863.

74. Praga M, Hernández E, Montoyo C, Andrés A, Ruilope L, Rodicio JL. Long-term beneficial effects of angiotensin-converting enzyme inhibition with nephrotic proteinuria. Am J Kidney Dis 1992; 20: 240-248.

75. Klahr S, Levey AS, Beck GJ, Caggiula AW, Hunsicker L, Kusek JW, Striker G et al. The effects of dietary protein restriction and blood pressure control on the progression of chronic renal disease. N Engl J Med 1994; 330: 877-884..

76. Rudberg S, Aperia A, Freyschuss U, Persson B. Enalapril reduces microalbuminuria in young normotensive Type I (insulin-dependent) diabetic patients irrespective of its hypotensive effect. Diabetologia 1990: 33: 470-476.

77. Mathiesen ER, Hommel E, Giese J, Parving H-H. Efficacy of captopril in postponing nephropathy in normotensive insulin dependent diabetic patients with microalbuminuria. Br Med J 1991; 303: 81-87.

78. Heeg JE, de Jong PE, van der Hem GK, de Zeeuw D. Efficacy and variability of the antiproteinuric effect of lisinopril. Kidney Int 1989; 36: 272-279.

79. Björck S, Nyberg G, Mulec H, Granerus G, Herlitz H, Aurell M. Beneficial effects of angiotensin converting enzyme inhibition on renal function in patients with diabetic nephropathy. Br Med J 1986; 293: 471-474.

80. Heeg JE, de Jong PE, van der Hem GK, de Zeeuw D. Reduction of proteinuria by angiotensin converting enzyme inhibition. Kidney Int 1987; 32: 78-83.

81. Björk S, Mulec H, Johnson SA, Nordén G, Aurell M. Renal protective effect of enalapril in diabetic nephropathy. Br Med J 1992; 304: 339-343.

82. Lewis EJ, Hunsicker LG, Bain RP, Rohde RD et al. The effect of angiotensin-converting enzyme inhibition on diabetic nephropathy. N Engl J Med 1993; 329: 1456-1462.

83. Kamper A-L, Strandgaard S, Leyssac PP. Late outcome of a controlled trial of enalapril treatment in progressive chronic renal failure. Hard end-points and influence of proteinuria. Nephrol Dial Transplant 1995; 10: 1182-1188.

84. Hannedouche T, Landais P, Goldfarb B, El Esper N, Fournier A, Godin M, Durand D, Chanard J, Mognon F, Suc J-M, Grünfeld J-P. Randomised controlled trial of enalapril and beta-blockers in non-diabetic chronic renal failure. Br Med J 1994; 309: 833-837

85. Giatras I, Lau J, Levey A, for the Angiotensin Converting Enzyme Inhibition and Progressive Renal Disease Study Group. Effect of angiotensin converting enzyme inhibitors on the progression of nondiabetic renal disease: a meta-analysis of randomized trials. Ann Int Med 1997: 127:337-345.

86. van Essen GG, Apperloo AJ, Rensma PL, Stegeman CA, Sluiter WJ, de Zeeuw D, de Jong PE. Are ACE-inhibitors superior to beta-blockers in retarding progressive renal function decline? Kidney Int 1997; 52, supp 63, S58-62.
87. Navis GJ, de Zeeuw D, de Jong PE. ACE-inhibitors: panacea for progressive renal disease? Lancet 1997;349:1852-1853.
88. Ruggenenti P, Perna A, Gherardi G, Garini G, Zoccali C, Salvadori M, Scolari F, Schena FP, Remuzzi G. Renoprotective properties of ACE inhibition in non-diabetic nephropathies with non-nephrotic proteinuria. Lancet 1999: 354: 359-364.
89. Gansevoort RT, Sluiter WJ, Hemmelder MH, de Zeeuw D, de Jong PE. Antiproteinuric effect of blood-pressure lowering agents: a meta-analysis of comparative trials. Nephrol Dial Transplant 1995; 10: 1963-1974.
90. Maki DD, Ma JZ, Louis TA, Kasiske BL. Long-term effects of antihypertensive agents on proteinuria and renal function. Arch Int Med 1995; 155: 1073-1080.
91. Weidmann P, Schneider M, Böhlen L. Therapeutic efficacy of different antihypertensive drugs in human diabetic nephropathy: an updated meta-analysis. Nephrol Dial Transplant 1995; 10 (supp 9): 39-45.
92. Peterson JC, Adler S, Burkart JM, Greene T, Hebert LA, Hunsicker LG, King AJ, Klahr S, Massry S, Seifter JL, for the MDRD Study group. Blood pressure control, proteinuria and the progression of renal disease. Ann Int Med 1995;123:754-762.
93. Mogensen CE, Keane WF, Bennett PH, Jerums G, Parving H-H, Passa P, Steffes MW, Striker GE, Viberti GC. Prevention of diabetic renal disease with special reference to microalbuminuria. Lancet 1995; 346: 1080-1084.
94. Lazarus JM, Bourgoignie JJ, Buckalew VM, Greene T, Levey AS, Milas NC, Paranandi L, Peterson JC, Porush JG, Rauch S, Soucie JM, Stollar C for the Modification of Diet in Renal Disease Study Group. Achievement and safety of a low blood pressure goal in chronic renal disease. Hypertension 1997;29:641-650.
95. de Jong PE, Navis GJ, de Zeeuw D. Renoprotective therapy: titration against proteinuria. Lancet 1999: 354: 352-353.

45. UPDATE OF THE LATEST INTERVENTION TRIALS IN HYPERTENSION AND TYPE 2 DIABETES

Lennart Hansson, M.D.
Clinical Hypertension Research, Department of Public Health and Social Sciences, University of Uppsala, P 0 Box 609, S- 751 25 Uppsala, Sweden.

INTRODUCTION

Patients with hypertension and type 2 diabetes mellitus constitute an important risk group. Their risk of cardiovascular morbidity and mortality is considerably higher than in non-diabetic patients with hypertension [1]. The concomitant appearance of arterial hypertension and type 2 diabetes has appropriately been referred to, by Mogensen, as "double jeopardy" [2].

In this context it is of considerable interest to assess the benefits that can be derived from antihypertensive treatment in such patients. Recently data has been made available from several large intervention trials in which type 2 diabetic patients have constituted either the entire study population or comprised an important part thereof. Seven such studies will be discussed briefly here: the Hypertension Optimal Treatment (HOT) Study [3], The United Kingdom Prospective Diabetes Study (UKPDS) [4,5], the Captopril Prevention Project (CAPPP) [6], the Appropriate Blood pressure Control in Diabetes (ABCD) Study [7], the Fosinopril Amlodipine Cardiovascular Events Trial (FACET) [8], the Systolic Hypertension in Europe (Syst-Eur) trial [9], the Swedish Trial in Old Patients with Hypertension-2 (STOP-Hypertension-2) [10] and the Heart Outcomes Prevention Evaluation (HOPE) trial [11].

In most of these trials there was a statistically significant trend towards lower rates of several cardiovascular endpoints the lower the blood pressure in the patients with type 2 diabetes. This finding supports the view recently expressed in the 1997 guidelines of the US Joint National Committee (JNC VI) that more ambitious goals of blood pressure lowering are needed for hypertensive diabetics [12] and a similar view was expressed in the 1999 guidelines for the management of hypertension, issued jointly by the World Health Organization and the International Society of Hypertension (WHO/ISH) [13].

Mogensen C.E. (ed.), THE KIDNEY AND HYPERTENSION IN DIABETES MELLITUS.
Copyright© 2000 by Kluwer Academic Publishers, Boston ● Dordrecht ● London. All rights reserved.

THE HOT STUDY

The objectives and design of the Hypertension Optimal Treatment (HOT) Study have been presented in detail before [14]. It is obviously well known that treatment of hypertension reduces cardiovascular morbidity and mortality [15-19]. It is, however, also known that treated hypertensive patients, in spite of receiving antihypertensive treatment, are at greater risk of suffering cardiovascular complications than matched normotensive subjects [20,21]. It is possible, and even likely, that the reason for this could be that quite frequently the treated blood pressure has not been lowered down to strictly normotensive levels [22]. Against this view warnings have been issued that, because of a J-shaped relationship between blood pressure and risk, a too vigorous reduction in blood pressure may be associated with increased cardiovascular risk [2325]. The latest addition to the J-curve discussion was the presentation of the Rotterdam Study data in elderly men and women, which did not find a J-shaped relationship between blood pressure and the risk of myocardial infarction [26]. However, without any doubt this issue needed to be addressed in a randomized and prospective trial and this was the major reason for conducting the HOT Study.

A total of 18,790 hypertensive patients, aged 50-80, with diastolic blood pressure in the range $\geq$ 100 to $\leq$ 115 mm Hg were included in the HOT Study. Patients were recruited in 26 different countries in Europe, the Americas and Asia [14]. The average duration of the study was 3.8 years and the total number of patient-years was 71,050 [3].

Patients were randomized to one of three diastolic blood pressure target groups: $\leq$ 90, $\leq$ 85 or $\leq$ 80 mm Hg in a trial using the PROBE-design (prospective, randomized, open with blinded endpoint evaluation) [27].

Antihypertensive therapy was initiated in all patients with the long-acting vascular selective dihydropyridine-derived calcium antagonist felodipine in a dose of 5 mg once daily. Additional therapy and dosage increments in four further steps were prescribed in order to reach the randomized target [13]. Angiotensin converting enzyme (ACE) inhibitors or beta-blockers were added in step 2 and dosage titrations were used in steps 3-5, with the possibility of adding a diuretic in step 5 [14].

The subgroup of patients with type 2 diabetes at baseline comprised 1501 patients. In this subgroup a statistically significant trend was found: the lower the target blood pressure the lower the incidence of major cardiovascular events, i.e. fatal plus non-fatal stroke and myocardial infarction plus other cardiovascular mortality (Table 45-1). The risk of major cardiovascular events (strokes and myocardial infarctions, fatal and non-fatal + other cardiovascular mortality) was reduced by 40% by being randomized to target group $\leq$ 80 mm Hg rather than target group $\leq$ 90 mm Hg (Figure 45-1). It is worth keeping in mind that the difference in achieved diastolic blood pressure between these two groups was only 4 mm Hg. In other words, even a small further reduction of blood pressure in hypertensive patients with type 2 diabetes, receiving virtually identical antihypertensive therapy, had a profound effect on cardiovascular risk. In fact, effective lowering of blood pressure to levels of $\leq$ 80 mm Hg in diastolic blood pressure virtually abolished the excess cardiovascular risk attributable to diabetes. Further detailed analyses of the data on patients with type 2 diabetes mellitus in the HOT Study are in preparation (Hansson L et al. To be published).

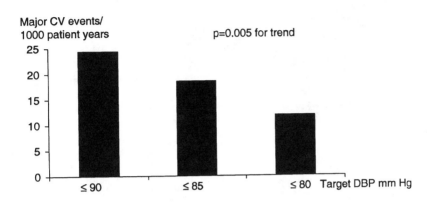

Fig. 45-1. Major cardiovascular events (Fatal and non-fatal strokes and myocardial infarcts plus other cardiovascular mortality) in patients with diabetes mellitus at randomization in the HOT Study in relation to diastolic blood pressure target group.

Table 45-1. Major cardiovascular events in patients with diabetes mellitus at baseline in relation to target blood pressure group in the HOT Study.

Target DBP mmHg	Number of patients	Patients with event*	Events per 1000 Patient-years*
≤ 90	501	45	24.1
≤ 85	501	34	18.6
≤ 80	499	22	11.9

p-value for trend = 0.005.
[Hansson L et al. To be published.]

THE UKPDS STUDY

The United Kingdom Prospective Diabetes Study (UKPDS) was a long-term multicenter trial conducted at British hospitals [4,5]. Its purpose was to assess the value of "tight" versus "less tight" control of blood sugar and blood pressure on cardiovascular risks.

For the assessment of effective control of blood pressure it recruited 1148 hypertensive patients with type 2 diabetes. They were randomized to "less tight" blood pressure control (n=390, 34%), aiming at a blood pressure of <180/105 mm Hg or "tight" blood pressure control (n=758, 66%), aiming at <150185 mm Hg [4].

The efficacy of atenolol (n=358, 31%) and captopril (n=400, 35%) in reducing risk of macrovascular and microvascular complications was compared and both compounds were found to be equally effective in this regard [5]. The "tight" control of blood pressure group, treated with captopril or atenolol, achieved significantly lower levels of blood pressure, (144/82 mm Hg on average), than the patients in the "less tight" group, who were mainly treated with diuretics.

When "tight" control of blood pressure was compared to "less tight" control, significantly lower rates of most cardiovascular complications were achieved by "tight" control (Table 45-2) [4]. In terms of reducing cardiovascular risks the benefits of "tight" control of blood pressure were always more beneficial than tight control of blood glucose, as assessed by HbAlc, and for stroke "tight" metabolic control was actually associated with a worsening of prognosis as compared to "less tight" control [4,5].

Table 45-2. Risk reduction in percent in the group with "tight" vs "less tight" control of blood pressure in the UKPDS Study.

	Risk reduction(%)	p-value
Any diabetes related complication	24	0.0046
Diabetes related death	32	0.019
Stroke	44	0.013
Microvacular disease	37	0.0092
Heart failure	56	0.0043
Retinopathy progression	34	0.0038
Deterioration of vision	47	0.0036

[Based on reference 4]

THE CAPPP STUDY

The Captopril Prevention Project (CAPPP) aimed at comparing an angiotensin converting enzyme (ACE) inhibitor-based antihypertensive regimen with a conventional regimen, based on diuretics and/or beta-blockers, as regards the preventive effect against cardiovascular morbidity and mortality [6]. ACE inhibitors have been widely used in the treatment of high blood pressure and have been listed as first-line therapy for hypertension in several national and international guidelines, e.g. the most recent ones from the World Health Organization and the International Society of Hypertension (WHO/ISH) [12]. Yet there existed no randomized intervention trial data with ACE inhibitors in hypertension to show that such treatment reduces cardiovascular morbidity or mortality before the CAPPP Study [6].

A total of 11,018 hypertensive patients were studied in a prospective, randomized, open, blinded-endpoint evaluation (PROBE) trial [27] conducted at 475 health centres in Sweden and Finland. Patients aged 25-66 years with diastolic blood pressure ≥ 100 mm Hg were included.

All primary cardiovascular events (fatal and non-fatal myocardial infarction and stroke plus other cardiovascular mortality) were not different in the two groups, the relative risk being 1.03, [6]. Of particular interest was the finding that the incidence of diabetes mellitus was significantly lower in the ACE inhibitor group, a finding with obvious long-term risk implications.

In the patients with type 2 diabetes at baseline (n=572) the ACE inhibitor-based regimen was significantly better than conventional treatment in preventing a number of cardiovascular complications (Table 45-3) [6].

Table 45-3. Relative risks of cardiovascular events in patients with diabetes at baseline in the CAPPP Study.

	Relative risk with 95% confidence intervals	p-value
Primary endpoints*	0.59 (0.38-0.91)	0.019
Fatal cardiovascular events	0.48 (0.21-1.10)	0.085
Stroke, fatal and non-fatal	1.02 (0.55-1.88)	0.95
Myocardial infarctions, fatal and non-fatal	0.34 (0.17-0.67)	0.002
All fatal events	0.54 (0.31-0.96)	0.034
All cardiac events	0.67 (0.46-0.96)	0.030
* Primary endpoint was a combination of fatal and non-fatal strokes and myocardial infarctions plus other cardiovascular mortality.		

[Based on reference 6]

THE ABCD STUDY

A subgroup analysis from Appropriate Blood Pressure Control in Diabetes Trial (ABCD) was published in 1998 showing that hypertensive diabetic patients had a significantly lower risk of myocardial infarction when treated with the ACE inhibitor enalapril than the calcium antagonist nisoldipine [7]. While this may well be a correct observation, it is unusual to publish endpoint data from a sub-study when the results of the main study are still unknown. For this reason it would seem appropriate to reserve final judgement until the results of the main ABCD Study have been reported.

THE FACET STUDY

The Fosinopril versus Amlodipine Cardiovascular Events Trial (FACET) was published in 1998 [8]. It appeared to show that diabetic patients treated with the ACE inhibitor fosinopril had a significantly lower risk of major cardiovascular events than patients treated with the calcium antagonist amlodipine [8]. Unfortunately this trial is plagued by several inconsistencies. The results of the FACET trial have been reported on at least three occasions, in 1996 [29], in 1997 [30] and in 1998 [8]. It is disturbing that the conclusions differ between the three versions that have been published. In 1996 the conclusions of a poster on FACET were that only the group of hypertensive diabetic patients who received combined treatment with fosinopril and amlodipine had a significant reduction of cardiovascular risk [29]. The second version, also published as a poster, a year later, concluded that "the results suggest that fosinopril is more effective than amlodipine in preventing cardiovascular events" [30]. As noted above, the third version claimed that fosinopril was significantly better than amlodipine [8]. The addition of new authors, doubts about the randomization process and the discrepancies discussed above suggest that the results of the FACET study should be interpreted with caution [31].

THE SYST-EUR TRIAL
The Systolic Hypertension in Europe showed that antihypertensive treatment with the dihydropyridine-derived calcium antagnonist nitrendipine significantly reduced cardiovascular morbidity in elderly hypertensive patients with isolated systolic hypertension, as compared to placebo [19]. A sub-study of Syst-Eur showed that the patients with isolated systolic hypertension ($\geq$ 160/<95 mm Hg) and type 2 diabetes mellitus had at least as great benefits of antihypertensive treatment as the non-diabetics [9]. It is worth noting that a subgroup analysis of the first large intervention trial in patients with isolated systolic hypertension, the Systolic Hypertension in the Elderly Program (SHEP) [16] also showed positive effects in the diabetic subgroup when comparing antihypertensive treatment with a diuretic as compared to placebo [32].

THE STOP-HYPERTENSION 2 STUDY
The Swedish Trial in Old Patients with Hypertension-2, published in November 1999 [10] studied 6614 elderly patients (age 70-84 years, average 76) hypertensive ($\geq$ 180 mm Hg systolic and/or $\geq$ 105 mm Hg diastolic blood pressure) [10]. They were randomized to either of three therapeutic alternatives: beta-blockers and/or diuretics, calcium antagonists (felodipine or isradipine) or ACE inhibitors (enalapril or lisinopril) [10].

The three therapeutic alternatives were shown to be equally effective in lowering blood pressure and in preventing the primary endpoint (cardiovascular mortality) as well as the combined endpoint of fatal and non-fatal strokes + fatal and non-fatal myocardial infarctions + other cardiovascular mortality [10].

In the subgroup of 719 patients with type 2 diabetes mellitus at baseline (to be published) there were no significant differences regarding mortality between the three therapies, although the calcium antagonists were numerically more effective - about 20% - than the betablockers/diuretics and the ACE inhibitors in preventing cardiovascular mortality (Table 45-4). On the other hand the ACE inhibitors were most effective in preventing myocardial infarction in the hypertensive patients with type 2 diabetes (Hansson L et al. To be published).

Table 45-4. Relative risks, with 95% confidence intervals, of cardiovascular mortality in 719 patients with type 2 diabetes mellitus in the STOP-Hypertension-2 trial

CaA vs Conventional:	Relative risk 0.78 (95% Cl 0.50 - 1.25)
ACEI vs Conventional:	Relative risk 0.91 (95% Cl 0.59 - 1.40)
ACEI vs CaA:	Relative risk 1. 19 (95% Cl 0.75 - 1.89)

CaA =		Calcium antagonists (felodipine or isradipine).
ACEI =		Angiotensin Converting Enzyme Inhibitors (enalapril or lisinopril)
Conventional	=	Beta-blockers (atenolol or metoprolol or pindolol) or Hydrochlorothiazide plus amiloride (Moduretic).

[Hansson L et al. To be published.]

THE HOPE TRIAL

In HOPE patients with high cardiovascular risk, previous stroke, previous myocardial infarction, diabetes mellitus etc. were randomized to either placebo or ACE inhibition in addition to their other medications [11]. Statistically significant reductions in cardiovascular morbidity (25%) were observed in the patients randomized to ACE inhibitor treatment. This was possibly a specific effect related to the ACE inhibitor treatment. However, it might also be linked to the 2 mm Hg lower level of blood pressure obtained in this group. It is of interest to note that in the 1501 patients with type 2 diabetes in the HOT Study (see above) a 4 mm Hg difference in diastolic blood pressure was associated with a 50% lower risk of major cardiovascular events [3].

CONCLUSIONS

The benefits of effective lowering of blood pressure in hypertensive patients with type 2 diabetes were clearly demonstrated in the HOT Study [3] and later the same year confirmed in the UKPDS Study [4,5]. It appears that the choice of antihypertensive medication is of secondary importance if diastolic blood pressures around 80 mm Hg or lower can be achieved by intensive antihypertensive treatment [3,4].

On the other hand CAPPP showed clearly better results with an ACE inhibitor-based therapeutic regimen than treatment based on diuretics and/or beta-blockers [6]. The levels of blood pressure achieved in CAPPP were higher than those in HOT and UKPDS and it is conceivable that in such a situation an ACE inhibitor may offer advantages over conventional treatment, an advantage that disappears if blood pressure is normalized as in the HOT and UKPDS trials. This would be in agreement with the benefits of ACE inhibition in patients with type 1 diabetes mellitus in whom captopril was significantly better than placebo in preventing the development of end-stage renal failure or a doubeling of serum creatinine, provided that the diastolic blood pressure was above 95 mm Hg [33].

The doubts about the safety of calcium antagonist have disappeared following convincing studies in which no excess risk could be shown. The usefulness of this class of agents in hypertensive patients with diabetes was obvious in the HOT Study [3], in the diabetic subgroup in the Syst-Eur trial [9] and in the STOP-Hypertension-2 trial [10] in which the calcium antagonists even appeared to be about 20% more effective than ACE inhibitors and diuretics/beta-blockers (n.s.) in preventing cardiovascular mortality.

It can be concluded that hypertensive patients with type 2 diabetes benefit significantly from antihypertensive treatment in terms of having reduced cardiovascular mortality and morbidity, particularly when their blood pressure is lowered effectively, i.e. down to strictly normotensive levels.

REFERENCES

1. Stamler J, Vaccaro 0, Neaton JD, Wentworth D. Diabetes, other risk factors, and 12-yr cardiovascular mortality for men screened in the multiple risk factor intervention trial. Diabetes care 1993;16:434-444.

2. Mogensen C E. Editorial: Combined high blood pressure and glucose in type 2 diabetes: double jeopardy. BMJ 1998; 317:693-694

3. Hansson L, Zanchetti A, Carruthers SG, Dahlöf B, Eimfeldt D, Ménard J, Julius S, Rahn KH, Wedel H, Westerling S for the HOT Study Group. Effects of intensive blood pressure lowering and low-dose aspirin in patients with hypertension. Principal results of the Hypertension Optimal Treatment (HOT) randomised trial. Lancet 1998;351:1755-1762.

4. UK Prospective Diabetes Study Group. Tight blood pressure control and risk of macrovascular and microvascular complications in type 2 diabetes: UKPDS 38. BMJ 1998;317:703-713.

5. UK Prospective Diabetes Study Group. Efficacy of atenolol and captopril in reducing risk of macrovascular and microvascular complications in type 2 diabetes: UKPDS 39. BMJ 1998;317:713-720.

6. Hansson L, Lindholm L H, Niskanen L, Lanke J, Hedner T, Nikiason A, Luomanmdki K, Dahlöf B, de Faire U, Mérlin C, Kariberg B E, Wester P 0, Björck J-E for the Captopril Prevention Project (CAPPP) Study Group.Effect of angiotensin-converting-enzyme Inhibition compared with conventional therapy on cardiovascular morbidity and mortality in hypertension: the Captopril Prevention Project (CAPPP) randomised trial. Lancet 1999;353:611-616.

7. Estacio RO, Jeffers BW, Hiatt WR, Biggerstaff SL, Gifford N, Schrier RW. The effect of nisoldipine as compared with enalapril on cardiovascular outcomes in patients with non-insulin dependent diabetes and hypertension. NEJM 1998;338:645-652. 1 5

8. Tatti P, Pahor M, Byington RP, Di Mauro P, Guarisco R, Strollo G, Strollo F. Outcome results of the Fosinopril versus amlodipine cardiovascular events randomized trial (FACET) in patients with hypertension and NIDDM. Diabetes Care 1998;21:597-603.

9. Tuomilehto J, Rastenyte D, Birkenhdger WH, Thijs L, Antikainen R, Buipitt CJ, Fletcher AE, Forette F, Goldhaber A, Palatini P, Sarti C, Fagard R for the Systolic Hypertension in Europe Trial lnvestiagtors. Effects of calcium-channel blockade in older patients with diabetes and systolic hypertension. N Engi J Med 1999:340:677-684.

10. Hansson L, Lindholm LH, Ekbom T, Dahlöf B, Lanke J, Scherst6n B, Wester P-0, Hedner T, de Faire U, for the STOP-Hypertension-2 study group. Randomised trial of old and new antihypertensive drugs in elderly patients: cardiovascular mortality and morbidity the Swedish Trial in Old Patients with Hypertension-2 study. Lancet 1999;354:1751-1756.

11.   The Heart Outcomes Prevention Evaluation Study Investigators.   Effects of an angiotensin-converting-enzyme inhibitor, ramipril, on death from cardiovascular causes, myocardial infarction, and stroke in high risk patients. NEJM 2000; (to be published January 20, 2000).

12.   Joint National Committee on Prevention, Detection, Evaluation, and Treatment of High Blood Pressure.   The sixth report of the Joint National Committee on Prevention, Detection, Evaluation, and treatment of High Blood Pressure. Arch Intern Med 1997; 1 57:2413-2446.

13.   Guidelines Sub-Committee. 1999 World Health Organization - International Society of Hypertension guidelines for the management of hypertension.   BLOOD PRESSURE 1999;8(suppi l):1-36.

14.   The HOT Study Group.   The Hypertension Optimal Treatment (HOT) Study - A prospective study of the optimal therapeutic goal and the value of low-dose aspirin in antihypertensive treatment. BLOOD PRESSURE 1993;2:113-119. 1 6

15.   Collins R, Peto R, MacMahon S, Hebert P, Fiebach N H, Eberiein K A, Godwin J, Qizilbash N, Taylor J 0, Hennekens C H. Blood pressure, stroke, and coronary heart disease. Part 2, short-term reductions in blood pressure: over-view of randomised drug trials in their epidemiological context. Lancet 1990;335:827-838.

16.   SHEP Cooperative Research Group.   Prevention of stroke by antihypertensive drug treatment in older persons with isolated systolic hypertension: final results of the systolic hypertension in the elderly program. JAMA 1991;265:3255-3264.

17.   Dahlöf B, Lindholm L H, Hansson L, Scherstén B, Ekbom T, Wester P-0. Morbidity and mortality in the Swedish trial in Old Patients with Hypertension (STOPHypertension). Lancet 1991;338:1281-1285.

18.   MRC Working Party.   Medical Research Council trial of treatment of hypertension in older adults: principal results. Brit Med J 1992;304:405-412.

19.   Staessen J A, Fagard R, Thijs L, Celis H, Arabidze G G, Birkenhdger W H, Buipitt C J, de Leeuw P W, Dollery C T, Fletcher A E, Forette F, Leonetti G, Nachev C, O'Brien E T, Rosenfeld J, Rodicio J L, Tuomilehto J, Zanchetti A, for the Systolic Hypertension in Europe (Syst-Eur) Trial Investigators.   Randomised double-blind comparison of placebo and active treatment for older patients with isolated systolic hypertension.   Lancet 1997;350:757-764.

20.   Lindholm L, Ejlertsson G, Scherstein B. High risk of cerebro-cardiovascular morbidity in well treated male hypertensives.   A retrospective study of 40-59-year-old hypertensives in a Swedish primary care district. Acta Med Scand 1984;216:251-259.

21.   Isles C G, Walker L M, Beevers D G, Brown 1, Cameron H L, Clarke J, Hawthorne V, Hole D, Lever A F, Robertson J W K, Wapshaw J A. Mortality in patients of the Glasgow Blood Pressure Clinic. J Hypertens 1986;4:141-156.

22.   Hansson L. Editorial: How far should blood pressure be lowered? What is the role of the J-curve? Am J Hypertension 1990;3:726-729. 1 7

23.   Stewart 1 McD G. Relation of reduction in pressure to first myocardial infarction in patients receiving treatment for severe hypertension. Lancet 1979;i:861-865.

24.   Cruickshank J M, Thorp J M, Zacharias F J. Benefits and potential harm of lowering high blood pressure. Lancet 1987;1:581-584.

25.   Alderman, M H, Ooi W L, Madhavan S, Cohen H. Treatment-induced blood pressure reduction and the risk of myocardial infarction. JAMA 1989;262:920-924.

26.   van den Hoogen PCW, van Popele NM, Feskens EJM, van der Kuip DAM, Grobbee DE,Hofman A, Witteman JCM. Blood pressure and risk of myocardial infarction in elderly men and women: the Rotterdam Study. J Hypertens 1999;17:1373-1378.

27.   Hansson L, Hedner T, Dahlof B. Prospective Randomized Open Blinded End-point (PROBE) Study: A novel design for intervention trials. BLOOD PRESSURE= 1992; 1: 1 13 -119.

28.   Hansson 1, Zanchetti A et al. for the HOT Study Group. Effects of aggressive lowering of blood pressure in patients with hypertension and type 2 diabetes.The Hypertension Optimal Treatment - HOT - Study. 1999 (in preparation).

29.   Tatti P, Guarisco R, Di Mauro P, Strollo F. Reduced risk of major cardiovascular events with the association of two antihypertensive drugs in a non-insulin dependent diabetic population. American Diabetes Association Annual Meeting. San Fransisco, June 8-11, 1996 (poster).

30.   Tatti P, Pahor M, Byington RP, Di Mauro P, Guarisco R, Strollo F. Results of the Fosinopril Amlodipine Cardiovascular Events Trial (FACET) in hypertensive patients with non-insulin dependent diabetes mellitus (NIDDM). American Heart Association 70th Scientific Meeting. Orinado, November 9-12, 1997 (poster). antagonists. J Hypertens 1998;16:119-124.

31.   van Zwieten PA, Hansson L. Calcium antagonists and safety: the turning of the tide. BLOOD PRESSURE 1999;8:5-8. 1 8

32.   Curd J D, Pressel S L, Cutler J A, Savage P J, Applegate W B, Black H, Camel G, Davis B R, Frost P H, Gonzalez N, Guthrie G, Oberman A, Rutan G H, Stamler J for the Systolic Hypertension in the Elderly Program Cooperative Research Group. Effect of diuretic-based antihypertensive treatment on cardiovascular disease risk in older diabetic patients with isolated systolic hypertension. JAMA 1996;276:1886-1892.

33.   Lewis E J, Hunsicker L G, Bain R P, Rohde R D, for the Collaborative Study Group. The effect of angiotensin-converting-enzyme inhibition on diabetic nephropathy. N Engl J Med 1993;329:1456-1462.

46. SCIENTIFIC BASIS FOR NEW GUIDELINES FOR THE TREATMENT OF HYPERTENSION IN TYPE 2 DIABETES

Klavs Würgler Hansen, Per Løgstrup Poulsen and Carl Erik Mogensen
Medical department M, Aarhus Kommunehospital. Aarhus University Hospital, DK-8000 Aarhus

INTRODUCTION

In 1993 the American Diabetes Association (ADA) stated that antihypertensive treatment should be started in diabetes (type 1 or 2) if blood pressure exceeded 140/90 mmHg, with the goal of reduction to less than 130/85 mmHg [1]. Exactly the same values are proposed in 1999 not only by ADA, but also JNC VI and WHO/ISH [2-4]. The 1993 strategy for antihypertensive treatment in diabetic patients was based on 1) extrapolation from the very large intervention studies in non-diabetic patients 2) knowledge from epidemiological studies in (largely) type 2 diabetic patients but without evidence from prospective studies in type 2 diabetic patients. Between 1993 and 1999 a number of large important intervention studies in type 2 diabetes have been published, the results of the majority were available for incorporation in the above mentioned guidelines.

This chapter will discuss whether the present guidelines indeed are evidence based or fail to implement the full body of available information.

THE BASIS FOR GUIDELINES BEFORE 1993

The major epidemiological studies available in 1993 were the Framingham and MRFIT diabetic cohorts. In the very large MRFIT cohort the cardiovascular mortality was increased by a factor 2 to 4 (depending on number of additional risk factors) in diabetic patients and a clear association with systolic blood pressure was demonstrated with no threshold value [5].

It is less clear why a goal of < 130/85 mmHg was chosen in 1993. Probably this was based on the general assumption that the goal should be lower in diabetic patients because of diabetes per se is an important cardiovascular risk factor. The exact value 130/85 mmHg may be a consequence of the JNC stratification of a normal (<140/90 mmHg) blood pressure into high normal (140-130/90-85 mmHg), normal (130-120/85-80 mmHg) and optimal (<120/80mmHg) blood pressure. From a definition point of view

Mogensen C.E. (ed.), THE KIDNEY AND HYPERTENSION IN DIABETES MELLITUS.
Copyright© 2000 by Kluwer Academic Publishers, Boston ● Dordrecht ● London. All rights reserved.

diabetic patients should at least obtain a blood pressure which could be designated as normal i.e. < 130/85 mmHg.

THE BASIS FOR GUIDELINES IN 1999

The major studies in type 2 diabetic patients are listed in table 46-1 and can be separated in 1) placebo controlled studies 2) trials looking for the optimal blood pressure goal 3) trials comparing different antihypertensive drugs 4) trials exploring the effect of ACE-inhibitors in normotensive patients with one additional cardiovascular risk factor including microalbuminuria. The key data for some of these studies are presented on table 46-2.

Placebo controlled studies in isolated systolic hypertension
1) SHEP (1996) [6]
2) Syst-Euro (1999) [7]

Trials exploring the optimal blood pressure goal
3) UKPDS:38 (1998) [8]
4) HOT (1998) [9]

Trials exploring the optimal drug
5) UKPDS:39 (beta blockers vs ACE-inhibitors) (1998) [11]
6) FACET (dihydropyridin calcium antagonists vs ACE-inhibitors) (1998) [13]
7) ABCD (dihydropyridin calcium antagonists vs ACE-inhibitors) (1998) [14]
8) CAPPP (betablockers/diuretics vs ACE-inhibitors) (1999) [12]
9) STOP-2 (betablockers/diuretics vs ACE-inhibitors vs dihydropyridin calcium antagonists) (1999) [15]

Trials exploring the effects of ACE-inhibitors in normotensive microalbuminuric patients
9) Ravid (1993) [17]
10) Steno Type 2 study (1999) [18]
11) HOPE (2000) [19]

Table 46-1. Important trials with antihypertensive drugs in type 2 diabetic patients in the period 1993-1999.

PLACEBO CONTROLLED STUDIES IN HYPERTENSIVE TYPE 2 DIABETIC PATIENTS

Both the SHEP [6]and Syst-Euro [7] trials were placebo controlled studies in isolated systolic hypertensive patients with a secondary publication of the results from the diabetic subpopulation (about 10 % diabetic patients). The SHEP study was based on thiazide diuretics and Syst-Euro on a calcium channel blocker (nitrendipine), with the option of supplementation with ACE inhibitors or diuretics. In both studies the incidence of CVD events in the placebo arm was about the double in diabetic patients compared with non-diabetic patients. The relative risk reduction for cardiovascular events in the SHEP study was similar (about 30 %) in both diabetic and non-diabetic patients. The active antihypertensive treated diabetic patients in the SHEP study had their risk for CVD events reduced to a level comparable with <u>untreated</u> (placebo) patients without diabetes. In contrast the Syst-Euro trial showed a very high risk reduction (about 70 %) in diabetic patients compared with non-diabetic patients (30 %).

Table 46-2: HYPERTENSION IN NIDDM, CLINICAL STUDIES (continue on next pages)

Study	Inclusion criteria: Age Blood pressure	number drug priority	Target	Baseline	Achieved	Major CV events per 1000 patient years	Myocardial infarction	Stroke	Cardiovascular Mortality
HOT (Lancet 351, 1755-62, 1998) Duration: 3.8 years	Age (50-80) Mean 61.5 years Diast. BP 100-115	(n=501) (n=501) (n=499) felodipine; ACE-inhib, β-blockers	≤90 ≤85 ≤80	175/105 174/105 173/105	148/85 146/83 144/81	24.4 18.6 11.9*	7.5 4.3 3.7	9.1 7.0 6.4	11.1 11.2 3.7*
SHEP (JAMA, 265, 3255-3264, 1991) (JAMA, 276, 1886-1892, 1996) Duration: 4.5 years	Age >60 Years, Mean 71 years Systolic BP≥160 Diastolic BP< 90	Placebo: (n=300)		170/75	≈155/72	63	26	29	Major coronary heart disease events: 32
		Active: (n=283) thiazide, atenolol	BP> 180: <160 BP160-179: Reduction >20	170/77	≈145/70	43*	15*	19	18*

Study	Population	Treatment	Criteria	Baseline BP	Achieved BP	Endpoint 1	Endpoint 2	Stroke	Mortality
Syst-Euro (Lancet, 350,757-764, 1997) (N Eng J Med, 340:677-684, 1999) Duration: 2 years	Age >60 years Mean 70 years Syst.BP 160-219 Diast.BP < 95	Placebo (n246)		≈ 174/86	≈161/84	All CV end points. 58	Cardiac events: 27	Stroke: 27	CV mortality: 26
		Active (n≈246) nitrendipine enalapril, thiazide	Syst < 150 or Reduction > 20	≈ 174/86	≈151/79	22*	12	8	8*
UKPDS (BMJ 317,703-713, 1998) Duration: 8.4 years	Age (25-65) Mean 56 years BP≥160/90 Previously treatment: BP150/85	Less tight (n=390)	<180/105	160/94	154/87	Any diabetes rel. end point (ev./1000 years) 67.4	Myocardial infarction 23.5	Stroke 11.6	Micro vascular disease 19.2
		Tight(n=758) captopril or atenolol, furosemid	<150/85	159/94	144/82	50.9*	18.6	6.5*	12.0**
CAPPP (Lancet 353,611-616 1999) Duration: 6.1 years	Age 25-66 Mean 55 years Diast. BP.≥100	Conventional AHT (diuretics, β-blockers) n =263	Diast. BP ≤90	163/97	151/85	All CV end-poins	Myocardial infarction	Stroke	
		Captopril n =309	Diast. BP ≤90	164/97	154/86	Relative risk 0.59*	Relative risk 0.34*	Relative risk 1.0	

HOPE (Lancet 355: 253-59, 2000) Dur: 4.5 years	> 55 yr mean 65 years Establis-hed CVD+diabetes or diabetes + one risk factor (smo-king, hyper-tension, dyslipe-demia or microal-buminu-ria)	Placebo (n=1769)		142/ 79	143/ 77	Com-bined CV end-points	Myo-cardial infarc-tion	Stro ke	CV morta-lity
		Ramipril (n=1808)		142/ 80	140/ 77	relative risk 0.75*	Rela-tive risk 0.78*	Re-la-tive risk 0.67 *	Rela-tive risk 0.63*

*Denotes statistical significant difference when compared with placebo or less intensive treated group.

As a consequence the risk for CVD events in hypertensive diabetic patients in the Syst-Euro trial, was reduced to the level for antihypertensive treated patients without diabetes. This promising results of the Syst-Euro study should be evaluated on the background that this was a placebo controlled study i.e. the study drug (nitrendipine) is clearly much more efficient (in both diabetic and non-diabetic patients) than placebo for prevention of complications related to hypertension.

OPTIMAL BLOOD PRESSURE GOAL

The tight blood pressure control part of the UKPDS study [8] showed a significant reduction of any diabetes related end point, macrovascular disease (except myocardial infarction), diabetes related death and of retinal complications. The baseline blood pressure was 160/94 mmHg and the aim in the tight blood pressure control arm was < 150/85 mmHg (achieved 144/82 mmHg) and the aim in the less tight control arm was < 180/105 mmHg (achieved 154/87 mmHg). In the tight control group 29 % needed 3 or more antihypertensive drugs.

In the HOT study [9] baseline blood pressure (measured automatically with the Visomat OZ, oscillometric device) was 173/105 mmHg (L. Hansson, personal communication) and in the diabetic subgroup the frequency of major CVD events was gradually decreased with lower diastolic target blood pressure without evidence of a J curve phenomenon. The frequence of major CVD events in the group with target <80 mmHg (achieved 144/81mmHg) was 11.9/1000 patients/year, which was significantly lower than the event rate (24.4/1000 patients/year) in the group with target < 90 mmHg (achieved 148/85 mmHg). The usual interpretation is an effect of reduction of blood pressure per se in the diabetic subpopulation (not seen in the total study population). However in the < 80 mmHg group, the number of diabetic patients treated with ACE inhibitors in addition to the main drug felodipine is unknown and it could be argued that part of the observed beneficial effect possibly should be ascribed to a drug effect in addition to a mere blood pressure lowering effect. It should be noted that despite an attempt to reach the target < 80 mmHg, the achieved blood pressure for more than half the patients in this group was > 80 mmHg leaving the question open whether the protocol target (< 80 mmHg) or the achieved target (< 85 mmHg) should be the goal for guidelines. In addition it should be mentioned as a caveat that the HOT study did not use ordinary auscultatory blood pressure measurements but an automatic device which in a subsequently published validation study [10] was shown to underestimate the diastolic blood pressure significantly by 0.9 mmHg and underestimated the systolic blood pressure by 6.4 mmHg. If these differences, as stated, were independent of the level of blood pressure, it could be argued that the true targets were a diastolic blood pressure of < 81, <86 and < 91 mmHg respectively and that the achieved blood pressure in the group with target < 81 mmHg was 150/82 mmHg.

OPTIMAL DRUG

In UKPDS a beta blocker [11] was compared with an ACE-inhibitor with no difference in the outcome. It is perhaps surprising that even the frequency of sudden death was similar. A larger proportion of patients on betablockers (35 %) than on ACE-inhibitors (22 %) terminated treatment due to possible side effects. In the betablocker group weight gain was significantly higher throughout the study (3.4 versus 1.6 kg) and HBA_{1c} significantly higher for the first four years (7.5 versus 7.0 %). In the CAPPP study [12] analysis of the diabetic subpopulation showed large risk reduction (66%) for myocardial infarction in the captopril versus the conventional (thiazide,beta blocker) group. Even total mortality was lower in captopril treated patients.

Although some methodological problems exist, two studies comparing dihydropyridin calcium antagonists with ACE-inhibitors both reported increased frequency of cardiovascular disease in the calcium antagonist group [13,14]. In the STOP-2 study [15] no difference for the primary end point (fatal CV disease) was seen, when conventional drugs (diuretics/betablockers) were compared with ACE-inhibitors or dihydropyridin calcium antagonists. This also held for the diabetic subpopulation. In the total population myocardial infarction and congestive heart failure was significant less frequent in the ACE-inhibitor group than in the calcium antagonist group. Specific analysis for diabetic patients has now been performed (see chapters 5 and 45).

At this moment dihydropyridin calcium antagonist is not recommended as monotherapy in diabetes. The results of the ALLHAT study is awaited for clarification of the issue [16].

ACE-INHIBITORS IN MICROALBUMINURIC PATIENTS

Ravid has shown a reduction of the frequency of diabetic nephropathy by ACE-inhibitor treatment in normotensive lean microalbuminuric type 2 diabetic patients [17]. With a multiple intervention approach, including ACE inhibitor treatment irrespective of blood pressure the same was shown in the Steno type 2 study, however with no difference in the fall rate of GFR [18]. In the Steno type 2 study the baseline blood pressure was about 147/86 mmHg and the achieved blood pressure was 136/78 mmHg in the intensive treated group compared with 144/81 mmHg in the group receiving standard care.

In the recent HOPE study [19] diabetic patients without heart failure were included if 1) they had established CVD *or* 2) possess one risk factor which could be smoking, hypertension, dyslipedemia or microalbuminuria. The main end point was a combination of cardiovascular mortality, myocardial infarction or stroke. This composite end point was clearly reduced in diabetic patients included in study because of a previous cardiovascular event whereas no significant effect was seen for diabetic patients without previous cardiovascular events. Since the inclusion criteria are multiple and not mutually exclusive, it is impossible from the present data to draw any conclusions with respect to effect on the main composite end point of ACE-inhibition in microalbuminuric type 2 diabetic patients without previous cardiovascular event or without hypertension.

The effect of ACE inhibition in the total population was much more prominent in patients with the highest quartile of baseline systolic blood pressure, however, in diabetic patients the effect was seemingly independent of the baseline blood pressure level [19].

SUMMARY

Trials published in 1993-99 has underscored the paramount importance of tight blood pressure control, which can reduce both macro-and microvascular complications. The actual goal for diastolic blood pressure should be < 80 mmHg or < 85 based on the interpretation of the HOT study. Unfortunately this study had diastolic blood pressure as intervention and target value, however the main clinical problem in type 2 diabetic patients is isolated systolic hypertension comprising about 2/3 of the hypertensive population [20]. The baseline and achieved blood pressure in the presented studies is far above 140 mmHg and 130 mmHg respectively (fig 46-1), and recommendations to obtain a systolic blood pressure < 130 mmHg is still not evidence based, but relies on epidemiological results. In the UKPDS study major CVD events declined with lower systolic blood pressure (10 % reduction for a 10 mmHg reduction of blood pressure) without any threshold value [21]. Thus the principle of "the lower the better" is reinforced by the UKPDS study, but results from epidemiological studies are less important than results from intervention studies as basis for treatment guidelines. On top of the practical problems of achieving a goal of < 130 systolic in type 2 diabetic patients is the problem of "white coat hypertension" or "isolated clinic hypertension". This problem is particular important for the older population with systolic hypertension. In the Syst-Euro trial the systolic day time average blood pressure was 20 mmHg lower than the systolic clinic blood pressure [22]. Analysis of a subpopulation of the Syst-Euro population in which ambulatory blood pressure was performed demonstrated (in the

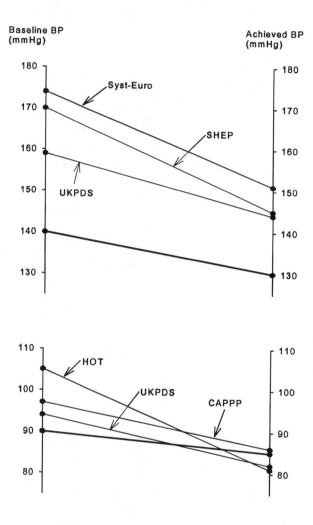

Fig. 46-1. Baseline and achieved blood pressure in five large intervention trials in hypertensive type 2 diabetic patients: The Syst-Eur and SHEP trials included patients with isolated systolic hypertension. The CAPPP and HOT studies were based on diastolic hypertension. The levels for intervention (<140/90 mmHg) and goal (<130/85 mmHg) proposed by most international guidelines are presented for comparison (heavy black lines).

placebo group) a much clearer association between cardiovascular events and ambulatory blood pressure (mainly night value) than clinic blood pressure [22].

For this reason it seems at the moment not justified to recommend a reduction of systolic blood pressure to < 130 mmHg in all type 2 diabetic patients. The actual guidelines from several internal and national institutions are shown in table 46-3 for comparison.

Table 46-3. Present (1999) international and national guidelines for antihypertensive treatment in type 2 diabetes. All guidelines recommend intensive BP reduction for patients with nephropathy. (goal < 130-125/80-75 mmHg)

Institution or Society	Intervention	Goal
WHO/ISH [4] JNC IV [3]	BP > 140/90 (consider intervention if high normal BP i.e. 140-130/90-85)	BP< 130/85
ADA [2]	BP > 140/90	BP< 130/85
BHS [22]	BP > 140/90	BP < 140/80
European Policy Group [23]	BP > 140/90	BP< 140/85

It is difficult to argue against ACE-inhibitors as first line drugs except in patients with ischemic heart disease (which perhaps should be treated with both ACE-inhibitors and beta blockers).

Present evidence suggest ACE-inhibitor treatment in all patients with microalbuminuria irrespective of blood pressure with the purpose of delaying the progression to diabetic kidney disease. Hopefully further analysis of the HOPE data and future studies will contribute to the discussion whether ACE-inhibitors should be recommended to all patients with type 2 diabetes and one additional risk factor.

REFERENCES
1   Consensus Statement. Treatment of hypertension in Diabetes. Diabetes Care 1993; 16: 1394-1397
2   American Diabetes Association. Standards of medical care for patients with diabetes mellitus. Diabetes Care 1999; 22: Suppl.1:S32-S41.
3   The Joint National Commitee on Detection, Evaluation, and Treatment of High Blood Pressure. The sixth report of the joint national committee on detection, evaluation, and treatment of high bloood pressure. Arch Intern Med 1997; 157: 2413-2446
4   1999 Guidelines for the management of hypertension: Memorandum from a World Health Organization/International Society of Hypertension meeting. Guidelines sub-committee. J Hypertens 1999; 17:151-183

5   Stamler J,Vaccaro O, Neaton JD, Wentworth D for the multiple risk factor intervention trial research group. Diabetes, other risk factors, and cardivascular mortality for men screened in the multiple risk factor intervention trial. Diabetes Care; 16: 434-44

6   Curb JD, Pressel SL, Cutler JA, Savage PJ, Applegate WB et al for the Systolic Hypertension in the Elderly Programme Cooperative Research Group. JAMA 1996; 23: 1886-1892

7   Tuomilehto J, Rastenyte D, Birkenhäger WH, Thijs L, Antikainen R, Bulpitt CJ, Fletcher AE, Forette F, Goldhaber A, Palatini P, Sarti C, Fagard R for the systolic hypertension in europe trial investigators. Effects of calcium-channel blockade in older patients with diabetes and systolic hypertension. N Eng J Med 1999; 340: 677-684

8   UK Prospective Diabetes Study Group. Tight blood pressure control and risk of macrovascular and microvascular complications in type 2 diabetes: UKPDS 38. BMJ 1998; 317: 703-713

9   Hansson L, Zanchetti A, Carruthers SG, Dahlöf B, Julius S, Ménard J, Rahn KH, Wedel H, Westerlin S. Effects of intensive blood -pressure lowering and low-dose aspirin in patients with hypertension: principal results of the Hypertension Optimal Treatment (HOT) randomised study. Lancet 1998; 13: 1755-1762

10   Lithell H, Berglund L. Validation of an oscillometric blood pressure measuring device: A substudy of the HOT study. Blood Pressure 1998; 7: 149-152

11   UK prospective Diabetes Study Group. Efficacy of atenolol and captopril in reducing risk of macrovascular and microvascular complications in type 2 diabetes: UKPDS 39. BMJ 1998; 317: 713-720

12   Hansson L,Lindholm LH, Niskanen L, Lanke J,Hedner T, Niklason A, Luomanmäki K, Dahlöf B, de Faire U, Mörlin C, Karlberg BE, Wester PO, Björck JE. Effect of angiotensin-converting-enzyme inhibition compared with conventional therapy on cardiovascular morbidity and mortality in hypertension: the Captopril Prevention Project (CAPPP) randomised trial. Lancet 1999;353:611-616.

13   Tatti P, Pahor M, Byington RP, Mauro PD, Guarisco R, Strollo G, Strollo F. Outcome results of the fosinopril versus amlodipine cardiovascular events randomised trial (FACET) in patients with hypertension and NIDDM. Diabetes Care 1998; 21: 597-603

14   Estacio RO, Jeffers BW, Hiatt WR, Biggerstaff SL, Gifford N, Schrier RW. The effect of nisoldipine as compared with enalapril on cardiovascular outcomes in patients with non-insulin-dependent diabetes and hypertension. N Eng J Med 1998; 338: 645-653

15   Hansson L, lindholm LH, Ekbom T, Dahlöf B, Lanke J, Scherstén B, Wester P-O, Hedner T, de Faire U for the STOP-hypertension-2 study group- Lancet 1999; 354: 1751 1756

16   Davis BR, Cutler JA, Gordon DJ, Furberg CD, Wright JT, Cushman WC, Grimm RH, Larosa J, Whelton PK, Perry M, Alderman MH, Ford CE, Oparil S, Francis C, Proschan M, Pressel S, Black HR, Hawkins CM for the ALLHAT research group. Rationale and design for the antihypertensive and lipid lowering treatment to prevent heart attack trial (ALLHAT). Am J Hypertens 1996; 9: 342-360

17   Ravid M, Savin H, Jutrin I, Bental T, Katz B, Lishner M. Long-term stabilizing effects of angiotensin-converting enzyme inhibition on plasma creatinine and on proteinuria in normotensive type II diabetic patients. Ann Intern Med 1993; 118: 577-581

18   Gæde P, Vedel P, Parving H-H, Pedersen O. Intensified multifactorial intervention in patients with type 2 diabetes and microalbuminuria: the Steno type 2 randomised study. Lancet; 353: 617-622

19   The Heart Outcomes Prevention Evaluation (HOPE) Study Investigators. Effects of ramipril on cardiovascular and microvascular outcomes in people with diabetes mellitus: results of the HOPE study and MICRO-HOPE substudy. Lancet, 2000; 355: 253-259

20   Tarnow L, Rossing P, Gall M-A, Nielsen FS, Parving H-H. Prevalence of arterial hypertension in diabetic patients before and after the JNC-V. Diabetes Care 1994; 17: 1247-1251

21   Turner RC, Millns H, Neil HAW, Stratton IM, Manley SE, Matthews DR, Holman for the United Kingdom prospective Diabetes Study Group. Risk factors for coronary artery disease in non-insulin dependent diabetes melitus: United Kingdom prospective diabetes study (UKPDS:23). BMJ 1998; 316: 823-828

22   Staessen JA, Thijs L, Fagard R, O'Brien ET, Clement D, Leeuw PW, Mancia G, Nachev C, Palatini P, Parati G, Tuomilehto J, Webster J for the Systolic Hypertension in Europe Trial Investigators. Predicting cardiovasvular risk using conventional vs ambulatory blood pressure in older patients with systolic hypertension. JAMA 1999; 282: 539-546

23   Ramsay LE, Williams B, Johnston GD, MacGregor GA, Poston L, Potter L, Poulter NR, Russel G for the British Hypertension Society. Guidelines for the management of hypertension: report of the third working party of the British Hypertension Society. J Hum Hypertens 1999; 13: 569-592

24   European Diabetes Policy Group 1999. A desktop guide to type 2 diabetes mellitus. Diabetic Med 1999; 16: 716-730

REGULATORY CONSIDERATIONS IN THE DEVELOPMENT OF THERAPIES FOR DIABETIC NEPHROPATHY AND RELATED CONDITIONS

G. Alexander Fleming
Senior Vice President, Regulatory Affairs, Worldwide Clinical Trials, MD 20815, Washington D.C

INTRODUCTION

The importance of regulation in the drug development process is well appreciated, but the principles and practices of the major regulatory agencies overseeing therapeutic development are much less understood even by well-informed academicians. This chapter is intended to provide a better understanding of the regulatory framework and processes that are pertinent to therapeutic development in general and the advancement of therapies for diabetic nephropathy and related conditions in particular. While this attempt reflects the perspective and focus of a former evaluator in the United States Food and Drug Administration (FDA), the important roles of other national and supranational authorities cannot be over-stated for what has become a shared, global enterprise.

HISTORY OF THERAPEUTIC REGULATION

The modern history of therapeutic evaluation and regulation began around the early 1900s though some historians will point to precursor events that occurred as early as in feudal times [1]. The FDA developed out of legislative responses to a series of safety disasters involving a variety of food and drugs (1906 Food and Drug Act), a deadly formulation of sulfanilamide that included ethylene glycol (1938 Food, Drug, and Cosmetic Act), and thalidomide (The Amendment of 1962 to the Food, Drug, and Cosmetic Act) [2]. Ironically, it was the thalidomide tragedy that provoked a codification of scientific methods in the pharmaceutical regulatory process at the FDA [3]. The irony stems from the fact that thalidomide was not licensed in the US and very few thalidomide-induced birth defects occurred in the US [1]. Furthermore, Congress

Mogensen C.E. (ed.), THE KIDNEY AND HYPERTENSION IN DIABETES MELLITUS.

responded to this safety issue without giving the FDA additional powers to enforce drug safety. Authority to enforce safety was in place since 1938. Instead, the Agency was for the first time given formal authority to require that effectiveness be scientifically demonstrated (based on "substantial evidence") before a pharmaceutical could be approved. The 1962 Amendment Food, Drug, and Cosmetic Act specifies that "The term substantial evidence means evidence from adequate and well-controlled studies"[4,5]. This provision is the legal cornerstone of modern therapeutic regulation and has been interpreted by the FDA in fine detail. Among other things, this dictum has led to a general requirement for two, usually placebo-controlled, studies of appropriate size and duration for the indication being sought as the basis of a New Drug Application (NDA) approval.

Until the mid-twentieth century, Europe was the site of most pharmaceutical development. During the era that produced humankind's first synthetic wonder drugs beginning with aspirin and closing with the production of penicillin, governmental regulation in Europe developed in a quieter, less visible fashion than was the case in the USA. In general, the European approach to pharmaceutical licensing involved less legal formality. The licensing processes of European countries depended heavily on the advice of experts, primarily academicians, outside of government. Relatively small bureaucracies were established to administer the licensing process, but scientific and technical expertise was largely provided from appointed committees and individual consultants.

Different political and social conditions in the USA from the turn of the century to the present produced a different approach to therapeutic regulation in that country. Aggressive journalism and the Roosevelt New Deal predilection for large, protective government programs were among the major influences. The FDA evolved into a very large government agency that progressively acquired much of the necessary expertise to evaluate and regulate therapies of all kinds including pharmaceuticals, blood and other biologic products, medical devices, and veterinary medicine products. Related to its origin in the Department of Agriculture, the FDA is also responsible for the regulation of foods.

RECENT DEVELOPMENTS IN THERAPEUTIC REGULATION
The final decade of the millennium has produced as much change in the world of therapeutic development and regulation as occurred during the preceding 50 years. Cataclysmic changes in electronic communication, geopolitics, trade, consumerism, and science are among the obvious explanations. A growing perception in the 1970's and 80's of a "drug gap", i.e. pharmaceuticals' taking longer to become available in the USA than in Europe, led to the involvement of Congress. This culminated in the passage of the Prescription Drug Users' Fee Act (PDUFA) [6,7] in 1992 and the Food and Drug Modernization Act (FDAMA) of 1997 [8]. These laws codified existing practices and defined a host of new responsibilities and managerial approaches. Self-initiated changes

within the FDA, already underway before the above legislation, were just as important in reshaping the Agency's drug evaluation processes. FDA's Good Review Practice (GRP) initiative began in the early 1990's and continues as an effort to define, evolve, and support the understanding and practice of scientifically sound approaches by evaluators—in and outside of government—including those within commercial organizations [9,10].

The emergence of a united Europe induced an equally important result. Faced with the formidable challenge of reconciling the wide range of different political systems, laws, and cultures across their continent, the Europeans became the architects of the harmonisation process. Harmonisation used in this context is simply defined as the process of achieving the maximal amount of agreement possible among parties with diverse positions. In practice this involves striving to reach complete agreement on each specific issue, but when this is not possible, to identify the most specific expression that all parties can accept. Some of the earliest applications of this approach occurred in the realm of good clinical practice (GCP). GCP refers to an accepted body of principles and practices by which biomedical research is conducted. Representatives from Nordic countries wrote the first GCP document and the European Union (EU) and later the World Health Organization (WHO) followed. Interestingly, while the FDA had developed an even more extensive body of GCP regulations and guidances over its history, the Agency had no single, integrated GCP document.

The harmonization movement within the pharmaceutical world produced the immensely important International Conference on Harmonisation of Technical Requirements for the Registration of Pharmaceuticals for Human Use (ICH) [11]. ICH began around 1990 and will continue for the foreseeable future. It has brought together representatives of the pharmaceutical regulatory authorities and the pharmaceutical industries from Europe, Japan, and the United States. The objective of ICH is to achieve a single set of requirements in the areas of manufacturing, animal testing, and clinical trials that are acceptable to all three authorities for new drug approval. Prior to ICH, developers of pharmaceuticals had to contend with three major sets of expectations and requirements, which on some issues differed substantially. By 1997, ICH had reconciled an enormous number of issues. The ICH process and progress is represented conceptually in figure 47-1. ICH documents have been adopted by the FDA as guidances and to some extent enacted as regulations in Europe and Japan. The finalized documents from the clinical area (referred to as Efficacy) are listed in table 47-1. Figure 47-2 reflects a way of categorizing these documents and relating them to a sequence of steps involved in pharmaceutical development. Equally important documents have been produced for pharmaceutical chemistry and manufacturing (referred to as Quality) and preclinical evaluation (referred to as Safety). Full texts of all these documents can be found on the FDA/CDER homepage [2]. While ICH is intended to provide guidance for pharmaceutical developers, many of these ICH products are discourses on scientific principles and practices for all involved or interested in the development of therapies.

A.

Lack of Regulatory Harmonisation in 1990

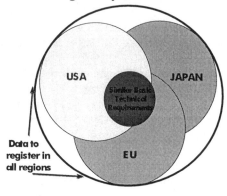

B.

Approaching the Harmonisation Target in 2000

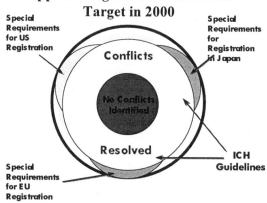

Figure 47-1. The degree of concordance among the three major regulators' requirements for pharmaceutical development are depicted prior to ICH (A) and as the original objectives of ICH were achieved in 1997 (B).

THE EVOLVED MODERN PRINCIPLES OF THERAPEUTIC EVALUATION

The ICH movement and important initiatives at the FDA and other regulatory organizations have led to the concept that good scientific principles and practices of pharmaceutical evaluation should be understood and utilized by <u>all</u> those involved in the development of therapies [12]. ICH, FDA, and other regulators have produced a body of official regulations and guidances that reflect these principles and good practices. The pharmaceutical industry is the expressed intended audience, but these writings have clear relevance to academicians and regulatory officials themselves. The FDA itself has embarked on a formal process to detail good practice standards for its own reviewers with its GRP initiative. GRP, while intended for official evaluators, provides yet another source of good principles and practices for anyone who assesses pharmaceutical safety and efficacy.

Reviews of principles for designing clinical trials and evaluating their data abound [13,14]. Others are more directly applied to the regulatory context [15,16]. Some of these regulatory principles are summarised below:

Finalised ICH Clinical Guidelines

Code	Topic
E1	The Extent of Population Exposure to Assess Clinical Safety for Drug Intended for Long-term Treatment of Non-Life-Threatening Conditions
E2A	Clinical Safety Data Management: Definitions and Standards for expedited Reporting
E2B	Clinical Safety Data Management: Data Elements for Transmission of Individual Case Safety Reports
E2C	Clinical Safety Data Management: Periodic Safety Update Reports for Marketed Drugs
E3	Structure and Content of Clinical Study Reports
E4	Dose-Response Information to Support Drug Registration
E5	Ethnic Factors in the Acceptability of Foreign Clinical Data
E6	Good Clinical Practice: Consolidated Guideline
E7	Studies in Support of Special Populations: Geriatrics
E8	General Considerations for Clinical Trials
E9	Statistical Considerations in the Design of Clinical Trials
E10	Choice of Control Group in Clinical Trials
M3	Non-Clinical Safety Studies for the Conduct of Human Clinical Trials for Pharmaceuticals
S6	Safety Studies for Biotechnology-Derived Products

Table 47-1. The titles of the ICH clinical area (Efficacy) guidances

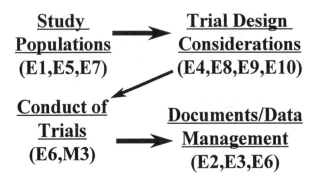

**Efficacy Topics:
Categories of Documents**

Figure 47-2. Guidances from the clinical area (Efficacy) are arranged in four categories. Each category corresponds to the step in the pharmaceutical development process at which it is typically of greatest consideration

BENEFIT/RISK RELATIONSHIP
The final regulatory decision about whether or not to sanction the availability of a therapy is based on the perceived balance of benefits and risks that the therapy affords for the population of patients for whom it is intended. The availability of other therapies, the expected course of not treating the condition and other considerations will influence the amount of risks that can be accepted for the benefits provided. Ultimately a licensing decision for a therapy relies on the knowledge and judgement of experts in and outside of government. Collectively, these experts must provide an understanding of all the relevant scientific, clinical, ethical, legal, and administrative issues that are involved.

EFFECTIVENESS
The estimate of a therapy's effectiveness, i.e. ability to produce health benefits in the intended patient or user population, is determined by all experience in which relevant biologic responses to the therapy and, sometimes, related therapies are measured. The range of data afforded by this experience form a hierarchy of value ranging from that provided by the most rigorously controlled study to the single anecdotal report. Effectiveness is an overall conclusion to be distinguished from efficacy, which characterizes the positive results of single experiments (ranging from *in vitro* studies to

large clinical trials). Regulatory authorities may state, *a priori*, minimally acceptable outcomes necessary for claiming effectiveness, but this is a preliminary estimate based on assumptions about the quality of the data and safety outcomes, which cannot be confirmed until all studies have been completed and analyzed.

Circumstances can alter the magnitude of response or the response itself that regulators will ultimately accept as adequate to show effectiveness. An important attribute of a regulatory authority is to abide by its commitments to accept specified outcomes as indicative of effectiveness. This imperative must be balanced by the equally important need to take into account important scientific developments that may occur over the considerable amount of time involved in developing a therapy.

Not uncommonly, therapeutic development and regulatory approval must rely on outcomes that predict clinical benefits, i.e. surrogate endpoints, instead of the demonstration of direct clinical benefits themselves. In many cases, use of surrogate endpoints may be the only practical means by which therapies for chronic diseases and conditions can be developed. Blood glucose and cholesterol levels are well know examples of surrogates by which many therapies for diabetes and hyperlipidemia were developed and more recently have been confirmed as producing clinical benefits. The selection of surrogates should reflect an expert consensus, but this approach is not infallible. Probably the best know example of a surrogate that was used to justify marketing approval and was later discredited is from the development of agents for suppression of ventricular arrhythmias. The Cardiac Arrhythmia Suppression Trial (CAST) [17] evaluated the survival benefit conferred by treatment with one of three agents. These therapies were approved on the basis of efficacy in reducing frequency of ventricular arrhythmias following myocardial infarction. Instead of the anticipated reduction of cardiac deaths, CAST revealed that all three therapies were associated with an excess of total mortality compared to placebo. This experience does not invalidate the surrogate approach. It only shows the value of confirming clinical benefit for therapies that were approved on the basis of surrogate outcomes. When viewed from a broad perspective, the benefits to patients that have resulted from the use of surrogates in therapeutic development far exceeds the harm that this approach has caused.

Because surrogate outcomes reflect human judgements based on the best available information at a point in time, additional data may alter the estimated value of a surrogate and thereby change the acceptability of the surrogate as a primary efficacy outcome. In effect, an authority might reject a previously accepted surrogate outcome that has been discredited, or it might accept a surrogate measure as a primary outcome that has since been validated.

SAFETY

In no case is therapeutic safety absolute. A safety profile can be estimated only for the dose, disease, and population in which it has been tested. The safety risks predicted by preclinical and clinical experience that can be accepted to justify further human exposure—investigational or as approved clinical use—depend on the severity of the disease itself, availability of therapeutic alternatives, and ultimately the benefit that the treatment affords.   In general, an adequate definition of a therapy's safety profile requires far greater numbers of patients and duration of treatment than is required to define effectiveness. Given the extent and duration of investigation that is reasonable to require of developers before a therapy can be approved for its indicated use, only relatively frequently occurring adverse reactions can be detected prior to marketing (typically no lower than a .05% incidence).   Detection during marketed use of rare but serious toxicities such as major organ failure can alter a therapy's benefit to risk relationship enough to warrant restrictions on the use of the therapy or even withdrawal of its marketing approval.

Ongoing evaluation of a new therapy's safety beyond the date of its marketing approval is therefore essential. In some cases, large controlled trials are required, as a condition for approval, to be performed in the post approval period.   Such studies are most likely to be required when unresolved safety issues persist and the therapy is intended for chronic use in large populations. Large post approval studies may also be used to demonstrate major benefits, such as positive effects on survival, which could not practically be shown in pre-approval studies.   Reporting by health providers and patients of toxicity associated with therapies is a very important source of information for further refining the estimates of their safety profiles.   Such reports must be carefully compiled and evaluated by the marketer and regulatory authority alike, especially during the first years of marketing but for an indefinite time beyond this initial period as well. Finally, epidemiological approaches can also be used to better define issues of safety and effectiveness.

ANIMAL TESTING

Despite the increasing importance of *in vitro* methodologies, animal testing is the primary means of evaluating the desired and toxic effects of a potential human therapy prior to introduction of the therapeutic agent into humans. Ethical understandings dictate that some evidence of a therapy's efficacy as well as safety be obtained prior to exposing humans to a new compound. Wholly satisfactory animal models for evaluating safety and efficacy rarely exist. For some therapies, such as vaccines and antidepressants, indirect surrogate measures in animals or even *in vitro* approaches are all that can be used to predict clinical benefit prior to human exposure. Animal models may over predict as much as under predict clinical benefits of treatments for humans. The development of therapies for diabetes has frequently been associated with seemingly appropriate animal models that strongly suggested human efficacy, which nonetheless could not be confirmed in human trials.

For general toxicology evaluation, larger animals such as dogs and non-human primates tend to better approximate human intermediary and drug metabolism than small animals.   Large animals are less feasibly used for providing the large numbers of animals required for examining multiple doses and gender differences. On the other hand, the much shorter life span and faster metabolism of small animals provide a means of simulating life long exposure to a candidate therapy. Small animals such as mice and rats may therefore provide better or at least complementary models for exploring long term toxicity including carcinogenicity. Because of considerable size and metabolic differences among experimental animals and humans, it is important to relate toxic effects across species to exposure, i.e., the amount of the therapeutic agent that animals from each species "sees" over time. This exposure to the therapeutic agent is generally expressed as the blood concentration of the agent integrated over a given period of time.

The significance for humans of a therapy's toxic effects in animals requires interpretation in every case. Known differences in drug metabolism or sensitivity between the test animal and humans may help to allay concerns about the potential for toxicity in humans. However, some findings in animals even at very large multiples of the anticipated human exposure cannot be dismissed. It must be understood that high exposures to a therapy are used in animals, in part, to compensate for the relatively short duration of exposure that can be obtained in animals compared to chronic use in humans. On the other hand, for a multitude of reasons, the absence of a toxic effect in animals does not exclude the possibility of the toxic effect in humans. Experimental animals are generally more uniform genetically, are studies under highly controlled conditions, and results are very unlikely to have any value in predicting rare, idiosyncratic toxicity in humans.

The practice of providing animal toxicology data in the official physician product information though common is of dubious value because of the inability of most physicians to interpret such data. Ultimately, all that matters are human safety data, but these may not become available until years of human use have elapsed. Some long term issues like carcinogenicity are almost never systematically addressed with human data. Animal toxicology data should be seen as only supplementary to data from human experience. The role of animal toxicology testing is primarily for protecting the safety of subjects and patients involved in pre-approval clinical investigation. By and large, the data from controlled clinical trials are the basis of determining a therapy's benefit to risk relationship and forming the body of information aimed at guiding patients and physicians in its safe and appropriate use when the therapy is first approved.

THE LEARN AND CONFIRM PARADIGM

Ethical and scientific considerations require that therapeutic development proceed carefully through a series of measured steps within the well know four phases of therapeutic investigation. Earliest investigation is spent in understanding how the healthy human body handles and tolerates the therapeutic agent. Subsequent studies start to show what the agent does to the body. At this point, hypotheses begin to form (or sharpen, if preclinical data had initiated them) about how the agent could be used to provide health benefits. A hypothesis that a therapy could provide a heath benefit warranting regulatory approval is provided by at least one and usually several small to medium sized, well controlled clinical studies. This hypothesis is confirmed with one and usually two more large studies that not only confirm efficacy (effectiveness) but provide enough patients to estimate the safety profile for the therapy's intended use. On the basis of the totality of data from all these clinical and preclinical studies, the regulatory authority with the help of experts determines if the therapy's benefit to risk relationship is acceptable. Thus, therapeutic development proceeds through cycles of learning and confirming--starting when or frequently before a therapy is identified and proceeding into and through the period of marketed use. The learn and confirm concept [18] expresses the epistemological basis of therapeutic development. That is, knowledge about a therapy is gained by repetitively advancing hypotheses and systematically testing them. In the fullness of time, knowledge about the benefits and risks of a therapy asymptotically approaches but never reaches complete understanding.

The FDA, by its interpretation of its legally defined authority, has set a fairly rigorous standard for demonstration of effectiveness. To warrant marketing approval, the FDA in most cases has required that at least two well controlled studies show differences in primary efficacy outcomes that are statistically significant (generally defined as $p < .05$). The Agency has more recently shown a willingness to accept a single, well designed large trial with a treatment effect on the primary outcome, which is highly statistically significant. In effect, the significance level of such a trial should reach the equivalent composite significance of two independent trials each with significance at the $p = .05$ level, i.e., a significance level of $p < .0025$ [3]. In general, however, two trials (each with somewhat different designs) are to be preferred over a single trial. Two trials reduce the possibility of an unperceived systematic error or bias in the design or interpretation of a single study leading to an incorrect conclusion. The FDA has also accepted single studies to justify new drug approvals under other conditions. These include when a survival benefit has been clearly demonstrated, when no other therapy is available for a life threatening disorder, and when the disorder affects a very small population.

REGULATORY FLEXIBILITY

Therapeutic regulatory authorities must continue to balance their two major responsibilities: to facilitate the development of therapies that are desperately needed and to protect the public from unsafe, ineffective, or inadequately labeled therapies. The dictum, *primum non nocere*, is not tenable in this context. Nearly everyone recognizes that no therapy, approved or under investigation, is without risks. To strike a reasonable balance between these imperatives, regulators have to approve therapies before the risks are definitively established. To require such information prior to approval would, at a minimum, deprive patients of needed therapy for a period of time. In many cases, this requirement would deter therapeutic developers from ever seeking new therapies for chronic diseases. As part of an overall approach to managing risks, regulators are more and more taking into account the actual medical practice and other conditions under which a new therapy will be used. For example, the regulators must ask how consistently will patients be adequately monitored for toxicity known to be caused by the therapy. The concern of regulators about a therapy's significant toxicity will not be diminished by the availability of a highly effective monitoring test if the test is unlikely to be regularly used in everyday practice. Thus, regulators must weigh a number of considerations on a case by case basis as to just what body of evidence is required prior to proceeding with a given study and, finally, what is needed for marketing approval. A particularly difficult problem is to weigh modest therapeutic benefit for many or most patients against a severe risk for a very few patients.

PERSISTING DIFFERENCES IN APPROACHES TO THERAPEUTIC EVALUATION

While ICH and other initiatives have achieved considerable agreement among the major regulatory authorities and therapeutic developers about the principles with which they evaluate therapies, significant differences exist in how the regulatory authorities execute their responsibilities. As an example, the European and FDA approaches to new drug approval differ significantly. The various national regulatory agencies and the European Union's relatively new European Agency for the Evaluation of Medicinal Products (EMEA) and the Committee on Proprietary Medicinal Products (CPMP) have relatively small staffs of review professionals. The EMEA and CPMP rely heavily on outside academic consultants for general advice and to produce expert reports (evaluations) of licensing applications. These reports are the basis of licensing recommendations made by committees, which are also composed of outside experts. In contrast, the FDA is staffed with a large number of full-time reviewing professionals who have training and experience within their assigned areas of responsibility. While the FDA does utilize outside experts on its advisory committees and occasionally in situations where internal expertise may require supplementation, the drug review process is performed by and licensing decisions are made by FDA scientists and clinicians.

Another significant difference between the environments in Europe and the USA is the closer involvement of the national governments within the EU in determining prices of pharmaceuticals. This involvement does not occur within the evaluation process itself, but it has a very important impact on that process. In the US, the FDA without any economic consideration, licenses pharmaceuticals and other therapies. That is not to say that other parts of the U.S. government do not have a strong interest in and influence on therapeutic pricing, but the FDA does not provide any support for these determinations. In Europe, however, therapeutic developers are asked by the regulatory authorities themselves to provide data from trials that directly compare the clinical and economic outcomes of the new therapy with an established therapy. The European approach is ultimately to evaluate efficacy (and presumably safety) relative to existing therapies. At the FDA, the emphasis is on establishing absolute efficacy, that is, a treatment's effect compared to placebo. In effect, the FDA requires only that a therapy be shown to work, not that it necessarily work equally well as, or better than, an existing therapy. The European approach is more burdensome than that of the FDA for a therapy that is intended to provide efficacy equivalent only to that of the standard therapy. In general, many more patients are required to adequately power an active-controlled study than a placebo study to achieve the same conclusion, i.e., the therapy can be approved.

These different regulatory prospectives of Europe and the U.S. on control groups are harmonized to a large extent in the ICH E10 document. All experts will agree that a placebo control group is very valuable, if not indispensable, even for studies that also involve comparisons of active therapies. There is also universal agreement that use of a placebo group is unethical in trials that involve conditions in which harm will occur if therapy is withdrawn. This issue then comes down to deciding when a placebo group is ethically, or for some other reason, not acceptable in the evaluation of a potential useful therapy. Traditionally, the FDA has emphasized the absolute benefit to risk relationship as the appropriate means of testing and approving therapies and consequently has had a stronger stomach for placebo studies than their colleagues in Europe. However, the FDA has never sanctioned the use of placebo-controlled trials in clearly inappropriate situations such as the treatment of acute infectious diseases or treatable oncological disease. The list of conditions for which placebo trials can be justified is shrinking as more and more data substantiate the long-term benefits of treating chronic diseases such as hypertension, diabetes, and hyperlipidemia. This progress in clinical investigation and therapeutics is enforcing a convergence from these two historically different regulatory perspectives.

Other important differences between European and US regulatory approaches are summarized in table 47-2.

REGULATORY SITUATION FOR DIABETES THERAPIES

Therapeutic development for diabetes therapies and related conditions has exploded in the post-DCCT era. The FDA's approach to regulation of therapies for diabetes drugs has also evolved [19]. While some significant compounds have been put into use for oral therapy of type 2 diabetes and recombinant insulin and insulin analogs provide some attractive features, a true therapeutic breakthrough has not occurred during this time [20]. Results of the Diabetes Control and Complications Trial (DCCT) and the United Kingdom Prevention of Diabetes Study (UKPDS) have stimulated greater awareness of the value of improving glycemic control and, to some extent, some success in achieving better glycemic control among type 1 and 2 patients. However, the average patient's glycemic control is far from acceptable. Diabetes complications will therefore continue to be a major cause of morbidity and mortality, and treatments for diabetic complications will be much needed for the foreseeable future.

For obvious reasons, development of therapies for diabetic complications is inherently more difficult than that for treatments of glycemic and other metabolic abnormalities of diabetes. Extraordinary amounts of time and resources have been invested in aldose reductase inhibitors, primarily as treatments for peripheral neuropathy but also for nephropathy and retinopathy. Convincing clinical benefits have yet to be shown for compounds in this therapeutic class [21,22]. Only one therapy for a diabetic complication of any kind is approved by the FDA, and few therapies, if any, are presently nearing the approval stage.

Table 47-2
Selected Differences in Pharmaceutical Regulation between the European Union and the United States

Aspect	United States	Europe
Typical level of ethical review	Institutional	Community or region
Level of review	Raw data	Reports and summaries
Standard control group	Placebo	Active treatment
Size of regulatory authority	Very large	Small
Basis of authority	Federal	Multinational and transnational
Economic considerations	Excluded from licensing process	Reflected in the kinds of studies that are required for licensing
Emphasis used in assuring data integrity	Verification that reported data match data in source documents	Evaluation of all systems and procedures involved in recording and handling data
Public access to data and basis of decision making	Limited only to proprietary information	Limited to expert and regulatory summaries

Examples are provided of typical differences in perspective and/or practice between Europe and the United States. Exceptions to these typical characterisations abound. Europe itself is not monolithic in its regulation and development of therapies.

Captopril (Capoten™ , Bristol-Myers Squibb Co.), an angiotensin converting enzyme inhibitor (ACEI) originally approved for treatment of hypertension was approved in early 1994 by the FDA for treatment of diabetic nephropathy [23]. The approval was based largely on results of a double-blind, placebo-controlled clinical trial that involved 409 patients at 30 centers in the United States and Canada. Captopril treatment was associated with a 50 percent reduction in the combined risk of death or of kidney failure requiring dialysis or a transplant compared to placebo. The trial was conducted in patients with type 1 diabetes who had proteinuria (24 hour urinary excretion >500 mg) and retinopathy. Subsequent trials have since demonstrated a benefit of captopril on progression to overt proteinuria in patients with 20-200 microgram/min. Thus, ACEI therapy has become standard therapy for patients with proteinuria of any degree in type 1 and 2 patients even though the original lower limit for proteinuria of 500 mg has not been modified in Captopril's approved indication. Moreover, ACEI therapy has become an attractive choice for treating hypertension uncomplicated by proteinuria in patients with diabetes largely because of the anticipation that this therapy will forestall the development of renal dysfunction as well as provide some other benefits [24].

Captopril's efficacy is substantial, but provides only about half that needed to completely forestall this complication. Complementary therapeutic approaches should be pursued to fully avert the development of nephropathy. Because captopril has become a standard therapy, the development of new therapies will be more challenging. The therapeutic window for subsequent treatments is considerably smaller since no nephropathy trial can be ethically conducted without ACEI therapy. For example, captopril therapy itself might fall short of producing statistically significant treatment effects in the same trials on which approval was based if a comparably effective background therapy had been used by most of the patients in the trial.

The other major obstacle for development of additional therapies aimed at preventing nephropathy is the strong secular trend in risk factor reduction for this complication. Improved glycemic and blood lipid control, decreased smoking, earlier detection and treatment of microalbuminuria all serve to lower the rate of progression to renal dysfunction and ESRD. Thus, the absolute treatment effect being pursued in the development of new therapies continues to shrink. It should be recognized, however, that a substantial number of patients will progress to disabling nephropathy despite the use of captopril therapy and all other currently recognized interventions. Captopril itself is not risk free. This therapy is recognized to cause anaphylactic-like reactions, angioedema, neutropenia/agranulocytosis, and increased proteinuria with occasional nephrotic syndrome. For all these reasons, additional anti-nephropathic therapies, particularly those that can be used preventatively in a general population, are very much needed.

AMINOGUANDINE: A CASE STUDY OF THERAPEUTIC DEVELOPMENT

The understanding led by Cerami, Brownlee and others that chronic exposure to high glucose concentration results in chemical modification of proteins has resulted in a major therapeutic target for preventing and treating diabetic complications. Cerami's sentinel work in this area also resulted in the identification of glycated hemoglobin (hemoglobin A_{1c}) as a diagnostic tool of immense importance not only to clinical therapeutics but to the development of therapies for glycemic control [25].

Aminoguanidine (Pimagedine, Alteon) is the first anti-glycation compound to be evaluated in clinical trials. Pimagedine has been shown to inhibit the formation of glycation end products (AGEs), which are strongly implicated in the development of micro- and macrovascular complications. Although the protective effects of pimagedine appear to be predominantly mediated by a reduction in pathologic glycation [26], this compound also functions as an inhibitor of nitric oxide synthase and oxidative stress, which are potential contributing factors to the development of tissue damage in diabetic patients [27]. In animal models of diabetes and diabetic complications, treatment with pimagedine resulted in the prevention or reduction of retinopathy [28,29] and the amelioration of albuminuria [30]. Pimagedine also prolonged the survival of diabetic rats made azotemic by renal ablation, suggesting that it has protective effects even in cases of existing renal damage [31]. Moreover, Pimagedine has demonstrated potential benefits against macroangiopathy, including anti-atherogenic effects in cholesterol-fed rabbits [32] and reduced infarct volume in a rat model of focal cerebral ischemia [33].

In a double-blind, placebo-controlled, 28-day trial, circulating hemoglobin advanced glycation end-products (AGE) levels were reduced significantly (by approximately 28%) in patients receiving an average dose of 1200 mg/day Pimagedine in contrast to no significant change in those receiving placebo [34]. To assess the efficacy of Pimagedine in diabetic patients with microvascular complications, three pivotal clinical trials have been initiated in North America. ACTION I (A Clinical Trial In Overt Nephropathy) was conducted in 690 patients with type 1 diabetes [35]. The results of ACTION I suggest that Pimagedine could provide important benefits to patients with early diabetic nephropathy. The treatment effect on time to doubling in serum creatinine, the pre-defined primary outcome measure, did not reach statistical significance. However, the study does provide other evidence that this therapy improves renal function. Reduction in proteinuria is the most compelling finding. Many experts may accept the treatment effect on proteinuria itself as a reflection of a significant clinical benefit. Statistically significant reductions in LDL cholesterol, and triglycerides, as well as lowered diastolic blood pressure were also seen. In addition, the data indicated favorable outcomes in measures of renal function, including creatinine clearance and filtration rate, as well as in the inhibition of the progression of retinopathy.

ACTION II was conducted in 599 patients with type 2 diabetes. However, an external monitoring committee recommended the discontinuation of this trial because of an insufficient risk/benefit ratio based upon data currently available at that time [36]. A third multicenter trial of patients with early diabetic nephropathy was undertaken in Europe, but was canceled due to slow enrollment and difficulty maintaining a placebo group. Finally, enrollment is also in progress for a trial of Pimagedine in type 1 and type 2 diabetic patients with end stage renal disease.

The development of Pimagedine therapy illustrates many of the principles expressed in the first part of this chapter. For example, the developers of this therapy evaluated the preclinical data and other considerations prior to making a decision about which therapeutic applications should be targeted. This therapy could conceivably be of value for a wide variety of conditions including aging itself. Pimagedine's developers decided that the condition for which the projected benefit to risk relationship was most acceptable is the prevention of progression from overt, but mild diabetic nephropathy to end stage renal failure. From the preclinical data, Pimagedine therapy could be seen to have some real and theoretical risks that would not be as well tolerated for conditions for which patients were at less risk from the disease itself. The choice of the patient population was influenced by other important considerations including the event rate for primary outcomes and the biology of the disease and the intervention itself. These considerations would determine the size and duration of the trial.

The designs of the major Pimagedine nephropathy studies reflected considerable confidence in this therapeutic approach. These sizable, very long, and costly studies were designed to definitively (as much as is possible to do prior to marketing) demonstrate the benefit risk relationship of the therapy. The developers had clear direction for designing the study. They drew on the model of the captopril study, which had been used to successfully win a nephropathy indication for that drug. Disappointingly, the primary outcome results fell just short of achieving statistical significance in ACTION I. Why? The relatively small effect on general renal function and progression to end-stage renal disease is clearly related to the originally unanticipated, almost universal use of captopril therapy by patients in this trial. This illustrates a hazard for any long-term trial. The imposition of a new standard background therapy during the course of a trial, just as occurred in this case, decreases the absolute magnitude of efficacy that can be achieved in the trial. Use of a background therapy undermines the biostatistical power of a trial to demonstrate a treatment effect of the new therapy. The data suggest that Pimagedine, as monotherapy would have about the same effects on renal function and proteinuria as captopril. Similarly, captopril would likely be shown to have marginal efficacy if it were re-examined as add-on therapy to background Pimagedine treatment.

The Pimagedine situation presents some regulatory quandaries. The ACTION I trial failed to obtain statistical significance in the primary outcome, but an over all reading of the trial results as well as the circumstances of the trial would suggest to most experts that the therapy is efficacious. However, the FDA expects that the primary outcome will be convincingly affected by the new therapy in order to approve it. Picking other outcomes in a non pre-specified way after the trial is completed is considered an exploratory approach that requires subsequent confirmation. The other major problem for Pimagedine is that the second trial, ACTION II, was intended to confirm the results of ACTION I. The two studies together would meet the FDA's "well controlled trials" requirement. Though in retrospect the lack of positive outcomes in ACTION II can be explained (patients had more advance disease and the presence of other co-morbidities), this leaves Pimagedine with at most one positive study. What are the sponsor and the FDA to do with results that fall short after a very large investment and good faith effort to provide a therapy that is much needed? One possible approach is discussed in the following section.

Until now, the clinical discussion of Pimagedine has been confined to therapeutic efficacy. Demonstrating effectiveness is only half the challenge for the developers of Pimagedine or any other therapy. To receive regulatory approval, the risks of the therapy have to be defined and the relationship of these risks to the benefits provided by the therapy has to be acceptable. Significant toxicity has been associated with Pimagedine therapy in ACTION I. The most notable observation was of crescentic glomerulonephritis associated with high anti-neutrophil cytoplasmic antibodies in three patients treated with the high dose of Pimagedine. No such cases were seen in the lower dose group, and the low dose treatment appears to provide benefits comparable to those achieved in the high dose group. Furthermore, what would appear to be a reliable monitoring procedure has been identified for discontinuing therapy before this syndrome can develop. A transient flu-like syndrome and mild anemia were also associated with therapy [37]. Because of the much increased danger from macrovascular complications faced by patients with overt nephropathy who progress to end stage renal disease, these risks from Pimagedine therapy may yet be acceptable. Some account must also be made of the fact that captopril itself is not without its own risks and cannot be used by every patient who is at high risk for developing end stage renal disease. Ultimately, it is the responsibility of the review scientists at the FDA and other regulatory authorities to weigh these considerations and determine whether the therapy should be approved or not and what additional information will be required in either case.

SURROGATES FOR DIABETIC NEPHROPATHY

As discussed above, regulatory authorities should appropriately modify requirements for therapeutic approval as scientific understanding evolves. These and other considerations ought to be taken into account in adjusting the requirements for therapies aimed at prevention and treatment of diabetic nephropathy. One possible approach is the use of well-accepted surrogate outcomes. Proteinuria is the leading candidate for this role in the case of Pimagedine and other therapies for nephropathy. In the original captopril trial, protein excretion was reduced by 30% in the first 3 months of captopril therapy, this reduction was maintained for the rest of the trial, and the effect on proteinuria correlated with the primary efficacy outcomes. A large body of evidence now supports the view that excreted protein itself is a tubular toxin [38]. Some experts now regard proteinuria as not only a reflection of dysfunction for all glomerulopathies, but as one of the common etiologic pathways on which all these diseases converge [39-44]. In streptozotocin-induced diabetic rats, the albuminuric-lowering effects of both Pimagidine and ACEI have recently been associated with normalisation of glomerular protein kinase C. These data suggest that despite entirely different mechanisms of action, the renoprotective effects of these agents likewise converge at a common biochemical pathway [45]. Reduction of protein excretion regardless of cause could thereby be justified as a therapeutic objective [46]. By extension, protein excretion could be accepted as a reasonable surrogate if not outright clinical outcome on which a nephropathy indication could be based. The FDA has also implemented a provision for, in effect, provisionally approving a life saving therapy on the basis of one or more surrogate outcomes. As a condition of approval, the sponsor is obligated to finish or conduct a study in the post-approval period, which confirms the therapy's clinical benefit.

If the FDA will accept that proteinuria is in itself a clinically relevant beneficial outcome, as many experts will now testify, then the Agency should be willing to accept that a second pivotal Pimagedine trial could be run with proteinuria as the primary outcome. Such a trial could be expected to show a treatment difference in this outcome in 6-12 months. Acceptance of a relatively short study as a second pivotal trial would be a reasonable adjustment in agency expectations given the need for additional anti-nephropathic therapies and the implausibility of conducting a repetition of the ACTION I study. In essence, an additional short term trial with proteinuria as the primary efficacy endpoint would serve as the second pivotal study. This second trial could also be continued long enough to assess a clinical endpoint, e.g., creatinine clearance or time to dialysis. Clearly, it would be very difficult to continue a control group beyond approval, but the controlled trial could be extended up to the time of approval. That might result in data from up to 18 to 24 months' additional experience and possibly a confirmation of preserved creatinine clearance as approval comes. Other confirmatory approaches could be considered. Following the original treated cohorts using historical comparisons might suffice to confirm that Pimagedine therapy ultimately provides clinical benefits though the shortcomings of this approach are well know.

Those with a more conservative perspective will still insist that developers of new therapies be required to show effects on the same kind of outcomes like time to doubling of serum creatinine and progression to End stage renal disease (ESRD) studied in the captopril. Though some evaluators within FDA may hold this view, senior FDA officials have informally indicated willingness to accept biostatistically significant treatment effects on renal function such as creatinine clearance, as sufficient for justifying approval. None of these approaches is practical for developing therapies for prevention or earlier intervention. Because of the accumulation of important, unsettled issues for developing nephropathy therapies, the FDA should hold an advisory committee hearing to provide resolution and clarity in this therapeutic area.

LONG-TERM SAFETY ISSUES

Evaluation of therapeutic safety has been discussed above, but further emphasis is warranted about the challenge of defining safety for therapies that will be used chronically. In the wake of a half dozen withdrawals of therapies from the U.S. market recently, a public debate continues about how soon therapies should be approved. The idiosyncratic hepatotoxicity that has plagued troglitazone, an insulin sensitizer for type 2 diabetes, is a good example of a very significant though relatively uncommon therapeutic safety problem that did not become clear until well after the therapy was widely used. Therapies that are developed for preventing development or progression of diabetic nephropathy carry this risk particularly when they entail unselective mechanisms of action or multiple biologic responses.

The primary responsibility for demonstrating safety is borne by the sponsor. The regulatory authorities play important supporting, evaluative, and verifying roles. The sponsor's and FDA's evaluation of therapeutic safety comes down to listening for and responding to signals. The word *signal* used in this context is meant to embrace the entire spectrum of information that bears on the risks or disadvantages of therapies. On one end of this spectrum are the cases of highly distinctive toxicities associated with virtually no other treatment and accepted by everyone as drug-induced or likely to be drug-induced. Choramphenicol's association with aplastic anemia is well known. Phenformin-induced lactic acidosis is another good example, though it took years of marketing before the relationship was detected [47]. The other end of the spectrum includes vague theoretical possibilities as well as single case reports of common adverse events associated with long-marketed therapies. There is less difficulty in dealing with the issues at the extremes of this spectrum. The largest challenge is to deal with the signals in the middle of the spectrum. It is these signals that may ultimately reflect effects that have huge consequences in the aggregate, such as was revealed by the CAST experience and could have not been appreciated without a controlled trial.

CONCLUSIONS

Of diabetic microvascular complications, nephropathy is the most important in terms of mortality and economic impact. Diabetic nephropathy is the most common cause of end stage renal disease and dialysis dependency in the industrialized world. The importance of this disorder and the rapidly expanding knowledge about its pathophysiology warrant the attention that it has been shown in this book and numerous other efforts. Clearly, much remains to be accomplished. The concerted efforts of patients, clinicians, academicians, therapeutic developers, regulators, and politicians are necessary to achieve effective preventions and treatments within the next decade.

REFERENCES

1. See: A. S. C. Ross, *The Assize of Bread*, Economic History Review, Second Series, vol. 9, 332-42, 1956.
2. R. Temple. Development of Drug Law, Regulations, and Guidance in the United States. In Principles of Pharmacology, Basic Concepts and Clinical Applications, Revised Reprint. Pp 1643-1664. Editor Paul L. Munson with Co-editors Robert A. Mueller and George R. Bresse. Chapman and Hall, New York, 1994
3. R. E. McFadyen, *Thalidomide in America: A Brush with Tragedy*. Clio Medica : 11, no. 2, 79-93, 1976.
4- United States Food, Drug, and Cosmetic Act: Section 505(d).
5. Guidance for Industry Providing Clinical Evidence of Effectiveness for Human Drugs and Biological Products Additional copies are available from: the Drug Information Branch (HFD- 210), Center for Drug Evaluation and Research (CDER), 5600 Fishers Lane, Rockville, MD 20857.
6. Prescription Drug Users Fee Act of 1992; United States Public Law Number 102-57, 106 Stat. 4491, October 29, 1992.

7.   R. Sheila, S. Kaitin, K. Kaitin, the Prescription Drug User Fee Act of 1992: A 5-year experiment for industry and the FDA, Pharmacoeconomics 121: 126, 1996.

8.   Food And Drug Administration Moderization Act Of 1997; United States Public Law Number 105-15, 111 Stat. 2296, Page 2295 October 1, 1997.

9.   R.Temple, *Development of Drug law, Regulations, and Guidance in the United States.*

10.   B. Barton, and G.A. Fleming, *Good Clinical Practice: Any Changes Expected in the USA?* Drug Information Journal, 28: 1115-1117, 1994

11.   J. Showalter,   International Conference on Harmonization. The Journal of Biology & Business 1(2): 90-93.

12.   G.A.Fleming, *Beyond Drug Evaluation: The Science of Drug Evaluation, Molecular Medicine* 2:5, 1996.

13.   S.J.Pocock. Clinical trials: a Practical Approach. John Wiley, New York, 1983.

14.   L.M. Friedman, C.D. Furberg, D.L. DeMets. Fundamentals of Clincial Trials. Second Edition. PSG, Boston, 1985.

15.   R. Temple. A regulatory authority's opinion about surrogate endpoints. In Nimmo WS, Tucker GT, eds. Clinical Measurement in Drug Evaluation. Vol. 3, p. 21. Chichester: John Wiley and Sons, Ltd, 1995.

16.   R. Temple. Difficulties in evaluating positive control trials. Proceedings of the American Statistical Association, Biopharmaceutical Section, 1983.

17.   The Cardiac Arrhythmia Suppression Trial Investigators. Effect of the anti-arrhythmic moricizine on survival after myocardial infarction. New England Journal of Medicine. 327: 227-233, 1992.

18.   L. B. Sheiner. Learning versus confirming in clinical drug development. J Clin Pharm Ther, 61(3):275-291, 1997

19.   G.A. Fleming. American Heart Journal 138: S338-S345, 1999

20.   G.A. Fleming, S. Jhee, R. Coniff, H. Riordan, M. Murphy, N. Kurtz, N.Cutler. *In Optimizing Therapeutic Development in Diabetes.* Greenwich Medica Media, London, pp. 47-60, 1999.

21.   The Sorbinil Retinopathy Trial Research Group: A randomized trial of sorbinil, an aldose reductase inhibitor in diabetic retinopathy, Arch Ophthalmol 108:1234-1244, 1990.

22.   M. Foppiano, G. Lombardo,   Worldwide pharmacovigilance systems and tolrestat withdrawal. Lancet 1997; 349: 399-400.

23.   E.J. Lewis, L.G. Hunsicker, R.P. Bain, & R.D. Rohde, for the Collaborative Study Group. The effect of angiotensin-converting-enzyme inhibition on diabetic nephropathy. New England Journal of Medicine,329(20):1456-1462, 1993.

24.   Heart Outcomes Prevention Evaluation (HOPE) Study Investigator. Effects of ramipril on cardiovascular and microvascular outcomes in people with diabetes mellitus: results of the HOPE study and MICRO-HOPE substudy Lancet 355, 253-259, 2000.

25.   G.A. Fleming, S,Jhee, R. Coniff, H,Riordan, M. Murphy, N. Kurtz, N. Cutler. In Optimizing Therapeutic Development in Diabetes. Greenwich Medica Media, London, pp. ix-x, 1999.

26.   T. Soulis-Liparota, M, Cooper, D. Papazoglou, B. Clarke, G. Jerums. Retardation by aminouanidine of development of albuminuria, mesangial expansion, and tissue fluorescense in streptozotocin-induced diabetic rat. Diabetes 40(10): 1328-1334.

27. C.W. Yang, C.C.Yu, Y.C. Ko, C.C. Huang. Aminoguanidine reduces glomerular inducible nitric oxide synthase (iNOS) and transforming growth factor-beta 1 (TGF_beta 1) mRNA expression and diminshes glomerulosclerosis in NZB/W F1 mice. Clin Exp Immunol 1998; 113(2): 258-264.

28. H.P.Hammes, M. Brownlee, D. Edelstein, M. Saleck, S. Martin, K. Federlin. Aminoguanidine inhibits the development of accelerated diabetic retinopathy in the spontaneous hypertensive rat. Diabetologia 1994; 37(1):32-35.

29. H.P. Hammes, D. Strodter , A. Weiss, R.G. Bretzel, K. Federlin, M. Brownlee. Secondary intervention with aminoguanidine retards the progression of diabetic retinopathy in the rat model. Diabetologia 1995; 38(6): 656-660.

30. D. Edelstein, M. Brownlee,. Aminoguanidine ameliorates albuminuria in diabetic hypertensive rats. Diabetologia 1992; 35(1): 96-97.

31. E.A. Friedman, D.A. Distant, J.F. Fleishhacker, T.A. Boyd, K. Cartwright. Aminoguanidine prolongs survival in azotemic-induced diabetic rats. AM J Kidney Dis 1997; 30(2): 253-259.

32. S. Panagiotopoulos, R.C. O'Brien, R. Bucala, M.E. Cooper, G. Jerums.. Aminoguanidine has an anti-atherogenic effect in the cholesterol-fed rabbit. Atherosclerosis 1998; 136(1): 125-131.

33. G.A. Zimmerman, M. Meistrell 3rd, O. Bloom, K.M.Cockroft, M. Bianchi, D. Risucci, J. Broome, P. Farmer, A. Cerami, H. Vlassara, et al. Neurotoxicity of advanced glycation endproducts during focal stroke and neuroprotective effects of aminoguanidine. Proc Natl Acad Sci USA 1994; 92(9): 3744-3748.

34. Makita Z, Vlassara H, Rayfield E, Cartwright K, Friedman E, Rodby R, Cerami A, Bucala R, Hemoglobin-AGE: a circulating marker of advanced glycosylation. Science 1992: 258(5082): 651-653.

35. G. Appel, K. Bolton , B. Freedman, J-P. Wuerth, K. Cartwright. Pimagedine (PG) Lowers Total Urinary Protein (TUP) and Slows Progression of Overt Diabetic Nephropathy in Patients with Type 1 Diabetes Mellitus. Abstract: American Society of Nephropathy Annual Meeting [A0786] 1999.

36. Script No.2320. Side Effects with Alteon's pimagedine. March 25, 1998, p. 24.

37. F. Whittier, B. Spinowitz, J-P. Wuerth, K. Cartwright. Pimagedine safety profile in patients with type I diabetes mellitus. Abstract: American Society of Nephropathy Annual Meeting [A0941] 1999.

38. M.E. Thomas, N.J. Brunskill, K.P. Harris, E Bailey, J.H. Pringle, P.N. Furness, J. Walls Proteinuria induces tubular cell turnover: A potential mechanism for tubular atrophy. Kidney International: 55(3):890-8. 1999.

39. The GISEN Group (Gruppo Italiano di Studi Epidemiologici in Nefrologia. Randomised placebo-controlled trial of effect of ramipril on decline in glomerular filtration rate and risk of terminal renal failure in proteinuric, non-diabetic nephropathy Lancet 349: 1857-63, 1997.

40. P.L. Kimmel, G.J. Mishkin, W.O. Umana. Captopril and renal survival in patients with human immunodeficiency virus nephropathy. American Journal Of Kidney Diseases 28: 202-8, 1996.

41. S.Wakai, K. Nitta, K. Honda, S. Horita, H Kobayashi, K.Uchida, W.Yumura, H. Nihei. Relationship between glomerular epithelial cell injury and proteinuria in IgA nephropathy. Nippon Jinzo Gakkai Shi 40(5):315-21, 1998.

42.   F. Locatelli, D. Marcelli, M. Comelli, D. Alberti, G. Graziani, G. Buccianti, B. Redaelli, A. Giangrande. Proteinuria and blood pressure as causal components of progression to end-stage renal failure. Northern Italian Cooperative Study Group. Nephrology Dialysis Transplant, 11(3):461-7, 1996.

43.   G. Remuzzi. Renoprotective Effect of ACE Inhibitors: Dissecting the Molecular Clues and Expanding the Blood Pressure Goal. American Journal of Kidney Diseases 34: 951-954. 1999

44.   K. Sharma, B.O. Eltayeb, T.A. McGowan, et al. Captopril induced reduction of serum levels of transforming growth factor-ß1 correlates with long-term renoprotection in insulin-dependent diabetic patients. American Jounal of Kidney Disease 34:818-823, 1999

45.   T.M. Osicka, Y. Yu, S Panagiotopoulos, et al. Prevention of albuminuria by aminoguanidine or ramipril in streptozoticin-induced diabetic rats is associated with the normalization of glomerular protein kinase C. Diabetes 49: 87-93, 2000.

46.   W.F. Keane, G. Eknoyan. Proteinuria, Albuminuria, Risk, Assessment, Detection, Elimination (PARADE): A Position Paper of the National Kidney Foundation American Journal of Kidney Disease 33:1004-1010, 1999.

47.   Califano J. Order of the Secretary, U.S. Department of Health, Education and Welfare, Suspending Approval. Re: New Drug Applications for Phenformin: NDA 11-624, NDA 12-752, NDA 17-127; 17 July, 1977. Phenformin: removal from general market. FDA Drug Bulletin 7(3):14-16, 1997.

NOTES

1)   Thalidomide was not approved by the FDA until July, 1998, for the treatment of the debilitating and disfiguring lesions associated with erythema nodosum leprosum (ENL), a complication of Hansen's Disease, commonly known as leprosy. The approval carried stringent measures to minimize use during pregnancy.

2)   http://www.fda.gov/cder

3)   Biostatistical significance does not directly equate to clinical meaningfulness. A highly statistically significant effect can theoretically be reached with a treatment effect that is not clinically meaningful, especially if large numbers of patients are studied. However, when the primary efficacy outcome(s) and the biostatistical plan for the registration grade studies have been prospectively stated by the sponsor and agreed to by the FDA, an outcome with a significance level of $p<.05$ is implicitly understood if not explicitly stated to indicate a clinically meaningful effect. Frequently, the sponsor, with the FDA's concurrence, will state the magnitude of a clinically meaningful effect *a priori*. The study is then sized to provide a stated probability that the study will, at a stated p value, be able to reject the null hypothesis (i.e. exclude that the demonstrated treatment effect is less than that considered to be clinically meaningful).

48. THE RENIN ANGIOTENSIN SYSTEM IN THE PAHTOGENESIS OF DIABETIC COMPLICATIONS

Bryan Williams, MD FRCP
Professor of Medicine, University of Leicester School of Medicine, Clinical Sciences Building, Leicester Royal Infirmary, PO Box 65 Leicester, UK.

INTRODUCTION

The Renin Angiotensin System (RAS) is traditionally viewed as an endocrine system primarily involved in the regulation of systemic blood pressure and salt and water homeostasis. However, angiotensin II, the effector molecule of the RAS has many actions beyond its effects on blood pressure regulation. In this regard, the actions of angiotensin II can be viewed as either haemodynamic or non-haemodynamic and in many instances these actions are complementary or synergistic in their capacity to cause tissue injury. Moreover, the concept of angiotensin-mediated haemodynamic and non-haemodynamic actions has led to the hypothesis that therapeutic inhibition of the RAS may provide protection of vulnerable target organs beyond that expected of blood pressure alone, largely via the inhibition of the non-haemodynamic actions of angiotensin II.

This chapter will briefly overview the RAS and then focus on the many actions of angiotensin II and their potential relevance to the pathogenesis of diabetic complications including nephropathy and retinopathy.

OVERVIEW OF THE RENIN ANGIONTENSIN SYSTEM

The classic renin-angiotensin system is viewed as an endocrine system in which renin is secreted by the juxtaglomerular apparatus within the kidney and acts on its specific substrate angiotensinogen, produced by the liver, to generate Ang I. The Ang I is then acted on by angiotensin converting enzyme (ACE), predominantly within the pulmonary circulation, to generate Ang II. Ang I and II are subsequently degraded by various enzyme systems to yield angiotensin [1-7], Ang III or Ang IV (Fig 48-1) [1].

Renin is 38kDa aspartyl protease that shows high substrate specificity for angiotensinogen and is produced by smooth muscle like cells (the macula densa) within a unique anatomical structure adjacent to renal glomeruli; the juxtaglomerular apparatus (JGA). Within the JGA, renin is produced as a 45kDa pre-prorenin and released as renin after a two stage cleavage of the signal sequence and the prosegement. Renin secretion from the kidney is influenced by many factors such as; renal nerve activity (increased sympathetic nerve activity increases renin release) , renal perfusion pressure (renal ischaemia increases renin release), sodium balance (decreased renal distal tubular delivery of sodium increases renin release and *vice versa*) and various hormones, including Ang II (increased Ang II suppresses renin release).

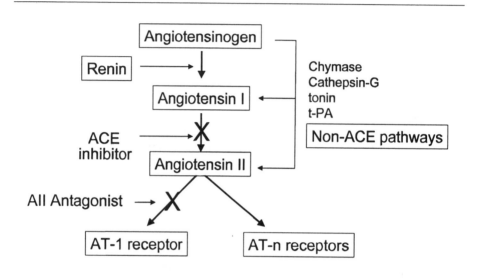

Figure 48-1. The classical and alternative pathways for Angiotensin II generation

Angiotensinogen is a 60 kDa protein and is the only substrate from which Ang II is ultimately generated. Angiotensinogen is predominantly produced in the liver but it is also expressed in many other tissues including; brain, fat, heart, kidney, lung and fibroblasts. Renin acts on angiotensinogen to release Ang I. This molecule has little biological activity and primarily functions as the precursor peptide for the generation of Ang II via the action of ACE.

Angiotensin Converting Enzyme (ACE) is a zinc metalloproteinase that cleaves two peptides (histidine and leucine) from the carboxy terminal end of the decapeptide Ang I to yield the octapeptide Ang II. However, it is important to note that the actions of ACE are not specific for Ang I. ACE, also termed kininase II, is involved in the enzymatic inactivation of bradykinin. Thus, the therapeutic inhibition of ACE will not only decrease the production of Ang II, it will also inhibit the degradation of bradykinin and other peptides normally subject to kininase II degradation ie. substance P, neurokinins, and leutinising hormone. The potentiation of kinins by ACE-inhibition may have clinical effects via the hypothetical beneficial actions of bradykinin on the vascular endothelium and the undesirable induction of a dry irritating cough in a significant number of patients treated with ACE-inhibitors.

THE CONCEPT OF A TISSUE RENIN ANGIOTENSIN SYSTEM

The aforementioned classical RAS implies that the majority of angiotensin II is generated within the vascular compartment. Considerable evidence suggests, however, that angiotensin II can also be generated within the extravascular compartment, ie. locally within tissues [1,2]. This has given rise to the concept of a "circulating" and a "tissue" RAS. Most of the essential elements of the RAS (ie. renin and angiotensinogen) can be detected and synthesised in many tissues, and there is evidence that the expression and activity of the RAS in these various tissues may be "locally" and independently regulated. This may be particularly important in tissues such as the kidney (see N Hollenberg chapter) in which high levels of angiotensin Ii are generated. Moreover, in such tissues, inhibition of systemic angiotensin II production does not necessarily imply inhibition of tissue angiotensin II production. This may have important implications if locally generated angiotensin II is important in the pathogenesis of tissue injury in diabetes.

MULTIPLE PATHWAYS OF ANGIOTENSIN II GENERATION

It is now clear that the RAS is not the only mechanism whereby Ang II can be generated from angiotensinogen. Various non-renin angiotensinogenases exist that are capable of generating both Ang I and Ang II directly from angiotensinogen, without involvement of renin or ACE. These enzymes include: i) A chymostatin Ang II generating enzyme (CAGE) that can locally generate appreciable quantities of Ang II from angiotensinogen. ii) Chymases (serine proteinases), many of which have been identified in various human tissues including the heart. iii) Other enzymes not traditionally considered to be relevant to the RAS, ie. tissue plasminogen activator, cathepsin G and tonin, also have the capacity to generate Ang II directly from angiotensinogen without involvement of renin or ACE (Fig.48-2) [1]. Once again, this concept may be important from a therapeutic perspective as it is most unlikely that total blockade of angiotensin II production can be achieved by ACE-inhibition alone.

ANGIOTENSIN II RECEPTORS

The emergence of highly selecetive and specific angiotensin II receptor antagonists along with molecular cloning of the angiotensin II receptors has led to a tremendous interest and growth in our knowledge about the function and complexity of the angiotensin II receptors [3]. A full review of the angiotensin II receptors is outside the scope of this chapter, suffice it to say that; at least four sub-types of the angiotensin II receptor exist ($_{AT1-4}$). Two main Ang II receptor subtypes have been classified in man; AT_1 and AT_2. AT_1 receptors have a classic peptide receptor structure with seven transmembrane spanning helices, coupled to G-proteins (G_i and G_q) for intracellular signalling. AT_1 receptors are widely distributed and almost all of the recognised cardiovascular actions of Ang II cited below appear to be mediated via the AT_1 receptor. The function of the AT_2 receptor is less well delineated although this receptor is not as ubiquitously expressed as the AT_1 receptor and is often only transiently expressed during tissue development and repair suggesting it may have a role in cell growth regulation.

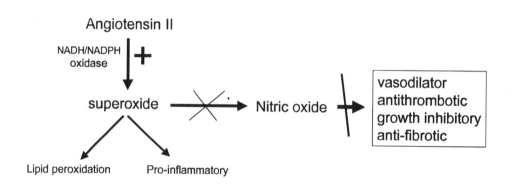

Figure 2: The effect of angiotensin II-induced superoxide production via NADH/NADPH oxidase: Quenching of nitric oxide, lipid peroxidation and a pro-inflammatory stimulus.

BIOLOGICAL ACTIONS OF ANGIOTENSIN II

Ang II-induced cell contraction:
Ang II contracts vascular smooth muscle and induces vasoconstriction. There is variability in the sensitivity of different vascular beds to Ang-II induced vasoconstriction; renal and mesenteric beds being the most sensitive and arteries being more sensitive than veins. Angiotensin II also contracts glomerular mesangial cells and thus can directly influence the glomerular surface area for filtration. Ang II also acts synergistically with other vasoconstrictors ie. arginine vasopressin (AVP) and noradrenaline to induce vaso- or glomerular constriction. Thus, Ang II increases vasoconstriction directly and also potentiates the vasoconstrictor actions of AVP and the sympathetic nervous system. .

Ang II-induced Cell Growth:
Ang II is a growth factor for vascular smooth muscle cells, cardiac myocytes and glomerular mesangial cells [4,5]. Angiotensin II also promotes the synthesis and release of potent vascular smooth muscle cell and mesangial cell mitogens such as platelet derived growth factor (PDGF) which may mediate some of its growth promoting actions. Not surprisingly therefore, Ang II has been implicated in the pathogenesis of abnormal cardiovascular growth responses leading to: i) remodelling of resistance vessels thereby perpetuating a chronic increase in peripheral vascular resistance and blood pressure, ii) left ventricular hypertrophy and remodelling, and iii) intimal hyperplasia.

Ang II-induced Matrix synthesis:
Increased vascular and renal matrix deposition is the hallmark of diabetic vascular and glomerular disease. Angiotensin II stimulates increased matrix protein synthesis in blood vessels, the heart and the glomerular mesangium [6,7]. Matrix accumulation in these sites has important consequences, leading to reduced vascular compliance, impaired cardiac function (particularly diastolic dysfunction) and glomerulosclerosis. It seems likely that Ang II-induced matrix accumulation in these sites is due, at least in part, to stimulation of TGFβ production - a potent cytokine involved in the regulation of matrix accumulation. Moreover, Ang II receptors have been identified on cardiac fibroblasts suggesting that it may be directly involved in the regulation of matrix synthesis. Furthermore, Ang II stimulates the release of aldosterone which has also been implicated in the pathogenesis of cardiovascular and renal matrix accumulation.

The effects Angiotensin II on Endothelial function:
The vascular endothelium plays a key role in regulating cardiovascular and renal function and growth [8]. It produces powerful vasoconstrictor and growth promoting substances such as Endothelin-1, and vasodilator substances such as nitric oxide (NO), bradykinin, prostacyclin (PGI$_2$) and endothelial derived hyperpolarising factor (EDHF). In health, there is low level constitutive production of NO, maintaining a state of active vasodilatation and anti-proliferation. In many cardiovascular disorders, including hypertension, diabetes and renal failure, the function and/or integrity of the endothelium is disturbed. This disturbance is characterised by increased endothelial permeability to albumin and other macromolecules, decreased production and/or increased destruction of NO and the development of a pro-thrombotic endothelial surface. These developments are key to the subsequent pathogenesis of cardiovascular and renal complications in patients with diabetes and hypertension.

Angiotensin II has the potential to influence many key aspects of endothelial function, including: NO and Endothelin-1 (ET-1) production, endothelial permeability and endothelial growth ie. angiogenesis.

Ang II, Nitric Oxide destruction and Superoxide production:
NO has very important actions on cardiovascular and renal function. These actions include; i) Regulation of vascular tone, blood pressure and regional blood flow via its vasorelaxing action on vascular smooth muscle. ii) A direct antiproliferative action on

vascular smooth muscle and glomerular mesangial cells (hence increased vascular smooth muscle or glomerular mesangial proliferation when the endothelium is dysfunctional or damaged). iii) Potent antithrombotic actions by inhibiting platelet adhesion to the endothelium.

NO is constitutively produced by the endothelium via the enzyme nitric oxide synthase (NOS) but is labile with a half life of only a few seconds. Ang II may directly influence NO levels by inducing the production of superoxide radicals. Angiotensin II acting via AT_1 receptors activates a NADP/NADPH oxidase in vascular smooth muscle and glomerular mesangial cells [9,10]. This enzyme generates superoxide which inactivates NO and increases lipid peroxidation.

Thus Ang II acting via the AT_1 receptor could potentially induce endothelial dysfunction by enhancing NO destruction by reactive oxygen species. This is a very important concept with regard to the role of angiotensin II in the development of diabetic vascular complications. There is compelling evidence of increased oxidant stress associated with the diabetic state and increased consumption of antioxidant activity [11]. The pro-oxidant properties of angiotensin II will serve to further stress the antioxidant reserve of cardiovascular and renal tissues. This will in turn remove one of the main natural restraints to local growth factors (ie. NO) and thereby exacerbate tissue injury. In my view, this is potentially the most important mechanism whereby angiotensin II may be particularly toxic to vascular and renal cells in patients with diabetes mellitus (figure 48-2].

Ang II and Endothelial Permeability:
Ang II has been implicated in the pathogenesis of increased endothelial permeability, another important manifestation of endothelial dysfunction in patients with diabetes. Ang II increases the production of vascular endothelial growth factor (VEGF) by human vascular smooth muscle via the AT_1 receptor [12]. VEGF is one of the most potent vascular permeabilising factors thus far identified and a powerful angiogenic peptide that has been strongly implicated in the pathogenesis of microangiopathy in diabetes mellitus [13-16].

Ang II and Endothelial Proliferation/Angiogenesis:
The proliferation of endothelial cells and the development of new microvessels is the hallmark of diabetic microangiopathy. Angiotensin II directly stimulates cultured endothelial proliferation, seemingly via the AT_1 receptor. Furthermore, Ang II-induced VEGF production via the AT_1 (see above) may also be important in the regulation of endothelial growth, angiogenesis and the pathogenesis of microangiopathy [13-19].

POTENTIAL ROLE OF ANGIOTENSIN IN THE PATHOGENESIS OF DIABETIC COMPLICATIONS
There is now a wealth of data supporting a direct (blood pressure independent) role for Ang II in the pathogenesis of diabetic nephropathy and microangiopathy. As discussed above, Ang II has the potential to exert numerous actions on kidney function and

structure. Ang II modulates glomerular filtration by influencing afferent and efferent glomerular arteriolar tone and by a direct effect on mesangial cells to modulate the glomerular ultrafiltration coefficient, largely via its action on mesangial contraction [20,21]. Ang II may also influence glomerular permeability to protein via its effects on glomerular haemodynamics and a direct action on the glomerular sieving coefficient. Ang II also stimulates renal sodium reabsorbtion via direct effects on the proximal tubule and via stimulation of aldosterone secretion [20]. Furthermore, as indicated above, Ang II is important in the regulation of cellular growth and differentiation, both in the development of the normal kidney and the pathogenesis of renal disease [22,23]. In the latter regard, Ang II has also been shown to be important in the pathogenesis of renal interstitial fibrosis, perhaps in part, via the induction of TGFβ expression [24,25]. Beyond, the kidney, the capacity of Ang II to induce angiogenesis has also been implicated in the pathogenesis of retinal neovascularisation in diabetes mellitus [17,18,26].

The relative importance of systemically-derived versus locally generated Ang II in the pathogenesis of tissue injury remains controversial [1,2]. Nevertheless, it is intriguing that all of the necessary substrates and enzymes for Ang II generation are expressed in cells within the renal glomerulus and the eye [17,22]. Moreover, their expression appears to increase in association with the development of diabetic nephropathy and retinopathy [17].

The most compelling evidence in support of an important role for Ang II in the pathogenesis of diabetic nephropathy and retinopathy comes from clinical studies which demonstrate the efficacy of angiotensin converting enzyme inhibitors (ACE-inhibitors) in protecting against the progression of diabetic nephropathy and perhaps also retinopathy [26-30].

Many of the aforementioned actions of Ang II, are not direct effects but depend on the capacity of Ang II to stimulate the release of a cascade of cytokines from resident cells. For example, the fibrogenic action of Ang II in the renal interstitium may, at least in part, be dependent on the Ang II-induced release of TGFβ [25]. Ang II also increases the production of PDGF and TGFβ by vascular and renal tissues.. It is unknown which Ang II receptor subtype is involved in PDGF and TGFβ upregulation, but it seems likely that this effect is also mediated via the AT_1 receptor. It is also conceivable that some of the actions of Ang II on the renal glomerulus and the retina in diabetic subjects, are due to Ang II-induced release of VEGF [15,19]. Ang II is a potent stimulus for VEGF mRNA expression and peptide production [12]. This action is Ang II concentration dependent and rapid in onset and is mediated via the AT_1 receptor because this effect is inhibited by losartan, a highly specific and selective AT_1 receptor antagonist [12].

The action of Ang II to increase VEGF production could be relevant to the pathogenesis of diabetic nephropathy and retinopathy. The renin angiotensin system (RAS) has been shown to be activated in renal tissues and within the eye in diabetes mellitus [17,22]. It has been suggested that local activation of the RAS in these circumstances may contribute to glomerular and interstitial structural (mesangial and interstitial matrix accumulation) and functional changes (increased permeability to protein) and retinal neovascularisation and capillary leakage. Although some of these pathological developments relate to the pressor actions of RAS activation, it is clear that Ang II may induce tissue injury via pressor-independent actions (see above). Mindful of the potent actions of VEGF, it is tempting to speculate some of these effects of the pressor-independent effects RAS activation could result from Ang II-induced VEGF production within the renal glomerulus and the retina. In the kidney, it is unclear what the deleterious effects of increased VEGF production might be, because the renal actions of VEGF remain speculative. Nevertheless, evidence implicating VEGF in the pathogenesis of diabetic retinal neovascularisation is much more substantial. Concentrations of VEGF are raised in the vitreous humour of patients with proliferative diabetic retinopathy [31]. It is plausible that intraocular Ang II generation may be an important stimulus for increased VEGF production and the resulting retinal neovascularisation [18].

THERAPEUTIC IMPLICATIONS

ACE inhibition has been shown to be very effective in retarding the development and progression of diabetic nephropathy and possibly also retinopathy. It seems likely that these benefits are, at least in part, independent of the protective effect of blood pressure lowering. However, the potential for angiotensin II to potentiate haemodynamically mediated tissue injury in the kidney or the eye is very compelling. If as seems likely, ACE inhibition is insufficient, even when given in high doses, to prevent angiotensin II generation, the possibility of directly inhibiting the angiotensin receptors has obvious appeal. However, what if some of the benefit of ACE-inhibition ie. nephroprotection, is not mediated via inhibition of the RAS, but via potentiation of bradykinin? This raises the possibility that the ultimate therapeutic assault on the RAS may involve ACE-inhibition in combination with AT_1 receptor blockade. I think this is a likely therapeutic approach in the future for patients with early or established evidence of progressive diabetic nephropathy.

In conclusion, the scientific rationale and clinical trial data strongly suggests that effective inhibition of the RAS is important in protecting diabetic patients from progressive microvascular injury. Some of this benefit is undoubtedly related to the associated blood pressure reduction and the favourable impact of RAS blockade on microvascular haemodynamics. Nevertheless, the pro-inflammatory, growth promoting, pro-fibrotic, non-haemodynamic actions of angiotensin II are also worthy of blockade.

REFERENCES

1.   Campbell DJ. Circulating and tissue renin angiotensin systems. J Clin Invest 1987, 79: 1-6.
2.   Lee MA, Bohm M, Paul M, Ganten D. Tissue renin angiotensin systems and their role in cardiovascular diseases. Circulation. 1993; 87: 7-13.
3.   Unger T, Chung O, Csikos T, et al. Angiotensin receptors. J. Hypertension. 1996. 14: (suppl. 4) S95-S103.

4.   Berk BC, Vekshtein V, Gordon HM, Tsuda T. Angiotensin II stimulated protein synthesis in cultured vascular smooth muscle cells. Hypertension 1989; 13: 305-314.

5.   Naftilan AJ, Gilliland GK, Eldridge CS, Kraft AS. Induction of the proto-oncgene c-jun by angiotensin II. Mol Cell Biol. 1990. 10:5536-5540.

6.   Himeno H, Crawford DC, Hosoi M, Chobanian AV, Brecher P. Angiotensin II alters aortic fibronectin independently of hypertension. Hypertension, 1991; 23: 823-826.

7.   Bardy N, Merval R, Benessiano J, Samuel J-L, Tedgui A. Pressure and Angiotensin II synergistically induce aortic fibronectin expression in organ culture model of rat aorta. Circ Res. 1996, 79: 70-78.

8.   Griendling K, Ollerenshaw JD, Minieri CA, Alexander RW. Angiotensin II stimulates NADH and NADPH activity in cultured vascular smooth muscle cells. Circ Res, 1994; 74: 1141-1148

9.   Rajagopaian S, Kurz S, Munzel T, Tarpey M, Freeman BA, Griendling KK, Harrison DG. Angiotensin II mediated hypertension in the rat increases vascular superoxide production via membrane NADH/NADPH oxidase activation. J Clin Invest, 1996; 97:1916-1923

10. Arnal JF, Michel JB, Harrison DG. Nitric oxide in the pathogenesis of hypertension. Curr Opin Nephrol Hypertens. 1995, 4: 182-188.

11. Tesfamariam B. Free radicals in diabetic endothelial dysfunction. Free Radical Biol & Med. 1994, 16: 383-391.

12. Williams B, Baker A-Q, Gallacher B, Lodwick D. Angiotensin II increases vascular permeability factor gene expression by human vascular smooth muscle. Hypertension. 1995. 68: 160-167.

13. Ferrara N, Houck K, Jakeman L, Leung DW. Molecular and biological properties of the vascular endothelial growth factor family of proteins. Endocr. Rev. 1992. 13: 18-22.

14. Williams B. Vascular permeability/endothelial growth factors: A potential role in the pathogenesis and treatment of vascular diseases. Vasc. Med. 1996. 1: 251-258.

15. Williams B. Factors regulating the expression of vascular permeability/vascular endothelial growth factor by human vascular tissues. Diabetilogia. 1997. 40: S118-S120.

16. Iijima K, Yoshikawa N, Connolly DT, Nakamura H. Human mesangial cells and peripheral blood mononuclear cells produce vascular permeability factor. Kidney Int. 1993. 44: 959-966.

17. Danser AHJ, Van Den Dorpel NA, Deinum J, etal. Renin, pro-renin and immunoreactive renin in vitreous fluid from eyes with and without diabetic retinopathy. J. Clin. Endocrinol. Metab. 1989. 68: 160-167.

18. Williams B. Angiotensin II, VEGF, and diabetic retinopathy. Lancet. 1998. 351: 837-838.

19. Williams B. A potential role for angiotensin II-induced vascular endothelial growth factor expression in the pathogenesis of diabetic nephropathy. *Mineral and Electrolyte Metab.* 1998, 24: 400-405.

20. Blantz RC and Gabbai FB. Effect of angiotensin II on glomerular haemodynamics and ultrafiltration coefficient. Kidney Int. 1987. 31 (suppl. 20): 108-111.

21. Zatz R, Dunn BR, Meyer TW, Brenner B. Prevention of diabetic glomerulopathy by pharmacological amelioration of glomerular capillary hypertension. J. Clin. Invest. 1986. 77: 1925-1930.

22. Lai KN, Leung JCK, Lai KB, To WY, Yeung VTF, Lai FMM. Gene expression of the renin-angiotensin system in human kidney. J. Hypertension. 1998. 16: 91-102.

23. Tufro-McReddie A, Romano LM, Harris JM, Ferder L, Gomez A. Angiotensin II regulates nephrogenesis and renal vascular development. Am. J. Physiol. 1995. 269: F110-F115.

24.   Cooper ME, Allen TJ, Macmillan PA, Clarke BE, Jerums G, Doyle AE. Enalapril retards glomerular basement membrane thickening and albuminuria in the diabetic rat. Diabetilogia. 1989. 32: 326-328.

25.   Gilbert RE, Cox A, Wu LL, Allen TJ, Lennart Hulthen U, Jerums G, Cooper ME. Expression of transforming growth factor β1 and type IV collagen in the renal tubulointerstitium in experimental diabetes: Effects of ACE inhibition. Diabetes. 1998. 47: 414-422.

26.   Chaturvedi N, Sjolie A-K, Stephenson JM, et al. Effects of lisinopril on progression of retinopathy in normotensive people with type I diabetes. Lancet. 1998. 351: 285-231.

27.   Lewis EJ, Hunsicker LG, Bain RP, Rohde RD (the collaborative study group). The effect of angiotensin converting enzyme inhibition of diabetic nephropathy. N.Eng.J.Med. 1993. 329: 1456-1462.

28.   Kasiske B, Kalil R, Ma J, Liao M, Keane W. Effect of antihypertensive therapy on the kidney on in patients with diabetes: a meta-regression analysis. Ann. Int.Med. 1993. 118: 129-138.

29.   Laffel LM, McGill JB, Gans DJ. The beneficial effect of angiotensin converting enzyme inhibition with captopril on diabetic nephropathy in normotensive IDDM patients with microalbuminuria: North American Microalbuminuria Study Group. Am. J. Med. 1995. 99: 497-504.

30.   The EUCLID study group. Randomised placebo controlled trial of lisinopril in normotensive patients with IDDM and normoalbuminuria or microalbuminuria. Lancet. 1997. 349: 1787-1792.

31.   Aiello LP, Avery RL, Arrigg PG, et al. Vascular endothelial growth factor in ocular fluid of patients with diabetic retinopathy and other retinal disorders. N. Eng. J. Med. 1994. 331: 1480-1487.

49. MICROALBUMINURIA, BLOOD PRESSURE AND DIABETIC RENAL DISEASE: ORIGIN AND DEVELOPMENT OF IDEAS

C.E. Mogensen
Medical Department M, Diabetes and Endocrinology, Aarhus Kommunehospital, Aarhus University Hospital, Aarhus, Denmark

(Modified from Diabetologia, 1999; 42: 263-285, with permission)

INTRODUCTION

Microalbuminuria and diabetic renal disease are closely linked [1-14] and are associated with increasing blood pressure and often antecedent hyperfiltration [1]. Microalbuminuria usually indicates the beginning of diabetic nephropathy as opposed to overt nephropathy characterized by clinical proteinuria according to generally defined standards [14-15] but it has an even broader impact because it is also often found in essential hypertension as first described by Parving et al. [16]. This indicates that it is involved in early renal and vascular disorders which can predict advancing renal disease as well as the progression of cardiovascular disease [17]. This concept of prediction however is becoming increasingly difficult to pursue because many patients are treated with anti-hypertensive drugs and other types of interventions when microalbuminuria is diagnosed; such measures often return albumin excretion to normal [17-19]. Further in population-based studies microalbuminuria is not uncommon, especially in elderly people where it is also strongly related to cardiovascular disease and mortality, as in both in Type 1 (insulin-dependent) and Type 2 (non-insulin-dependent) diabetes mellitus [20-29]. Whether it should be considered as a part of the metabolic syndrome is still doubtful as it relates more specifically to high blood pressure and glucose intolerance rather than to obesity [333, 30]. In diabetic pregnancy, an increase of microalbuminuria predicts complications [7, 31].

Thus microalbuminuria can be considered as an early sign of damage not only of the kidney but also the cardiovascular system [17, 18, 28, 32]. For intervention strategies to prevent or reverse the abnormality, also with perspectives of hard endpoints, it is crucial to define and recognize pathogenetic risk factors involved in the aetiology of disease [33-41]. It is, however, equally important to consider early signs of disease and microalbuminuria usually indicates detectable renal structural damage [42-49].

Mogensen C.E., (ed)., THE KIDNEY AND HYPERTENSION IN DIABETES MELLITUS .

Table 49-1 Studies related to nephromegaly, hyperfiltration and microalbuminuria

Phenomenon	Nephromegaly	Hyperfiltration	Immune-measurement of albumin	Microalbuminuria Type 1 diabetes
Early observation	Paris 1849 C. Bernard [62]	Belgium/Italy Switzerland [276-278]	Upsala [99]	London, Aarhus [100, 283, 284]
Subsequent studies and observations	Several pathologists [63]	Denmark [279, 280]	London, RIA [282]	Follow-up: London, Copenhagen, Aarhus [73, 105, 106]
Newer studies	Aarhus 1973 [67, 68], Copenhagen 1991 [275]	Boston [70], Stockholm [71], London [281]	Aarhus [283, 284]	Many studies [290, 349, 350,351, 381]
Confirmed and/or clinical significant	Munich 1998 [69]	Confirmed [362] but clinical assessment may be too cumbersome	Rapid procedures Aarhus [102-104] Guidelines [285-287]	Important guidelines [287]. Cyclosporine damage [324]

If we can diagnose and intervene with effective strategies at an earlier stage, e. g. at hyperfiltration [50-56] or guided by provocation tests [57, 58] or with very early risk factors we might be able to further improve prognosis.

Very early risk factors to be considered could be pre-natal, such as genetic elements, birth-weight and familial predisposition to renal and vascular disease. The interrelation of risk factors seems to some extent, however, to have confused the medical community for years. This also applies to de facto pathogenetic importance of hyperglycaemia per se, not only because of poor recognition of hyperglycaemia before the glycated haemoglobin-era, but also the failure to recognize that the two important risk factors, e.g. high blood pressure and increased blood glucose concentrations, must be considered together. These are fundamental risk factors for cardiovascular disease also, and in diabetes, hyperlipidaemia could be of equal or even greater importance [59] Considered together, the long-term occurrence over the years of high blood glucose and high blood pressure is highly indicative of the development of renal disease, other microvascular lesions and also macrovascular disease. Conversely, low blood pressure may be protective, even with long-standing diabetes and somewhat poor glycaemic control.

Another confounding issue has been the seemingly independent development of retinopathy and renal disease in some situations. Some studies have failed to recognize that morphological diagnosis of renal disease is often lacking in epidemiological studies, in contrast to visible retinopathy, although clinically meaningful microvascular disease usually develops in a very concordant fashion [60, 61].

This review discusses how pertinent concepts of diabetic renal disease have developed over the years (Tables 49-4). It also focuses on earlier diagnosis based on exact measures such as ambulatory blood pressure, provocation tests and precise monitoring of glomular filtration rate (GFR) as well as other renal function tests to define the earliest possible stage predictive of incipient or overt disease (Table 49-5). Several new theoretical concepts are mentioned briefly (Table 49-6) and potential endpoints are discussed (Table 49-7).

Table 49-2 Glomerulopathy, epidemiology, syndrome X and significance of near-normal

Phenomenon	Glomerulopathy and proteinuria	Epidemiology of microalbuminuria and mortality	Metabolic syndrome or syndrome X	Significance of long-term glycaemic control
Early observation	Kimmelstiel and Wilson, 1936 [292, 293]	London, Epidemiology [100] Aarhus, Mortality [112, 113]	Sweden 1923 [140] England 1939 [141-142] France 1949 [143] Italy 1965 [144]	Keiding 1952 [300] Providing the concept Pirart 1978 [84]
Subsequent studies	Several pathologists [294-297]	Aarhus [116] Fredericia [20] London [27]	Ferranini [32] Reaven [299] Hoorn Study [30]	Scandinavia [301] Gothenburg [222] Kumamoto [367]
Newer studies	Aarhus/ Minneapolis (Morphometry) [47, 298] Japan [127]	Mortality data firmly confirmed [113] Diabhycar [368] HOPE [369]	Concept used by many investigators, but correlation not too close [333].	DCCT [41, 349] Oslo/Aarhus [48] Gothenburg [302] Copenhagen [15] UKPDS [130]
Confirmed and/or clinical significant	Several reviews [147, 291]	Used now in all epidemiological and large trials [377,369,346,378]	Still somewhat ill defined [30,145]. Not measured clinically [370, 371].	Several guidelines (widely accepted, but AHT may be equally important)

NEPHROMEGALY AND HYPERFILTRATION

The origin of ideas often goes much further back than investigators in the research field acknowledge. Thus, nephromegaly had been observed more than a century before it was rediscovered. Claude Bernard [62], with quite another purpose in mind, observed pronounced nephromegaly in a patient with newly diagnosed diabetes who was in the care of M. Rayer in a Parisian Hospital in the 1840s and was examined after a sudden and unexpected death. The nephromegaly seen in the post mortem examination corresponds closely with new observations. Between 1848 and 1974 nephromegaly was not recognized clinically, although it seemed to be a common finding among pathologists [63]. It was described in textbooks in France even before Claude Bernard [64, 65]. Newer observations indicated considerable renal enlargement in experimental diabetes [66]. Nephromegaly was proposed as an index of long-term glycaemic control and could thus theoretically be used to document a possible relation between hyperglycaemia and later overt nephropathy [67-68]. This concept was recently further elaborated by the observation that diabetic patients with considerable nephromegaly were at greater risk of developing overt renal disease [69].

Table 49-3 The concept of renoprotection

Phenomenon	Protection by AHT. Incipient nephropathy (type 1)	Protection by AHT. Overt nephropathy (type 1)	Protection by AHT in microalbuminuira (Type 2)	ACE-I and renal protection
Early observation	Aarhus 1985 [190] Copenhagen [196, 197] Melbourne [198]	Aarhus, 1976-1982 [208, 211] Copenhagen [212-216] Gothenburg [217]	Melbourne [198] Several studies	Aarhus [308] Paris [195] Copenhagen [197] Melbourne [198]
Newer studies	Euclid [203, 303] Aarhus [177] Italy [304]	Many studies [219, 352, 353]	Several studies [305]	UKPDS (probably similar effect with beta-blockers) [131]
Confirmed and clinical significant	Several guidelines [287]	Several guidelines [287, 352]	Clinically used [305] Multifactorial intervention important [306]	Maybe more effective than ordinary AHT [379]

AHT, antihypertensive treatment

The functional abnormality, to some extent concomitant with nephromegaly, is hyperfiltration and intrarenal hypertension which was proposed to be of key pathogenetic relevance by Brenner and a key concept in nephrology [70]. Studies in diabetes indicate that hyperfiltration is of considerable importance [56] as evidenced by several follow-up studies, most convincingly by Rudberg et al. [71]. Some studies have failed to document correlations possibly because of too broad inclusion criteria, e. g. patients with newly diagnosed diabetes before insulin treatment [56]. These patients are known to have pronounced hyperfiltration that can be reversed with treatment [72]. The predictive role of hyperfiltration could be difficult to study now, because there is a more intensified control in diabetes, both before and after the development of microalbuminuria. Even so, hyperfiltration, associated with microalbuminuria and slightly raised blood pressure [73], is likely to be strongly predictive of renal disease, perhaps to some extent because hyperfiltration in parallel to nephromegaly is related to poor metabolic control [68, 74]. In contrast to microalbuminuria, hyperfiltration and nephromegaly are, however, rarely included in the clinical evaluation of patients, partly because their relevance under routine circumstances can be difficult to ascertain as the procedures involved are technically too demanding in a busy clinic. Regarding mechanisms, atrial natriuretic peptide could be involved both in hyperfiltration [74] and microalbuminuria [75, 76]. The genesis of hyperfiltration is, however, likely to be multifactorial [77]. Interestingly, in a recent 8-year prospective study (Dahlquist G. Personel communication) hyperfiltration again predicted abnormal albuminuria. Microalbuminuria was a very strong predictor of clinical proteinuria.

Table 49-4 Pathophysiological and genetic studies

Phenomenon	Complication genetically or metabolically determined?	Provocation tests (e.g. exercise)	24 h-amb. BP in diabetes	Dextran Ficoll and PVP clearance
Early observation	Siperstein 1973 [82]	Karlefors [146]	Rubler 1982 [160]	Uppsala [180]
Subsequent observations	Deckert [83] Aarhus [42]	Aarhus [150]	Aarhus [161]	Düsseldorf [181] Aarhus [2, 72] Liège [182]
Newer studies	London [309] Boston [310] Copenhagen [86] France [311] Minneapolis [325]	Only few studies [177, 312, 313]	Several studies [175]	Copenhagen [183] San Francisco [184]
Clinical significance	Renal complication metabolically determined and modulated by hypertension [365] Role of genetics?? [380]	Not widely used, but may be relevant in treatment trials [177, 314]	Should be used more (guidelines elaborated) [175]	Groningen [332] Litttle used [2]

PVP, polyvinyl-pyrrolidin

Table 49-5 *(continue on next page)*
STAGES IN THE DEVELOPMENT OF RENAL CHANGES AND LESIONS IN DIABETES MELLITUS (TYPE 1)

	Stage	Chronology	Main Structural changes or lesions	Glomerular filtration rate	Dextran clearance (% of GFR)
1	Acute renal hypertrophy-hyperfunction	Present at diagnosis of diabetes (reversible with good control)	Increased kidney size. Increased glomerular size	Increased by 20-50%	Normal
2	Normo-albuminuria (UAE<20 µg/min)	Almost all patients normo-albuminuric in first 5 years	On renal biopsy, increased BM thickness in some patients.	Increased by 20-50%	Normal
3	Incipient diabetic nephropathy, UAE 20-200 µg/min	Typically after 6-15 years (in ≈35% of patients)	Further BM-thickening and mesangial expansion, arrestable with AHT[d] *	Still supra-normal values, predicted to decline with development of proteinuria	Normal
4	Proteinuria, clinical overt diabetic nephropathy	After 15-25 years (in ≈35% of patients)	Clear and pronounced abnormalities *	Decline ≈10 ml/min/year with clear proteinuria[c]	Abnormal to high mol dextrans (non-specific and only with low GFR) [2]
5	End-stage renal failure	Final outcome, after 25-30 years or more	Glomerular closure and advanced glomerulopathy *	<10 ml/min	Not studied

BM = Basement membrane; UAE = Urinary albumin excretion rate; AHT = Antihypertensive treatment.
[a]The best clinical marker of early renal involvement; [b]Mostly ACE-inhibition + diuretics; [c]Without antihypertensive treatment
The classification was conceived and presented on ideas presented in ref. 2, and updated – Based on studies 1983-98 (refs. 2 and 14) . [d] Rudberg and Østerby et al [48]
Arteriolar hyalinosis and * increased interstitium

Table 49-5 *(continued)*
STAGES IN THE DEVELOPMENT OF RENAL CHANGES AND LESIONS IN DIABETES
MELLITUS (TYPE 1)

	Albumin excretion		Blood pressure	Reversible by strict insulin treatment	Arrestable or reversible by AHT
	Baseline UAE[a]	Exercise-induced UAE			
1	May be increased, but reversible	Increased, but reversible	Normal	Yes	No hypertension present. Microcirculatory changes modifiable
2	Normal by definition (12-20 µg/min may be abnormal)	Maybe abnormal after a few years	Normal (BP as in background population) Increase by 1 mmHg/year	Hyperfiltration reduced	Filtration fraction and UAE may be reduced [308]
3	Increase: ≈20%/year (of glomerular origin)	Abnormal aggravation of baseline UAE, related to BP-increase	Incipient increase, ≈3 mmHg/year (if untreated)	Microalbumin-uria stabilized, GFR also stable (if HbA_{1c} is reduced). Structural damage slower	Microalbuminuria reduced. Prevention of fall in GFR Arrestable by AHT[d]
4	Progressive clinical proteinuria[c] of glomerular origin	Pronounced increase in BP	High BP, increase by ≈5 mmHg/year (if untreated)	Higher fall in GFR with poor control	Progression reduced (aiming at 135/85 mmHg)
5	Often some decline due to decreasing GFR	Not studied	High (if untreated)	No	No

BM = Basement membrane; UAE = Urinary albumin excretion rate; AHT =
Antihypertensive treatment.
[a]The best clinical marker of early renal involvement; [b]Mostly ACE-inhibition + diuretics;
[c]Without antihypertensive treatment
The classification was conceived and presented on ideas presented in ref. 2, and updated –
Based on studies 1983-98 (refs. 2 and 14) . [d] Rudberg and Østerby et al. [48].

Table 49-6

Newer therapeutic concepts

	Aldose-reductose inhibition	Selective growth factor inhibition	Protein-kinase-C inhibition*	Angiotensin II receptor blockade*(**)	AGE-inhibition
Theoretical, basis, reference	Mau Pedersen [51]	Flyvbjerg, Ziaydeh [315, 316]	King et al. [317, 358]	Willemheimer [318, 359]	Cooper and Jerums [319]
Human studies	Mau Pedersen [51,52]	Few, Mau Pedersen [50]	Trials in progress	Studies conducted and in progress [247, 248, 354-357, 383-384]	In progress (Not promising – yet?)
Clinically used	No	Not yet	No	Widely used [318, 372]	No

*) May be related

**) Dual blockade may be useful [332, 372-382, 388].

Table 49-7

The endpoints: GFR-decline rate related to intermediary end-points in diabetic patients

Intermediary end-points	GFR-decline (young type 1 diabetic patients)	GFR-decline (middle-aged type 2 diabetic patients)
Microalbuminuria[a] (20-200 µg/min)	Decline in GFR[a] only seen with progression to proteinuria	Decline rate of GFR[a] usually not noteably different from normoalbuminuria
Proteinuria[b] (macroalbuminuria, >200 µg/min)	Clear decline in GFR[b] (Reduced by antihypertensive treatment)	Clear decline in GFR[c]. High mortality with increasing proteinuria
Blood pressure[b]	Controversy exists but a clear risk factor with co-existing abnormal albuminuria	Clear risk factor especially with co-existing abnormal albuminuria

Related to future mortality and ESRD with increasing power ([a]) ([b]) ([c])

ESRD, end-stage renal disease.

GENETIC OR FAMILIAL FACTORS

It has been suggested that there is a discrepancy between the development of renal disease and retinopathy in that retinopathy is much more common than nephropathy. It has possibly not been taken into consideration that the diagnoses of retinopathy is most often based on retinal photographs, that is morphology. By contrast renal disease is diagnosed by the occurrence of microalbuminuria or proteinuria and only rarely through renal biopsies. With morphological diagnosis the prevalence of the two microvascular lesions could be very similar. Actually, as shown by the Melbourne group, development of clinically important renal disease is strongly associated with the occurrence of retinopathy [60, 61]. Thus, the basis for considering susceptibility factors distinct from the development of renal disease and retinopathy could be weakly founded. In Type 2 diabetes the appearence of retinopathy might be seen later but it clearly correlates with that of glomerulopathy [78]. It is nevertheless still surprising and so far unexplained that some Type 2 patients have proteinuria, but not retinopathy, according to standard evaluation [78].

Another key issue is that more than one risk factor must be present for the development of apparent clinical disease. Thus isolated hyperglycaemia might not suffice to develop overt renal disease, whereas two co-existing risk factors namely, hyperglycaemia and high blood pressure, must be present as underscored in the UK prospective diabetes study [79, 80]. Conversely the development of microalbuminuria is usually accompanied by the development of increased blood pressure. Therefore, there should be recognition of both risk factors. In long-term studies, in diabetic patients without clinically meaningful microvascular lesions, blood pressure is lower than in the general population which again supports the prerequisite of at least two risk factors in the genesis of renal disease [81].

Interestingly, clinical management was hampered for many years by the studies of Siperstein et al. [82] suggesting that morphological lesions can be present at or before the clinical diagnosis of diabetes. This would lend some support to genetic factors being decisive for the development of microvascular disease. A tempting, but dangerous conclusion would then be that the development of microvascular lesions is not responsive to better metabolic control but related to genetic "destiny" rather than to treatment failure [83]. These concepts were incorrect, at least for the kidney, as substantiated by the fundamental studies by R. Osterby who showed that structural lesions develop after diabetes has been present for some years [42-48]. Muscle basement membrane might be less suited to measurement [49].

In his long-term follow-up studies Pirart showed that for microvascular lesions and neuropathy, glycaemic control was important [84]. Several European intervention studies confirm the correlation between hyperglycaemia and the development of renal disease [85]. It was not, however, until the Diabetes Control and Complications Trial (DCCT) [41] was completed that this was widely accepted in the United States, an attitude which, in retrospect, could in many places have had a deleterious effect on clinical management before 1993. This could also apply to the management of Type 2 diabetic patients, in whom metabolic control quite often is not perfect, but this will clearly change after publication of the UK Prospective Diabetes Study [79]. This study also added hypertension as an even more important risk factor.

Studies on genetic predisposition should be considered in the context of several risk factors [15]. Thereby certain angiotensin-converting enzyme (ACE) genotypes have been shown to possibly affect progression [86], although data are diverse and might not relate to all Western populations [87, 88] as the effect can possibly only be seen in large meta-analyses [86]. In Type 2 diabetes there seems to be no such effect in Caucasians [86]. Familial predisposition to hypertension, also seen in affected patients, could still be important in a concordant, yet multifactorial, fashion [89, 90] and blood pressure can be treated once the patients become hypertensive. Recent work also suggests some racial and familial clustering of renal disease in black patients [91-92] but often such patient-material is small and familial clustering of environmental factors are just as likely [93].

An ambitious project has been proposed [336], possibly linking the very rare Finnish type of congenital nephrotic syndrome gene to diabetic nephropathy. The nephrin molecule is thought to be of utmost relevance. A multicenter project has been supported by a 15 million USD grant from the Novo Nordisk Foundation to unravel over 10 years the mechanisms of diabetic vascular disease [336]. Karl Trygveson, the main investigator and co-founder of the company, BioStratum (www.Biostratum.com). The consortium is February 2000, advertising in Science for investigators. An initial key issue may be new genetic markers and AGE-inhibitors?[400].

BIRTH WEIGHT, CV-DISEASE AND MICROALBUMINURIA

It has been suggested that low birth weight could be predictive of cardiovascular renal disease in diabetes and in the general population [94]. Abnormally high birth weight could also be a problem [95]. Small kidneys could relate to fewer glomeruli and an increase in the pressure gradient in existing tissue. This concept was not, however, supported by our studies on the relations between birth weight, renal and glomerular size [96]. Also in population-based studies we failed to find any correlation between microalbuminuria or raised albumin secretion and birth weight. Nor was there any correlation between blood pressure and birth weight [25]. Therefore, in the present Western world, it seems inconceivable that low birth weight could be an important determinant of essential hypertension or associated renal disease, in particular, because hypertension is highly prevalent in the Western population and found in perhaps 15-20 % of elderly people. Hypertension is more closely related to actual increased body mass index or abdominal adiposity. A relation between low birth weight and the much later development of diabetes and some element of cardiovascular disease might however exist in extreme situations in many poor countries [360], but this is may not be relevant to the management of patients in the Western world today [97, 98]. New post-hoc studies based on the so-called Barker Hypothesis continue to emerge [385-387, 395-398] (Explaining the French paradox?).

IMMUNE-BASED MEASUREMENT OF ALBUMINURIA IN LOW CONCENTRATIONS

Progress in medical research is often driven by new methodology and procedures, e.g. by more sensitive techniques. This was the case with the study of early development and early treatment of diabetes associated renal disease. The first study from 1961 describing measurements of albumin in normal urine was quite elaborate requiring pre-concentration of urinary albumin [99]. This completely changed after the introduction of radioimmuno-assays for albumin that often even required dilution of urine samples and led to the term microalbuminuria [100]. The introduction of such methods was important in the study of the early diabetes-associated renal impairment in cross-sectional and longitudinal studies. Radioimmuno-assays were, however, still laborious and time-consuming for clinical use and therefore it was an important step forward when immuno-turbidimetry and other immune precipitation tests were developed; this allowed processing of multiple samples of urine at high speed for use in clinical practice [12]. It was a major step forward in the clinical management of patients with diabetes and also those with essenial hypertension [17, 101].

Clinical management has benefited further from the introduction of effective and quick bedside and dipstick tests for measurement of albumin. The introduction of the Micral 1 and Micral 2 tests which are not quantitative was of major benefit [102, 103], with the Micral 2 test being very efficient and easy to use in the clinic [103].

In our clinical laboratory a very good quantitative correlation has been obtained through the measurement of the albumin:creatinine ratio by the DCA-2000 apparatus compared with measurement by immuno-turbidimetry [104]. Thereby it is possible to rapidly measure not only HbA1C but also albumin and creatinine [104], an ideal situation for small clinics where large-scale measurements of these compounds are not always necessary. We have thus experienced huge progress in our laboratory techniques from the initial extremely laborious methods in the early 1960s [99] to the very quick and efficient bedside tests of the 1990s [104], as well as excellent laboratory measurements.

MICROALBUMINURIA IN TYPE 1 DIABETES

Three independent groups have consistently shown that microalbuminuria predicts overt renal disease [73, 105, 106]. Consequently, it is now wide-spread clinical practice to screen for microalbuminuria, especially as it has subsequently been shown that intervention is effective (as described later). Follow-up studies of initial cohorts have also shown that microalbuminuria is strongly predictive of mortality from cardiovascular disease [107, 108]. In a recent study with shorter follow-ups, on a very large number of patients, the same phenomenon was observed [109]. In this study the observation of the deleterious effects of albuminuria was also, however, based on patients with clinical proteinuria, excluded in previous studies because of their well-known poor outcome.

The recent follow-up study from the DCCT [349] clearly confirms the initial observation in Europe [73, 105, 106]. 31% of microalbuminuric patients developed proteinuria after further 4 years of conventional insulin treatment [349].

In patients with long-standing diabetes and late microalbuminuria it can be assumed that microalbuminuria increases relatively slowly [110]. Therefore these patients perhaps have a somewhat different and more "benign" prognosis than "fast track" patients, diagnosed early on with microalbuminuria or proteinuria. Such interpretations could, however, still be problematic because we are not dealing with distinct entities but rather should regard the degree of albuminuria as a continuous variable (normo-micro-macro).

MICROALBUMINURIA IN TYPE 2 DIABETES

In a follow-up study first communicated in 1983 [111] it was shown that microalbuminuria in Type 2 diabetes is strongly predictive of an increased mortality risk [112]. This observation has since been confirmed in numerous studies [113]. Other factors could be associated with poor prognosis such as long-term hyperglycaemia and high blood pressure. Microalbuminuria seems though to be the strongest overall predictor of mortality as has also been found in non-diabetic population-based studies [81]. Interestingly, poor metabolic control has recently been shown to predict microalbuminuria [114, 115] and could also be a risk factor for its progression, whereas high blood pressure can be more important later on [114, 116-125]. Poor glycaemic control correlates with typical diabetic glomerular lesions [126]. More so-called "unspecific" lesions can also be observed but non-diabetic microalbuminuric controls are lacking, which is problematic. Indeed there might be some misclassification of patients in such studies because albuminuria usually decreases with antihypertensive treatment [126]. The "unspecific" lesions can also be considered as characteristic lesions in diabetic patients, again making exact classification problematic not necessarily in daily ordinary pathology practice but in scientific work which is to be tested by other investigators. Other studies have shown abnormalities in microalbuminuric Type 2 diabetic patients [127]. Among the many risk factors analysed [118-124] hyperglycaemia and hypertension seem to be of particular importance, as documented in initial studies on the relevance of higher albumin excretion rates in relation to other risk factors [8-10]. Thus again there is a requirement for two risks; hyperglycaemia and high blood pressure factors must combine to produce important clinical disease [114, 116]. Since microalbuminuria in Type 2 diabetes is a better predictor of cardiovascular than of microvascular disease other macrovascular disease factors must be taken into consideration. These include hyperlipidaemia whose reduction plays an important part in secondary prevention of cardiovascular disease in Type 2 diabetes.

The natural history of microalbuminuria in Type 2 diabetes has been surveyed recently [116]. Short-term intervention treatments are not usually very effective [119,125]. Long-term glycaemic control as in the Kumamoto study [40] and the UK prospective diabetes study [128-131] have, however, proven rather efficient especially when combined with long-term antihypertensive treatment [130,131]. Detailed accounts of microalbuminuria in the UK study are still awaited, but long follow-up is required.

DIFFERENCES BETWEEN TYPE 1 AND TYPE 2 DIABETES

More and more evidence suggests that the course of renal abnormalities is similar in Type 1 and Type 2 diabetes. Obviously, there are exceptions because patients with

Type 2 diabetes tend to be elderly and obese. This means hypertension is seen much earlier in Type 2 diabetes with subsequent renal damage. Another important point is that Type 2 diabetes can remain undiagnosed for many years and therefore some patients will have renal and retinal as well as cardiovascular damage at the first clinical diagnosis [29]. Risk factors for the development of renal disease include poor metabolic control and high, or increasing, blood pressure for both types. With microalbuminuria again glycaemic control and high blood pressure are important risk factors that can be controlled. In overt renal disease, there is a clear-cut correlation between blood pressure and decline in glomular filtration rate. There is also a correlation in Type 1 diabetes between glycaemic control and a decline in GFR [87, 88] but this is less clear in Type 2 diabetes where there seems to be no correlation between rate of decline of GFR and HbA$_{1C}$ [116].

Treatment modalities seem to be the same as confirmed by the UK prospective diabetes study [128-131]. An important point is that many patients with Type 2 diabetes have cardiovascular and cerebrovascular disease and might suffer premature mortality. Certainly, this can be modulated by early antihypertensive treatment as shown in several trials [132-138] (Table 49-8) and also by lipid lowering [139].

MICROALBUMINURIA IN POPULATION BASED STUDIES

Microalbumininuria is present in 5-10% in elderly populations [20, 28] and usually relates to hypertension but also to other risk markers of cardiovascular disease, such as abdominal obesity, hypertension and hyperuricaemia. The relation between microalbuminuria and early mortality in population-based studies was first documented 10-15 years ago [20, 27]. Accordingly microalbuminuria should be included in epidemiological studies with focus on cardiovascular and metabolic diseases. In essential hypertension, microalbuminuria is often diagnosed and predictive of cardiovascular and also of progressive renal disease [101]. This is relevant to "Syndrome X" where similar observations were made decades ago by Kylin in 1923, Himsworth in the 1930s, Vague in the 1940s, and Avogaro and Crepaldi in 1965 [140-144]. It is, however, still perhaps a too vaguely defined entity (not a diagnosis) [145] which often most strongly relates to simple obesity. In contrast microalbuminuria is more related to high blood pressure and diabetes as shown in the Hoorn Study [30] and should not be included in the so-called"syndrome". The HOPE Study [322] documented that ACE-I in patients with risk factors is effective especially in those with microalbuminuria.

The Fredericia Study is a Danish population-based study remarkable by including two generations. The first generation is a sub-group from a population-based study, which took place in the municipality of Fredericia, Denmark around 1981. The parent generation consisted of 228 subjects with diabetes and 223 control subjects to known diabetic subjects. The offspring generation was examined by Vestbo et al [377] and a significant relation between microalbuminuria in the parental generation and hypertension in the offspring both of type 2 diabetic population and the non-diabetic population was found. The offspring generation was examined again in 1997-98, and the results showed a preserved diurnal blood pressure profile and normal blood pressure level in non-diabetic offspring of type 2 diabetic subjects [334], though the offspring was characterised by features of the metabolic syndrome.

Table 49-8. Positive effect by AHT on cardiovascular end points in Type 2 diabetes

		FAVOURS:
1.	SHEP	Diuretics vs. placebo
2.	ABCD [135, 374]	ACE-I vs. CCB
3.	Facet [132]	ACE-I vs. CCB
4.	HOT [134]	Strict control (CCB-based)
5.	UKPDS [130]	Strict control (ACE-I + β-bl-based)
6.	SYST-EUR [133]	CCB (often with ACE-I) vs. placebo
7.	CAPPP [136]	ACE-I vs. conventional
8.	HOPE [322, 346]	ACE-I vs. placebo
9.	STOP-2 [326]	AHT, β-bl. and ACE-I vs. CCB
10.	ALLHAT* [401] (ACE-I and CCB)	Chlorthalidone vs. Doxozosin**
*ALLHAT expected to end year 2002.		
**Doxozosin-arm stopped [401].		
AHT; antihypertensive treatment, CCB; calcium channel blockers, β-bl; beta-blockers [373]		

PROVOCATION TESTS TO DETECT EARLY ABNORMALITIES IN RENAL FUNCTION

It was shown several years ago by Karlefors [146] that exercise induces a clear-cut increase in blood pressure, in particular, in diabetic patients with renal complications and blood pressure values in the upper normal range. We used this concept to describe and detect nascent changes in renal function prior to microalbuminuria and in certain patients quite a pronounced increase in albuminuria occurred during exercise, especially in those with preexisting microalbuminuria [147-150]. Increases in albuminuria are associated with raised blood pressure during exercise, an association that is quite strong. It is, however, not clear whether this test is predictive of advancing renal disease. Although the idea seems quite attractive, clear-cut follow-up studies have not been conducted. Therefore, in the clinical situation multiple baseline measurements are preferred to precisely define the degree of early renal involvement. To this end we measure the albumin creatinine ratio at each visit to the clinic [12]. It has also been proposed that tests that block tubular reabsorption, e. g. by lysine or other dibasic amino-acids be used but again these are too complicated for clinical use [151, 152] although, important physiological information on the nature of renal involvement in diabetes has thereby been obtained. By apparent complete blockade of tubular reabsorption, albumin excretion rises from 5 to approximately 300 µg/min, thus providing an estimate of transglomerular passage of albumin [57, 151]. In addition other provocation tests have been examined [153-157].

24-h AMBULATORY BLOOD PRESSURE MEASUREMENTS

Ambulatory blood pressure measurements were first developed in the 1960s by Sokolow's [158] and Pickering's group [159] and used in the 1980s by Rubler in diabetic patients [160]. The technique used was initially quite difficult and demanding not only for the patient but also the physician. With the introduction of more user-friendly equipment, such as the SpaceLabs apparatus, it is now common clinical practice to take ambulatory blood pressure measurements in situations where there is uncertainty as to the precise level of blood pressure, both before and during treatment [161-174]. An important confounding issue to be avoided is the situation-induced "white-coat" hypertension which is just as common in diabetic as in non-diabetic patients [175, 176]. This is also extremely important in clinical trials because fewer patients could be required to document treatment effects [162, 177]. More sophisticated questions might be answered by ambulatory blood pressure measurements. These include:

1) the effect of smoking which seems to increase blood pressure in diabetic patients in contrast to the paradoxical reduction in ambulatory blood pressure in non-diabetic patients [178];
2) the lower blood pressure in healthy women which is now well established but this conceivably protective biological feature is lost in diabetic patients [165];
3) the significance of a lack of nocturnal blood pressure "dips" in diabetic patients about which there are still some doubts [175].
4) Possible increase in night BP by strict metabolic control which we could by no means confirm [179].

In people with normoalbuminuria we have not found any major differences between those with and without diabetes and the phenomenon of dipping has been quite variable and not applicable in clinical settings [175]. It has, however, been reported that Type 1 diabetic patients on intensive insulin therapy to some extent lack nocturnal dipping which is not present in large series of patients [179].

It is important to record ambulatory blood pressure when describing the antihypertensive effect of drugs, e.g. angiotensin-converting enzyme inhibitors [162, 175, 178]. Thus, it is sometimes not possible, with the use of clinically based blood pressure, to detect a reduction in blood pressure that can only be unveiled during ambulatory blood pressure recordings. If it were not for these it could be argued that the inhibitors are renoprotective, even without any detectable effect on blood pressure. Thus by taking the ambulatory blood pressure we observed some blood pressure reduction in such patients, even in trials with relatively few patients [177]. Again, this illustrates the danger of limiting the concept of renoprotection, by excluding the beneficial effect of blood pressure reduction. Multiple blood pressure measurements with the most exact procedures are therefore essential.

DEXTRAN AND POLYMER CLEARANCE

Dextran clearance was introduced to describe the glomerular permeability to a large range of molecular sizes [180-182] and the principle was also used in diabetic patients [181]. When we introduced this technique in our laboratory for diabetic patients [2, 72] we saw no change in dextran clearance in patients with either newly diagnosed diabetes or long-standing diabetes when correcting for prevailing glomular filtration rate [72], since these patients are often hyperfiltering. In patients with microalbuminuria, Deckert [183], in contrast to other studies [184, 185], also failed to find any changes. We were, however, able to see changes in patients with advanced clinical proteinuria but only by long-term collection of urine after dextran infusion and use of very high-molecular weight dextran [2]. Thus in patients with advanced proteinuria only small permeability defects could be described, which could be a paradox because these patients were clearly proteinuric or even nephrotic. Possibly the dextran molecule is not suitable for this purpose, perhaps because it uncoils during the glomerular filtration process and charged dextrans possibly aggregate suggesting a falsely low clearance. The introduction of ficoll - a molecule with more fixed structure - could or could not provide new information on glomerular permeability to large molecules. Still, in the clinical situation, it is much easier and more practical (and better) to use endogenous plasma proteins as markers.

Newer studies, however, documented only limited change in ficoll clearance in proteinuric type 1 diabetic patients. As earlier described losartan reduced proteinuria, but had only a limited or a borderline effect on high molecular ficoll clearance [335].

RENAL AND OTHER ORGAN PROTECTION

To define risk markers for progressive renal as well as cardiovascular disease is clearly of interest academically but not necessarily of clinical importance as intervention might not always be possible. Theoretically, intervention should certainly be possible considering the two major risk factors, high blood pressure and hyperglycaemia. Renal protection, defined as any measure to prevent progression of renal impairment, could therefore include control of blood pressure and hyperglycaemia, based on observational risk factor studies, as poor glycaemic control is a major risk factor for progression from normo- to microalbuminuria [114, 115, 171]. In patients with microalbuminuria, glycaemic intervention is not, however, always clinically feasible, although highly desirable [15, 186-188]. The background could well be that patients with microalbuminuria previously have had poor metabolic control which could be inherently difficult to treat. In overt nephropathy, poor metabolic control is certainly associated with rapid progression [15, 87, 88]. Therefore during the entire course of renal involvement in diabetes good metabolic control is a main issue, likewise for the prevention of retinopathy, as well as, to some extent, cardiovascular disease, both in Type 1 and Type 2 diabetes. Table 49-7 describes the relation between intermediary end-points and the decline in glomular filtration rate. This is a dramatic development over the last 40 years as it has been argued that hypertension was "essential" to maintain sufficient organ perfusion and survival [35].

EARLY ANTI-HYPERTENSION TREATMENT TO PREVENT PROGRESSION IN RENAL DISEASE IN MICROALBUMINURIC PATIENTS:

In this context it is important to consider blood pressure as a continuous variable [189]. It cannot be argued that there is a clearly defined level representing high blood pressure unless long-term studies are conducted to observe correlation between blood pressure and development of cardiovascular and renal lesions. This applies to both Type 1 and Type 2 diabetes and the general population. Certainly diabetic patients could be more susceptible to renal damage than non-diabetic people or patients with essential hypertension, as related to blood pressure [18, 147].

This was the basis for our early intervention study in which microalbuminuric Type 1 diabetic patients with so-called "normal" blood pressure were enrolled in a clinical trial with a self-controlled approach [189-191]. In this study it was documented that antihypertensive treatment with beta-blockers could lead to regression of microalbuminuria. Further studies along this line showed that antihypertensive combination treatment in such patients is associated with declining albuminuria and slow progression (no decline in GFR) in early diabetic renal disease [192-194]. At present most diabetic patients are on combination therapy.

The benefit of this new therapy was clearly confirmed using angiotensin-converting enzyme inhibitors in the treatment of patients with microalbuminuria [195]. Numerous studies [196-203] have confirmed the effect of these inhibitors in Type 1 diabetes leading to regression of microalbuminuria, as also documented in a recent meta-analysis [203]. Interestingly, this effect is also seen in very early renal involvement in diabetes, such as in patients with mild microalbuminuria [177] between 20 and 70 μg per min. In this 2-year controlled clinical trial the progression expected was seen in the untreated control group with a mean increase rate between 15 and 20 %. With treatment using ACE-inhibition, there was a clear-cut reduction in albuminuria as seen in earlier studies in which the subjects had a higher degree of microalbuminuria. Therefore treatment could be effective quite early, just after the development of microalbuminuria as now advocated by recent guidelines [204]. In the study [177], the specific renal impact of ACE-inhibition was clearly documented. A fall in albuminuria correlated with a fall in filtration fraction. The long-term aim is, however, not regression of microalbuminuria per se, although this might be a reliable surrogate marker, but to prevent a decline in GFR. This requires long-term studies over 6-8 years. Indeed Mathiesen and co-workers [197] were able to show that the effect of ACE-inhibition is long lasting. Importantly, patients with clinical proteinuria had well-preserved GFR after a pause in treatment but only when ACE-inhibitors had been given over the previous 8 years. Without antihypertensive treatment, there was a clear-cut decline in GFR in those developing proteinuria. This is the first study to document a long-term preservation of GFR in Type 1 diabetes [197] as seen in Type 2 diabetes [200, 201]. Table 49-8 shows an outline of 10 controlled studies in microalbuminuric type 1 diabetic patients. Data include studies of 2 years duration or longer. Generally, microalbuminuria is reduced, but important new studies also indicate preservation of GFR and glomerular structure.

RENAL PROTECTION IN TYPE 1 DIABETES WITH OVERT NEPHROPATHY

There has been some discussion about the definition of renal protection in diabetes and in other renal diseases. In my view, a key point is that renal protection should mean GFR is better preserved by treatment, irrespective of its modality. It has been proposed that "renal protection" should be defined as a kind of treatment that preserves GFR, on top of the effect of blood pressure reduction. In my mind this definition is too narrow. Any kind of treatment that prevents a fall in GFR or reduces fall rates in GFR should be termed reno-protection. In many studies BP is not carefully recorded. A broader and weaker definition would be "reduction in proteinuria" since this nevertheless is often associated with the prevention of decline in GFR [151].

Initially, we studied early renal involvement in diabetes describing the now well-known phenomenon of hyperfiltration [1, 72, 205, 206]. Subsequently it was found pertinent to study the natural course of renal function changes in diabetic patients, especially in those with microalbuminuria and clinical proteinuria [207-210]. It became clear that a rise in blood pressure was associated with a fall per period of time in GFR in proteinuric patients and therefore anti-hypertensive trials were initiated with a self-controlled design. This was essential to gain optimal sensitivity in exploratory studies due to the limited number of patients [211].

It soon became clear that antihypertensive treatment with beta-blockers and diuretics and sometimes vasodilators was quite effective in preserving GFR [211-214] and in improving renal prognosis [215, 216]. These seem to be the first studies to document reno-protection (using the above definition) by antihypertensive treatment in diabetes specifically, and in fact, in renal disease in general. Later studies were conducted in other centres, in particular in Sweden [217] in patients with overt diabetic renal disease. All results suggested that the fall rate in GFR could be reduced by about 50 per cent from 10 ml $\cdot$ min^{-1} $\cdot$ year^{-1} to 5 ml $\cdot$ min^{-1} $\cdot$ year^{-1} or even more by more effective antihypertensive treatment and better glycemic control [15,214]. To some extent, this effect seems to be independent of the type of antihypertensive treatment and depends rather more on blood pressure reduction per se although there could be some disagreement [15]. The largest study so far conducted in overt renal disease in patients with Type 1 diabetes was the Collaborative Study in the United States [218]. Again this showed antihypertensive treatment to be effective in Type 1 diabetes. The study compared the use of ACE-inhibitors with other agents to control blood pressure. With a lower and more satisfactory degree of blood pressure attained during treatment, the effect with ACE-inhibitors and other agents was the same (Lewis, personal communication). In contrast with higher blood pressure the ACE-inhibitors seemed to be more efficient, although a strict cut-off has never been defined [219]. Importantly, in this study the ACE-i-graph obtained a significantly lower BP than the control group, a problem observed in several such trials. Such BP-differences may be crucial for observed renoprotection. In other studies it was found that the blood pressure level was important for the determination of the rate of decline in GFR and also some effect was observed by HbA1C as seen in other studies [15]. In Weidmann et al.'s meta-analysis [220] on proteinuria as a surrogate marker the effect of ACE-inhibition became progressively less as lowering of blood pressure was more intense [219]. In non-diabetic renal disease ACE-inhibition is also an important treatment strategy [221].

In my mind, it is clearly not productive to exclude, by definition, antihypertensive treatment as a reno-protective measure. I would prefer that all measures which protect against a decline in GFR be included in the definition both in diabetes and in other renal diseases. It is clear that antihypertensive treatment is important, however, in most renal diseases as suggested by our long-term studies in 1982 [211], subsequently confirmed [219], also for cardiovascular disease [130,131].

GLYCAEMIC CONTROL AND GLYCAEMIC MEASURES

It would seem plausible that diabetic lesions in the kidney and in the eyes, specific for diabetes, are caused by the diabetic state, especially hyperglycaemia. For many years, there was doubt however about this association, mainly because of difficulties in documenting long-term glycaemic control. The large-scale observational study conducted by Pirart and co-workers, however, showed a clear correlation between glycaemic control and the development of microvascular and neurological complications [84]. Intervention studies conducted in Scandinavia and elsewhere supported these observations [15] which were later confirmed by the DCCT as to the development of microvascular and possibly also macrovascular lesions. This formed the basis of the concept of glucotoxicity [41]. Nyberg et al. were the first to observe fairly stable GFR in patients with well-controlled metabolism [222] which was later confirmed [87,88]. They showed that the decline in the rate of GFR correlated with HbA1C and strong evidence for an earlier effect was obtained in the DCCT [41]. Thereafter, optimal glycaemic control became the elusive gold standard for care in Type 1 diabetes. Most experts would very much support this view, also for Type 2 diabetes, when intervention studies related to microvascular disease are positive [40] and there is also a clear correlation between glycaemic control and the development of complications in observational studies [186].

Over the past 25 years, we have observed a radical change in the management of patients, driven by new methods, such as home monitoring of blood glucose, insulin pumps, insulin pens, along with better monitoring of glycaemia, as well as better documentation of complications as measured by retinal photographs and microalbuminuria. Although insulin pumps were introduced around 1980 [223] and stimulated our hope for a practical way to achieve near-normoglycaemia [224-232], for many reasons they are used nowadays by fewer and fewer patients.

Pancreas transplantation, as a more radical approach towards euglycaemia, was proposed even earlier and was also thought to have great promise [233-235]. The idea and its considerable impracticality has been evaluated recently [236]. A new longterm study [237] suggested that the glomerular lesions in diabetic nephropathy could heal not after 5 but after 10 years of normoglycaemia effected by isolated pancreas transplantation. It should be noted that three of the eight patients in fact initially had normoalbuminuria, which in our experience (by strong contrast to the Minneapolis group) is associated with very limited lesions [47] and by definition such patients do not have nephropathy [14, 15]. Four patients had microalbuminuria and only one proteinuria, that is only one with overt nephropathy. Only open, nonsclerosed glomeruli were evaluated and no information on change in number of occluded glomeruli is available. Also analysis of interstitial expansion or vascular lesions would have been important considering necessary long-term treatment with Cyclosporin A. Biopsies were not taken from two patients at the follow-up because they had developed end-stage renal disease, so they were hardly normal again from any point of view. The follow-up rate of the very initial total cohort (at year zero) is not recorded. A fall in GFR (from 108 to 74 ml/min) was noted in patients that were followed for 10 years, hardly a sign of regression. It would be important to see this study confirmed but for practical reasons this is not to be expected. The study could have problematic implications if it were to create overoptimistic views on the usefulness of pancreas transplantations. Also it is noteworthy that pancreas transplantation does not always lead to a complete return to normal metabolism [238].

ANGIOTENSIN-CONVERTING ENZYME-INHIBITORS

Angiotensin-converting enzyme-inhibitors are antihypertensive agents which in several experimental studies [239], and also in human studies in diabetes [195], had a specific effect on renal function indicating reduction of trans-glomerular pressure. Thereby, a reduction in albuminuria has been shown by ACE-inhibitors; likewise, the rate of decline of GFR and even its arrest was seen in patients with microalbuminuria [197]. Therefore, the use of ACE-inhibitors has become a standard initial choice in early and late antihypertensive treatment of diabetic patients, but quite often combination therapy is required, also in clinical trials [196]. It is still debatable whether, with exactly the same effects on blood pressure, differences still remain between ACE-inhibitors and other anti-hypertensive agents though this argument has been resolved for beta-blockers, which exert the same beneficial action as ACE-inhibitors in Type 2 diabetes [131]. Nevertheless the debate seems to have been largely academic as usually ACE-inhibitors are quite efficient and only have a few side effects (no impact on glycaemia), at least early in the course of renal involvement in diabetes. In any case, the introduction of ACE-inhibitors has been a major step forward in diabetes care. We are still working on a new development combining ACE-inhibitors with diuretics and cardio-selective beta-blockers and even receptor antagonists as a potentially even more efficient treatment [194]. Years ago, it was suggested that antihypertensive treatment could impair renal circulation and thus be deleterious [35]. The small reduction in GFR along with reduced proteinuria is likely to be indicative of a beneficial effect [15]. Based on many studies, we now know that low blood pressure obtained by treatment or spontaneously is protective against the development of more advanced glomerulopathy and decline in GFR [219]. Renal vascular stenosis in diabetic patients very rarely imposes clinical problems [130, 131] and needs usually not be screened for before treatment [240]. A famous case report documented only few diabetic lesions in a post-stenotic kidney [323].

THE CONCEPT OF ANTIHYPERTENSIVE COMBINATION THERAPY IN DIABETES

Quite often in clinical practice antihypertensive combination therapy has to be used. This is not surprising considering the complex nature of high blood pressure in diabetes. With particular regard to renal involvement it could be advantageous to use ACE-inhibitors because of their effect on glomerular pressure [36, 239, 241]. Indeed, there could also be an additional effect on growth factors and cytokines by ACE-inhibition. Nevertheless, early on there may also be general hyperfusion related partly to cardiac involvement [242] that could be reduced by the use of beta-blockers. This concept of general vascular hyperperfusion in the genesis of vascular complications was proposed by Parving et al. [243]. In many Type 1 and Type 2 diabetic patients there are signs of sodium retention and therefore diuretic treatment could be beneficial.

Following these lines we have used a combination of beta-blockers and ACE-inhibitors [192, 193, 194] with diuretics as a basis therapy. This kind of treatment was effective in reducing albuminuria and persistent studies have shown long-term preservation of GFR in patients with early renal disease [194]. Therefore, this concept of treatment could prove important, also in the early management with only limited blood pressure increase. Very few side-effects are seen with early combination therapy where moderate doses can be used. Combinations including thiazides and beta-blockers are often used also in non-diabetics with only limited risk of developing glucose intolerance or diabetes with beta-blockers but the proven relative benefits seem clear [389].

Newer studies suggest excellent antihypertensive effect in type 2 diabetes with microalbuminuria by combining an ACE-inhibitor with an angiotensin receptor-blocker [332,382]. This combination was also used in other studies [327-330, 388].

RENAL INVOLVEMENT AND TREATMENT IN PATIENTS WITH TYPE 2 DIABETES AND PROTEINURIA

Patients in this category have a poor prognosis with a rapid decline in GFR, correlated with blood pressure, but not HbA1C [15, 244]. The prognosis is also poor because many patients develop cardiovascular disease which is the most common cause for the observed considerable increase in mortality. Black people have a considerable higher risk for disease progression compared to white people [390]. Therefore, it is important to conduct new trials in this area, indeed two major trials are in progress using treatment with an angiotensin-converting receptor blockade compared with standard treatment. In one study, treatment with calcium channel blockers is used in one arm. Some controversy has arisen recently regarding calcium channel blockers in diabetes [245, 246]. The results of large new trials are eagerly awaited, in the hope it will be possible to improve the care of these patients. In my mind, however, it is clear that early treatment, including screening of patients with microalbuminuria and well-preserved GFR would still be essential along with early antihypertensive treatment in general and better glycaemic control.

So far treatment with the receptor blocker Losartan has been effective in normoalbuminuric and microalbuminuric essential hypertensive patients [247]. In normoalbuminuric Type 1 diabetes, Losartan not only reduces blood pressure (in normotensive patients) but also hyperfiltration and insulin resistance and this is of potential benefit in Type 2 diabetes [248]. The clinical relevance remains though to be established.

THE NATURAL HISTORY OF DIABETIC RENAL DISEASE, A SOUND CONCEPT?

The term "the natural history of diabetic renal disease" has been widely used [249] but possibly it is no longer appropriate simply because we have and use many measures to change the course of renal disease in diabetic patients. The natural history can be a term used to describe the normal course in diabetic patients in purely observational studies. It is however, now clear that the course of renal disease strongly relates to glycaemic control with HbA1c lower than 7.5% microalbuminuria might not develop at all. Also when microalbuminuria is present there could be an effect of improved glycaemic control although this is difficult since control is often hard to achieve in these patients [188]. In overt renal disease several observational studies in Type 1 diabetes have shown that the rate of decline in renal function is correlated with HbA1C, which excludes the term "natural history" and obviously only applies to poorly treated patients. In the case of normal blood pressure the rate of decline in GFR is actually low and long-term studies have shown that survivors of long duration quite frequently have lower than normal blood pressure [81, 216].

RENAL BIOPSIES IN DIABETIC PATIENTS

Renal biopsies, introduced many years ago by Brun et al [343], have been used in several diabetic nephropathy research projects with very remarkable results [47,48, 298]. However, in clinical practise costly renal biopsies in diabetic patients practically never changes clinical treatments. Also as a prognostic tool, biopsies are hardly interesting from a clinical point of view. However, beneficial effect of antihypertensive treatment has been documented in a research project [48]. Non-diabetic lesion may be present in about 10 per cent of cases in type 2 diabetes [295, 296, 366] or even in 0 percent (chapter 19) and clinical consequences are uncertain or non-existing. Indication may vary and diabetic renal disease is hardly a reason for biopsy [399]. Calculation of cost/benefit is missing.

ALTERNATIVES TO MICROALBUMINURIA?

Microalbuminuria has emerged as a very powerful clinical predictor of overt renal and cardiovascular disease. This was recently confirmed in the post DCCT-study [349] and the HOPE-study [322, 346]. Although the correlation to structural changes may not be perfect, especially in type 2 patients, microalbuminuria certainly predicts clinical proteinuria in both types of diabetes, and in type 2 diabetes, also cardiovascular mortality. The power of microalbuminuria is strengthened by continous follow-up in the diabetes clinic. It should be mentioned that ACE-inhibition and other antihypertensive agents may normalize microalbuminuria so evaluation of the actual clinical situation should be done after discontinuation of therapy for one or two months. Early treatment has also proven to improve prognosis. However, it would be useful to have alternatives to microalbuminuria, especially in evaluation of the long-term fate of patients, but so far this has not been possible, as also discussed [381].

New technologies have also failed to replace microalbuminuria or to add accurate predictions of the disease. Identification of genes has so far been clinically too unreliable and in some studies no association is found. Other substances to be measured in urine and blood have not added any new developments. It has been proposed that extra-cellular-matrix molecules or products of glycation could be of importance, but this needs still to be confirmed. Measurements of cellular function in skin and lympocytes are interesting research tools as also discussed elsewhere in this volume, but not useful enough in clinical evaluation. Also new imaging technologies, such as eg. Positron-emission tomography and magnetic resonance imaging have not been useful although new studies may be required [367].

It has been proposed that increasing serum prorenin preceeds the unset of microalbuminuria, a highly interesting area that needs further investigation. However, the overlap between non-progressors and progressors is too large, and also it is too cumbersome to evaluate serum prorenin in the diabetes clinic. However, the observation is very interesting, also because dual blockade of the renal angiotensin system seems to be useful in clinical practise [332].

It can thus be concluded that there are no alternatives in the present situation. Microalbuminuria quite accurately predicts renal disease, especially with careful follow-up and measurements of albumin excretion rate in the clinics. Some American investigators are however, inclined to use much more invasive techniques such as renal biopsies [320,321]; writing in a title of a paper: "Can the insulin-dependent diabetic patients be managed without kidney biopsy".

CARDIOVASCULAR AND CEREBROVASCULAR ALONG WITH RENAL END-POINTS

Cardio- and also cerebro-vascular diseases are major causes of death in both Type 1 and Type 2 diabetes, especially when the kidney is affected. Although the concept of controlled clinical or therapeutic trial has evolved over the past 50 years [250-251], only a few large trials have been conducted in diabetes, the first being the UGDP (University Group Diabetes Program) [252] which is now, after the UKPDS [128-129], mainly of historical interest. No real large-scale controlled trials were done when introducing sulphonylureas [253], biguanides or insulin but this has changed now [128-129]. There has therefore been an increasing interest in cerebrovascular and cardiovascular end-points, especially in Type 2 diabetes with respect to effective modulation, mainly with antihypertensive treatment strategies, which show a beneficial effect (Table 49-8).

Most studies use ACE-inhibitors but it is noteworthy that any reduction in blood pressure seems to be important. Certain trials show ACE-inhibitors to be superior to calciumblockers and also conventional treatment [132, 135, 136]. Importantly, the UK prospective diabetes study showed a similar outcome using ACE-inhibitors and beta-blockers [128, 129]. Fewer side effects occurred with the use of ACE-inhibitors (Captopril was given only twice a day). This study also clearly showed that careful blood pressure monitoring and effective treatment reduce very considerably cardio and microvascular end-points (around 30 %). Therefore, antihypertensive treatment should be given great priority in the management of patients with Type 2 diabetes. The UK prospective diabetes study showed some effect of optimal glycaemic control but due to the nature of the trial this was not so evident. Combined euglycaemia (HbA,c = 6-7 %) and normotension is, however, highly protective when blood pressure is around 130/80 [79, 80].

META-ANALYSIS IN DIABETES

The meta-analysis approach was originally worked out in the physical and mathematical sciences [250, 251] but was soon used in medical studies to combine, for instance, data from trials and from observational cohorts, e.g. on the correlation between hard end-points such as mortality compared with risk factors such as blood pressure. Indeed studies with observations in many subjects have documented a clear linear correlation between hard end-points and blood pressure down to normal values.

Parving et al. did a modified meta-analysis of many small trials in the evaluation of progression of renal disease in Type 1 diabetic patients treated with ACE-inhibitors and non-ACE-inhibitors and found very similar progression rates during treatment [15, 214]. The analysis was before the Ed Lewis Study [218]. Most trials with microalbuminuric patients in Type 1 diabetes are of limited size and therefore it would be valuable to do meta-analysis also on such patients as done by Chaturvedi along with our group and others [203]. The beneficial effects on regression of microalbuminuria were better documented in this meta-analysis than in individual studies of homogeneous Type 1 diabetic patients. Table 49-8 shows results of a number of studies.

It is important to consider homogeneity before preceding with any meta-analysis otherwise the situation can be problematic such as in the metformin arm of the UK prospective diabetes study [129] in which a beneficial effect was found in newly diagnosed obese people with diabetes. Later on, in other patients with longer standing diabetes, poor glycaemic control and probably more advanced vascular damage, the beneficial effect of combination therapy (metformin plus sulphonylurea) was lost and an adverse effect was even noted. From a clinical point of view these two patient groups are different and in my view it is not relevant and even incorrect to make a meta-analysis in such a situation. There are, however, people who support the Petonian approach and believe that meta-analysis can be important even with non-homogeneity [254]. This has been questioned suggesting that meta-analysis does not always give the correct answer, especially if the question is not correctly formulated and patient material not homogeneous [255-261].

Table 49-9 (Continue on next page)

10 Controlled Studies of IDDM Microalbuminuric patients (duration of study ≥2y)

Study	Drugs	Baseline	Mean age: y	Mean BP	Duration of study, y
European Captopril Study (1994) [202]	Cap/Pla	46/46	32	124/77	2
North American Captopril Study (1995) [337]	Cap/Pla	70/73	33	120/77	2
EUCLID (1997) [338]	Lis/Pla	32/37	33	122/80	2
PRIMA (1997) [339]	Ram/Ram/Pla 1,25/5,0/-	18/19	-	?	2
Italian Microalbuminuria (1998) [340]	Lis/Nif/Pla	33/26/34	37	129/83	3
Mathiesen, Steno (1999) [197]	Cap+diu/Con	21/23	~29	126/77	8
ATLANTIS Paul O'Hare (Personal comm. 1999)	Ram/Ram/Pla 1,25/5,0/-	44/44/46	40	132/76	2
Melbourne DNSG [341]	Per/Nif/Pla	13/10/10	~30	132/77	2½
Padua/Aarhus (Low grade micro) (1998) [342]	Lis/Pla	32/28	41	124/83 131/81	2
Rudberg (1999) [48]	Ena/Met/Ref	7/6/9	~19	125/81	~3
Europe 9/North Am. 1	Mostly ACE-I	All 727 pts	19-40	127/79	2,8

Cap = Captopril, Lis = Lisinopril, Ram = Ramipril, Per = Perindopril, Ena = Enalapril, Meto = Metoprolol, Nif = Nifidipine, Con = Control group, Pla = Placebo, Ref: Reference group, DD: Diabetes duration

Table 49-9 (Continued)
10 Controlled Studies of IDDM Microalbuminuric patients (duration of study ≥2y)

Study	DD. y	Mean or median UAE µg/min	Effect on UAE of drug	Effect on BP	Effect of GFR	Note
European Captopril Study (1994) [202]	17	55	↓	↓	No	European arm
North American Captopril Study (1995) [337]	18	62	↓	↓	Creatinine cl. stable	North American arm
EUCLID (1997) [338]	13	~42	↓	↓?	?	Little/No effect on normo
PRIMA (1997) [339]	24	61	No	No	No	HbA1C = 7.4
Italian Microalbuminuria (1998) [340]	18	71	Lis ↓↓/Nif↓	L↓↓/Nif↓	S-crea: No	Effect with Nif
Mathiesen, Steno (1999) [197]	18	93	↓	?	Stable with Cap+Diu Diu	**Preservation of GFR by ACE-I**
ATLANTIS Paul O'Hare (1998) [348]	20	53	Ram 1,25+ 5 mg↓	↓	No	Not dose dependent HbA1C=1 1.0
Melbourne DNSG [341]	16	62	Per↓/Nif-	Tendency by Per/Nif ↓	No	No effect with Nif
Padua/Aarhus (Low grade micro) (1998) [342]	13,5 15,1	36 (range 20-70)	↓	↓(24h)	No	Effect in low micro related to FF
Rudberg (1999) [48]	11	~31	E↓/M↓/ref.-	No	No	**Preservation of structure by Ena/Met**
Europe 9/North Am. 1	16,7		Mainly ACE-I ↓	Mostly ↓		

Cap = Captopril, Lis = Lisinopril, Ram = Ramipril, Per = Perindopril, Ena = Enalapril, Meto = Metoprolol, Nif = Nifidipine, Con = Control group, Pla = Placebo, Ref: Reference group, DD: Diabetes duration

GUIDELINES BASED ON PATHOPHYSIOLOGICAL AND CLINICAL TRIALS

The World Health Organisation - International Society of Hypertension (WHO-ISH) Liaison Committee on hypertension was established in the mid-1970s and has subsequently produced several guidelines, the first in 1975 [262]. New guidelines have recently appeared [263] also related to hypertension in diabetes.

Several of these new guidelines have a similar approach [264-269]. There is a clear emphasis on early and effective antihypertensive treatment in patients with diabetes suggesting a lower threshold for the start of the treatment and also a lower blood pressure goal during treatment. Angiotensin-converting enzyme-inhibitors are often preferred as initial agents but combination therapy is often warranted.

In view of the recent observation that different types of drugs (ACE-I, beta-blockers, calcium channel blockers and diuretics) reduce cardiovascular risk in Type 2 diabetes there are different treatment options. In diabetic renal disease ACE-I is however important. The beneficial effects on regression of microalbuminuria were better documented in a meta-analysis than in individual studies of homogeneous Type 1 diabetic patients (table 49-9).

It is important to consider homogeneity before preceding with any meta-analysis otherwise the situation can be problematic such as in the metformin arm of the UK prospective diabetes study [129] in which a beneficial effect was found only in newly diagnosed obese people with diabetes.

The British Hypertension Society proposes [266]:

(1) "The threshold for antihypertensive treatment in Type 1 diabetes is $\geq$ 140/90 mmHg. The target blood pressure is < 130/80 mmHg, or lower (< 125/ 75 mmHg) when there is proteinuria $\geq$ 1 g/24 hours" and

(2) "Trials support treatment of all patients with Type 2 diabetes and blood pressure $\geq$ 140/90 mmHg, aiming for a target blood pressure < 130/80 mmHg. Blood pressures $\geq$ 140/80 mmHg on treatment should be considered sub-optimal" and

(3) "Thus there is evidence from outcome trials in hypertensive patients with diabetes for the efficacy and safety of ACE-inhibitors, betablockers, dihydropyridines, and low-dose thiazides.

The choice among these drug classes should be made using the criteria set out earlier for non-diabetic patients. Blood pressure control will usually require more than one antihypertensive drug, and about 30 % of hypertensive patients with diabetes need three or more agents in combination" [266]. A similar approach is seen in Table 49-9.

The problem is that it can be difficult to achieve such blood pressure especially in patients with proteinuria and overt renal disease and also in others with cardiovascular problems. Therefore, it is strongly advocated that treatment is started early, e.g. with development of microalbuminuria, even in patients with normal blood pressure.

Table 49-10. Proposed and potential strategies for the prevention and treatment of diabetic complications, with focus on nephropathy

Strategy	Helpful in diagnosis	Helpful in treatment
Analysis of Genetic factors [310,365]	No, but studies are needed.	At risk patients cannot yet be found. No Genetic modulation possible.
Familial factors [365]	To some extent (early diagnosis of hypertension)	No
Antiglycemic treatment [367,349]	Yes (HbA$_{1C}$ monitoring)	Yes clearly demanding and sometimes not feasible
Various types of AGE-inhibitors [319,400]	No	Some renal studies stopped Other studies started
Aldose reductase inhibitor [364]	No	No, renal studies stopped (?)
Growth factor inhibition [315]	No	Needs investigation
Protein kinase C inhibitors [317]	No	Needs investigation
Antihypertensive treatment [353,373]	Yes, often along with microalbuminuria and albuminuria or high BP	Yes, mainly ACE-I as basis for combination therapy
ACE-inhibitors [346]	No (genotyping not useful)	Yes, profoundly, especially in microalbuminuric patients
Lipid-lowering [375]	Yes, dyslipidemia	Probably, but needs further confirmation
Aspirine [134]	No	Probably (only for macrovasular disease)
C-peptide [361,394]	Sometimes	Further studies planned
Endothelial and Endo-peptidase inhibitors [392, 393]	No	Under investigation
Glycosaminoglycans [376]	No	Under investigation
Metalloproteinase [391]	No(?)	Under investigation

It has also been proposed that treatment should be started even before microalbuminuria [210]. Since complications are so closely associated with blood pressure increase (also in the normal range) this could easily be recommended in future guidelines as we now have effective treatment with limited side effects. More effective antihypertensive programmes seem to be essential [332].

Table 49-11. Trial in diabetes and microalbuminuria

		Principal Investigator	Completion
Microalbuminuria	DIABHYCAR Ramipril, small doses)	Marre	2001
	HOPE*, Microhope (Ramipril, moderate to high dose)	Yusuf/Gerstein	1999
	CALM** (Lisinopril and/or Candesartan)	Mogensen	2000
	DETAIL (Telmisartan)	Barnett	2003
	IRMA II (Irbesartan)	Arner	2000/2001
	Perindopril/ Indapamide	Mogensen/Viberti	2001
Non-diabetic (Microalbuminuria)	PREVEND*** (Fosinopril)	DeJong	2003
Macroalbuminuria	Renaal (Losartan)	Brenner	2001
	IDNT (Irbesartan)	Lewis	2000/2001
	ABCD2C (Valsartan)	Schrier	2003

* Already published
** Dual blockade
*** + statin treatment in a factorial design.

CONCLUDING REMARKS

This review describes observations in a number of areas related to diabetic renal disease and related topics. Over the past 30 years there has been a great change in the management of the patients with long-term diabetes as described by Lundbæk [270], based on the results of physiological and patho-physiological studies followed by clinical trials which have been quickly implemented into clinical practice and incorporated in revised guidelines. Not all ideas have proved successful although they might have provided important insight into the nature of the disease (table 49-10). Some erroneous concepts have, however, led to setbacks slowing down the introduction of effective treatment in patients.

These include a few very preliminary studies which suggested complications are predominantly genetically determined and therefore not readily modifiable. Considering complications to be generated primarily by a combination of glycaemic and haemodynamic factors (especially high blood pressure) – and not clearly genetically determined makes the treatment option much more attractive to the clinician [271, 272]. Table 49-11 provides a review on ongoing trials.

The role of low protein diet is not discussed but the potential nephrotoxic effect of dietary proteins was originally explored by Anitschkow and co-workers in St. Petersburg in 1913 [273]. This gave subsequently rise to the cholesterol research since rabbits were fed and they were not only exposed to a high protein but also a high fat diet. The protein contents of the diabetic diet is still discussed [53, 363] but the cholesterol issue in diabetes, later appeared to be even more important [375,376]. Interestingly, dietary intervention may also effect BP [274]

Acknowledgements. This review is dedicated to laboratory assistant Merete Moller, who over the years helped me and my co-workers in an extraordinary way to conduct the studies described herein. I am also most grateful to Anna Honoré for careful secretarial work and to Anette Andersen for reference management.

REFERENCES

1. Mogensen CE (1989) Hyperfiltration, hypertension, and diabetic nephropathy in IDDM patients. Based on the Golgi Lecture 1988, EASD meeting, Paris. Diabetes Nutrition & Metabolism 2: 227-244
2. Mogensen CE, Christensen CK, Vittinghus E (1983) The stages in diabetic renal disease. With emphasis on the stage of incipient diabetic nephropathy. Diabetes 32: 64-78
3. Mogensen CE, Chachati A, Christensen CK et al. (1985-6) Microalbuminuria: an early marker of renal involvement in diabetes. Uremia Investigation 9: 85-95
4. Mogensen CE (1987) Microalbuminuria as a predictor of clinical diabetic nephropathy. Kidney Int 31: 673-689
5. Mogensen CE (1990) Prediction of Clinical Diabetic Nephropathy in IDDM patients. Alternatives to microalbuminuria? Diabetes 37: 761-767
6. Mogensen CE, Marshall SM (1990) Early diagnosis of diabetic nephropathy. Twelve assertions on microalbuminuria and early nephropathy. In: Andreucci et al. (eds) International Yearbook of nephrology. Kluwer Academic Publ., Boston, Dordrecht, London pp 123-146
7. Mogensen CE, Hansen KW, Klebe J et al. (1991) Microalbuminuria: Studies in diabetes, essential hypertension, and renal diseases as compared with the background population. In: Grünfeld JP (ed) Advances in Nephrology, vol. 20. Mosby Year Book, Chicago, Illinois, pp 191-228
8. Mogensen CE, Hansen KW, Osterby R, Damsgaard EM (1992) Blood pressure elevation versus abnormal albuminuria in the genesis and prediction of renal disease in diabetes. Diabetes Care 15:1192-1204
9. Mogensen CE, Damsgaard EM, Froland A (1992) GFR-loss and cardiovascular damage in diabetes: A key role for abnormal albuminuria. Acta Diabetol 29: 201-213

10. Mogensen CE, Damsgaard EM, Froland A, Nielsen S, de Fine Olivarius N, Schmitz A (1992) Microalbuminuria in non-insulin-dependent diabetes. Clin Nephrol [Suppl 1138:S28-S39

11. Mogensen CE, Christensen CK, Christensen PD (1993) The abnormal albuminuria syndrome in diabetes. Microalbuminuria:Key to the complications. In: Belfiore F, Bergman RN, Molinatti GM (eds) Current Topics in Diabetes Research. Front Diabetes. Karger, Basel, pp 86-121

12. Mogensen CE, Poulsen PL, Heinsvig EM (1993) Abnormal albuminuria in the monitoring of early renal changes in diabetes. In: Mogensen CE, Standl E (eds) Concepts for the Ideal Diabetes Clinic. Diabetes Forum Series, Volume IV Walter de Gruyter, Berlin, New York, pp 289-313

13. Mogensen CE (2000) Diabetic nephopathy: Natural history and management. In: Ei Nahas (ed) Mechanisms and clinical management of progressive renal failure. Oxford University Press, Oxford, pp 211-240

14. Mogensen CE (1998) Preventing end-stage renal disease. Diabetic Medicine, 15: S51-S56

15. Parving H-H (1998) Renoprotection in diabetes: genetic and non-genetic risk factors and treatment. Diabetologia 41: 745-759

16. Parving H-H, Jensen HF-, Mogensen CE, Evrin PE (1974) Increased urinary albumin excretion rate in benign essential hypertension. Lancet 1: 1190-1192

17. Campese VM. Bianchi S, Bigazzi R (1999). Association between hyperlipidemia and microalbuminuria in essential hypertension. Kidney Int., 65(S71): S10-S13.

18. Christensen CK, Krussel LR, Mogensen CE (1987) Increased blood pressure in diabetes: Essential hypertension or diabetic nephropathy? Scand J Clin Lab Invest 47: 363-370

19. Pedersen EB, Mogensen CE (1976) Effect of antihypertensive treatment on urinary albumin excretion, glomerular filtration rate and renal plasma flow in patients with essential hypertension. Scand J Clin Lab Invest 36: 231-237

20. Damsgaard EM, Mogensen CE (1986) Microalbuminuria in elderly hyperglycaemic patients and controls. Diabetic Medicine 3: 430-435

21. Damsgaard EM, Froland A, Mogensen CE (1988) Albumin excretion above 15 μg/min is a strong predictor of death in elderly diabetics and non-diabetics. Diabetes Res Clin Pract 5 [Suppl ll:S9 (Abstract)

22. Damsgaard EM, Froland A, Jorgensen OD, Mogensen CE (1993) Prognostic value of urinary albumin excretion rate and other risk factors in elderly diabetic patients and non-diabetic control subjects surviving the first 5 years after assessment. Diabetologia 36: 1030-1036

23. Damsgaard EM, Froland A, Jorgensen OD, Mogensen CE (1990) Microalbuminuria as predictor of increased mortality in elderly people. BMJ 300: 297-300

24. Vestbo E, Damsgaard EG, Mogensen CE (1997) The relationship between microalbuminuria in first generation diabetic and non-diabetic subjects and microalbuminuria and hypertension in the second generation (a population based study). Nephrol Dial Transplant 12 [Suppl 2]: 32-36

25. Vestbo E, Damsgaard EM, Froland A, Mogensen CE (1996) Birth weight and cardiovascular risk factors in an epidemiological study. Diabetologia 39: 1598-1602

26. Vestbo E, Damsgaard EM, Froland A, Mogensen CE (1995) Urinary albumin excretion in a population based cohort. Diabet Med 12: 488-493

27. Yudkin JS, Forrest RD, Jackson CA (1988) Microalbumuminuria as predictor of vascular disease in non-diabetic subjects. Lancet ii:530-533

28.   Mølgaard H, Christensen PD, Hermansen K, Sørensen KE, Christensen CK, Mogensen CE (1994). Early recognition of sympathovagal dysfunction in microalbuminuria. Importance for cardiac mortality in diabetes? Diabetologia, 37:788-796.

29.   Olivarius de FN, Andreasen AH, Keiding N, Mogensen CE (1993) Epidemiology of renal involvement in newly-diagnosed middle-aged and elderly diabetic patients. Cross-sectional data from the population-based study "Diabetes care in General Practice", Denmark. Diabetologia 36: 1007-1016

30.   Jager A, Kostense PJ, Nijpels G, Heine RJ, Bouter LM, Stehouwer CDA (1998) Microalbuminria is strongly associated with NIDDM and hypertension but not with the insulin resistance syndrome: the Hoorn Study. Diabetologia 41: 694-700

31.   Ekbom P and the Copenhagen Pre-eclampsia in Diabetic Pregnancy Study Group (1999). Pre-pregnancy microalbuminuria predicts pre-eclampsia in insulin-dependent diabetes mellitus, The Lancet, 353: 377

32.   Ferrannini E (1993) The metabolic syndrome. In: Mogensen CE (ed) Target organ damage in the mature hypertensive. Science Press, London, pp 2.31-2.49

33.   Mogensen CE, Hansen KW, Mau Pedersen M, Christensen CK (1991) Renal factors influencing blood pressure threshold and choice of treatment for hypertension in IDDM. Diabetes Care 14: 13-26

34.   Mogensen CE, Mau Pedersen M, Hansen KW, Christensen CK (1992) Microalbuminuria and the organ-damage concept in antihypertensive therapy for patients with insulin--dependent diabetes mellitus. Journal of Hypertension 10:S43-S51

35.   Mogensen CE (1995) Diabetic Renal Disease: The Quest for Normotension - and Beyond. Diabetic Medicine 12: 756-769

36.   Mogensen CE (1995) Management of the diabetic patient with elevated blood pressure or renal disease. Early screening and treatment programs. In: Laragh JH, Brenner BM (eds) Albuminuria and Blood Pressure. Hypertension: Pathophysiology, Diagnosis, and management. 2nd ed., Raven Press Ltd. N. Y., pp 2335-2365

37.   Mogensen CE (1990) Prevention and treatment of renal disease in insulin-dependent diabetes mellitus. Semin Nephrol:260-273

38.   Mogensen CE (1994) Renoprotective role of ACE inhibitors in diabetic nephropathy. Brit Heart J 72 (l):38-45

39.   Mogensen CE (1994) Systemic blood pressure and glomerular leakage with particular reference to diabetes and hypertension. J Intern Med 235: 297-316

40.   Ohkubo Y, Kishikawa H, Araki E et al. (1995) Intensive insulin therapy prevents the progression of diabetic microvascular complications in Japanese patients with non-insulin-dependent diabetes mellitus: a randomized prospective 6-year study. Diabetes Research Clinical Practice 28: 103-117

41.   The Diabetes Control and Complications Trial Research Group (1993) The effect of intensive treatment of diabetes on the development and progression of long-term complications in insulin-dependent diabetes mellitus. New England Journal of Medicine 329: 977-986

42.   Osterby RH (1965) A quantitative estimate of the peripheral glomerular basement membrane in recent juvenile diabetes. Diabetologia 1: 97-100

43.   Osterby R (1971) Course of Diabetic Glomerulopathy. Acta Diabet Latina 8 (l):179-191

44.   Osterby R (1972) Morphometric studies of the peripheral glomerular basement membrane in early juvenile diabetes. Development of initial basement membrane thickening. Diabetologia 8: 84-92

45. Berg UB, Torbjornsdotter TB, Jaremko G, Thalme B (1998) Kidney morphological changes in relation to long-term renal function and metabolic control in adolescents with IDDM. Diabetologia 41:1047-1056

46. Osterby R (1990) Basement membrane morphology in diabetes mellitus. In: Ellenberg & Rifkin's Diabetes Mellitus, theory and practice, 4th ed., Elsevier, N. Y., Amsterdam, London, pp 220-233

47. Osterby R (1996) Lessons from kidney biopsies. Diabetes Metabol Rev 12:151-174

48. Rudberg S, Østerby R, Bangstad H-J, Dahlquiest G, Persson B (1999). Effect of angiotensin converting enzyme inhibitor or beta blocker on glomerular structural changes in young microalbuminuric patients with type 1 (insulin-dependent) diabetes mellitus. Diabetologia, 42: 589-595.

49. Williamson JR, Vogler NJ, Kilo C (1971) Structural abnormalities in muscle capillary basement membrane in diabetes mellitus. Acta Diabet Latina 8 [Suppl l]: 1 17-134

50. Mau Pedersen M, Christensen SE, Christiansen JS, Pedersen EB, Mogensen CE, Orskov H (1990) Acute effects of the somatostatin analogue on kidney function in Type 1 diabetic patients. Diabetic Med 7: 304-309

51. Mau Pedersen M, Christiansen JS, Mogensen CE (1991) Reduction of glomerular hyperfiltration in normoalbuminuric IDDM patients by 6 months of aldose reductase inhibition. Diabetes 40: 527-531

52. Mau Pedersen M, Mogensen CE, Christiansen JS (1995) Reduction of glomerular hyperfunction during short-term aldose reductase inhibition in normoalbuminuric, insulin-dependent diabetic patients. Endocrinology and Metabolism 2: 55-56

53. Mau Pedersen M, Mogensen CE, Schonau Jorgensen F, Moller B, Lykke G, Pedersen 0 (1989) Renal effects of limitation of high dietary protein in normoalbuminuric insulin-dependent diabetic patients. Kidney Int 36 [Suppl 271:S115-S121

54. MauPedersenM,WintherE,MogensenCE(1990)Reducing protein in the diabetic diet. Diabetes Metab 16:454-459

55. Mogensen CE (1986) Early glomerular hyperfiltration in insulin-dependent diabetics and late nephropathy. Scand J Clin Lab Invest 46: 201-206

56. Mogensen CE (1994) Glomerular hyperfiltration in human diabetes. Diabetes Care 17: 770-775

57. Mogensen CE, Solling K, Vittinghus E (1981) Studies on mechanisms of proteinuria using aminoacid-induced inhibition of tubular reabsorption in normal and diabetic man. Contr Nephrol 26: 50-65

58. Mogensen CE, Christensen CK, Christensen NJ, Gundersen HJG, Jacobsen FK, Pedersen EB, Vittinghus E (1981) Renal protein handling in normal, hypertensive and diabetic man. Contr Nephrol 24: 139-152

59. Turner RC, Millns H, Neil HA, Stratton IM, Manley SE, Matthews DR, Holman RR for the United Kingdom Prospective Diabetes Study Group (1998) Risk factors for coronary artery disease in non-insulin dependent diabetes mellitus: United Kingdom prospective diabetes study (UKPDS:23). British Medical Journal 316: 823-828

60. Mogensen CE, Vigstrup J, Ehlers N (1985) Microalbuminuria predicts proliferative diabetic retinopathy. Lancet II:1512-1513

61. Gilbert RE, Tsalamandris C, Allen TJ, Colville D, Jerums G (1998) Early nephropathy predicts vision-threatening retinal disease in patients with type 1 diabetes mellitus. Journal of the American Society of Nephrology 9: 85-89

62. Bernard C (1849) Compte Rendu de la Société du Biologie. Paris. Vol. 1: 80-81

63. Deckert D (1998) Historical aspects of diabetes and diabetic renal disease. In: Mogensen CE (ed) The Kidney and hypertension in diabetes mellitus. 4th ed., Kluwer Academic Publ., Boston, Dordrecht, London pp 1-6

64. Rayer P (1839) Traité des maladies des Reins et des altérations de la sécrétion urinaire, etudiées en elles-mêmes et dans leurs rapports avec les maladies des uretèthres, de la vessie, de la prostate, de l'urèthre, etc. Libraire de l'Académie Royale de médicine, Paris

65. Rayer P (1841)) Traité des maladies des Reins et des altérations de la sécrétion urinaire, etudiées en elles-mêmes et dans leurs rapports avec les maladies des uretèthres, de la vessie, de la prostate, de l'urèthre, etc. Libraire de l'Académie Royale de médicine, Paris

66. Ross J, Goldmann JK (1971) Effect of streptozotocin-induced diabetes on kidney weight and compensatory hypertrophy in the rat. Endocrinology. 88: 1079-1082

67. Mogensen CE, Andersen MJF (1973) Increased kidney size and glomerular filtration rate in early juvenile diabetes. Diabetes 22: 706-712

68. Mogensen CE, Andersen MJF (1975) Increased kidney size and glomerular filtration rate in untreated juvenile diabetics. Normalization by insulin treatment. Diabetologia ll: 221-224

69. Baumgartl HJ, Banholzer P, Sigl G, Haslbeck M, Standl E (1998) On the prognosis of IDDM patients with large kidneys. The role of large kidneys for the development of diabetic nephropathy. Nephrol Dial Transplant 13: 630-634

70. Hostetter TH, Rennke HG, Brenner BM (1982) The case for intrarenal hypertension in the initiation and progression of diabetic and other glomerulopathies. Am J Med 72: 375-380

71. Rudberg S, Persson B, Dahlquist G (1992) Increased glomerular filtration rate as a predictor of diabetic nephropathy - An 8-year prospective study. Kidney Int 41: 822-828

72. Mogensen CE (1971) Kidney function and glomerular permeability in early juvenile diabetes. Scand J Clin Lab Invest 28: 79-90

73. Mogensen CE, Christensen CK (1984) Predicting diabetic nephropathy in insulin-dependent patients. N Engl J Med 311: 89-93

74. Mau Pedersen M, Christiansen JS, Pedersen EB, Mogensen CE (1992) Determinants of intra-individual variation in kidney function in normoalbuminuric insulin-dependent diabetic patients: importance of atrial natriuretic peptide and glycaemic control. Clinical Science 83: 445-451

75. Eiskjær H, Mogensen CE, Schmitz A, Pedersen EB (1991) Enhanced urinary excretion of albumin and β-2 microglobulin in essential hypertension induced by atrial natriuretic peptide. Scand J Clin Lab Invest 51: 359-366

76. Lutterman JA, Vervoort G, Wetzels JFM, Berden JHM, Smits P (1998) Increased albuminuric response to infusion of atrial natriuretic peptide in normoalbuminuric Type 1 diabetes. Diabetologia 41:A39

77. Mau Pedersern M (1998) Early renal hyperfunction and hypertrophy in IDDM patients including comments on early intervention. In: Mogensen CE (ed) The Kidney and Hypertension in Diabetes Mellitus. Kluwer Academic Publ., Boston, Dordrecht, London, pp 383-392

78. Osterby R, Gall M-A, Schmitz A, Nielsen FS, Nyberg G, Parving H-H (1993) Glomerular structure and function in proteinuric type 2 (non-insulin-dependent) diabetic patients. Diabetologia 36: 1064-1070

79. Mogensen CE (1998) Combined high blood pressure and glucose in type 2 diabetes: double jeopardy (editorial). BMJ 317: 693-694

80. American Diabetes Association (1999) Implications of the United Kingdom Prospective Diabetes study Diabetes Care 22, Suppl. 1 S 27- S 31

81. Borch-Johnsen K, Nissen H, Henriksen E, Kreiner S, Salling N, Deckert T, Nerup J (1987) The natural history of insulin-dependent diabetes mellitus in Denmark: 1. Long-term survival with and without late diabetic complications. Diabet Med 4: 201-210

82. Siperstein MD, Unger RH, Madison LL (1968) Studies of muscle Capillary Basement Membranes in Normal Subjects, Diabetic and Prediabetic Patients. J Clin Invest 47: 1973-1999

83. Deckert T, Poulsen JE (1981) Diabetic nephropathy: fault or destiny? Diabetologia 21: 178-183

84. Pirart J (1978) Diabetes mellitus and its degenerative complications: a prospective study of 4,400 patients observed between 1947 and 1973. Diabetes Care 1: 168-188

85. Feldt-Rasmussen B, Mathiesen ER, Jensen T, Lauritzen T, Deckert T (1991) Effect of improved metabolic control on loss of kidney function in type 1 (insulin-dependent) diabetic patients: an update of the Steno studies. Diabetologia 34: 164-170

86. Tarnov L, Gluud C, Parving H-H (1998) Diabetic nephropathy and the insertion/deletion polymorphism of the angiotensin-converting enzyme gene. Nephrology Dialysis Transplantation 13: 410-412

87. Alaveras EAG, Thomas SM, Sagriotis A, Viberti GC (1997) Promotors of progression of diabetic nephropathy: the relative roles of blood glucose and blood pressure control. Nephrology Dialysis Transplantation 12: 71-74

88. Björck S, Blohmé G, Sylvén C, Mulec H (1997) Deletion insertion polymorphism of the angiotensin converting enzyme gene and progression of diabetic nephropathy. Nephrology Dialysis Transplantation 12: 67-70

89. Fagerudd JA, Tarnow L, Jacobsen P et al. (1998) Predisposition to essential hypertension and development of diabetic nephropathy in IDDM patients. Diabetes 47: 439-444

90. Rudberg S, Stattin E-L, Dahlquist G (1998) Familial and perinatal risk factors for micro- and macroalbuminuria in young IDDM patients. Diabetes 47:1121-1126

91. Cowie CC, Port F, Wolfe R, Savage PJ, Moll PP, Hawthorne VM (1989) Disparities in incidence of diabetic end-stage re-nal disease according to race and type of diabetes. N Engl J Med 321: 1074-1079

92. Freedman BI, Soucie JM, McCiellan WM (1997) Family history of end-stage renal disease among incident dialysis patients. J Am Soc Nephrol 8: 1942-1945

93. Borch-Johnsen K, Norgaard K, Hommel E, Mathiesen ER, Jensen JS, Deckert T, Parving H-H (1992) Is diabetic nephropathy an inherited complication? Kidney Int 41: 719-722

94. Barker DJP (1994) Mothers, babies and diseases in later life. BMJ Publishing Group

95. Nelson RG, Morgenstern H, Bennett P (1998). Birth weight and renal disease in Pima Indians with type 2 diabetes mellitus. American J Epidemiology, 148:650-656.

96. Nyengaard JR, Bendtsen TF, Mogensen CE (1996) Low birth weight - is it associated with few and small glomeruli in normal persons and NIDDM (non-insulin-dependent diabetes mellitus) patients? Diabetologia 39: 1634-1637

97. Ravelli ACJ, van der Meulen JHP, Michels RPJ, Osmond C, Barker DJP, Hales CN, Bleker OP (1998) Glucose tolerance in adults after prenatal exposure to famine. Lancet 351:173-177

98. Yudkin JS, Stanner S (1998) Prenatal exposure to famine and health in later life. Lancet 351: 1361-1362

99. Bergaard l, Risinger G (1961) Quantitative immunochemical determination of albumin in normal human urine. Acta Soc Med Upsaliensis 66: 217-222

100. Keen H, Chlouverakis C, Fuller J, Jarret RS (1969) The concomitants of raised blood sugar: studies in newly-detected hyperglycaemics. II. Urinary albumin excretion, blood pressure and their relation to blood sugar levels. Guy's Hospital Reports 118: 247-254

101. Bigazzi R, Bianchi S, Baldari D, Campese VM (1998) Microalbuminuria predicts cardiovascular events and renal insufficiency in patients with essential hypertension. J Hypertens 16: 1325-1333

102. Poulsen PL, Mogensen CE (1995) Evaluation of a new semiquantitative stix for microalbuminuria. Diabetes Care 18: 732-733

103. Mogensen CE, Viberti GC, Peheim E et al. (1997) Multicenter evaluation of the Micral-test II test strip, an immunologic rapid test for the detection of microalbuminuria. Diabetes Care 20:1642-1646

104. Poulsen PL, Mogensen CE (1998) Clinical evaluation of a test for immediate and quantitative determination of urinary albumin-to-creatinine ratio. Diabetes Care 21: 97-98

105. Parving H-H, Oxenboll B, Svendsen PA, Christiansen JS, Andersen AR (1982) Early detection of patients at risk of developing diabetic nephropathy. A prospective study of urinary albumin excretion. Acta Endocrinol (Copenhagen) 100:550-555

106. Viberti GC, Hill RD, Jarret RJ, Argyropoulos A, Mahmud U, Keen H (1982) Microalbuminuria as a predictor of clinical nephropathy in insulin-dependent diabetes mellitus. Lancet I:1430-1432

107. Mau Pedersen M, Christensen CK and Mogensen CE (1992) Long-term (18 year) prognosis for normo- and microalbuminuric type 1 (insulin-dependent) diabetic patients. Diabetologia 35:A60 (Abstract)

108. Messent JWC, Elliott TG, Hill RD, Jarrett RJ, Keen H, Viberti GC (1992) Prognostic significance of microalbuminuria in insulin-dependent diabetes mellitus: A twenty-three year follow-up study. Kidney International 41: 836-839

109. Rossing P, Hougaard P, Borch-Johnsen K, Parving H-H (1996) Risk factors for mortality in IDDM patients, a 10 years observational follow up study. BMJ 313: 779-784

110. Forsblom CM, Groop P-H, Ekstrand A, Groop LC (1992) Predictive value of microalbuminuria in patients with insulin-dependent diabetes of long duration. BMJ 305: 1051-1053

111. Mogensen CE (1983) Microalbuminuria in maturity onset, primarily type 2 (non-insulin-dependent) diabetes, predicts clinical proteinuria and early mortality. Diabetologia 26: 181 (Abstract)

112. Mogensen CE (1984) Microalbuminuria predicts clinical proteinuria and early mortality in maturity-onset diabetes. N Engl J Med 310: 356-360

113. Dinneen S, Gerstein HC (1997) The association of microalbuminuria and mortality in non-insulin-dependent diabetes mellitus. A systematic overview of the literature. Arch Intern Med 157:1413-1418

114. Tanaka Y, Atsumi Y, Matsuoka K, Onuma T, Tohjima T, Kawamori R (1998) Role of glycemic control and blood pressure in the development and progression of nephropathy in elderly Japanese NIDDM Patients. Diabetes Care 21:116-120

115. Forsblom CM, Groop P-H, Ekstrand A et al. (1998) Predictors of progression from normoalbuminuria to microalbuminuria in NIDDM. Diabetes Care 21:1932-1938

116. Schmitz A (1997) Microalbuminuria, blood pressure, metabolic control, and renal involvement. Longitudinal studies in white non-insulin-dependent diabetic patients. American Journal of Hypertension 10: 189S-197S

117. Schmitz A, Vaeth M, Mogensen CE (1994) Systolic blood pressure relates to the rate of progression of albuminuria in NIDDM. Diabetologia 37:1251-1258

118. Nielsen S, Schmitz O, Orskov H, Mogensen CE (1995) Similar insulin sensitivity in NIDDM patients with normo- and microalbuminuria. Diabetes Care 18: 834-842

119. Nielsen S, Schmitz O, Moller N, Porksen N, Klausen IC, Alberti KGMM, Mogensen CE (1993) Renal function and insulin sensitivity during simvastatin treatment in Type 2 (non-insulin-dependent) diabetic patients with microalbuminuria. Diabetologia 36:1079-1086

120. Nielsen S, Schmitz A, Rehling M, Mogensen CE (1997) The clinical course of renal function in NIDDM patients with normo- and microalbuminuria. J Intern Med 241: 133-141

121. Nielsen S, Schmitz A, Rehling M, Mogensen CE (1993) Systolic blood pressure determines the rate of decline of glomerular filtration rate in Type 2 (non-insulin-dependent) diabetes mellitus. Diabetes Care 16: 1427-1432

122. Nielsen S, Schmitz A, Poulsen PL, Hansen KW, Mogensen CE (1995) Albuminuria and 24-h ambulatory blood pressure in normoalbuminuric and microalbuminuric NIDDM patients: a longitudinal study. Diabetes Care 18: 1434-1441

123. Nielsen S, Schmitz A, Derkx FHM, Mogensen CE (1995) Prorenin and renal function in NIDDM patients with normo- and microalbuminuria. J Intern Med 238: 499-505

124. Nielsen S, Schmitz A, Bacher T, Rehling M, Ingerslev J, Mogensen CE (1999). Transcapillary escape rate and albuminuria in Type II diabetes. Effects of short-term treatment with low-molecular weight heparin. Diabetologia, 42:60-67.

125. Nielsen S, Schmitz A, Knudsen RE, Dollerup J, Mogensen CE (1994) Enalapril versus bendroflumethiazide in type 2 diabetes complicated by hypertension. Q J Med 87: 747-754

126. Fioretto P, Stehouwer CDA, Mauer M et al. (1998) Heterogeneous nature of microalbuminuria in NIDDM: Studies of endothelial function and renal structure. Diabetologia 41: 233-236

127. Inomata S, Osawa Y, Itoh M (1987) Analysis of urinary proteins in diabetes mellitus - with reference to the relationship between microalbuminuria and diabetic renal lesions. J Jpn Diabetes Soc 30: 429-436

128. UKPDS 33 (1998) An intensive blood glucose control policy with sulphonylureas or insulin reduces the risk of diabetic complications in patients with Type 2 diabetes. Lancet 352:837-853

129. UKPDS 34 (1998) Effect of an intensive blood glucose control policy with metformin on complications in Type 2 diabetic patients. Lancet 352: 854-865

130. Turner R, Holman R, Stratton 1 et al. for United Kingdom Prospective Diabetes Study Group (1998) Tight blood pressure control and risk of macrovascular and microvascular complications in type 2 diabetes: United Kingdom prospective diabetes study 38. BMJ 317: 703-713

131. Holman R, Turner R, Stratton I et al. for United Kingdom Prospective Diabetes Study Group (1998). Efficacy of atenolol and captopril in reducing risk of macrovascular and microvascular complications in type 2 diabetes: United Kingdom prospective diabetes study 39. BMJ 317: 713-720

132. Tatti P, Pahor M, Byington RP, Di Mauro P, Guarisco RG, Strollo G, Strollo F (1998) Outcome results of the fosinopril versus amlodipine cardiovascular events randomized trials (FACET) in patients with hypertension and NIDDM. Diabetes Care 21: 597-603

133. Tuomilehto J, Rastenyte D, Birkenhäger W, et al (1999) Effects of calcium-channel blockade in older patients with diabetes and systolic hypertension. N Engl J Med, 340: 677-84

134.   Hansson L, Zanchetti A, Carruthers SG et al. for the HOT Study Group (1998). Effects of intensive blood-pressure lowering and low-dose aspirin in patients with hypertension: principal results of the Hypertension Optimal Treatment (HOT) randomised trial. Lancet 351: 1755-1762

135.   Estacio RO, Jeffers BW, Hiatt RA, Biggerstaff SL, Gifford N, Schrier RW (1998) The effect of nisoldipine as compared with enalapril on cardiovascular outcomes in patients with non-insulin-dependent diabetes and hypertension. N Engl J Med 338: 645-652

136.   Hansson L, Lindholm LH, Niskanen L et al (1999). Principal results of the Captopril Prevention Project (CAPPP). Effect of angiotensin converting enzyme inhibition compared with conventional therapy on cardiovascular morbidity and mortality in hypertension. Lancet, 353: 611-616.

137.   Curb JD, Pressel SL, Cutler JA et al. (1996) Effect of diuretic-based antihypertensive treatment on cardiovascular disease risk in older diabetic patients with isolated systolic hypertension. Systolic Hypertension in the Elderly Program Cooperative Research Group. JAMA 276:1886-1892

138.   Malmberg K, Rydén L, Wedel H (1998) Calcium antagonists, appropriate therapy for diabetic patients with hypertension? Eur Heart J 19: 1269-1272

139.   Pyorala K, Olsson AG, Pedersen TR et al. (1997) Cholesterol lowering with simvastatin improves prognosis of diabetic patients with coronary heart disease. Diabetes Care 20:614-620

140.   Kylin E (1923) Studien über das Hypertonie-Hyperglykamie-Hyperurikaemie Syndrom. Zentralblatt fair Innere Medizin 7:105-112

141.   Himsworth HP (1939) Mechanisms of diabetes mellitus (Goulstonian Lecture). Lancet 2: 1-6, 65-68, 118-122, 171-175

142.   Himsworth HP (1949). The syndrome of diabetes mellitus and its causes. Lancet, March 19, 1949: 465-472

143.   Vague J (1949) Le diabéte de la femme android. Presse Med. Paris 57: 835-837

144.   Avogaro P, Creapaldi G (1965) Essential hypertension, hyperlipemia, obesity and diabetes. European Association for the Study of Diabetes. Diabetologia 1: 137 (Abstract)

145.   Jarrett RJ (1992) In defence of insulin: a critique of syndrome X. Lancet 340: 469-471

146.   Karlefors T (1966) Circulatory studies during exercise with particular reference to diabetes. Acta Med Scand 180 [Suppl 4491]:1-87

147.   Christensen CK (1991) The pre-proteinuric phase of diabetic nephropathy. Dan Med Bull 38:145-159

148.   Vittinghus E, Mogensen CE (1981) Albumin excretion and renal hemodynamic response to physical exercise in normal and diabetic man. Scand J Clin Lab Invest 41: 627-632

149.   Vittinghus E, Mogensen CE (1982) Graded exercise and protein excretion in diabetic man and the effect of insulin treatment. Kidney Int 21: 725-729

150.   Mogensen CE, Vittinghus E (1975) Urinary albumin excretion during exercise in juvenile diabetes. A provocative test for early abnormalities. Scand J Clin Lab Invest 35: 295-300

151.   Mogensen CE, Solling K (1977) Studies on renal tubular protein reabsorption: Partial and near complete inhibition by certain amino acids. Scand J Clin Lab Invest 37: 477-486

152.   Mogensen CE, Vittinghus E, Solling K (1975) Increased urinary albumin, light chain, and beta-2-microglobulin excretion after intravenous arginine administration in normal man. Lancet II:581-583

153.   Mogensen CE, Christensen NJ, Gundersen HJG (1978) The acute effect of insulin on renal haemodynamics and protein excretion in diabetics. Diabetologia 15: 153-157

154. Parving H-H, Christiansen JS, Noer I, Tronier B, Mogensen CE (1980) The effect of glucagon infusion on kidney function in short-term insulin-dependent juvenile diabetics. Diabetologia 19: 350-354

155. Parving H-H, Noer 1, Kehlet H, Mogensen CE. Svendsen PAa, Heding L (1977) The effect of short-term glucogen infusion on kidney function in normal man. Diabetologia 13: 323-325

156. Parving H-H, Noer 1, Mogensen CE, Svendsen PA (1978) Kidney function in normal man during short-term growth hormone infusion. Acta Endocrinol (Copenhagen) 89: 796-800

157. Mogensen CE, Vittinghus E, Solling K (1979) Abnormal albumin excretion after two provocative renal test in diabetes: Physical exercise and lysine injection. Kidney Int 16: 385-393

158. Hinman AT, Engel BT, Bickford AF (1962) Portable blood pressure recorder. Accuracy and preliminary use in evalutating intradaily variations in pressure. Am Heart J 63: 663--668

159. Richardson DW, Honour AJ, Fenton GW, Stott FH and Pickering GW (1964) Variation in arterial pressure throughout the day and night. Clin Sci 26: 445-460

160. Rubler S, Abenavoli T, Greenblatt HA, Dixon JF, Cieslik CJ (1982) Ambulatory blood pressure monitoring in diabetic males: A method for detecting blood pressure elevations undisclosed by conventional methods. Clin Cardiol 5: 447-454

161. Hansen KW, Christensen CK, Andersen PH, Mau Pedersen M, Christiansen JS, Mogensen CE (1992) Ambulatory blood pressure in microalbuminuric type 1 diabetic patients. Kidney Int 41: 847-854

162. Hansen KW, Klein F, Christensen PD et al. (1994) Effects of captopril on ambulatory blood pressure, renal and cardiac function in microalbuminuric type 1 diabetic patients. Diabetes Metab 20: 485-493

163. Hansen KW, Mau Pedersen M, Christensen CK, Christiansen JS, Mogensen CE (1992) Normoalbuminuria ensures no reduction of renal function in Type 1 (insulin-dependent) diabetic patients. J Intern Med 232: 161-167

164. Hansen KW, Mau Pedersen M, Christiansen JS, Mogensen CE (1993) Acute renal effects of angiotensin converting enzyme inhibition in microalbuminuric type 1 diabetic patients. Acta Diabetol 30: 149-153

165. Hansen KW, Mau Pedersen M, Christiansen JS, Mogensen CE (1993) Diurnal blood pressure variations in normoalbuminuric type 1 diabetic patients. J Intern Med 234: 175-180

166. Hansen KW, Mau Pedersen M, Christiansen JS, Mogensen CE (1994) Night blood pressure and cigarette smoking; disparate association in healthy subjects and diabetic patients. Blood Pressure 3: 381-388

167. Hansen KW, Mau Pedersen M, Marshall SM, Christiansen JS, Mogensen CE (1992) Circadian variation of blood pressure in patients with diabetic nephropathy. Diabetologia 35: 1074-1079

168. Hansen KW, Poulsen PL, Christiansen JS, Mogensen CE (1995) Determinants of 24-h blood pressure in IDDM patients. Diabetes Care 18: 529-535

169. Hansen KW, Poulsen PL, Mogensen CE (1994) Ambulatory blood pressure and abnormal albuminuria in type 1 diabetic patients. Kidney Int 45 [Suppl 45]:S134-S140

170. Hansen KW, Sorensen K, Christensen PD, Pedersen EB, Christiansen JS, Mogensen CE (1995) Night blood pressure: Relation to organ lesions in microalbuminuric type 1 diabetic patients. Diabet Med 12: 42-45

171.   Poulsen PL, Hansen KW, Mogensen CE (1994) Ambulatory blood pressure in the transition from normo- to microalbuminuria. A longitudinal study in IDDM patients. Diabetes 43: 1248-1253

172.   Poulsen PL, Ebbehoj E, Hansen KW, Mogensen CE (1997) 24-h blood pressure and autonomic function is related to albumin excretion within the normoalbuminuric range in IDDM patients. Diabetologia 40: 718-725

173.   Poulsen PL, Bek T, Ebbehoj E, Hansen KW, Mogensen CE (1998) 24-h ambulatory blood pressure and retinopathy in normoalbuminuric IDDM patients. Diabetologia 41: 105-110

174.   Staessen JA, Thijs L, Fagard R, O'Brien ET, Clement D, de Leeuw PW, Mancia G, Nachev C, Palatini P, Parati G, Toumilehto J, Webster J for the Systolic Hypertension in Europe Trial Investigators (1999). Predicting cardiovascular risk using conventional vs. ambulatory blood pressure in older patients with systolic hypertension. JAMA, 282: 539-546.

175.   Poulsen PL, Juhl B, Ebbehoj E, Klein F, Christiansen C, Mogensen CE (1997) Elevated ambulatory blood pressure in microalbuminuric IDDM patients is inversely associated with renal plasma flow. A compensatory mechanism? Diabetes Care 20: 429-432

176.   Pinkney JH, Denver AE, Yudkin JS (1997) Ambulatory blood pressure monitoring in diabetes: An analysis of its potential in clinical practice. Cardiovascular Risk Factors 7:175-183

177.   Poulsen PL, Ebbehoj E, Mogensen CE (1998) Early ACE-intervention in microalbuminuria: 24 h BP, renal function, and exercise changes. Nephrol Dial Transplant 13: 1056-1079

178.   Poulsen PL, Ebbehoj E, Hansen KW, Mogensen CE (1998) Effects of smoking on 24-h ambulatory blood pressure and autonomic function in normoalbuminuric insulin-dependent diabetes mellitus patients. Am J Hypertens 11: 1093-1099

179.   Poulsen PL, Hansen KW, Ebbehøj E, Knudsen ST, Mogensen CE (2000) No deleterious effects of tight blood glocuse control on 24-h ambulatory blood pressure in normoalbuminuric insulin dependent diabetes mellitus patients. J Clin Endocrinol Metab, 85: 155-58.

180.   Wallenius G (1954) Renal clearance of dextran as a measure of glomerular permeability. Acta Soc Med Upsaliensis [Suppl 4]

181.   Lins H, Jahnke K, Scholtan W (1959) Ober die Permeabilität makromolekularer Stoffe. In: Oberdisse K, Jahnke K (eds) Die Niere bei diabetischen und anderen Nephropathien in Diabetes Mellitus. Proceedings of the Ill. Congress of the International Diabetes Federation. Georg Thieme Verlag, Stuttgart, pp 203-206

182.   Lambert PP, Gassée JP, Askenasi R (1968) La perméabilité du rein aux macromolecules physiopathologie de la protéinurie. In: Lambert PP (ed) Acquisitions récentes de physiopathologie rénale. Editions Desoer S. A., Liège, Belgique, pp 181-214

183.   Deckert T, Kofoed-Enevoldsen A, Vidal P, Norgaard K, Andreasen HB, Feldt-Rasmussen B (1993) Size- and charge selectivity of glomerular filtration in type 1 (insulin-dependent) diabetic patients with and without albuminuria. Diabetologia 36: 244-251

184.   Myers BD, Nelson RG, Williams GW et al. (1 991) Glomerular function in Pima Indians with noninsulin-dependent diabetes mellitus of recent onset. J Clin Invest 88: 524-530

185.   Morelli E, Loon N, Meyer T, Peters W, Myers BD (1990) Effects of converting-enzyme inhibition on barrier function in diabetic glomerulopathy. Diabetes 39: 76-82

186.   Gaster B, Hirsch IB (1998) The effects of improved glycemic control on complications in type 2 diabetes. Archives of Internal Medicine 158: 134-140

187. Krolewski AS, Laffel LMB, Krolewski M, Quinn M, Warram JH (1995) Glycosylated hemoglobin and the risk of microalbuminuria in patients with insulin-dependent diabetes mellitus. N Engl J Med 332:1251-1255

188. Microalbuminuria Collaborative Study Group, UK (1995) Intensive therapy and progression to clinical albuminuria in patients with insulin dependent diabetes mellitus and microalbuminuria. BMJ 311: 973-977

189. Christensen CK, Mogensen CE (1985) The course of incipient diabetic nephropathy: Studies of albumin excretion and blood pressure. Diabetic Medicine 2: 97-102

190. Christensen CK, Mogensen CE (1985) Effect of antihypertensive treatment on progression of disease in incipient diabetic nephropathy. Hypertension 7:II-109-II-113

191. Christensen CK, Mogensen CE (1987) Antihypertensive treatment: long-term reversal of progression of albuminuria in incipient diabetic nephropathy. A longitudinal study of renal function. J Diabetes Complications 1: 45-52

192. Mau Pedersen M, Christensen CK, Hansen KW, Christiansen JS, Mogensen CE (1991) ACE-inhibition and renoprotection in early diabetic nephropathy. Response to enalapril acutely and in long-term combination wtih conventional antihypertensive treatment. Clin Invest Med 14: 642-651

193. Mau Pedersen M, Hansen KW, Schmitz A, Sorensen K, Christensen CK, Mogensen CE (1992) Effects of ACE inhibition supplementary to beta blockers and diuretics in early diabetic nephropathy. Kidney Int 41: 883-890

194. Mogensen CE, Pedersen M.M, Ebbehoj E, Poulsen PL, Schmitz A (1997) Combination therapy in hypertension-associated diabetic renal disease. International Journal of Clinical Practice [Suppl] 90: 52-58

195. Marre M, Chatellier G, Leblanc H, Guyenne T-T, Ménard J, Passa PH (1988) Prevention of diabetic nephropathy with Enalapril in normotensive diabetics with microalbuminuria. BMJ 297:1092-1095

196. Mathiesen ER, Hommel E, Giese J, Parving H-H (1991) Efficacy of captopril in postponing nephropathy in normotensive insulin-dependent diabetic patients with microalbuminuria. BMJ 303: 81-87

197. Mathiesen ER, Hommel E, Hansen HP, Smidt UM, Parving H-H. (1999) Randomised controlled trial of long term efficacy of captopril on preservation of kidney function in normtensive patients with insulin dependent diabetes and microalbuminuria. BMJ, 319; 24-25.

198. Melbourne Diabetic Nephropathy Study Group (1991) Comparison between perindopril and nifedipine in hypertensive and normotensive diabetic patients with microalbuminuria. BMJ 302:210-216

199. Barnes DJ, Cooper M, Gans DJ, Laffel L, Mogensen CE, Viberti GC (1996) Microalbuminuria Captopril Study Group. Captopril reduces the risk of nephropathy in insulin-dependent diabetic patients with microalbuminuria. Diabetologia 39: 587-593

200. Ravid M, Brosh D, Levi Z, Bar-Dayan Y, Ravid D, Rachmani R (1998). Use of enalapril to attenuate decline in renal function in normotensive, normoalbuminuric patients with type 2 diabetes mellitus. Ann Intern Med, 128: 982-988.

201. Ravid M, Brosh D, Levi Z, Bar-Dayan Y, Ravid D, Rachmani R (1998) Use of enalapril to attenuate decline in renal function in normotensive patients with type 2 diabetes mellitus. A randomized controlled trial. Ann Intern Med 128: 982-988

202. Viberti GC, Mogensen CE, Groop L, Pauls JF for the European Microalbuminuria Captopril Study Group (1994) Effect of captopril on progression to clinical proteinuria in patients with insulin-dependent diabetes mellitus and microalbuminuria. JAMA 271: 275-279

203.   Charturvedi N (1998) When should ACE inhibitors be used in IDDM patients? A combined analysis of clinical trials. Diabetologia 41:A5 (Abstract)

204.   Bennett PH, Haffner S, Kasiske BL et al. (1995) Screening and management of microalbuminuria in patients with diabetes mellitus - recommendations to the scientific advisory board of the national kidney foundation from an ad hoc committee of the council on diabetes mellitus of the national kidney foundation. Am J Kidney Dis 25:107-112

205.   Mogensen CE (1971) Glomerular filtration rate and renal plasma flow in short-term and long-term juvenile diabetes Scand J Clin Lab Invest 28: 91-100

206.   Mogensen CE (1971) Maximum tubular reabsorption capacity for glucose and renal hemodynamics during rapid hypertonic glucose infusion in normal and diabetic man. Scand J Clin Lab Invest 28: 101-109

207.   Mogensen CE (1976) Progression of nephropathy in longterm diabetes with proteinuria and effect of initial hypertensive treatment. Scand J Clin Lab Invest 36: 383-388

208.   Mogensen CE (1976) High blood pressure as a factor in the progression of diabetic nephropathy. Acta Med Scand [Suppl 602]:29-32

209.   Mogensen CE, Hansen KW, Mau Pedersen M, Christensen CK (1991) Renal factors influencing blood pressure threshold and choice of treatment for hypertension in IDDM. Diabetes Care 14[Suppl 4]:13-26

210.   Mogensen CE (1997) How to protect the kidney in diabetic patients: with special reference to IDDM. Diabetes 46 [Suppl 2]S104-SIll

211.   Mogensen CE (1982) Long-term antihypertensive treatment inhibiting progression of diabetic nephropathy. BMJ 285:685-688

212.   Parving H-H, Smidt UM, Andersen AR, Svendsen PAA (1983) Early aggressive antihypertensive treatment reduces rate of decline in kidney function in diabetic nephropathy. Lancet 1:1175-1179

213.   Parving H-H, Andersen AR, Schmidt UM, Hommel E, Mathiesen ER, Svendsen PAA (1987) Effect of antihypertensive treatment on kidney function in diabetic nephropathy. BMJ 294:1443-1447

214.   Parving H-H, Jacobsen P, Rossing K, Smidt UM, Hommel E, Rossing P (1996) Benefits of long-term antihypertensive treatment on prognosis in diabetic nephropathy. Kidney Int 49:1778-1782

215.   Parving H-H, Hommel E (1989) Prognosis in diabetic nephropathy. BMJ 299:230-233

216.   Mathiesen ER, Borch-Johnsen K, Jensen DV, Deckert T (1989) Improved survival in patients with diabetic nephropathy. Diabetologia 32: 884-886

217.   Björck S, Mulec H, Johnsen SA, Nordén G, Aurell M (1992) Renal protective effect of enalapril in diabetic nephropathy. BMJ 304: 339-343

218.   Lewis E, Hunsicker L, Bain R, Rhode R (1993) The effect of angiotensin-converting enzyme inhibition on diabetic nephropathy. N Engl J Med 329:1456-1462

219.   Weir MR, Dworkin LD (1998) Antihypertensive drugs, dietary salt, and renal protection: How low should you go and with which therapy? Am J Kidney Dis 32(l):1-22

220.   de Courten M, Bohlen L, Weidmann P (1994) Antihypertensive treatment of diabetic and nondiabetic renal disease: drug-specific differences in reducing proteinuria. J Hypertens 12 [Suppl 3]:S112

221.   Ruggenenti P, Perna A, Gherardi G, Gaspari F, Benini R, Remuzzi G on behalf of the Gruppo Italiano di Studi Epidemiologici in Nefrologia (GISEN) (1998) Renal function and requirement for dialysis in chronic nephropathy patients on long-term ramipril: REIN follow-up trial. Lancet 352:1252-1256

222.   Nyberg G, Blohmé G, Nordén G (1987) Impact of metabolic control in progression of clinical diabetic nephropathy. Diabetologia 30: 82-86

223. Pickup JC, Keen H, Parsons JA, Alberti KGMM (1978) Continuous subcutaneous insulin infusion: an approach to achieving normoglycaemia. BMJ 1: 204-207

224. Christensen CK, Christiansen JS, Christensen T, Hermansen K, Mogensen CE (1986) The effect of six months continuous subcutaneous insulin infusion on kidney function and size in insulin-dependent diabetics. Diabetic Medicine 3:29-32

225. Moller A, Rasmussen L, Ledet T, Christiansen JS, Christensen CK, Mogensen CE, Hermansen K (1986) Lipoprotein changes during CSII treatment in IDDM patients Scand J Clin Lab Invest 46: 471-475

226. Thuesen L, Christiansen JS, Sorensen KE et al. (1986) Exercise capacity and cardiac function in type 1 diabetic patients treated with continuous subcutaneous insulin infusion. A controlled study. Scand J Clin Lab Invest 46: 779-784

227. Hermansen K, Moller A, Christensen CK et al. (1987) Diurnal plasma profiles of metabolise and hormone concentration in insulin-dependent diabetic patients during conventional insulin treatment and continuous subcutaneous insulin infusion. A controlled study. Acta Endocrinol (Copenhagen) 114: 433-439

228. Mogensen CE (1988) Therapeutic interventions in nephropathy of IDDM. Diabetes Care 11 [Suppl 1]:10-15

229. Jakobsen J, Christiansen JS, Christensen CK, Hermansen K, Schmitz A, Mogensen CE (1988) Autonomic and somatosensory nerve function after two years of continuous subcutaneous insulin infusion in type 1 diabetes. Diabetes 37: 452-455

230. Hermansen K, Schmitz 0, Boye N, Christensen CK, Christiansen JS, Alberti KGMM, Orskov H, Mogensen CE (1988) Glucagon responses to intravenous arginine and oral glucose in insulin-dependent diabetic patients during six months conventional or continous subcutaneous insulin infusion. Metabolism 37: 640-644

231. Schmitz A, Christiansen JS, Christensen CK, Hermansen K, Mogensen CE (1989) Effect of pump versus pen treatment on glycemic control and kidney-function in longterm uncomplicated insulin-dependent diabetes-mellitus (IDDM). Dan Med Bull 36:176-178

232. Mogensen CE, Hansen KW (1990) Preventing or postponing renal disease in insulin-dependent diabetes by glycemic and nonglycemic intervention. In: Klinkmann H, Smeby LC (eds) Terminal Renal Failure: Therapeutic Problems, Possibilities, and Potentials. Contrib Nephrol, Karger, Basel78:73-101

233. Kelly WD, Lillehei RC, Merkel FK, Idezuki Y, Goetz FC (1967) Allotransplantation of the pancreas and duodenum along with the kidney in diabetic nephropathy. Surgery 61: 827

234. Dubernard JM, Traeger J, Neyra P, Touraine JL, Tranchant D, Blanc-Brunat N (1978) A new method of preparation of segmental pancreatic grafts for transplantation. Trials in dogs and in man. Surgery 84: 633

235. Sutherland DER, Dunn DL, Goetz FC et al. (1989) A 10year experience with 290 pancreas transplants at a single institution. Ann Surg 210: 274-285

236. Manske CL (1999) Risks and benefits of kidney and pancreas transplantation for diabetic patients. Diabetes Care, 22 (S2): B114-120

237. Fioretto P, Steffes MW, Sutherland DER, Goetz FC, Mauer M (1998) Reversal of lesions of diabetic nephropathy after pancreas transplantation. N Engl J Med 339: 69-75

238. Nyberg G, Hoidaas H, Brekke IB, Hartmann A, Nordén G, Olausson M, Osterby R (1996) Glomerular ultrastructure in kidneys transplanted simultaneously with a segmental pancreas to patients With type 1 diabetes. Nephrol Dial Transplant ll: 1029-1033

239. Zatz R, Dunn BR, Meyer TW, Anderson S, Rennke HG, Brenner BM (1986) Prevention of diabetic glomerulopathy by pharmacological amelioration of glomerular capillary hypertension. J Clin Invest 77: 1925-1930

240. Williams B, Cooper ME, McNally PG (1998) Antihypertensive treatment in NIDDM with special reference to abnormal albuminuria. Addendum regarding renovascular hypertension and renal artery stenosis (especially NIDDM). In: Mogensen CE (ed) The Kidney and Hypertension in Diabetes Mellitus. Kluwer Academic Publ, Boston, Dordrecht, London, pp 432-434

241. Mogensen CE (1992) Angiotensin converting enzyme inhibitors and diabetic nephropathy. Their effects on proteinuria may be independent of their effects on blood pressure. Editorial. BMJ 304: 327-328

242. Thuesen L, Christiansen JS, Falstie-Jensen N, Christensen CK, Hermansen K, Mogensen CE, Henningsen P (1985) Increased myocardial contractility in short-term Type 1 diabetic patients: an echocardiographic study. Diabetologia 28:822-826

243. Parving H-H, Viberti GC, Keen H, Christiansen JS, Lassen NA (1983) Haemodynamic factors in the genesis of diabetic microangiopathy. Metabolism 32: 943-949

244. Gall M-A, Borch-Johnsen K, Hougaard P, Nielsen FS, Parving H-H (1995) Albuminuria and poor glycemic control predicts mortality in NIDDM. Diabetes 44: 1303-1309

245. Abernethy DR, Schwartz JB (1999). Calcium antagonist drugs. New Engl J Med, 341: 1447-57.

246. Mogensen CE (1999) Drug treatment for hypertensive patients in special situations: Diabetes and hypertension. Clin Exp Hypertens, 21(5-6): 895-906.

247. Nielsen S, Dollerup J, Nielsen B, Jensen HA, Mogensen CE (1997) Losartan reduces albuminuria in patients with essential hypertension. An enalapril controlled 3 months study. Nephrol Dial Transplant 12:19-23

248. Nielsen S (1998) Losartan modifies glomerular hyperfiltration and insulin sensitivity in type 1 diabetes. Diabetologia 41[Suppl l]:A5 (Abstract)

249. Krolewski AS, Warram JH, Christlieb AR, Busick EJ, Kahn CR (1985) The changing natural history of nephropathy in type 1 diabetes. Am J Med 78: 785-794

250. The controlled therapeutic trial [editorial] (1948) BMJ 2: 791-792

251. Chalmers I (1998) Unbiased, relevant and reliable assessments in health care. BMJ 317:1167-1168

252. University Group Diabetes Program (1970) A study of the effects of hypoglycemic agents on vascular complications in patients with adult-onset diabetes. Diabetes 19 [Suppl 2]: 747-830

253. Creutzfeldt W (1994) The discovery of the oral treatment of diabetes mellitus with sulphonylureas. In: Mogensen CE, Standl E (eds) Research methodologies in Human Diabetes, part 1. Walter de Gruyter, Berlin, New York, pp 11-20

254. Peto R, Collins R, Gray R (1995) Large-scale randomized evidence: large, simple trials and overviews of trials. J Clin Epidemiol 48(l): 23-40

255. Thompson SG, Pocock SJ (1991) Can meta-analyses be trusted? Lancet 338: 1127-30

256. Thomson SG (1994) Why sources of heterogeneity in metaanalysis should be investigated. BMJ 309: 1351-1355

257. Feinstein AR (1995) Meta-analysis: statistical alchemy for the 21st century. J Clin Epidemiol 48: 71-79

258. Spitzer WO (1995) The challenge of meta-analysis (Editor's Keynote Address). J Clin Epidemiol 48:1-4

259. Victor N (1995) The challenge of meta-analysis: Discussion. Indications and contraindications for meta-analysis. J Clin Epidemiol 48: 5-8

260. Sharp SJ, Thomson SG, Altman DG (1996) The relation between treatment benefit and underlying risk in metaanalysis. BMJ 313: 1550-1551

261. Lelorier J, Geneviève G, Benhaddad A, Lapierre J, Derderian F (1997) Discrepancies between meta-analyses and subsequent large randomized controlled trials. New Engl J Med 337: 536-542

262. WHO-ISH (1975) Effectiveness of treatment of mild hypertension. WHO Geneva CVD/75.5

263. 1999 WHO/ISH Hypertension Guidelines (1999) J Hypertens, 17:151-83

264. The Sixth Report of the Joint National Committee on Prevention, Detection, Evaluation, and Treatment of High Blood Pressure (1997) Arch Intern Med 157: 2413-2446

265. Recommendations et références médicales de l'annees. Diagnostic et traitement de l'hypertension artérielle essentielle de l'adulte de 20 A 80 ans (1998) Journal des Maladies Vasculaires (Paris) 23, 3: 204-231

266. Ramsey LE, Williams B, Johnston GD, MacGregor GA, Poston L, Potter JF, Poulter NR, Russell G. British Hypertension Society Guidelines for Hypertension management 1999: Summary (1999). BMJ, 319: 630-635

267. American Diabetes Association (1999) Standards of medical care for patients with diabetes mellitus. Diabetes Care 21:S23-S31

268. American Diabetes Association (1999) Diabetic nephropathy. Diabetes Care 21:S50-S53

269. National High Blood Pressure Education Program Working Group on Hypertension and Renal Disease (1996) 1995 Update of the working group reports on chronic renal failure and renovascular hypertension. Arch Intern Med 156:1938-1947

270. Lundbæk K (1953) Long-term diabetes. The clinical picture in diabetes mellitus of 15-25 years' duration with a follow-up of a regional series of cases. Munksgaard, Copenhagen and Lange, Maxwell & Springer Ltd., London, New York

271. Cooper ME (1998) Pathogenesis, prevention and treatment of diabetic nephropathy. Lancet 352: 213-219

272. Parving H-H (1998) Is antihypertensive treatment the same for NIDDM and IDDM patients? Diabetes Research and Clinical Practice 39 [Suppl]:S43-S47

273. Anitschkow N, Chalatow S (1913) Uber experim. Cholesterinsteatose, Zentralbl. f. alg Pathol u. pathol Anst Bd 24: 379-403

274. Appel LJ, Moore TJ, Obarzanek E, Vollmer WM, Svetkey LP, Sacks FM, Bray GA, Vogt TM, Cutler JA, Windhauser MM, Lin P-H, Karanja N for the DASH Collaborative Research Group (1997). A clinical trial of the effects of dietary patterns on blood pressure. New Engl J Med, 336: 1117-1123.

275. Feldt-Rasmussen B, Hegedüs L, Mathiesen ER, Deckert T (1991). Kidney volume in type 1 (insulin-dependent) diabetic patients with normal or increased urinary albumin excretion: effect of long-term improved metabolic control. Scand J Clin Lab Invest, 51: 31-36

276. Cambier P (1934) Application de la théorie de Rehberg a l'etude clinique des affections rénales et du diabete. Annales Médicine 35: 273-299

277. Fiaschi E, Grassi B, Andres G (1952). La funzione renal nel diabete mellito. Rassegna di Fisiopatologia Clinica & Terapeutica 24: 373-410

278. Stadler G, Schmid R, Wolff MV (1960) Funktionelle Mikroangiopathie der Nieren beim behandelten Diabetes mellitus im Kindesalter. Dtsch Med Wochenschr 85: 346

279. Ditzel J, Schwartz M (1967) Abnormally increased glomerular filtration rate in short-term insulin-treated diabetic subjects. Diabetes 16: 264

280. Mogensen CE (1972) Glomerular filtration rate and renal plasma flow in long-term juvenile diabetics without proteinuria. BMJ 4: 257-259

281. Yip WJ, Jones LS, Wiseman JM, Hill C, Viberti GC (1996) Glomerular hyperfiltration in the prediction of nephropathy in IDDM. Diabetes 45:1729-1733

282. Keen H, Chlouverakis C (1963) An immunoassay method for urinary albumin at low concentrations. Lancet ii: 913

283. Miles DW, Mogensen CE, Gundersen I-UG (1970) Radioimmunoassay for urinary albumin using a single antibody. Scand J Clin Lab Invest 26: 5-11

284. Mogensen CE (1971) Urinary albumin excretion in early and long-term juvenile diabetes. Scand J Clin Lab Invest 28: 183-193

285. Mogensen CE (1995) Management of early nephropathy in diabetic patients. Ann Rev Med 46: 79-93

286. Mogensen CE (1988) Management of diabetic renal involvement and disease. Lancet I:867-870

287. Mogensen CE, Keane WF, Bennett PH et al. (1995) Prevention of diabetic renal disease with special reference to microalbuminuria. Lancet 346:1080-1084

288. Keen H, Chlouverakis C (1964) Urinary albumin excretion and diabetes mellitus. Lancet ii: 1 155

289. Mogensen CE, Vestbo E, Poulsen PL et al. (1995) Microalbuminuria and potential confounders. A review and some observations on variability of urinary albumin excretion. Diabetes Care 18:572-581

290. Mogensen CE, Poulsen PL (1994) Epidemiology of microalbuminuria in diabetes and in the background population. Curr Opin Nephrol Hypertens 3: 248-256

291. Borch-Johnsen K, Wenzel H Viberti GC, Mogensen CE (1993) Is screening and intervention for microalbuminuria worthwhile in patients with insulin dependent diabetes? BMJ 306:1722-1725

292. Kimmelstiel P, Wilson C (1936) Intercapillary lesions in the glomeruli of the kidney. Am J Pathol 12: 83-95

293. Kimmelstiel P (1959) On Diabetic Glomerulosclerosis. Diabetes Mellitus. Proceedings of the III Kongress of the International Diabetes Federation. Georg Thieme Verlag, Stuttgart, pp 178-184

294. Gellman DD, Pirani C, Soothill JF, Muehrcke RC, Kark RM (1959) Diabetic nephropathy: a clinical and pathological study based on renal biopsies. Medicine 38: 321

295. Schwartz MM, Lewis EJ, Leonard-Martin T, Lewis JB, Batlle D and the Collaborative Study Group (1998). Renal pathology patterns in type 2 diabetes mellitus: relationship with retinopathy. Nephrol Dial Transplant, 13: 2547-2552.

296. Olsen S, Mogensen CE (1996) How often is Type 2 diabetes mellitus complicated with non-diabetic renal disease? A material of renal biopsies and an analysis of the literature. Diabetologia 39: 1638-1645

297. Thomsen CAA (1965) The Kidney in Diabetes Mellitus. A Clinical and Histological Investigation Based on Renal Biopsy Material. Munksgaard, Copenhagen

298. Mauer SM, Steffes MW, Ellis EN, Sutherland DER, Brown DM, Goetz FC (1984) Structural functional relationships in diabetic nephropathy. J Clin Invest 74: 1143-1155

299. Reaven GM (1997) The kidney: An unwilling accomplice in Syndrome X. Am J Kidney Dis 30: 928-931

300. Keiding NR, Root HF, Marble A (1952) Importance of control of diabetes in prevention of vascular complications. JAMA 150:964-969

301. Wang PH, Lau J, Chalmers TC (1993) Meta-analysis of effects of intensive blood-glucose control on late complications of type 1 diabetes. Lancet 341: 1306-1309

302. Mulec H, Blohmé G, Grande B, Björck S (1998) The effect of metabolic control on rate of decline in renal function in insulin-dependent diabetes mellitus with overt diabetic nephropathy. Nephrol Dial Transplant 13: 651-655

303. Chaturvedi N, Sjolie A-K, Stephenson JM et al. and the EUCLID Study Group (1998) Effect of lisinopril on progression of retinopathy in normotensive people with type 1 diabetes. Lancet 351: 28-31

304. Crepaldi G, Carta Q, Deferrari G et al. and The Italian Microalbuminuria Study Group in IDDM (1998) Effects of lisinopril and nifedipine on the progression to overt albuminuria in IDDM patients with incipient nephropathy and normal blood pressure. Diabetes Care 21: 104-110

305. Cooper M, McNally P (1998) Antihypertensive treatment in NIDDM, with special reference to abnormal albuminuria. In: Mogensen CE (ed) The kidney and hypertension in diabetes mellitus, 4th ed., Kluwer Academic Publ., Boston, Dordrecht, London, pp 419-434

306. Gæde P, Vedel P, Parving H-H, Pedersen O (1999) The Steno Type 2 study: Intensive multifactorial intervention delays the progression of micro- and macroangiopathy in microalbuminuric Type 2 diabetic patients. Lancet 353; 617-622.

307. Anderson S (1998) Pathogenesis of diabetic glomerulopathy: The role of glomerular hemodynamic factors. In: Mogensen CE (ed) The kidney and hypertension in diabetes mellitus, 4th ed., Kluwer Academic Publ., Boston, Dordrecht, London, pp 297-306

308. Mau Pedersen M, Schmitz A, Pedersen EB, Danielsen H, Christiansen JS (1988) Acute and long-term renal effects of angiotensin converting enzyme inhibition in normotensive, normoalbuminuric insulin-dependent diabetic patients. Diabetic Med 5: 562-569

309. Viberti GC, Keen H, Wiseman MJ (1987) Raised arterial pressure in parents of proteinuric insulin-dependent diabetics. BMJ 295: 515-517

310. Doria A, Warram JH, Krolewski AS (1995) Genetic susceptibility to nephropathy in insulin-dependent diabetes: from epidemiology to molecular genetics. Diabetes Metab Rev 11: 287-314

311. Marre M (1999) Genetics and the predictions of complications in type 1 diabetes. Diabetes Care, 22: B53-B58

312. Mogensen CE (1998) Exercise and the kidney in diabetes. In: The Kidney and hypertension in diabetes mellitus, 4th ed., Kluwer Academic Publ., Boston, Dordrecht, London, pp 191-198

313. Mogensen CE, Schmitz A, Christensen CK (1988) Comparative Renal Pathophysiology Relevant to IDDM and NIDDM Patients. Diabetes 4(5):453-483

314. Tuominen JA, Ebeling P, Koivisto VA (1998) Long-term lisinopril therapy reduces exercise-induced albuminuria in normoalbuminuric normotensive IDDM patients. Diabetes Care 21: 1345-1348

315. Flyvbjerg A, Hill C, Logan A (1999). Pathophysiological role of growth factors in diabetic kidney disease: Focus on innovative therapy. Trends in Endocrinology and Metabolism, 10: 267-272.

316. Wolf G, Ziyadeh FN (1999). Molecular mechanisms of diabetic renal hypertrophy. Kidney Int, 56: 393-405.

317. King GL, Ishii H, Koya D (1997). Diabetic vascular dysfunction: A model of excessive activation of protein kinase C. Kidney Int., 52:S77-S85.

318. Willenheimer R, Dahlöf B, Rydberg E, Erhard L (1999). AT_1-receptor blockers in hypertension and heart failure: clinical experience and future directions. European Heart Journal, 20: 997-1008

319. Friedman EA (1999). Advanced glycation end-products in diabetic nephropathy. Nephrol Dial Transplant, 14 (s3): 1-9.

320. Chavers BM, Bilous RW, Ellis EN, Steffes MW, Mauer M (1989) Glomerular lesions and urinary albumin excretion in type 1 diabetes without overt proteinuria. N Engl J Med 320:966-970

321. Fioretto P, Steffes MW, Mauer M (1994) Glomerular structure in nonproteinuric IDDM patients with various levels of albuminuria. Diabetes 43:1358-1364

322. The Heart Outcomes Prevention Evaluation Study Investigators (2000) Effects of an angiotensin-converting-enzyme inhibitor, ramipril, on death from cardiovascular causes, myocardial infarction and stroke in high-risk patients. New Engl J Med, 342:145-53.

323. Berkman J, Rifkin H. (1973) Unilateral nodular diabetic glomeruloschlerosis (Kimmelsteil-Wilson). Report of a case. Metabolism Clin Exp 22; 715-722.

324. Parving H-H, Tarnow L, Nielsen FS, Rossing P, Mandrup-Poulsen T, Osterby R, Nerup J (1999). Cyclosporine nephrotoxicity in type 1 diabetic patients. A 7-year follow-up study. Diabetes Care, 22: 478-83.

325. Fioretto P, Steffes MW, Barbosa J, Rich SS, Miller ME, Mauer M (1999). Is diabetic nephropathy inherited? Studies of glomerular structure in type 1 diabetic sibling pairs. Diabetes, 48: 865-869.

326. Hansson L, Lindholm LH, Ekbom T, Dahlöf B, Lanke J, Scherstén B, Wester P-O, Hedner T, de Faire U for the STOP-Hypertension-2 study Group (1999). Randomised trial of old and new antihypertensive drugs in elderly patients: cardiovascular mortality and morbidity the Swedish Trial in Old Patients with Hypertension-2 study. Lancet, 354: 1751-56.

327. Azizi M, Guyene T-T, Chatellier G, Wargon M, Ménard J (1997). Additive effects of losartan and enalapril on blood pressure and plasma active renin. Hypertension, 29: 634-640.

328. Hamroff G, Katz SD, Mancini D, Blaufarb I, Bijou R, Patel R, Jondeau G, Olivari M-T, Thomas S, Le Jemtel TH (1999). Addition of angiotensin II receptor blockade to maximal angiotensin-converting enzyme inhibition improves exercise capacity in patients with severe congestive heart failure. Circulation, 99: 990-992.

329. Hebert LA, Falkenheim ME, Nahman NS, Jr Cosio FG, O'Dorisio TM (1999). Combination ACE inhibitor and angiotensin II receptor antagonist therapy in diabetic nephropathy. Am J Nephrol, 19: 1-6.

330. Ruilope LM, Aldigier JC, Ponticelli C, Oddoustock P, Botteri F, Mann JF on behalf of the European Group for the Investigation of Valsartan in Chronic Renal Disease (2000). Valsartan and benazepril in chronic renal disease. Journal of Hypertension, 18:89-95.

331. Hemmelder MH, de Jong P, de Zeeuw D (1998). A comparison of analytic procedures for measurement of fractional dextran clearances. J Lab Clin Med, 132:390-403.

332. Mogensen CE. (2000) Intervention strategies for microalbuminuria: The role of angiotensin II antagonists, including dual blockade with ACE-I and a receptor blocker. Journal of the Renin-Angiotensin Aldosterone System (JRAAS), 1, 63.

333. Nielsen S, Jensen MD (1999). Relationship between urinary albumin excretion, body composition, and hyperinsulinemia in normotensive glucose-tolerant adults. Diabetes Care, 10: 1729-1733.

334. Hauerslev CF, Vestbo, E, Frøland A, Mogensen CE, Damsgaard EM. (2000). Normal blood pressure and preserved diurnal variation in offspring of type 2 diabetic patients characterised by the features of the Metabolic Syndrome. Diabetes Care, 23:283-89.

335. Andersen S, Parving H-H, Blouch K, Deckert M, Myers BD (1999). Angiotensin II receptor blockade and barrier function in diabetic nephropathy. J Am Soc Nephrol 10: 125A.

336. Tryggvason K. (1999). Unraveling the mechanisms of glomerular ultrafiltration: Nephrin, a key component of the slit diaphragm. J Am Soc Nephrol 10: 2440-45.

337. Laffel LMB, McGill JB, Gans DJ on behalf of the North American Microalbuminuria Study Group. (1995). The beneficial effect of angiotensin-converting-enzyme inhibition with captopril on diabetic nephropathy in normotensive IDDM patients with microalbuminuria. Am Journ Med, 99: 497-504.

338. The Euclid Study Group. (1997). Randomised placebo-controlled trial of lisinopril in normotensive patients with insulin-dependent diabetes and normoalbuminuria or microalbuminuria. Lancet, 349: 1787-92.

339. Bojestig M, Karlberg B, Verho M and the Prima Study Group (1997). ACE inhibition during two years did not improve urinary excretion in normotensive microalbuminuric patients. Diabetologia, 1998; 41:A544.

340. Crepaldi G, Carta Q, Deferrari G, Mangili R, Navalesi R, Santeusanio F, Spalluto A, Vanasia A, Villa GM, Nosadini R for the Italian Microalbuminuria Study Group in IDDM (1998). Diabetes Care, 21:104-110.

341. Jerums G on behalf of the Melbourne Diabetic Nephropathy Study Group, Melbourne, Australia (1998). Ace inhibition vs. calcium-channel blockade in normotensive type 1 and type 2 diabetic patients with microalbuminuria. Nephrology Dial Trans, 13: 1065-66.

342. Ebbehøj E, Poulsen PL, Nosadini R, Fioretto R, Fioretto P, Crepaldi C, Mogensen CE (1998). Early ACE-I intervention in microalbuminuria: 24h BP, renal function and exercise changes. Abstract of the 34th Annual Meeting of the EASD Barcelona, Spain 8-12 Sept. 1998. Diabetologia, 41(1).

343. Brun C, Gormsen H, Hilden T, Iversen P, Raaschou F (1953). Diabetic nepropathy. Kidney biopsy and renal function tests. Am J Med, 15: 187-97.

344. Deinum J, Rønn B, Mathiesen E, Derkx FHM, Hop WCJ, Shalekamp MADH (1999). Increase in serum prorenin precedes onset of microalbuminuria in patients with insulin-dependent diabetes mellitus. Diabetologia, 42: 1006-1010.

345. Luetscher JA, Kraemer FB, Wilson DM, Schwartz HC, Bryer-Ash M (1985). Increased plasma inactive renin in diabetes mellitus. N Engl J Med, 312: 1412-17.

346. Heart Outcomes Prevention Evaluation (HOPE) Study Investigators (2000). Effects of ramipril on cardiovascular and microvascular outcomes in people with diabetes mellitus: results of the HOPE study and MICRO-HOPE substudy. Lancet, 355: 253-59.

347. McCarty MF (1998) A central role for protein kinase C overactivity in diabetic glomerulosclerosis: implications for prevention with antioxidants, fish oil, and ACE inhibitors. Medical Hypotheses, 50: 155-65.

348. O'Hare JP, Michael A, Viberti GC on behalf of the ATLANTIS Study Group. (1998). Ramipril reduces albumin excretion rate in normotensive IDDM patients with microalbuminuria. Diabetologia, 41(S1): A284

349. The Diabetes Control and Complications Trial/Epidemiology of Diabetes Interventions and Complications Research Group. (2000). Retinopathy and nephropathy in patients with type 1 diabetes four years after a trial of intensive therapy. N Engl J Med, 342: 381-9.

350. Warram JH, Scott LJ, Hanna LS, Wantman M, Cohen SE, Laffel LMB, Ryan L, Krolewski AS (2000). Progression of microalbuminuria to proteinuria in type 1 diabetes. Non-linear relationship with hyperglycemia. Diabetes, 49: 94-100.

351. The Microalbuminuria Collaborative Study Group (1999). Predictors of the development of microalbuminuria in patients with type 1 diabetes mellitus: a seven year prospective study. Diabetic Med, 16: 918-925.

352. Trocha AK, Schmidtke C, Didjurgeit U, Mülhauser I, Bender R, Berger M, Sawicki PT (1999). Effects of intensified antihypertensive treatment in diabetic nephropathy: mortality and morbidity results of a prospective controlled 10-year study. Journ Hypert, 17: 1497-1503.

353. Breyer J, Berl T, Bain RP, Rohde RD, Lewis EJ and the Collaborative Study Group (1999). Effect of intensive blood pressure control on the course of type 1 diabetic nephropathy. Am Journ of Kidney Dis, 34: 809-817.

354. Andersen S, Tarnow L, Rossing P, Hansen BV, Parving H-H (2000). Renoprotective effects of angiotensin II receptor blockade in type 1 diabetic patients with diabetic nephropathy. Kidney Int, 57: 601-606.

355. Brenner BM, Cooper ME, de Zeeuw D, Grunfeld JP, Keane WF, Kurokawa K, McGill JB, Mitch WE, Parving H-H, Remuzzi G, Ribeiro AB, Schluchter MD, Snavely D, Zhang Z, Simpson R, Ramjit D, Shahinfar S for the Renaal Study Investigators (2000). The Losartan Renal Protection Study - Rationale Study (Reduction of endpoints in NIDDM with the angiotensin II antagonist Losartan). Submitted.

356. Rodby RA, Rohde RD, Clarke WR, Hunsicker LG, Anzalone DA, Lewis EJ for the Collaborative Study Group (2000). The Irbesartan Type II Diabetic Nephropathy Trial: Study Design and Baseline Patient Characteristics. Submitted.

357. Muirhead N, Feagan BF, Mahon J, Lewanczuk RZ, Rodger NW, Botteri F, Oddou-Stock P, Pecher E, Cheung R (1999). The effects of valsartan and captopril on reducing microalbuminuria in patients with type 2 diabetes mellitus: A placebo-controlled trial. Curr Ther Research, 60: 650-

358. Flyvbjerg A, Hill C, Grønbaek H, Logan A (1999). Effect of ACE-inhibition on renal TGF-beta Type II receptor expression in experimental diabetes in rats. J Am Soc Nephrol, 10: 679A

359. Price DA, Porter LE, Gordon M, Fisher NDL, De'Oliveira JMF, Laffel LMB, Passan DR, Williams GH, Hollenberg NK (1999). The paradox of the low-renin state in diabetic nephropathy. J Am Soc Nephrol, 10: 2382-2391.

360. Hoy WE, Rees M, Kile E, Mathews JD, Wang Z (1999). A new dimension to the Barker hypothesis: low birthweight and susceptibility to renal disease. Kidney Int, 56: 1072-77.

361. Wahren J and Johansson BL (1998). Ernst-Friedrich-Pfeiffer Memorial Lecture. New aspects of C-peptide physiology. Horm Metab Res, 30: A2-5

362. Soper CPR, Barron JL, Hyer SL (1998). Long-term glycaemic control directly correlates with glomerular filtration rate in early type 1 diabetes mellitus before the onset of microalbuminuria. Diabetic Medicine, 15: 1010-14.

363. Barsotti G, Cupisti A, Barsotti M, Sposini S, Palmieri D (1998). Dietary treatment of diabetic nephropathy with chronic renal failure. Nephrology Dialysis Transp 13(S8): 49-52.

364. Oates J, Mylari BL (1999). Aldose reductase inhibitors: therapeutic implications for diabetic complications. Exp. Opin Invest Drugs, 8: 2095-2119.

365. Fogarty DG, Rich SS, Hanna L, Warram JH, Krolewski AS. (2000). Urinary albumin excretion in families with type 2 diabetes is heritable and genetically correlated to blood pressure. Kidney Int, 57: 250-57.

366. Christensen PK, Gall M-A, Parving H-H (2000). The course of GFR in albuminuric type 2 diabetic patients with or without diabetic glomerulopahty. Diabetes Care, supl. 2, B14-20

367. Schichiri M, Kishikawa H, Ohkubo Y, Wake N (2000). Long-term results of the Kumamoto Study on optimal diabetes control in type 2 diabetic patients. Diabetes Care, 23(s2): B21-30

368. Marre M, Lièvre M, Vasmant D, Gallois Y, Hadjadj S, Reglier J-C, Chatellier G, Mann J, Viberti GC, Passa P on behalf of the DIABHYCAR Study Group (2000). Determinants of elevated urinary albumin in the 4,937 type 2 diabetic subjects recruited for the DIABHYCAR Study in Western Europe and North America. Diabetes Care, 23(s2) B40-49.

369. Gerstein HC, Mann JFE, Pogue J, Dinneen SF, Hallé JP, Hoogwerf B, Joyce C, Rashkow A, Young J, Zinman B, Yusuf S on behalf of the HOPE Study Investigators (2000). Prevalence and determinants of microalbuminuria in high-risk diabetic and nondiabetic patients in the Heart Outcomes Prevention Evaluation Study. Diabetes Care, 23(s2): B35-40.

370. Sørensen TIA (2000. The changing lifestyle in the world:body weight and what else? Diabetes Care, 23(s2): B1-5.

371. Shaw JE, Zimmet PZ, McCarty D, de Courten M (2000). Type 2 diabetes worldwide according to the new classification and criteria. Diabetes Care, 23(s2): B5-11.

372. Burnier M, Brunner HR (2000). Angiotensin II receptor antagonists. Lancet; 355: 637-45.

373. Lièvre M, Gueyffier F, Ekbom T, Fagard R, Cutler J, Schron E, Marre M, Boissel J-P for the INDANA Steering Committee (2000). Efficacy of diuretics and beta-blockers in diabetic hypertensive patients: results from a meta-analysis. Diabetes Care; 23(s2): B65-72

374. Estacio RO, Jeffers BW, Gifford N, Schrier RW (2000). Effect of blood pressure control on diabetic microvascular complications in patients with hypertension and type 2 diabetes. Diabetes Care, 23(s2): B54-65.

375. Steiner G (2000). Lipid intervention trials in diabetes. Diabetes Care; 23(s2): B49-54.

376. Gambaro O, Vanderwo FJ (2000). Glycosaminoglycans – use in treatment of diabetic nephropathy (Review), JASN, 11: 359-368.

377. Pinto-Sietsma S-J. Janssen WMT, Hillege HL, Navis G, de Zeeuw D, deJong PE (2000) Urinary albumin excretion is associated with renal functional abnormalities in a non-diabetic population: Striking similarities with diabetes. JASN (in press).

378. Mulder J, Pinto-Sietsma SJ, Janssen WMT, Hillege HL, de Zeeuw D, deJong PE (1999). Smoking behaviour and urinary albumin excretion in the general population. JASN, 10:175A

379. Chan JCN, Ko GTC, Leung DHY, Cheung RCK, Cheung MYF, So W-Y, Swaminathan R, Nicholls MG, Critchley AJH, Cockram CS (2000). Long-term effects of angiotensin-converting enzyme inhibition and metabolic control in hypertensive type 2 diabetic patients. Kidney Int. 57: 590-600.

380. Bain SC, Chowdhury TA (2000). Genetics of diabetic nephropathy and microalbuminuria. J R Soc Med, 93: 62-66.

381. Mogensen CE (2000). Letter to the Editor: IDDM, prediction of worsening nephropathy. Submitted.

382. Mogensen CE, Neldam S, Tikkanen I, Oren S, Viskoper R, Watts RW, Cooper ME for the CALM Study Group (2000). Role of dual blockade of the renin-angiotensin system in hypertensive, microalbuminuric, non-insulin dependent diabetes: The CALM Study. BMJ, Submitted.

383. Porush JG (2000). The benefits of angiotensin II receptor antagonists in high-risk hypertensive patients with diabetes. Eur Heart J Supplements, 2(suppl. B): B22-B27.

384. Peters H, Ritz E (1999). Dosing angiotensin II blockers – beyond blood pressure. Nephrol Dial Transplant, 14: 2568-70.

385. Eriksson JG, Forsén T, Tuomilehto J, Winter PD, Osmond C, Barker DJP (1999). Catch-up growth in childhood and death from coronary heart disease: longitudinal study. BMJ, 318: 427-31.

386. Forsén T, Eriksson JG, Toumilehto J, Osmond C, Barker DJP (1999). Growth in utero and during childhood among women who develop coronary heart disease: longitudinal study. BMJ, 319: 1403-7.

387. Barker DJP (1999). Commentary: Intrauterine nutrition may be important. BMJ, 318: 1477-78

388. Schmitt F, Natov S, Martinez F, Lacour B, Hannedouche TP (1996). Renal effects of angiotensin I-receptor blockade and angiotensin convertase inhibition in man. Clinical Science, 90: 205-213.

389. Gress TW, Nieto FJ, Shahar E, Wofford MR, Brancati FL for the Atherosclerosis Risk in Communities Study (2000). Hypertension and antihypertensive therapy as risk factors for type 2 diabetes mellitus. NEJM, 342: 905-11.

390. Krop JS, Coresh J, Chambless LE, Shahar E, Watson RL, Szklo M, Brancati FL (1999). A community-based study of explanatory factors for the excess risk for early renal function decline in blacks vs. whites with diabetes. Arch Intern Med, 159: 1777-83.

391. Ebihara S, Nakamura T, Shimada N, Koide H (1998). Increased plasma metalloproteinase-9 concentrations precede development of microalbuminuria in non-insulin-dependent diabetes mellitus. Am J Kidney Dis, 32: 544-50.

392. Tikkane T, Tikkanen I, Rockell MD et al. (1998). Dual inhibition of neutral endopeptidase and angiotensi-converting enzyme in rats with hypertension and diabetes mellitus. Hypertension, 32: 778-85.

393. Turner AJ, Murphy LJ (1996). Molecular pharmacology of endothelin converting enzyme. Biochem Pharmacol 51: 91-102.

394. Johansson B-L. Borgt K. Fernqvist-Forbes E, Kernell A, Odergren T, Wahren J (2000). Beneficial effects of C-peptide on incipient nephropathy and neuropathy in patients with type 1 diabetes mellitus. Diabetic Med, 17: 1-9.

395. Lucas A, Fewtrell MS, Cole TJ (1999): Fetal origins of adult disease – the hypothesis revisited. BMJ, 319: 245-9.

396. Dwyer T, Blizzard L, Morley R, Ponsonby A-L (1999). Within pair association between birth weight and blood pressure at age 8 in twins from a cohort study. BMJ, 319:1325-9.

397. Hattersley AT, Tooke JE (1999). The fetal insulin hypothesis: an alternative explanation of the association of low birthweight with diabetes and vascular disease. Lancet, 353: 1789-92.

398. Poulter NR, Chang CL, MacGregor AJ, Snieder H, Spector TD (1999). Association between birth weight and adult blood pressure in twins: historical cohort study. BMJ, 319: 1330-3.

399. Fuiano G, Mazza G, Comi N, Caglioti A, De Nicola L, Iodice C, Andreucci M, Andreucci VE (2000). Current indications for renal biopsy: a questionnaire-based survey. Am J Kidney Dis, 35: 448-457.

400. Khalifah RG, Baynes JW, Hudson BG (1999). Amadorins: novel post-Amadori inhibitors of advanced glyaction reactions. Biochem Biophys Res. Commun, 257: 251-8.

401. Messerli FH (2000). Implication of discontinuation of Doxozosin arm of ALLHAT. Lancet, 355: 863-64.

INDEX